Refractive Surface Ablation
PRK, LASEK, Epi-LASIK, Custom, PTK, and Retreatment

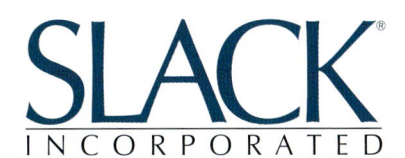

Refractive Surface Ablation

PRK, LASEK, Epi-LASIK, Custom, PTK, and Retreatment

EDITED BY

PAOLO VINCIGUERRA, MD
DEPARTMENT OF OPHTHALMOLOGY
ISTITUTO CLINICO HUMANITAS
MILAN, ITALY

FABRIZIO I. CAMESASCA, MD
DEPARTMENT OF OPHTHALMOLOGY
ISTITUTO CLINICO HUMANITAS
MILAN, ITALY

SLACK
INCORPORATED
Delivering the best in health care information and education worldwide

www.slackbooks.com

ISBN-13: 978-1-55642-713-8
ISBN-10: 1-55642-713-1

Copyright © 2007 by SLACK Incorporated

All rights reserved. No part of this book may be reproduced, stored in a retrieval system or transmitted in any form or by any means, electronic, mechanical, photocopying, recording or otherwise, without written permission from the publisher, except for brief quotations embodied in critical articles and reviews.

The procedures and practices described in this book should be implemented in a manner consistent with the professional standards set for the circumstances that apply in each specific situation. Every effort has been made to confirm the accuracy of the information presented and to correctly relate generally accepted practices. The authors, editor, and publisher cannot accept responsibility for errors or exclusions or for the outcome of the material presented herein. There is no expressed or implied warranty of this book or information imparted by it. Care has been taken to ensure that drug selection and dosages are in accordance with currently accepted/recommended practice. Due to continuing research, changes in government policy and regulations, and various effects of drug reactions and interactions, it is recommended that the reader carefully review all materials and literature provided for each drug, especially those that are new or not frequently used. Any review or mention of specific companies or products is not intended as an endorsement by the author or publisher.

SLACK Incorporated uses a review process to evaluate submitted material. Prior to publication, educators or clinicians provide important feedback on the content that we publish. We welcome feedback on this work.

Published by: SLACK Incorporated
                6900 Grove Road
                Thorofare, NJ 08086 USA
                Telephone: 856-848-1000
                Fax: 856-853-5991
                www.slackbooks.com

Contact SLACK Incorporated for more information about other books in this field or about the availability of our books from distributors outside the United States.

Library of Congress Cataloging-in-Publication Data

Refractive surface ablation : PRK, LASEK, epi-LASIK, custom, PTK, and retreatment / edited by Paolo Vinciguerra.
    p. ; cm.
 Includes bibliographical references and index.
   ISBN-13: 978-1-55642-713-8 (hardcover : alk. paper)
   ISBN-10: 1-55642-713-1 (hardcover : alk. paper)
 1. Eye--Refractive errors--Laser surgery. 2. Cornea--Laser surgery. I. Vinciguerra, Paolo.
   [DNLM: 1. Refractive Errors--surgery. 2. Cornea--surgery. 3. Keratectomy, Laser--methods. 4. Ophthalmologic Surgical Procedures--methods. WW 340 R332 2006]

RE926.R44 2006
617.7'1--dc22

2006021958

For permission to reprint material in another publication, contact SLACK Incorporated. Authorization to photocopy items for internal, personal, or academic use is granted by SLACK Incorporated provided that the appropriate fee is paid directly to Copyright Clearance Center. Prior to photocopying items, please contact the Copyright Clearance Center at 222 Rosewood Drive, Danvers, MA 01923 USA; phone: 978-750-8400; website: www.copyright.com; email: info@copyright.com

Printed in the United States of America.

Last digit is print number: 10   9   8   7   6   5   4   3   2   1

Dedication

This book is dedicated to the two women of my life: my mother, Maria and my wife, Maria Teresa.

My mother forged my character, encouraging my spirit of observation, humility, respect for work, for men, and attention to what is really important, forgetting appearances.

She motivated me to pursue and achieve goals without complaining or minding fatigue. Above all, she gave always me intense love. She believed in me even when it was not easy to do.

My wife, Maria Teresa, also always believed in me, regardless of appearances and difficulties.

As my fiancée, she helped me to overcome the problems of graduating, to start my professional life, never hindering my professional or research choices, even when they limited my free time or possible income.

As my wife, her presence has always been discrete but essential in hard as well as in happy times. As a pharmachologist, she always encouraged my thoroughness in research, revised my studies, and motivated me to pursue even difficult paths when they could possibly lead to better results. Her suggestions have been precious. She often understands everything in just a second.

You can easily realize how these two allies make all my endeavours easy.

—PV

To my wife, Delia, and my children, Matteo and Alessandro, for their love and support regardless of all the time I dedicate to my work.

To four men that believed in me: Alberto Weiss, William C. Chandler—Past International President Lions Club International, Maurizio Mauri, and Paolo Vinciguerra.

—FIC

Contents

Dedication v
Acknowledgments ix
About the Editor xi
Contributing Authors xiii
Introduction xv
Foreword—Steven E. Wilson, MD xvii

Section I: Patient Selection and Preoperative Management: Understanding Surface Ablation

Chapter 1: Topography in Surface Ablation 3
Paolo Vinciguerra, MD; Luca Maestroni, MD

Chapter 2: Useful Information for the Refractive Surgeon: Aberrometry and Its Application to Vision Care 17
Raymond A. Applegate, OD, PhD

Chapter 3: Clinical Application of Differential Wavefront Aberrometry 27
Phil Buscemi, OD; Harkaran S. Bains

Chapter 4: Understanding Wavefront: Microns vs Diopters 33
Stephen D. Klyce, PhD

Chapter 5: Patient Selection for Surface Ablation 41
Paolo Vinciguerra, MD; Luca Maestroni, MD

Chapter 6: Biomechanics of Surface Ablation and LASIK 59
Jennifer R. Lewis, PhD; Cynthia J. Roberts, PhD

Section II: General Principles

Chapter 7: General Principles in Surface Ablation 75
Paolo Vinciguerra, MD; Fabrizio I. Camesasca, MD; Maria Ingrid Torres Munoz, MD

Chapter 8: Smoothing in Excimer Refractive Surgery 83
Paolo Vinciguerra, MD; Fabrizio I. Camesasca, MD

Chapter 9: Evaluation and Development of Ablation Profiles 91
Paolo Vinciguerra, MD; Fabrizio I. Camesasca, MD

Section III: Surface Ablation

Chapter 10: Treatment of Myopia 97
Fabrizio I. Camesasca, MD; Paolo Vinciguerra, MD; Alessandro Randazzo, MD

Chapter 11: Treatment of Astigmatism 107
Paolo Vinciguerra, MD; Fabrizio I. Camesasca, MD; Guido Nizzola, MD; Daniel Epstein, MD, PhD

Chapter 12: Treatment of Hyperopia 121
Paolo Vinciguerra, MD; Fabrizio I. Camesasca, MD

Chapter 13: Treatment of Presbyopia 129
Fabrizio I. Camesasca, MD; Paolo Vinciguerra, MD; Maria Ingrid Torres Munoz, MD

Chapter 14: Topographically Guided Transepithelial PRK for Refractive and Therapeutic Purposes 133
Leopoldo Spadea, MD; Angela Di Gregorio, MD

Chapter 15: The Role of Amino Acids in Corneal Healing: A New Method for Evaluating Cellular Density and Extracellular Matrix Distribution 143
Maria Ingrid Torres Munoz, MD; Paolo Vinciguerra, MD; Fabrizio I. Camesasca, MD; Fabio Grizzi, PhD; Francesco Saverio Dioguardi, MD; Nicola Dioguardi, MD

Section IV: The Evolution of Surface Ablation: LASEK, Epi-LASIK, and Custom Ablation

Chapter 16: LASEK 151
Thomas V. Claringbold II, DO; Lee Shahinian Jr, MD

Chapter 17: Butterfly LASEK 159
Paolo Vinciguerra, MD; Fabrizio I. Camesasca, MD

Chapter 18: LASEK With Custom Ablation and Smoothing 163
Paolo Vinciguerra, MD; Fabrizio I. Camesasca, MD

Chapter 19: Refractive, Aberrometric, and Pachymetric Stability and Patient's Satisfaction in Refractive Status and Vision Profile After Customized Treatment 169
Mario R. Romano, MD

Chapter 20: Advanced Surface Ablations for Myopia: Epi-LASIK 175
Vikentia J. Katsanevaki, MD, PhD; Maria I. Kalyvianaki, MD; Irini I. Naoumidi, PhD; Ioannis G. Pallikaris, MD, PhD

Chapter 21: LASEK and Epi-LASIK Excimer Surface Ablation 181
Elena Albè, MD; Dimitri T. Azar, MD

Chapter 22: Wavefront Customized PRK: Zyoptix 189
Stefano Baiocchi, MD, PhD; Marco Lazzarotto, MD; Claudia Sforzi, MD, PhD; Aldo Caporossi, MD

Chapter 23: No Alcohol LASEK vs PRK: A Comparative Study 199
Leopoldo Spadea, MD; Arianna Fiasca, MD

Chapter 24: *In Vivo* Confocal Microscopy: Clinical Relevance in Refractive Surgery
and in Epithelial Flap-Based Surface Ablation Techniques 205
Leonardo Mastropasqua, MD; Mario Nubile, MD; Manuela Lanzini, MD

Chapter 25: Corneal Wound Healing Response in LASEK 219
Marcelo V. Netto, MD; Rajiv R. Mohan, PhD; Renato Ambrósio Jr, MD; Steven E. Wilson, MD

Section V: Management of Complications

Chapter 26: Photorefractive Keratectomy: Complications During the Epithelial and Stromal Healing Phases 229
Aldo Caporossi, MD; Marco Lazzarotto, MD; Tomaso Caporossi, MD; Stefano Baiocchi, MD, PhD

Chapter 27: Reducing the Risk for Post-LASIK Ectasia 237
Daniel Epstein, MD, PhD; Paolo Vinciguerra, MD

Chapter 28: Diagnosis of Decentered Treatment 243
Paolo Vinciguerra, MD; Alessandro Randazzo, MD

Chapter 29: The Use of Mitomycin C in Surface Ablation 247
Francesco Carones, MD

Section VI: Phototherapeutic Keratectomy: Making Possible the Impossible

Chapter 30: Custom Phototherapeutic Keratectomy With Intraoperative Topography 255
Paolo Vinciguerra, MD; Fabrizio I. Camesasca, MD

Chapter 31: Long-Term Follow-Up of Ultrathin Corneas After Surface Retreatment
With Phototherapeutic Keratectomy 265
Paolo Vinciguerra, MD; Maria Ingrid Torres Munoz, MD; Fabrizio I. Camesasca, MD; Fabio Grizzi, PhD; Cynthia Roberts, PhD

Chapter 32: Nomograms for Surface Laser Correction 271
Guy M. Kezirian, MD, FACS

Section VII: The Refractive Surgery Patient: After Surgery

Chapter 33: Cataract Extraction With Intraocular Lens Implant After Refractive Surgery 281
Paolo Vinciguerra, MD; Pietro Rosetta, MD; Nadia Incarnato, MD

Chapter 34: Pharmacological Modulation of Corneal Wound Healing After Surface Ablation 291
Edoardo Midena, MD; Catia Gambato, MD; Alessandra Ghirlando, MD

Chapter 35: Corneal Surface Analysis After Photorefractive Keratectomy 299
Sebastiano Serrao, MD, PhD; Marco Lombardo, MD

Chapter 36: Very High Frequency Digital Ultrasound: Artemis 2 Scanning in Corneal Refractive Surgery 315
Dan Z. Reinstein, MD, MA(Cantab), FRCSC; Ronald H. Silverman, PhD; Timothy J. Archer, BA(Oxon)

Chapter 37: The Fractal Geometry of Human Corneal Stroma 331
Fabio Grizzi, PhD; Carlo Russo, PhD; Maria Ingrid Torres Munoz, MD; Francesco Saverio Dioguardi, MD; Nicola Dioguardi, MD

Appendix A: Pre- and Intraoperative Instrumental Diagnostics 337
Paolo Vinciguerra, MD; Fabrizio I. Camesasca, MD

Appendix B: LASEK Information for Patients 339
Thomas V. Claringbold II, DO; Lee Shahinian Jr, MD

Index *345*

Acknowledgments

The Editors would like to thank all the members of the Department of Ophthalmology of the Istituto Clinico Humanitas, Rozzano, Milano—Italy, for their generous support, day by day.

Thank you wholeheartedly: Marco Gramigna, Giorgio Gaspari, Pietro Rosetta, Elena Bernasconi, Ingrid Torres, Carlo Castellani, Alessandro Randazzo, Alessandra Di Maria, Rosario Urso, Eleonora Greco, Maria Grazia Quaranta, Nadia Incarnato, Elena Albè, Riccardo Scotti, Adriana Sergio, Paolo Gironda Veraldi, Raffaella Ricci, Antonio Battistini, Marco Criscito, Massimo Vitali, and Monia Moretti.

A particular thank to Hideo and Motoki Ozawa and the NIDEK Co, Ltd. Without their support several diagnostic and surgical advancements, this book would not have been possible. They have always openly welcomed any potential improvement to their technology and equipment with brave foresight.

Special thanks to the Trans-Edit Group, Milan, Italy (www.transeditgroup.it), for postediting on all the chapters written by Italian authors.

A warm thankyou to Dan Epstein, MD, PhD, for his numerous, precious suggestions during the preparation of this book.

About the Editors

Paolo Vinciguerra, MD began his studies on refractive surgery in 1986. Since that time, he has been constantly involved with projecting and developing excimer laser applications to refractive surgery, first with Aesculap Meditech (1989 to 1990), then with NIDEK (1991 to present). He has authored several patents: cross-cylinder ablation method for the correction of astigmatism, recentering mask technique ablation profiles for custom ablation, artificial eye for testing excimer ablation, custom ablation transition zone for custom ablation, computerized system for the analysis of corneal stroma with confocal microscopy and fractal analysis, development-integrated topographer/aberrometer/autorefractometer/pupillometer, as well as a variety of surgical instruments.

Dr. Vinciguerra has developed several original refractive surgery techniques: cross cylinders in hyperopic-myopic and high astigmatism, recentering mask technique, presbyopia technique, phototherapeutic keratotomy (PTK), smoothing after refractive surgery, a specific masking fluid for smoothing after PTK and PRK, Butterfly LASEK, variable aspheric transition zone, retreatment technique for hyperopic eyes, custom ablation transition zone, definition of new topographic indexes for automated evaluation of corneal optical quality, use of Scheimpflug camera in refractive surgery, and a new system for the preoperative evaluation of cataractous eyes that underwent previous refractive surgery with index of complexity and identification of the most appropriate IOL to be implanted. He has also developed several original surgical instruments.

Dr. Vinciguerra is Chairman of the Ophthalmology Department of the Istituto Clinico Humanitas, Rozzano, Milano, Italy. He is Consultant for the Italian High Council for Health since 2003, is member of the Italian Committee for Continuing Medical Education, has been Visiting Professor with the Ohio State University, and is actively involved with several Italian and International Ophthalmological Societies. He has received five ASCRS and two ISRS-AAO Best Paper Prizes, the International Society of Refractive Surgery Award for scientific contribution in 1988, the American Academy of Ophthalmology Achievement Award Certificate in 2003, and the Lans Lecture Award of the International Society of Refractive Surgery in 2005.

Since 2000, he promotes and chairs the international refractive surgery meeting Refr@ctive.online.

Dr. Vinciguerra has held and participated in manifold courses worldwide on refractive surgery and published numerous scientific papers and books on refractive surgery

Fabrizio Ivo Camesasca, MD was Fellow to Research with the Helen Keller Eye Research Foundation, Birmingham, Alabama, in 1988 to 1990, and achieved the Educational Commission for Foreign Medical Graduates Licensure in 1989. Besides his ophthalmological career, he was involved with the planning and start-up of the Istituto Clinico Humanitas, one of the largest general hospitals in Milan, Italy, from 1993 to 1998. He is Vice-Chairman of the Ophthalmology Department of Istituto Clinico Humanitas, has worked with Dr. Paolo Vinciguerra since 1999, and has been involved with refractive surgery since 2000.

In 2000, he received the American Academy of Ophthalmology Achievement Award Certificate. He is a member of the Italian Committee for Continuing Medical Education, and of the Scientific Committee for the Italian Ophthalmological Society.

Dr. Camesasca has been the scientific secretary of the international refractive surgery meeting Refr@ctive.online since 2000.

Dr. Camesasca has held several courses worldwide and has published numerous scientific articles and book chapters on refractive, cataract, and retinal surgery.

Contributing Authors

Elena Albe`, MD
Ophthalmology Department
Istituto Clinico Humanitas
Milan, Italy

Renato Ambrósio Jr, MD
Department of Ophthalmology
University of São Paulo
São Paulo, Brazil
Instituto de Olhos Renato Ambrósio
Rio de Janeiro, Brazil

Raymond A. Applegate, OD, PhD
Professor and Borish Chair of
  Optometry
College of Optometry
University of Houston
Houston, Texas

Timothy J. Archer, BA(Oxon)
St. Thomas' Hospital
Kings College
London, United Kingdom

Dimitri T. Azar, MD
Field Chair of Ophthalmic Research
Professor and Head
Department of Ophthalmology and
  Visual Sciences
Illinois Eye and Ear Infirmary
University of Illinois at Chicago
Chicago, Illinois

Harkaran S. Bains
NIDEK Technologies America
Greensboro, North Carolina

Stefano Baiocchi, MD, PhD
Department of Ophthalmological and
  Neurosurgical Sciences
University of Siena
Siena, Italy

Phil Buscemi OD
President
MedOps
Greensboro, North Carolina

Aldo Caporossi, MD
Director
Department of Ophthalmological and
  Neurosurgical Sciences
University of Siena
Siena, Italy

Tomaso Caporossi, MD
Department of Ophthalmological and
  Neurosurgical Sciences
University of Siena
Siena, Italy

Francesco Carones, MD
Carones Ophthalmology Center
Milan, Italy

Thomas V. Claringbold II, DO
Chief Ophthalmologist
MidMichigan Physicians Group
Assistant Clinical Professor
Michigan State University
Clare, Michigan

Angela Di Gregorio, MD
Eye Clinic
S. Salvatore Hospital
University of L'Aquila
L'Aquila, Italy

Francesco Saverio Dioguardi, MD
Laboratori di Medicina Quantitativa
Istituto Clinico Humanitas IRCCS
  Rozzano
M. Rodriguez Foundation Scientific
  Institute for Quantitative Measures in
  Medicine
Milan, Italy

Nicola Dioguardi, MD
Laboratori di Medicina Quantitativa
Istituto Clinico Humanitas IRCCS
  Rozzano
M. Rodriguez Foundation Scientific
  Institute for Quantitative Measures in
  Medicine
Milan, Italy

Daniel Epstein, MD, PhD
Department of Ophthalmology
University Hospital
Zurich, Switzerland

Arianna Fiasca, MD
Eye Clinic
Department of Surgical Sciences
L'Aquila University
Italy

Catia Gambato, MD
Department of Ophthalmology
University of Padova
Padova, Italy

Alessandra Ghirlando, MD
Department of Ophthalmology
University of Padova
Padova, Italy

Fabio Grizzi, PhD
Laboratori di Medicina Quantitativa
Istituto Clinico Humanitas IRCCS
  Rozzano
M. Rodriguez Foundation Scientific
  Institute for Quantitative Measures in
  Medicine
Milan, Italy

Nadia Incarnato, MD
Ophthalmology Department
Istituto Clinico Humanitas
Milan, Italy

Vikentia J. Katsanevaki, MD, PhD
University of Crete Medical School
Vardinoyannion Eye Institute of Crete
Crete, Greece

Maria I. Kalyvianaki, MD
University of Crete Medical School
Vardinoyannion Eye Institute of Crete
Crete, Greece

Guy M. Kezirian, MD, FACS
SurgiVision Consultants, Inc.
Scottsdale, Arizona

Stephen D. Klyce, PhD
Professor of Ophthalmology and
  Anatomy/Cell Biology
Louisiana State University Medical
  Center School of Medicine
Adjunct Professor of Biomedical
  Engineering
Tulane University
New Orleans, Louisiana

Manuela Lanzini, MD
Ophthalmology Clinic
University "G. D'Annunzio"
Chieti-Pescara, Italy

Marco Lazzarotto, MD
Department of Ophthalmological and
  Neurosurgical Sciences
University of Siena
Siena, Italy

Jennifer R. Lewis, PhD
Ohio State University
Department of Ophthalmology
Biomedical Engineering Center
Columbus, Ohio

Marco Lombardo, MD
SerraoLaser
Rome, Italy

Luca Maestroni, MD
Department of Ophthalmology
Istituto Clinico Humanitas
Milan, Italy

Leonardo Mastropasqua
University "G. D'Annunzio"
Department of Medicine and Aging Sciences
Section of Ophthalmology
Chieti-Pescara, Italy

Edoardo Midena, MD
Professor of Ophthalmology
Department of Ophthalmology
University of Padova
Padova, Italy

Rajiv R. Mohan, PhD
The Cole Eye Institute
The Cleveland Clinic Foundation
Cleveland, Ohio

Maria Ingrid Torres Munoz, MD
Department of Ophthalmology
Istituto Clinico Humanitas
Milan, Italy

Irini I. Naoumidi, PhD
University of Crete Medical School
Vardinoyannion Eye Institute of Crete
Crete, Greece

Marcelo V. Netto, MD
The Cole Eye Institute
The Cleveland Clinic Foundation
Cleveland, Ohio
Department of Ophthalmology
University of São Paulo
São Paulo, Brazil

Guido Nizzola, MD
Poliambulatorio Chirurgico Modenese
Modena, Italy

Mario Nubile, MD
Ophthalmology Clinic
University "G. D'Annunzio"
Chieti-Pescara, Italy

Ioannis G. Pallikaris, MD, PhD
Associate Professor of Ophthalmology
Department of Ophthalmology
University of Crete—Medical School
Crete, Greece

Alessandro Randazzo, MD
Department of Ophthalmology
Istituto Clinico Humanitas
Milan, Italy

Dan Z. Reinstein, MD, MA(Cantab), FRCSC
London Vision Clinic
London, United Kingdom
Weill Medical College of Cornell University
New York, NY
St Thomas' Hospital
Kings College
London, United Kingdom

Cynthia J. Roberts, PhD
Ohio State University
Department of Ophthalmology
Biomedical Engineering Center
Columbus, Ohio

Mario R. Romano, MD
Ophthalmology Department
S. Sebastiano Hospital
Caserta, Italy

Pietro Rosetta, MD
Department of Ophthalmology
Istituto Clinico Humanitas
Milan, Italy

Carlo Russo, PhD
Laboratori di Medicina Quantitativa
Department of Ophthalmology
Istituto Clinico Humanitas, IRCCS, Rozzano
M. Rodriguez Foundation Scientific Institute for Quantitative Measures in Medicine
Milan, Italy

Sebastiano Serrao, MD, PhD
SerraoLaser
Rome, Italy

Claudia Sforzi, MD, PhD
Department of Ophthalmological and Neurosurgical Sciences
University of Siena
Siena, Italy

Lee Shahinian, Jr, MD
Clinical Professor of Ophthalmology
Stanford University School of Medicine
Los Altos, California

Ronald H. Silverman, PhD
Weill Medical College of Cornell University
New York, New York

Leopoldo Spadea, MD
Associate Clinical Professor of Ophthalmology
Eye Clinic
Department of Surgical Sciences
L'Aquila University
Italy

Steven E. Wilson, MD
The Cole Eye Institute
The Cleveland Clinic Foundation
Cleveland, Ohio

Introduction

We have written this book because of our enthusiasm and satisfaction with surface ablation throughout the years. The worldwide resurgence of surface ablation is remarkable, and is related to the advantages provided by new lasers, which have solved several limitations of old lasers (ie, small optical zones). These limitations have occasionally induced severe complications, an important issue in these years of constantly increasing litigation. Thus, we believe that the time is ripe for a complete textbook on surface ablation.

Writing a book on surface ablation refractive surgery has been both exciting and challenging. Translating the everyday practice into written information elicits a review process of personal beliefs and experiences. We have tried to capture all the details of the logical process, starting when a patient enters our office and asks for refractive correction and ending almost 12 months after surgery, when the situation can be regarded as stable.

Surface ablation refractive surgery techniques have received very close attention from the emergence of the technique to the introduction of LASIK. Thereafter, the interest of surgeons, mostly in the United States, has been dedicated to stromal techniques. Nevertheless, use of surface ablation has continued with constant updates and advancements of its technical components and clinical expertise. A wide critical review of these advancements, their integration, and results has been lacking until now, while such information is certainly available for LASIK. Recently, surface ablation has received renewed and increasing attention thanks to the introduction of new technical approaches, such as LASEK and Epi-LASIK, aimed at reducing patient pain—one of the major drawbacks of PRK.

This book has been structured to provide a step-by step, complete, and exhaustive text on surface ablation. Its main sections take the reader from the very beginning to advanced topics in surface ablation:

* Initially, patient selection and preoperative management are discussed, as well as the bases for understanding surface ablation.
* Surface ablation differs profoundly from intrastromal ablation in several relevant aspects, the most important of which, in our opinion, is the reparative response. In PRK, this response is mostly sensitive to the obtained corneal curvature gradient, while in LASIK, an important role is played by biomechanical forces. This book presents these features of surface ablation with evaluation of profiles, nomograms, and the key role of final surface smoothing.
* Treatment of every refractive defect is examined in detail:
  * Myopia, with attention to transition zone and induction of spherical aberration.
  * Astigmatism, and the problem of the uncorrected meridian.
  * Hyperopia, with problems related to increase of corneal prolate curvature.
  * Presbyopia, presenting the different approaches available.
* Recent evolutions and advancements in surface ablation (ie, LASEK, Epi-LASIK, and custom ablation) are illustrated by experts. Particular attention is dedicated to the differences among the techniques and to the advantages of each technique.
* The most complicated parts of the surgeon's work are examined: diagnosis and management of complications (ie, diagnosis of true vs false decentration) and consequent treatment as well as analysis, diagnosis, and treatment of patients with small optical zones, etc.
* Special attention and an entire section are dedicated to phototherapeutic keratectomy (PTK) with the latest technical updates, transepithelial PTK, and intraoperative topographical evaluation.
* Finally, long-term patient management and special problems in patients who have undergone surface ablation (ie, cataract extraction and IOL implantation) are discussed.

This book can be used as a guidebook for refractive surgeons who wish to increase their knowledge of surface ablation with basic information on all the above-mentioned steps. In addition, special advanced sections are provided for refractive surgeons who are experts in surface ablation and intend to examine specific topics in detail. Custom ablation has one overriding aim—all surgeons would like to optimize the corneal surface without excessive tissue consumption. We have provided a step-by-step illustrated analysis of optical zone optimization accompanied by tissue-saving strategies. The introduction of custom ablation and intraoperative topography has widened the horizons of PTK, now a powerful tool for the treatment of complications and corneal abnormalities. An especially complex topic, the analysis of postoperative visual complaints (ie, halos and night vision problems), has also received attention. The book provides an advanced analysis of diagnostic techniques (ie, topography and pachymetry) and an approach for possible surgical management.

Our most sincere gratitude goes to all the colleagues and experts who have generously shared their knowledge with us and with all our readers.

Paolo Vinciguerra
Fabrizio I. Camesasca
Milan, Italy, May 2006

Foreword

What is the role of surface ablation in your refractive surgery practice? Whether your procedure of choice is PRK, LASEK, or Epi-LASIK, research from many investigators published over the past decade has conclusively demonstrated that surface ablation is the procedure of choice for many patients, and that these procedures may be used successfully as the primary procedure for the correction of most refractive errors. Similarly, treatment with PTK is frequently optimal therapy for patients with corneal diseases such as recurrent corneal erosion or eyes with refractive surgery complications such as buttonhole flaps or irregular astigmatism.

There are many factors and nuances regarding application of surface ablation and prevention and treatment of complications that the refractive surgeon must fully appreciate to enhance the outcomes of surface ablation procedures. Paolo Vinciguerra and Fabrizio I. Camesasca have brought many of the world's experts together in *Refractive Surface Ablation: PRK, LASEK, Epi-LASIK, Custom, PTK, and Retreatment* to provide concise, but thorough, chapters on every aspect of PRK, LASEK, Epi-LASIK, and PTK. From patient selection and preoperative planning, to application treatments for specific refractive errors, to detailed descriptions of the surgical techniques, to prevention and management of complications, every aspect of surface ablation is detailed in this comprehensive book. Not only should every refractive surgeon have a copy of this book for reference, but it should also be required reading for all trainees in cornea and refractive surgery. As we near the 20-year anniversary of the introduction of excimer laser refractive and therapeutic surgery, it is indeed fortunate that we have such a comprehensive treatise detailing the application of several of the most important procedures. The editors and authors are to be congratulated for providing such a valuable resource.

Steven E. Wilson, MD
Professor of Ophthalmology
Director of Corneal Research
The Cole Eye Institute
Cleveland Clinic Foundation
Cleveland, Ohio

SECTION I

PATIENT SELECTION AND PREOPERATIVE MANAGEMENT: UNDERSTANDING SURFACE ABLATION

CHAPTER 1

TOPOGRAPHY IN SURFACE ABLATION

Paolo Vinciguerra, MD; Luca Maestroni, MD

Keratoscopy

Keratoscopy is based on the reflection of luminous rings projected by a dedicated apparatus (keratoscope).

ACQUISITION

Correct data acquisition is fundamental to achieve a reliable examination. Great attention must be paid to the correct positioning of the head as well as ensuring the patient focuses on the luminous sight, that the lachrymal film is well laminated, and that the rings are in focus.

In relation to the keratoscope, a frontal position is certainly the most comfortable but not the best for acquisition; indeed, it would be better to turn the head so that the patient fixes on the luminous ring with abduction of the examined eye, moves to the left while the right eye is being analyzed, and then moves towards the right while the left eye is being analyzed. This way, the shadow of the nose is reduced and the slight lowering of the upper eyelid due to convergence is eliminated, thus increasing the range of the area covered by the rings (Figure 1-1). With deep set eyes, it would be expedient to increase the thickness of the instrument's forehead rest; the resulting hyperdistention of the head reduces the shadow cast over the cornea from the frontal bone and allows more extensive exploration of the upper sectors.

Keratoscopy provides morphological information, hence each evaluation must be performed based on the appearance of the corneal rings.[1]

The regularity and the continuity of keratoscope rings are an indicator of good surface quality at each point; the lachrymal film and corneal epithelium give good reflection, ensuring the specularity of the cornea. Such characteristics are only compromised in the most evident stages of altered curvature with corneal ectasy. A descemetocele with focal opacification, hypercurvature to such an extent as to alter the lamination of the lachrymal film, or the formation of a leukoma at the apex of the cone, appear as irregular and/or broken rings. Data processing in such cases is not reliable, and the keratoscopic image is the only one capable of providing accurate information (Figures 1-2 and 1-3).[1]

EVALUATION

A regular reflection may only be produced by a surface with a constant radius of curvature. In a normal cornea, the rings appear concentric, well delineated, and defined. Irregularities indicate an abrupt variation in curvature.[1-3]

Contrast is an important parameter in keratoscopic evaluation. This is generated by perfect corneal transparency, and any reduction in contrast reflects a reduction in corneal transparency.

The topographic map is calculated based on the distance between the rings. This detail is very important in keratoscopic evaluation. The closer the rings, the greater the curvature of the surface undergoing analysis. On the contrary, widely spaced rings are indicative of a flat surface. Analysis of the overall curvature is just as important as localized variations. Often, in the initial stages of keratoconus, it is difficult to observe keratoscopic distortions, since the slight localized narrowing of the rings, an indicator of increased curvature of the anterior corneal surface, may go undetected, especially with an inexperienced or distracted observer.

The distance between the rings becomes fundamental in the evaluation of corneal leukomas of whatever origin. As already mentioned, topographic extrapolation in such cases is frequently unreliable given the irregularity and the incompleteness of the rings, and it may not be simple to understand whether corneal opacity is raised or depressed. Simple evaluation of the behavior of the rings will show whether opacity is raised

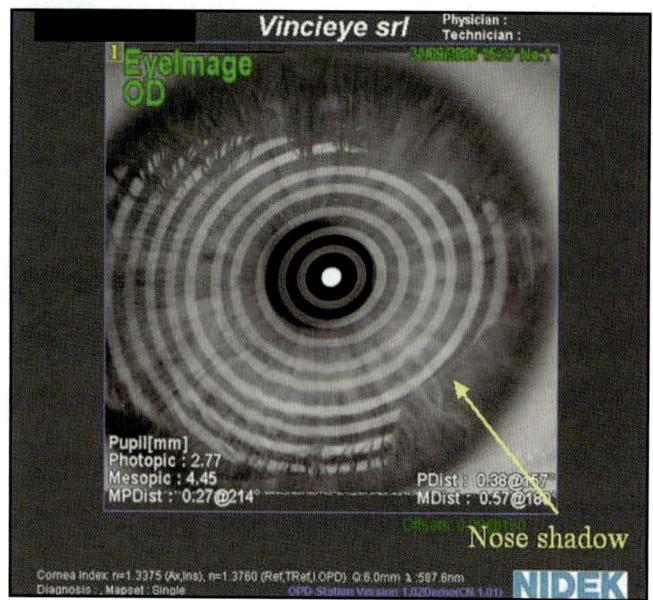

Figure 1-1. Astigmatism case with area shadowed by the nose. The operator needs to properly turn the patient's head to achieve the widest possible keratoscopic reflex in order to have a reliable topographic map.

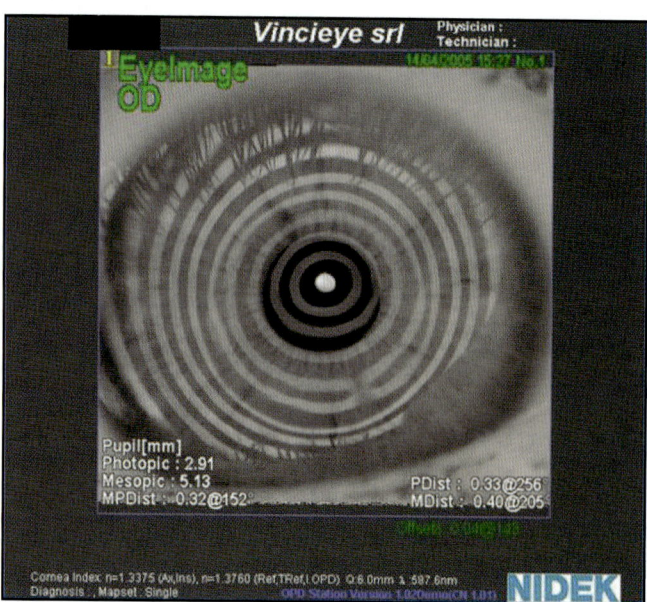

Figure 1-2. Keratoscopic image, a case of haze post-PRK. Rings are interrupted with irregular margins. It can be easily realized that vision in this eye is poor.

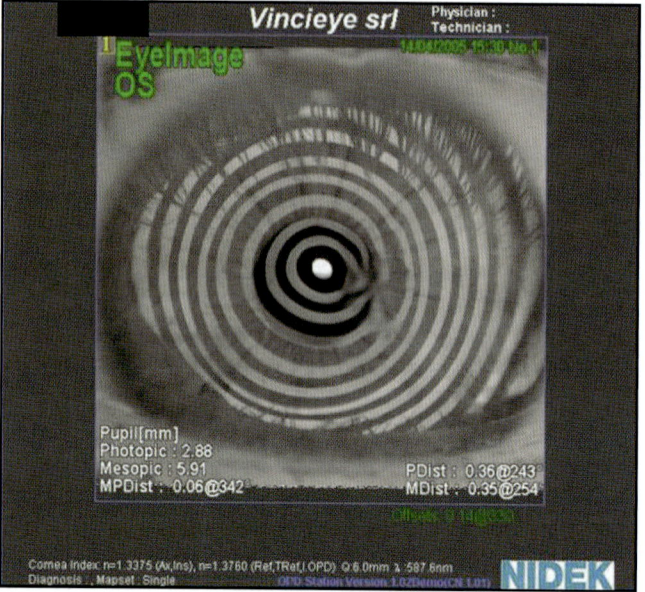

Figure 1-3. Fellow eye of Figure 1-1, keratoscopic image, haze and irregular cornea post-PRK. In a case like this, where correct attribution of consecutive rings is difficult, the topography map may not fully represent the ring alterations and thus corneal surface deformation.

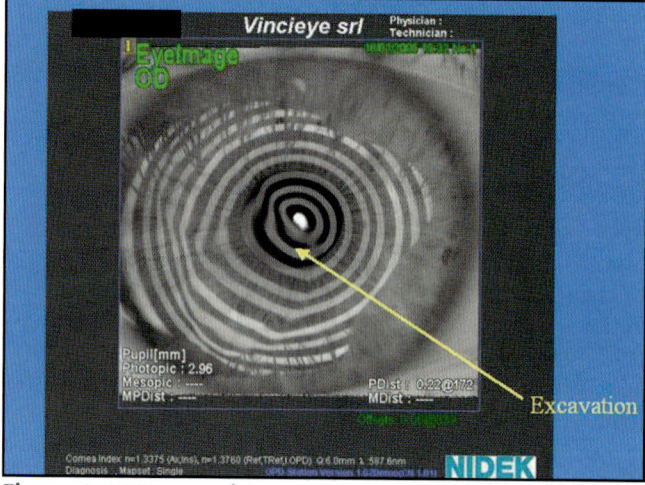

Figure 1-4. An eye after a corneal abscess with a profound excavation highlighted by wide, irregular rings.

(converging rings in the vicinity of leukomatous formations), level, or depressed (divergent rings in the vicinity of lesions) (Figures 1-4 through 1-10).

Variations in the distance between rings from the center to the periphery provides an estimate of corneal eccentricity; in a prolate cornea (more curved at the center, flatter at the margin) the distance between rings increases moving from the center to the periphery, in an oblate cornea (flatter at the center, more curved at the margin) the rings are closer at the periphery than at the center.

Abrupt changes in curvature, as in cases of keratoconus, imply a significant increase in eccentricity and account for any associated deficiency of vision.

Evaluation of the keratoscopic examination may point out processing errors in the evaluation of hypercurved surfaces; when two rings are very close, the software may ignore one, considering the subsequent ring directly.

The map calculation will be effected by this, and curvature will be underestimated, resulting in a cornea which appears more "normal" than it is in reality.

As already mentioned, the keratoscope projects luminous concentric rings, hence the reflected rings must also be round; in the case of corneal astigmatism, the cornea has a

Topography in Surface Ablation 5

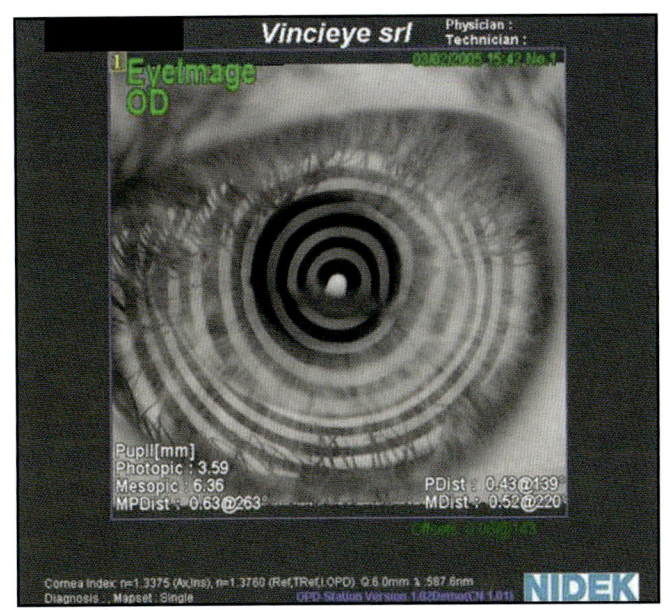

Figure 1-5. A corneal flap stria in a LASIK eye.

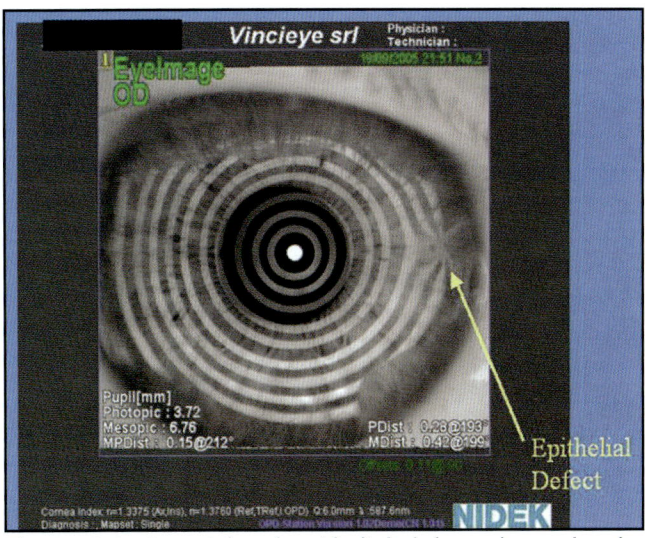

Figure 1-6. A peripheral epithelial defect, shown by the incomplete, irregular rings.

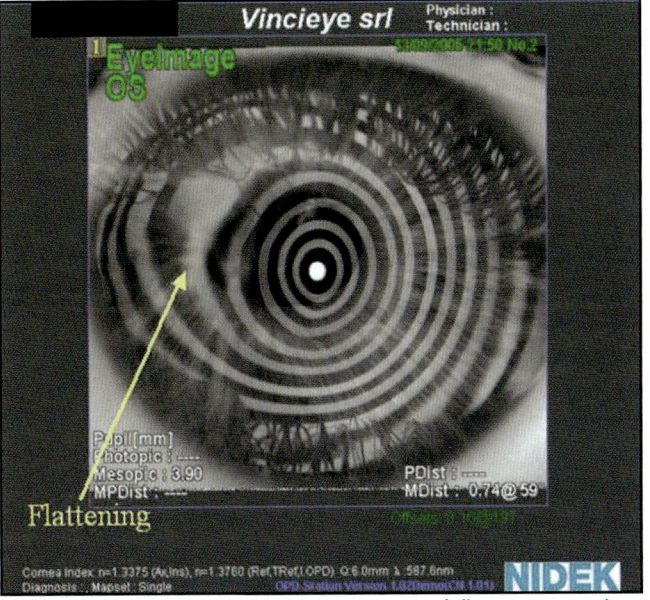

Figure 1-7. Severe post-traumatic corneal flattening, inducing marked hyperopic astigmatism.

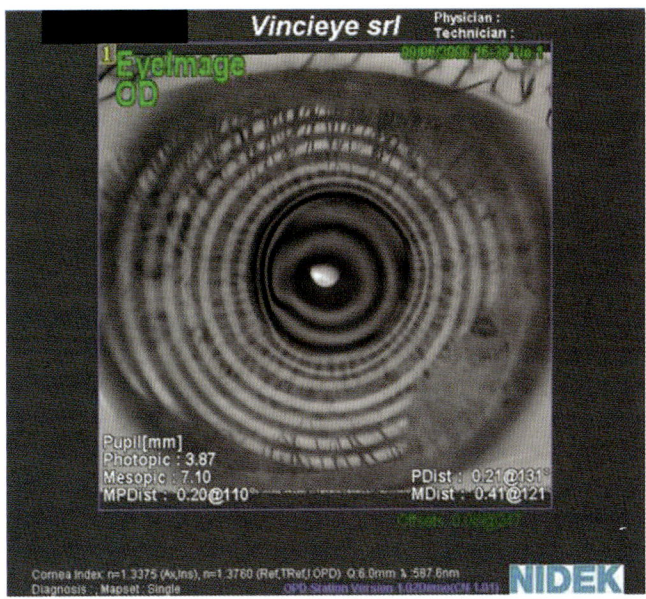

Figure 1-8. Postcorneal abscess deformation. The central cornea has been severely flattened, and the rings are so deformed to be unprocessable. Such a flattening, being limited to a small area with surrounding preserved corneal stroma, can be successfully treated by PTK. The processing software may not accept such a wide first, inner ring. Other times, the ring may be too small to be located within the central, whiter reflex. Ring detection, in these cases, must be carefully verified by the operator.

more oval rather than spherical conformation; consequently, it reflects ovals, not rings. Depending on the characteristics of the astigmatism (with or against the rule, regular or irregular, large or small bow-tie), there will be compression of the rings on one meridian with respect to the other, and focal or diffuse variations will be observed.

Another important aspect to be considered in a keratoscopic reading is the symmetry of the rings. Complete symmetry over the entire examined field is observed in emmetropic individuals or those affected by spherical refractive errors (myopia or hypermetropia), and the rings appear round and concentric.

Linear symmetry is typical of individuals affected by congenital regular astigmatism. The rings appear oval and there is only perfect symmetry along the two main meridians. The symmetry of the rings, whether complete or linear, is of fundamental importance because it indicates the possibility for correcting any refractive errors using lenses.

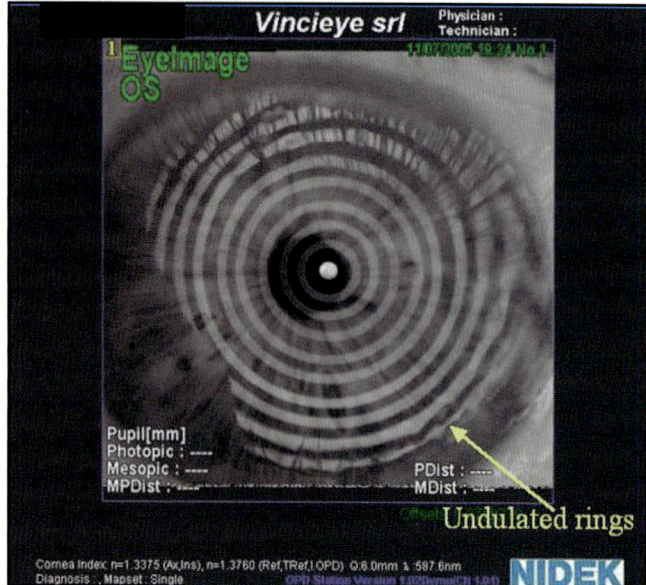

Figure 1-9. Undulated peripheral rings. This is an artifact due to dry corneal surface. After instillation of artificial tears, the reflex will be regular, complete and the keratoscopy processable.

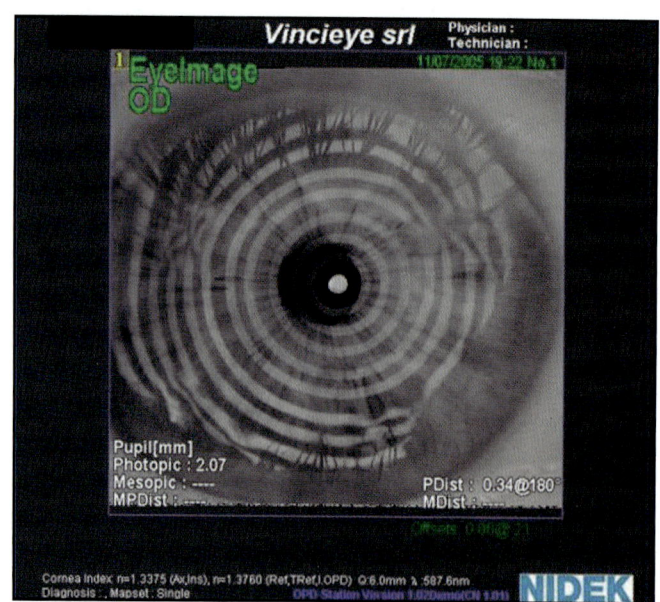

Figure 1-10. In this case, the irregularities, much more diffuse and profound, are due to corneal opacities and surface irregularity.

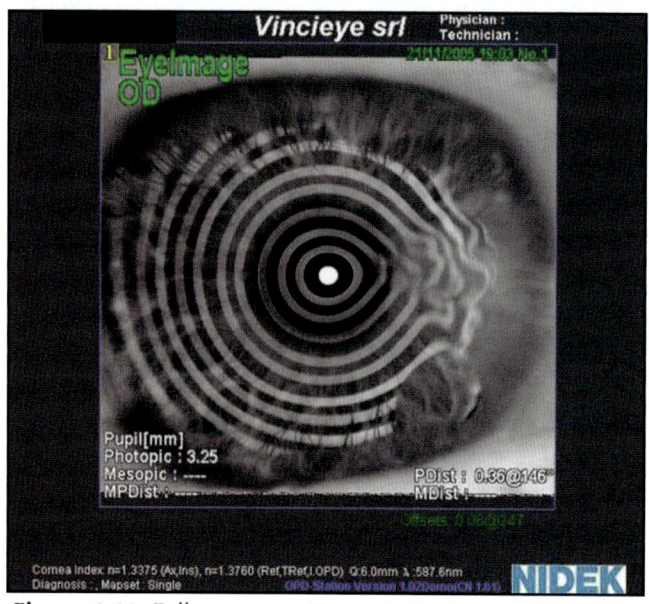

Figure 1-11. Fellow eye to Figure 1-10. A pterygium case. In this case, when the pupil enlarges in scotopic conditions, an irregular portion of cornea will be involved and vision will become poor.

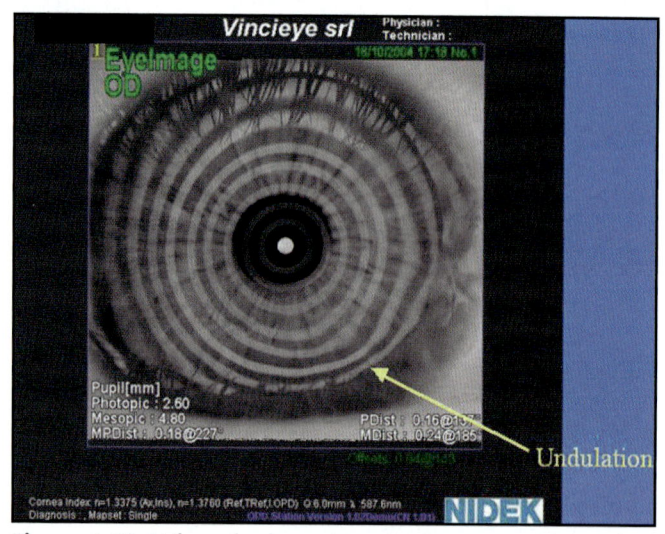

Figure 1-12. When the keratoscopic rings are undulated as in this case, the variation in dioptrical power is extremely high and is concentrated in a small portion of the cornea. Ring detection in such cases may be inaccurate and not rendering in detail the important deformation.

Complete asymmetry is observed in abnormal corneas and compromises visual acuity and the possibility to correct refractive errors proportionally linked to its extent. The rings may be irregular or even absent in some areas, and show abrupt changes in the distances between one another (Figures 1-11 and 1-12).

Analysis of the complete examination will provide indications useful for recognizing congenital astigmatism, which is generally detected by regular rings closer on the more myopic (or less hypermetropic) meridian, giving a series of concentric ovals that are irregular and astigmatic in shape, where the asymmetry indicates a high variation in the curvature per unit of surface, and which may be a manifestation of a progressive corneal disease.

To assess how much a corneal alteration of whatever origin and extent influences a patient's visual acuity and quality of vision, it is essential to know the spatial relationship with the pupillary foramen. Generally, this rule especially applies to keratoconus, where the apex of the ectasia is frequently decentered and where relatively slight astigmatism may be greatly incapacitating with respect to defects of greater extent,

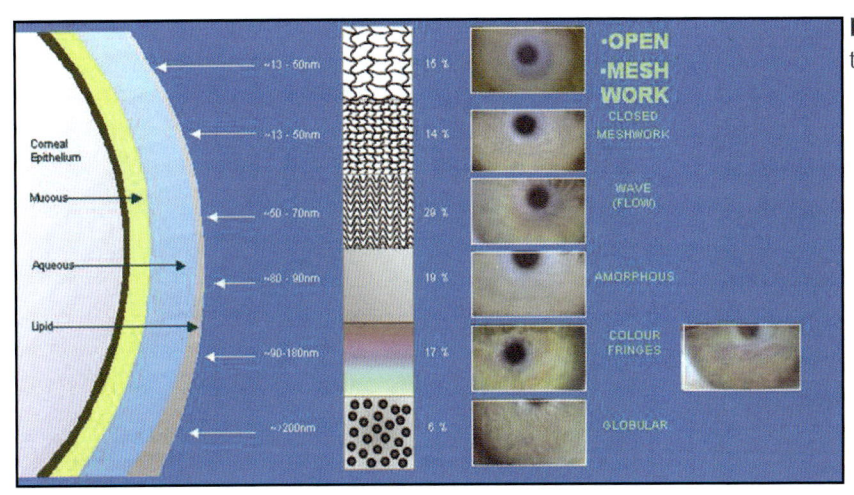

Figure 1-13. Preocular tear film lipid patterns. (Courtesy of Keeler.)

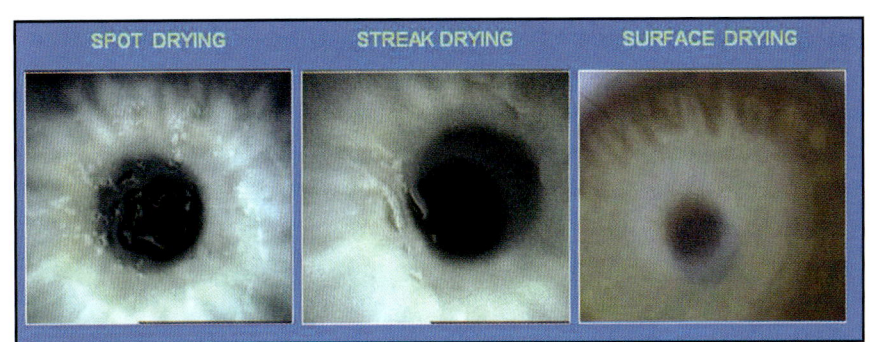

Figure 1-14. Normal pre-soft lens drying patterns. (Courtesy of Keeler.)

depending on their localization and the pupillary diameter of the individual in question.

Lachrymal Film

The colorimetric corneal map, with whatever algorithm it is calculated, provides information on the curvature of the anterior corneal surface and the lachrymal film at any given time. However, in the vast majority of cases, it does not indicate the cause giving rise to any anomalies and, above all, may frequently be misleading due to the presence of artefacts. Thus, keratoscopy constitutes an essential complement, since it allows proper analysis of the lachrymal film which, as is well known, is indispensable for good reflection of the luminous mires and constitutes one of the major sources of artefacts. Keratoscopy is a dynamic examination and is, hence, an irreplaceable tool for evaluating lamination of the lachrymal film, a similarly dynamic process.[1]

In many cases, the patient simply blinking is sufficient to establish whether a given alteration is due to poor lamination of the tear film, the presence of filaments, or mucous aggregates or secretions.

Anomalies of the corneal or conjunctival surfaces or disorders affecting the eyelids or tear ducts frequently compromise the lamination processes (Figures 1-13 and 14). In such cases, there is frequently supernatant accumulation in the lower sectors, which can distort the corneal curvature data shown by topography.

If there is any corneal hypercurvature, as in the case of keratoconus, the lachrymal film may level out the surface, making the curvature homogeneous and causing the pathology to go unrecognized or be underestimated.

On the other hand, in the case where corneal tissue is lacking for whatever reason, the tear film may act as plaster, filling the defect, which may then go unnoticed during processing.

A further advantage of keratoscopy is constituted by the possibility of a three-dimensional evaluation of the corneal surface and the lachrymal film, permitted by illumination of the keratoscope cone over multiple, even lateral, planes. This allows better evaluation of the area of defective lamination or stagnation, which has significant importance in giving rise to visual fluctuations.

The practice of acquiring keratoscopic and other images, and evaluating the computer results without knowing under what conditions they were surveyed and from which images they were calculated, should be prohibited. Alterations in the lachrymal film may give topographic patterns similar to keratoconus, whereby static evaluation of just the colorimetric map may give rise to gross diagnostic errors.

Corneal Topography

This is computerized keratoscopy processing that constitutes the gold standard for measuring the curvature of the anterior corneal surface.[1-3]

In refractive patients, careful topographic analysis is indispensable for various reasons. First, it is ideal for identifying corneal disorders such as keratoconus, which, in the initial stages, does not give rise to any clinical manifestations and is not identifiable any other way. Also, nonprogressive localized

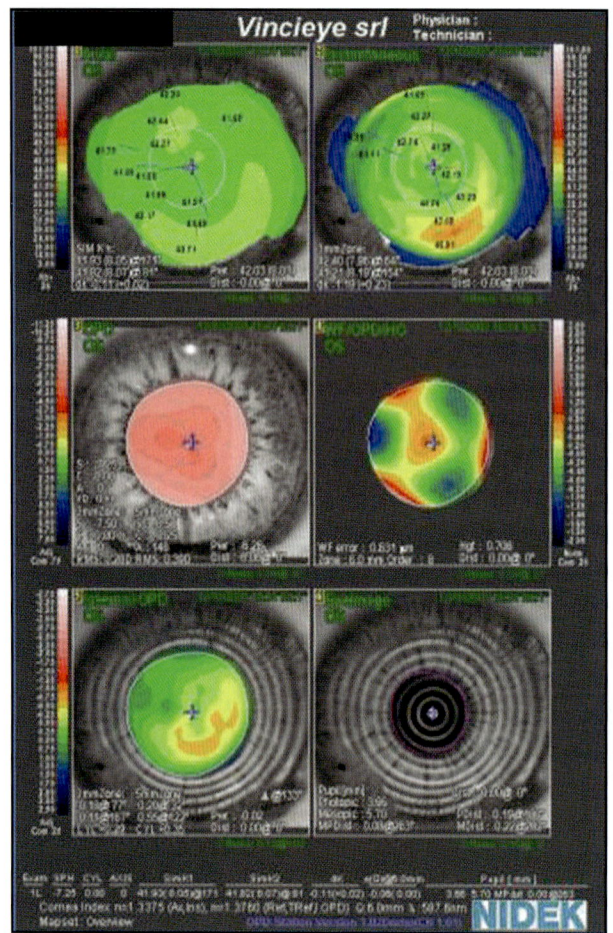

Figure 1-15. A normal keratometry could not highlight the presence of this peripheral keratoconus.

hypercurvature, such as forme fruste keratoconus, may not be detected by means of simple objective slit-lamp examination but may lead to serious and irreversible alterations of corneal structure if it progresses to corneal thinning for refractive purposes.

Progressive or fruste keratoconus represents the most obvious case where topography is of crucial importance, but all corneal disorders involving local or more widespread alteration of the curvature of the anterior surface may be identified and documented by means of this examination (Figures 1-15 through 1-21).

Even in nondisease conditions, corneal curvature represents an important preoperative parameter, especially in hypermetropies, where the possibility of obtaining good results depends on the curvature obtained. Indeed, if eccentricity becomes too accentuated, a pattern similar to keratoconus is created with inevitable consequences for visual quality.

Another situation where corneal topography has been shown to be irreplaceable is with reversible corneal deformations brought on by contact lenses (warpage). A very high percentage of potential candidates for refractive surgery use contacts and exhibit varying extents of warpage. Its presence may only be detected by means of corneal mapping, and at the risk of a bad outcome, all surgery should be suspended until

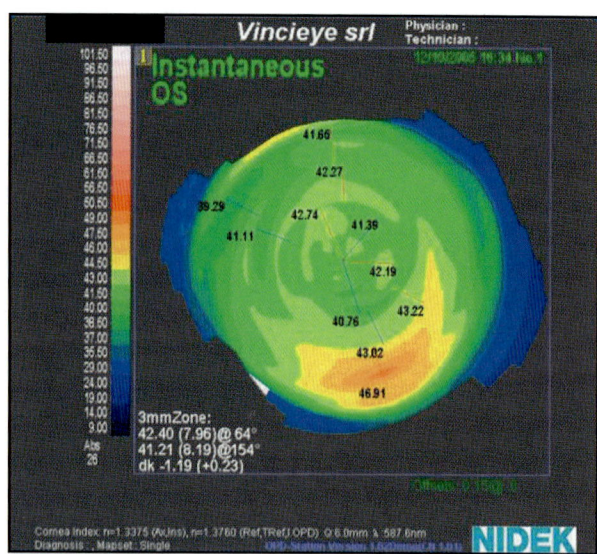

Figure 1-16. Same eye as Figure 1-13, instantaneous algorithm.

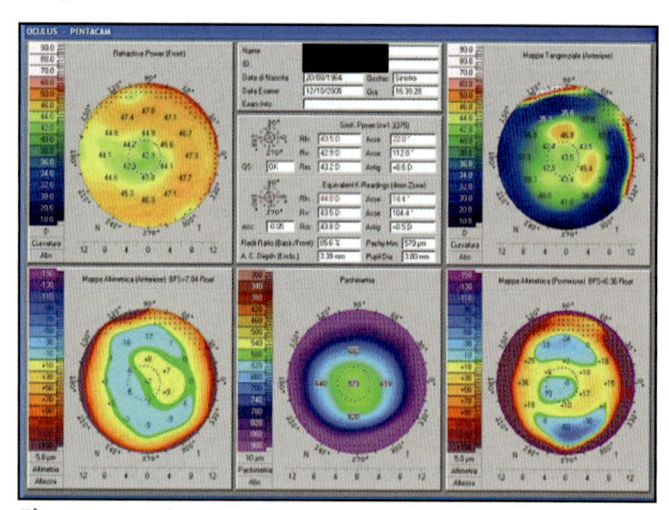

Figure 1-17. Same eye as Figure 1-13, Pentacam evaluation. Anterior altimetric map, below left, shows an island pattern. Note also the difference in thickness (below, center) between superior and inferior cornea (682 vs 620).

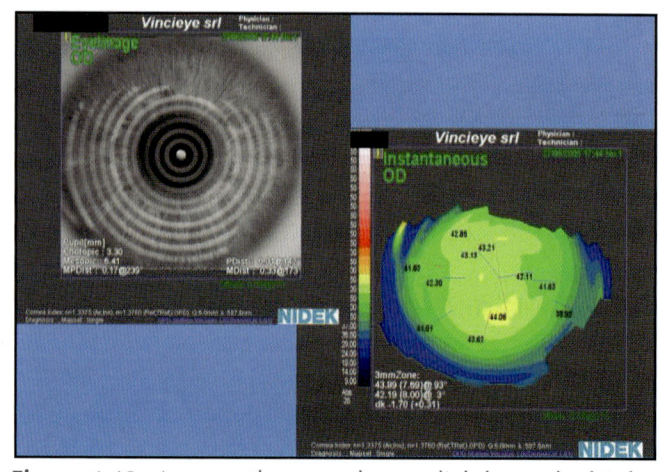

Figure 1-18. Apparently normal eye, slightly marked inferior curvature.

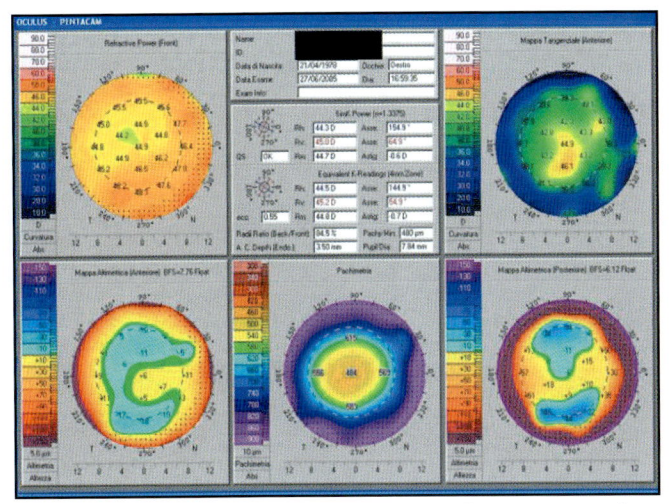

Figure 1-19. Same eye as Figure 1-16, Pentacam evaluation. Pachymetry map highlights a minimal thickness of 480 μm.

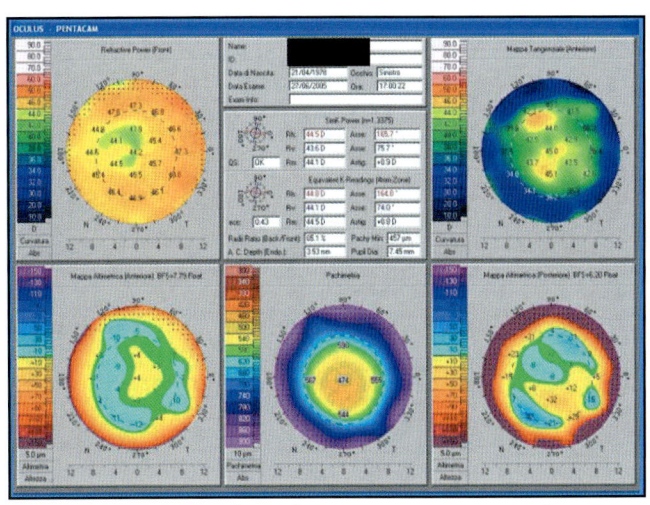

Figure 1-20. Contralateral eye in Figure 1-16, Pentacam evaluation. Note minimal thickness of 457 μm, located inferiorly. Posterior elevation map shows that posterior surface is more curved inferiorly.

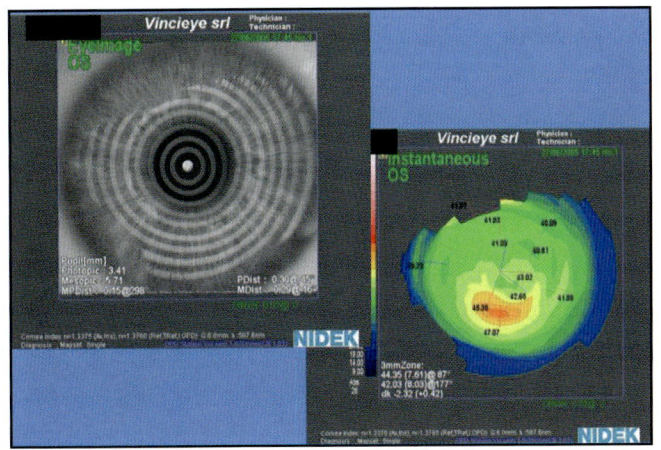

Figure 1-21. Same eye as Figure 1-18. Instantaneous algorithm confirms the presence of a conus.

the normal corneal profile is completely restored (Figures 1-22 through 1-34). Furthermore, warpage may frequently simulate a keratoconus, and differential diagnosis requires the prolonged suspension of using lenses and the subsequent repetition of the examination, which in the case of warpage, will highlight the restored regularization of the corneal profile (Figures 1-35 and 36). This process may require some time, even up to 6 months.

Corneal topography may be calculated according to various mathematical formulae, known as algorithms, and analyzes the shape of the anterior surface, not the dioptric power. Given the historic origins of keratometry, even for curvature maps, the unit of measurement that has been adopted is the diopter, which in physics measures optical power and not curvature. For this reason, ANSI (American National Standard Institute) has recently introduced the "keratometric diopter" as the unit of measurement for the curvature of the anterior corneal surface (which is equivalent to the curvature of a sphere with a radius of curvature of 8 mm 337.5 D/8 mm).[4]

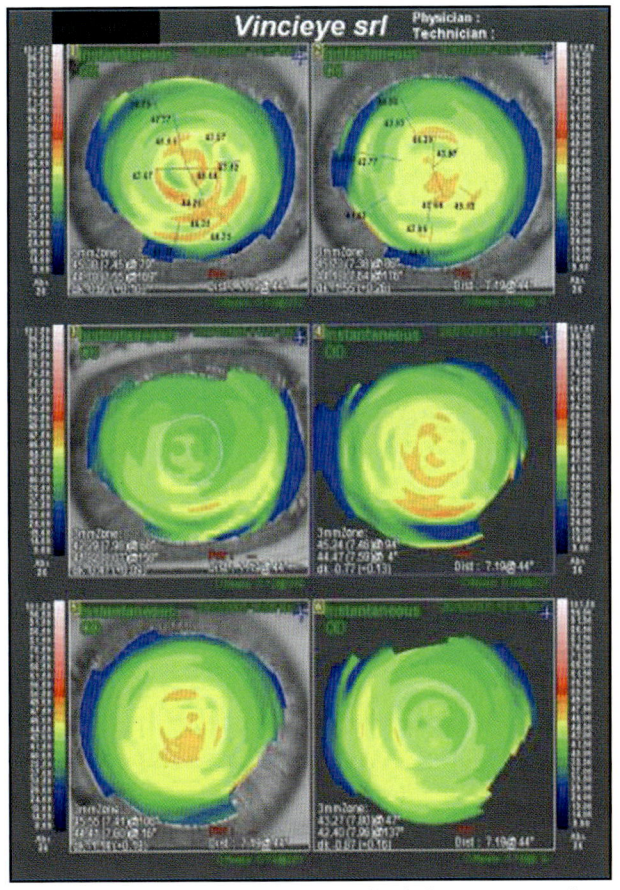

Figure 1-22. Keratoconus masked by contact lens warpage. In this series of instantaneous topographies, a contact-lens-induced warpage progressively disappears in right eye (top left, top right, center left) and left eye (center right, bottom left, bottom right), with appearance of true keratoconus-related asymmetry of curvature.

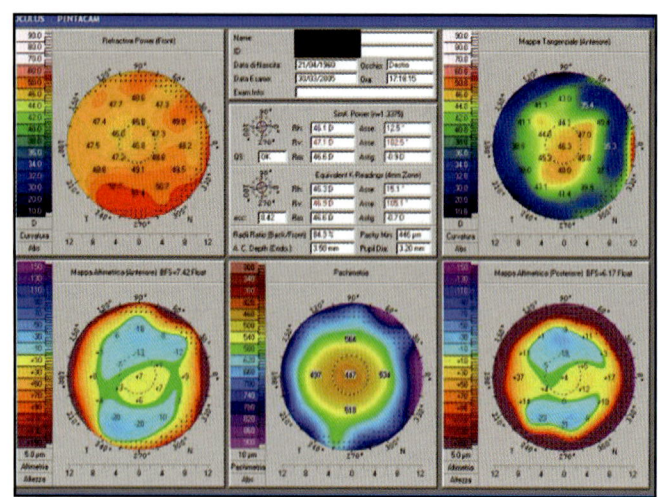

Figure 1-23. Same case as Figure 1-22, RE Pentacam evaluation. Note the island pattern (bottom left) in the anterior altimetric map, the thin cornea in the pachymetric map (447 mu, bottom center), and the almost-island pattern on the posterior altimetric map.

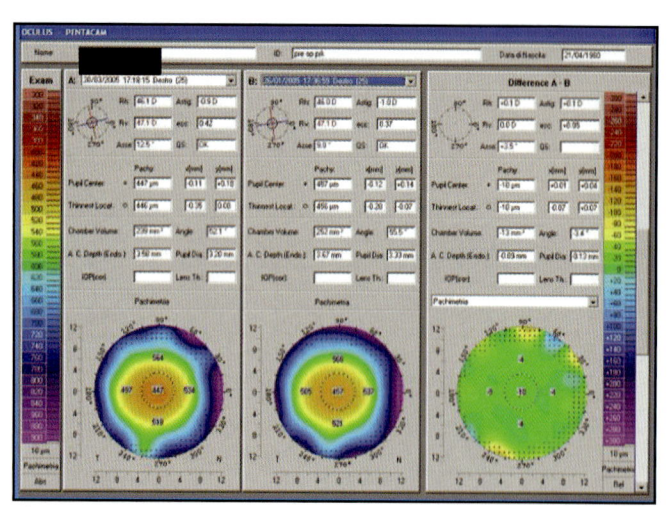

Figure 1-24. Differential map of RE in Figure 1-22 showing that in 2 months, the pachymetry map decreased centrally by 10 μm.

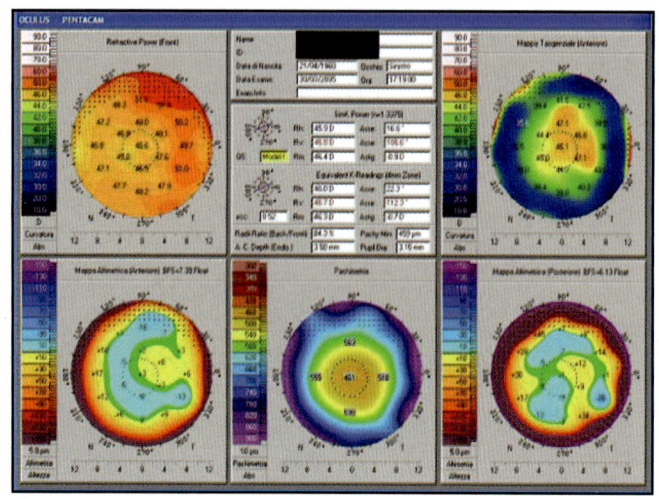

Figure 1-25. Same case as Figure 1-22, LE Pentacam evaluation. Note the island pattern (bottom left) in the anterior altimetric map as well as in the posterior altimetric map.

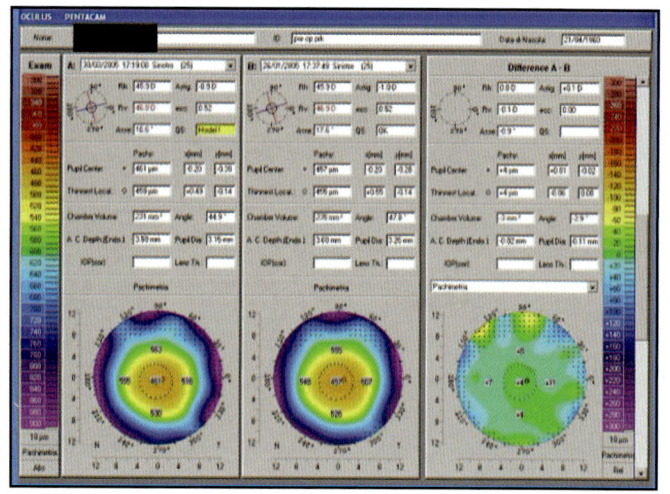

Figure 1-26. Differential map of LE in Figure 1-22 showing that in 2 months, the pachymetry map increased centrally by 4 μm. Stopping contact lens use changes thickness but not pachymetric pattern.

The parameters of greatest interest are curvature, slope, and height (absolute or relative to a reference surface); the aforesaid parameters are distinct but related to one another.[4]

Until a few years ago, topographic reconstruction was performed exclusively through the use of axial algorithms. Axial curvature is defined as the reciprocal of the distance of a point on the corneal surface from the topographic axis along the cornea meridian, normal to the point itself.

Nowadays, it is aided by instantaneous, altimetric, and aberrometric analyses, allowing the attainment of more detailed and, without doubt, more reliable information.

It has been known for some time that due to the method of calculation, axial mapping involves a significant degree of approximation that increases proportionally with the distance from the corneal vertex (hence from the topographic axis). For this reason, it is generally considered poorly reliable and even more so out of the area of the central 3 mm.

Since many corneal disorders, at least in the initial stages, may manifest themselves exclusively in paracentral or peripheral areas, the need to explore these areas more reliably and in further detail seems obvious.

The instantaneous or tangential algorithm calculates curvature based on the tangent to the anterior corneal surface in each point analyzed, whereby the analysis is not influenced by the distance from the center, and the map has good reliability even in peripheral areas. For this reason, it has become the gold standard for topographic analysis in numerous disorders, including keratoconus.

Tangential mapping, along with height mapping, provides information pertaining to the curvature and slope of the cornea respectively, while axial and aberrometric mapping evaluate the optical effect the cornea exerts on ocular diopter. Actually, axial topography is an approximation derived from tangential topography (although broader and more uniform)

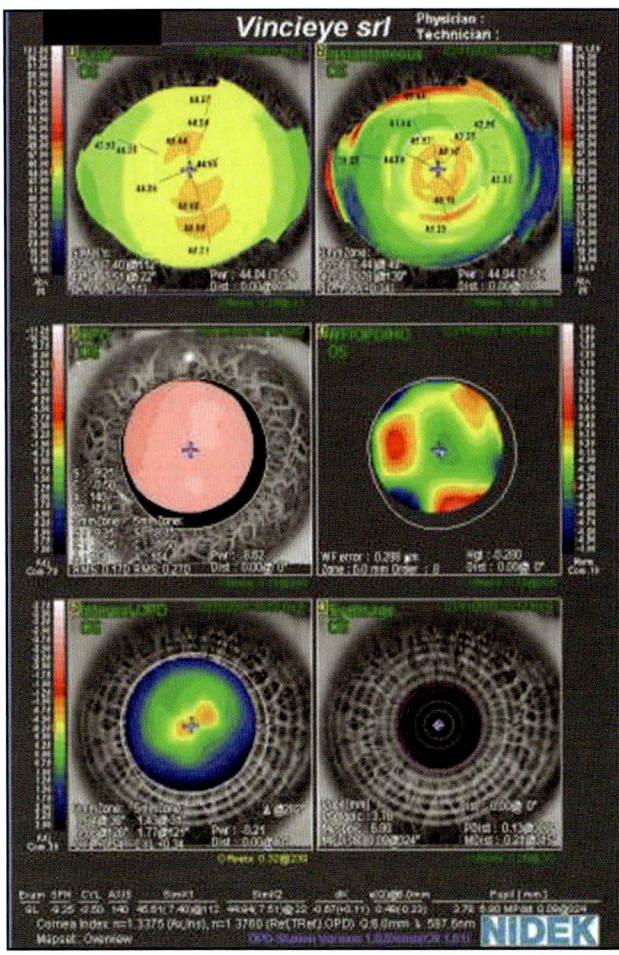

Figure 1-27. Contact lens-induced warpage (LE). Central flattening divides the astigmatic bow-tie in two. Instantaneous algorithm map shows contact lens leaning on corneal surface, not corresponding with true lens border.

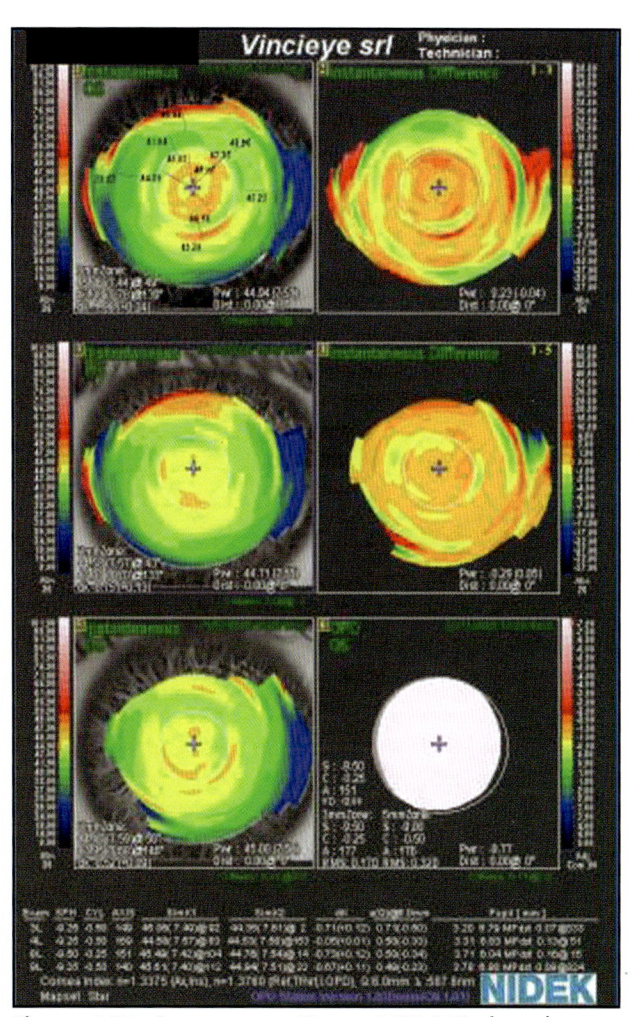

Figure 1-28. Same eye as Figure 1-27 (LE), from bottom to top, left, progressive change of pattern after contact lens withdrawal. On the left column, differential maps.

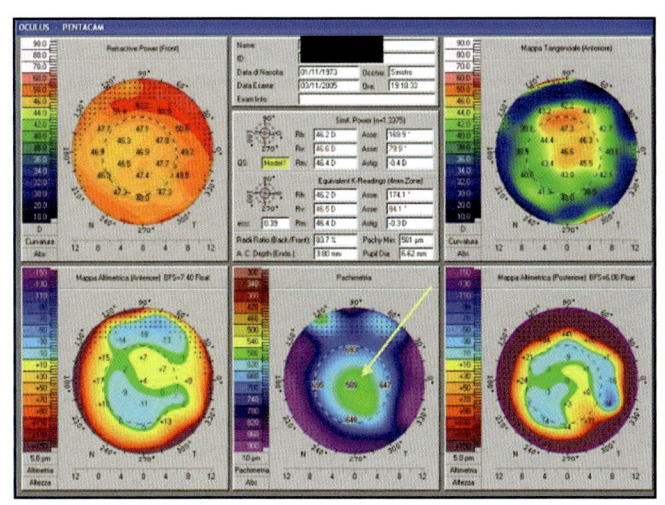

Figure 1-29. Same eye as Figure 1-27 (LE), Pentacam evaluation. The thinnest point on the pachymetric map (589 μm, arrow) does not correspond to the highest point on anterior altimetric or most curved point on tangential map (instantaneous, top right). The thinnest area is slightly decentered inferotemporally. This is compatible with forme-fruste keratoconus.

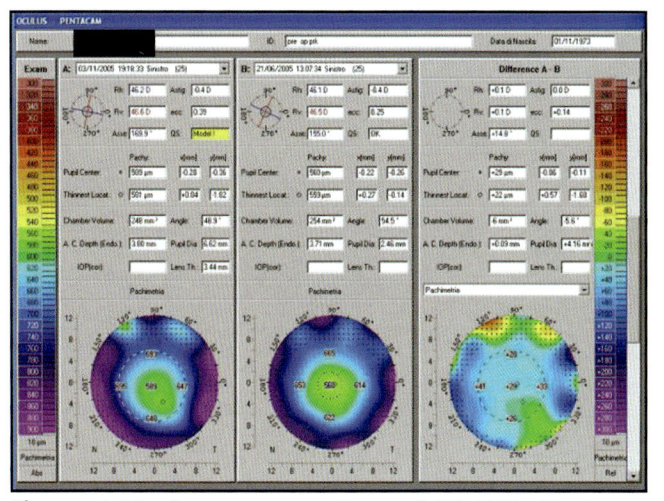

Figure 1-30. Same eye as Figure 1-27 (LE), Pentacam pachymetric differential map. After contact lens withdrawal, thickness has increased by 29 μm.

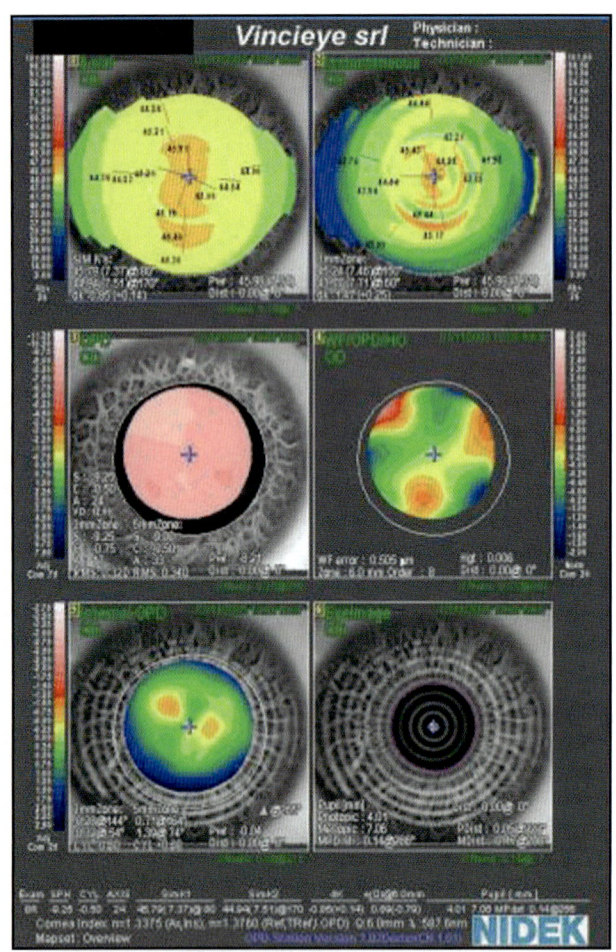

Figure 1-31. Contralateral eye in Figure 1-27 (RE).

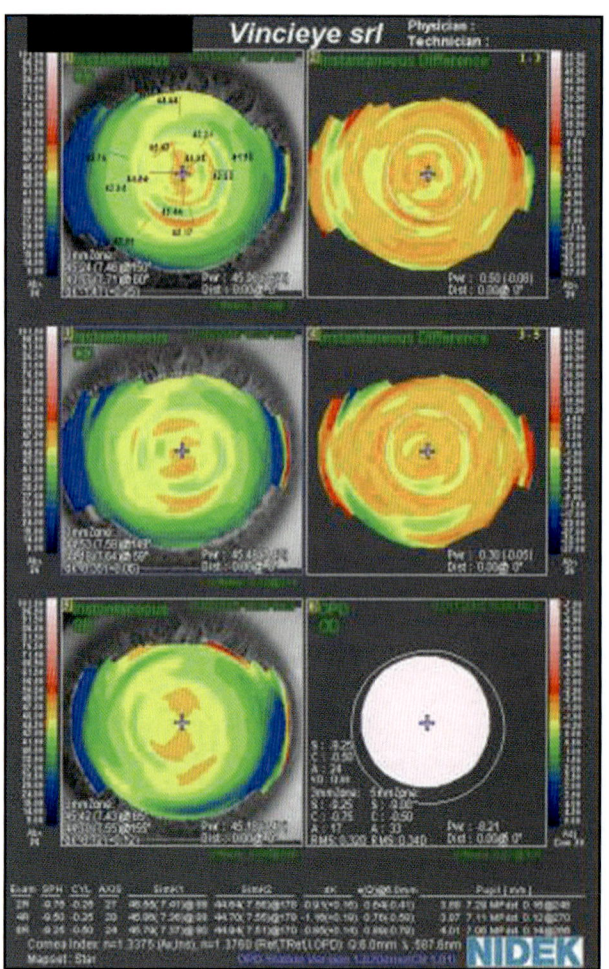

Figure 1-32. Same eye as Figure 1-31 (RE), after contact lens withdrawal, left, bottom to top, the true astigmatic pattern—without central separation of the bow-tie—progressively emerges. On the left side the differential maps.

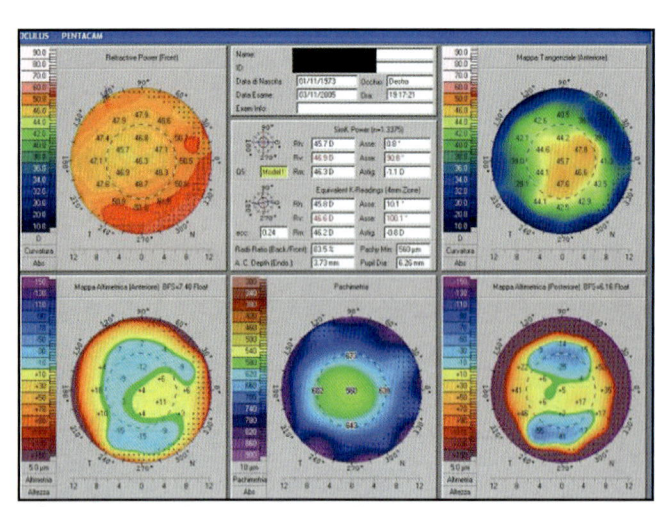

Figure 1-33. Same eye as Figure 1-31 (RE), Pentacam evaluation. Island pattern on anterior altimetric map, not on posterior altimetric.

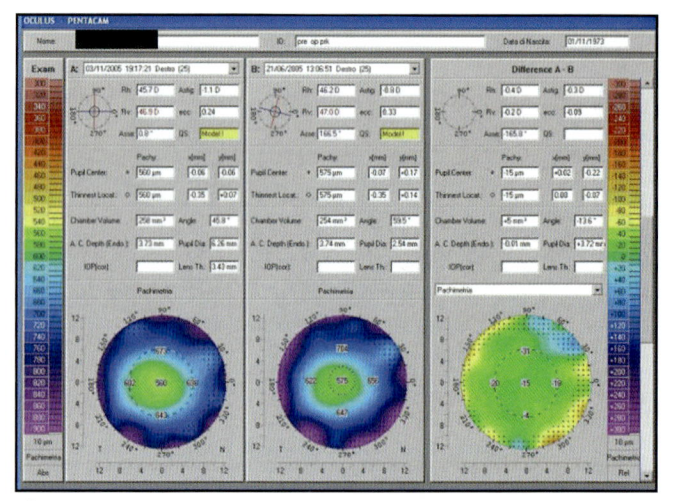

Figure 1-34. Same eye as Figure 1-31 (RE), Pentacam pachymetric differential map. After contact lens withdrawal, thickness has decreased by 15 μm.

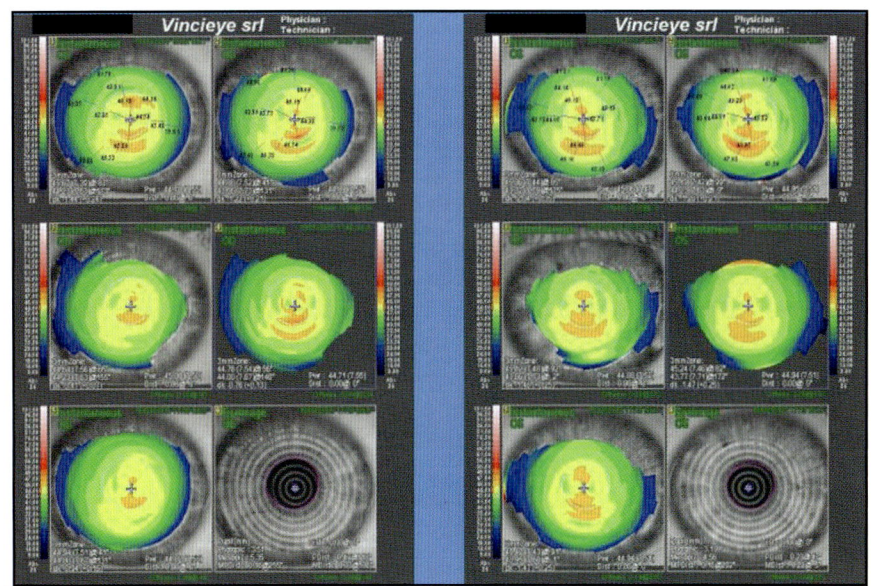

Figure 1-35. Contact lens warpage: RE and LE. The astigmatic bow-tie in this case has the inferior part cut by the warpage, and after lens withdrawal, from top to bottom, it progressively resumes a normal conformation. A custom ablation performed on the basis of the initial topography would have corrected a fictitious coma.

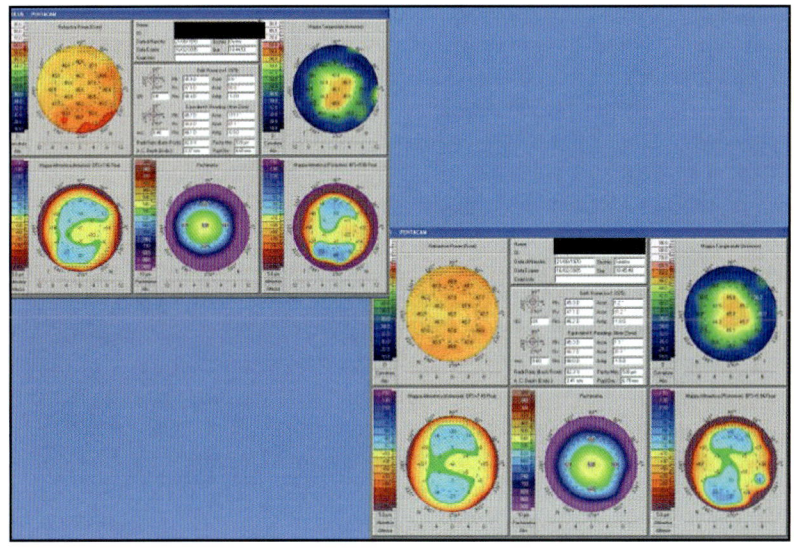

Figure 1-36. Same eyes as Figure 1-35, Pentacam evaluation. The anterior altimetric pattern is cookie like in both eyes, indicative of a normal eye.

that certainly makes it lose much information in relation to curvature. It is still used out of habit and because it allows highlighting regular astigmatic bow-ties and their axes with greater clarity, which may be useful in aiding the prescription of eyeglasses.

The real innovation in corneal diagnostics is constituted by height mapping, which measures not the curvature, but the height of any given point (ie, its position in space) and its elevation, or rather the position of any given point with respect to a reference surface.

Height algorithms may be calculated from reflection topographs, and in this case, data are obtained by deduction of corneal curvature or by means of projection equipment.[4,6]

Corneal height may not be shown directly on a map due to problems of scale. The variations in corneal height being surveyed are in the order of microns, while the area under investigation (ie, the entire corneal surface) extends for many millimeters.

An easily understood equivalent situation occurs with the view of the earth from a satellite, where the earth's surface extends for many thousands of kilometers and impedes perception of the height of the mountains that are "only" a few thousand meters in height.

The solution devised for geographical mapping (ie, showing elevation relative to sea level by means of a colorimetric scale) has also been adopted for corneal topography, and in this case, sea level has been substituted by a spherical reference surface (best fit sphere [BFS]). With this method, the areas located below the BFS appear in blue, those above in red, and those in the same plane in green, with color intensity increasing in proportion to the distance from the BFS itself.

This method for describing the cornea is very different from the usual corneal curvature map. First, the most curved and most flattened meridians appear inverted, since the most curved meridian will fall below "sea level," while the most flattened will be above the reference sphere. Thus, the classic astigmatic bow-tie, visible in axial, tangential, and height algorithms, appears blue along the most refractive meridian and red along the least refractive.

Having described how an astigmatic cornea appears, it should be added that a nonastigmatic cornea does not appear, as one might expect, homogeneous in terms of height and color. Because a normal cornea is not spherical, but prolate (ie, more curved at the center than at the margins), the map will show a central round red area surrounded by a blue median peripheral ring, in turn surrounded by a red ring at the extreme margin.

Height mapping is indispensable for identifying ectasic areas; with the instantaneous algorithm, an ectasic area appears red just as the most refractive meridian appears in irregular astigmatism. Instead, the two conditions are clearly differentiated by height topography, where the asymmetric bow-tie visible by instantaneous mapping in the case of irregular astigmatism appears blue since it is located on the most curved meridian and falls below the sphere of reference (BFS). An ectasic area is rather like a mountain that rises above sea level and hence appears red.

In order to best use the information provided, one should not be limited to a hasty glance at the map in the search for gross alterations such as a red stamp caused by an obvious keratoconus. Instead, it is necessary to follow a precise analytical procedure.

As already underlined, topographic interpretation may not be left out from keratoscopic analysis. Only the keratoscopic data can tell whether a particular alteration is due to the lachrymal film, to the erroneous processing of different anatomical parts such as the eyelids or conjunctival surfaces, or a true corneal disorder and, therefore, whether we are viewing a reliable map or an invention of the computer.

It would be appropriate for the acquisition of the images—a delicate and extremely important stage—to be entrusted to skilled operators, if not the ophthalmologist. That way, information would be obtained on the dynamics of the lachrymal film which would be lost with a single photogram.

The first step in reading a map is evaluating the scale in which it is drawn. The 3 colorimetric scale types available on all topographs are *absolute*, *normalized*, and *adjustable*.

With the *absolute* scale, each color corresponds to a fixed dioptric value, and the steps are further at the extremes of the scale, and closer (1.5 D) between 35.0 and 51.0 D, which are the values most commonly encountered, while out of this interval, the chromatic variation is every 5.0 D.

The *normalized* scale associates the darkest red with the most curved point and the most intense blue with the flattest point; the width of the steps depends on how much the "peak" rises over the "plane" (ie, the dioptric range between maximum and minimum curvature).

The *adjustable* scale allows the operator to select the width of the dioptric interval necessary for the chromatic variation.

The absolute scale is undoubtedly the most commonly used, since it is much more reproducible and more readily interpreted. Furthermore, it allows good comparison of maps obtained at different times, even using different equipment.

The adjustable map is useful for highlighting small dioptric variations which might be overlooked with larger intervals, but narrowing the chromatic interval increases the risk of overestimating each small variation in slope given the high color contrast generated. Furthermore, by selecting narrower "steps," especially with corneas having inhomogeneous curvature, there may be numerous unevaluated areas since they are off-scale, whereby better definition of detail is at the expense of the overall view.

The normalized scale has very variable resolution; it is comparable to the absolute scale if the corneal dioptric range is large but better if the slopes are not very steep. However, comparison with subsequent examinations is very difficult. Furthermore, very different corneas may take on very similar appearances.

It is generally always better to first analyze the absolute map, which rapidly provides a reliable overall view and is not subject to interpretational errors due to the colorimetric scale. To resolve and measure slight variations in curvature with greater precision, it may sometimes be useful to obtain an adjustable map.

Having processed the map, it is necessary to evaluate whether processing is complete or whether there are any unprocessed areas in order to move on to careful analysis of the corneal profile, the homogeneity of curvature, the presence of any patterns associated with refractive defects, abrupt changes in slope, and any unprocessed areas.

A normal cornea has a prolate profile that is more curved at the center than at the edge; in the absolute scale, the central area will appear yellow or green, and the color will gradually diminish until reaching the blue of the flatter edge.

The progressiveness of the chromatic variation is an index of the homogeneity of the corneal surface and of the mildness of the variations in slope. Therefore, evaluation of the tangential topograph allows a good estimate of corneal eccentricity.

The presence of different colors in adjacent areas should always be evaluated with extreme care, just as the nonprocessing of parts of the examination.

An area with a concentration of very different dioptric values is frequently an indicator of a corneal disorder and when included within a pupillary field, gives rise to refractive defects that are difficult to correct, seriously affecting vision quality. In this sense, a useful compliment is provided by the indices calculated by the software, which express in numerical terms what is visually expressed by topography. In the aforementioned case of an irregular corneal surface with abrupt changes in curvature, this is highlighted by a chromatically inhomogeneous map with correspondingly anomalous surface asymmetry index (SAI), coefficient of variation of corneal power (CVP), and standard deviation of corneal power (SDP) values.

The failure to process parts of the field under examination is frequently caused by corneal surface irregularities requiring careful assessment by means of keratoscopy.

Analysis of corneal morphology is very useful in defining refraction; for example, the identification of an astigmatic bow-tie will provide valuable indications as to the extent, axis, and regularity of the refractive defect and on the most appropriate corrective method.

The evaluation of the pupil, and its relationship with any alterations of the corneal surface, is of fundamental importance.

It is obvious that a topographic irregularity of any origin will have an effect on visual acuity proportional to its closeness to the center of the pupil.

In keratoconus, the spatial relationship between the ectasia and the pupillary foramen has extreme clinical significance; the aberrations and the astigmatism generated by the conus, even when of relatively modest extent, can be very incapacitating, even more than greater dioptric defects, depending on their location and the pupillary diameter of the individual under examination. In this sense, the recently marketed topographs allowing the execution of pupillometries and pupillographies have proved themselves extremely valuable.

Rather frequently, it is impossible to obtain good corrected visual acuity in patients with negative objectivity due to eye disorders. In such cases, the importance of a corneal topograph is frequently overlooked since one of the greatest sources of optical aberrations and loss of visual acuity is the cornea.

Keratorefractive Indices

Corneal morphology, on which optical characteristics depend, may be described by numerical indices and thus compared to a model cornea or a range of values defined as normal.

Each topograph calculates distinct indices, whereby differences may be encountered by using different equipment. Nonetheless, they are very useful for summarily quantifying and analyzing a defined aspect of corneal optical quality. Generally, the values for each cornea analyzed are compared with the mean values for a sample of normal corneas and considered within the norm when included between ±2 SD, suspect when between ±3 SD, and altered when out of the aforementioned ranges.

The most commonly used indices include:

* **Sim-K** (simulated keratometry) and the keratometric value of the cornea under examination.
* **Astigmatism**: This is expressed as a function of the pupillary diameter, like corneal toricity expressed in diopters of an area centered on the corneal vertex with a diameter equal to that of the pupil (normally, the most significant diameters used are 3 and 5 mm). It represents the extent and the axis of the regular astigmatic component of the cornea. A difference in axis or power between the two pupillary diameters indicates an irregular astigmatism that cannot be corrected by glasses.
* **Average pupillary power**: This is the mean axial curvature, expressed in diopters, of a 3-mm diameter centered on the entry pupil, giving greater weight to the central corneal points. It represents the spherical equivalent of the aforementioned area. It is a useful parameter for describing mean curvature in very irregular corneas where, given the heterogeneity, simple morphological analysis is insufficient for understanding the true curvature.
* **Asphericity**: This is one of the parameters with greatest importance given that it describes the corneal profile and the difference in curvature between the center and the periphery. It indicates the degree to which the cornea is prolate or oblate. Corneal asphericity is determined by examining the asphericity of the conicoid most similar to the corneal segment of interest. It may be expressed through four different indices, which are the shape factors p and SF, the eccentricity e, and the asphericity coefficient Q, which express exactly the same information and which are easily interconverted between one another by means of simple calculation formulae. In a prolate cornea, p varies from 0 to 1, while in an oblate cornea, it is greater than 1. $Q = p - 1$, hence a prolate ellipse ranges between -1 to 0, while an oblate surface is > 0; $e < 0$ indicates an oblate surface, a normal cornea (prolate) has eccentricity values of around 0.5.
* **Spherical aberration**: The longitudinal spherical aberration (LSA) expressed in diopters within a corneal area of 4.5 mm centered on the center of the pupil. It expresses the difference between marginal and paraxial power.
* **Irregularity of curvature:** This is expressed (in diopters) as the standard deviation or mean square deviation of the instantaneous curvature with respect to the BFS.
* **Surface asymmetry (SAI)**: This is one of the first indices to have been introduced in corneal topography, and represents the asymmetry of instantaneous curvature of the surfaces of the two hemimeridians opposing along each meridian. In the ideal cornea, it is equal to 0. In the case of asymmetry, the mean instantaneous curvature of the flatter hemisphere is colored blue, the most curved is red, and the SAI indicates the difference between the two.

References

1. Vinciguerra P, et al. Atlante di topografia corneale. *Fogliazza*. 1995.
2. Koch DD, Haft EH. Introduction to corneal topography. In: *An Atlas of Corneal Topography*. Thorofare, NJ: SLACK Incorporated; 1993.
3. Bogan SJ, Waring GO, Ibrahim O: classification of normal corneal topography based on computer assisted videokeratography. *Arch Ophthalmol*. 1990;108:945-949.
4. McRae SM, Krueger RR, Applegate R. *Customized Corneal Ablation*. Thorofare, NJ: SLACK Incorporated; 2001.
5. Sher NA, Bowers RA, Zabel RW, et al. Clinical use of the 193 nm excimer laser in the treatment of corneal scars. *Arch Ophthalmol*. 1991;109:491-498.
6. McRae SM, Krueger RR, Applegate R. *Customized Corneal Ablation*. Thorofare, NJ: SLACK Incorporated; 2001.

CHAPTER 2

Useful Information for the Refractive Surgeon: Aberrometry and Its Application to Vision Care

Raymond A. Applegate, OD, PhD

This chapter provides a basic and useful understanding of whole eye and corneal aberrometry and its application to vision care for the practicing refractive surgeon. The implications of aberrometry for vision care require an understanding of what is meant by the word "vision," the components that drive retinal image quality, and what fundamentally limits vision. The chapter is written in sections and subsections that can stand alone allowing the reader to gloss over areas they are comfortable with and read sections of particular interest.

What Is Meant by the Term Vision?

As a starting point, it is worth defining what a clinician means when referring to *vision* and what the patient means when they talk about their vision. Clinically, we typically use the word vision as a substitute for high contrast photopic visual acuity; however, vision is a very complex set of abilities that include contrast detection, color vision, motion discrimination, stereopsis, localization, visual field, etc. Within acuity alone there is high contrast photopic letter acuity, high contrast mesopic acuity, high contrast scotopic acuity, low contrast photopic acuity, low contrast mesopic acuity, low contrast scotopic acuity, dynamic acuity, vernier acuity, grating acuity, etc. While different measures of acuity are correlated to each other, each type of acuity reveals different aspects of vision that can be useful. For example, in an elderly population, a loss of low contrast mesopic acuity is predictive of a future loss in high contrast photopic acuity.[1] Another example is that the metrics of retinal image quality determined from whole eye aberrometry are not particularly good at predicting high contrast photopic acuity in eyes with normal to better than normal vision but are predictive of low contrast mesopic acuity.[2]

Contrast how clinicians typically define vision with what a refractive surgery patient means when they arrive at the office and despite having 6/6 high contrast photopic acuity offer a heartfelt chief complaint, "I don't see as well as I used to." The patient wants to know why (Figure 2-1). They want validation that they are not crazy, even though they may still be seeing 6/6. They want us to fix what "we" broke. Aberrometry is a powerful tool that can help us understand and fix what "we" or a colleague broke.

The Optical Quality of the Retinal Image

The optical quality of the retinal image is principally defined by diffraction, whole eye wavefront error (wave aberration), scatter, and chromatic aberration. It is important to keep in mind that of these components, diffraction and wave aberration, are fundamentally pupil diameter dependent. Refractive surgery can induce scatter; however, if surgery is performed at the standard of care, scatter is generally not a lasting vision limiting effect. On the other hand, as an individual ages, scattering becomes an increasingly important factor defining retinal image quality and should not be ignored. Clinically viable instruments are currently being built and tested that will help differentiate scatter from wavefront error defects.[3-7] Given the aging population, the ability to differentiate scatter from wavefront error defects will increase in clinical importance. Chromatic aberration is caused by the dispersive properties of the ocular media and, therefore, is little impacted by refractive surgery. The component of retinal image quality that is most affected by surgical intervention is the wave aberration of the eye.

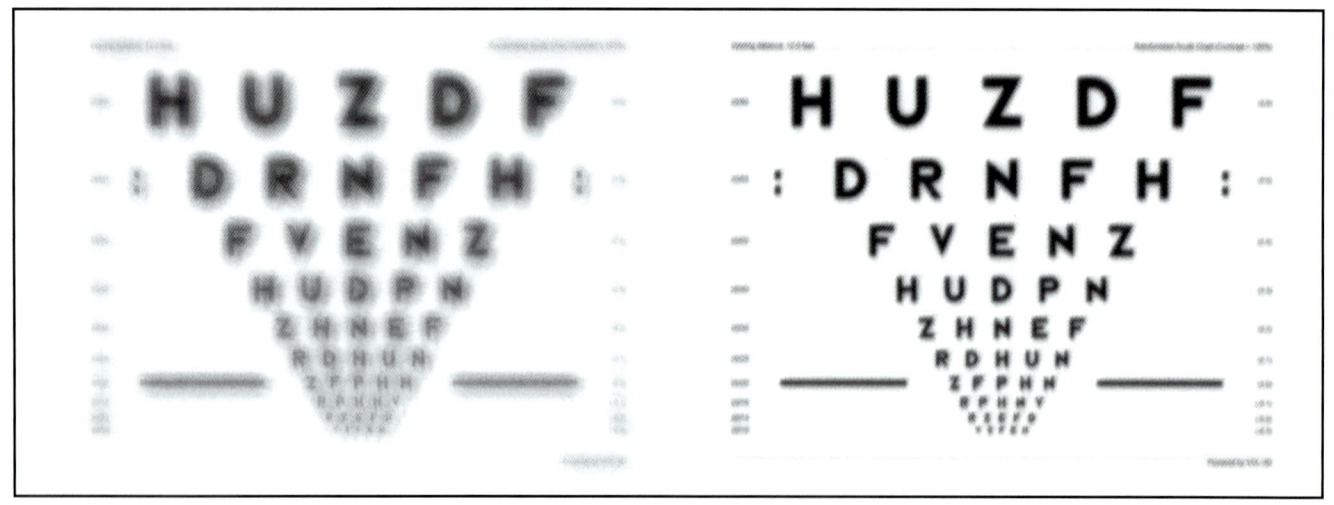

Figure 2-1. Left: Retinal image simulation of a refractive surgery patient best corrected who can read the 6/6 line and knows that their vision was better prior to surgery than after. Pupil diameter is 3 mm. High-order RMS wavefront error over a 3-mm pupil is 0.23 µm. Right: Retinal image simulation of a typical age-matched normal eye best corrected with 6/4.5 acuity. Pupil diameter is 3 mm. High-order RMS error over a 3-mm pupil is 0.09 µm. Horizontal bar marks the 6/6 line. Simulations were performed through a 3-mm pupil using Visual Optics Laboratory (v 6.72 Sarver and Associates, Inc). (Courtesy of R.A. Applegate, OD, PhD.)

Diffraction

Diffraction was defined by Sommerfeld in 1894[8] as any deviation of light rays from a rectilinear path that cannot be interpreted as reflection or refraction. Diffraction effects are pupil size dependent. The diffraction effects induced by pupil diameter are easily viewed by observing how increasing pupil diameter decreases the diameter of the point spread function (PSF) in a perfect eye (no wavefront aberrations -such an optical system is often referred to as diffraction limited).

Why Use the PSF to Illustrate Diffraction Effects?

The PSF (Figures 2-2 and 2-3) defines how any optical system (including the eye) images a point of light. How an optical system images a point of light is fundamentally important. Objects are made up of an infinite number of points. The PSF of the eye describes how each object point is imaged onto the retina. Consequently, the PSF is one of the fundamental methods for describing the optical quality of an imaging system such as the eye. Figure 2-3 displays a set of monochromatic PSFs for an aberration-free eye (diffraction limited) for pupil diameters ranging between 1 and 8 mm. Notice in Figure 2-3 that the best image of an object point in an **aberration-free eye** is obtained when the pupil is the largest.

The angular size of a monochromatic PSF (angular size of the Airy's disk) is defined as follows:

$$\theta = \frac{1.22\lambda}{a}$$

Where:
θ = the angular extent in radians
λ = the wavelengths of light
a = the diameter of the pupil

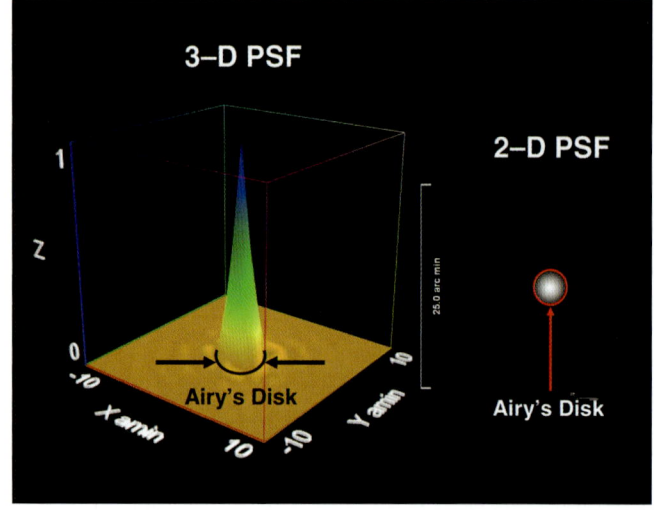

Figure 2-2. A three-dimensional (left) and two-dimensional representation of a PSF for an aberration-free eye, 1-mm pupil diameter. Plotted is the relative amount of light varying from no light (0 on the Z scale) to the most light (1) as a function of the angular distance in arc minutes in the x and y directions of the graph. The circle described when the illuminance distribution first hits 0 is the Airy's disk (marked by arrows). This figure was generated using Visual Optics Laboratory (v 6.72 Sarver and Associates, Inc). (Courtesy of R.A. Applegate, OD, PhD.)

To give a clinical sense of the impact of diffraction on acuity for different pupil diameters, Figure 2-4 displays retinal simulations of standard logMAR acuity charts for four different pupil diameters ranging from 1 to 8 mm.

Clinical implications of diffraction include the following:
* Diffraction fundamentally defines the resolution limit of retinal image quality in an eye with no wavefront error.

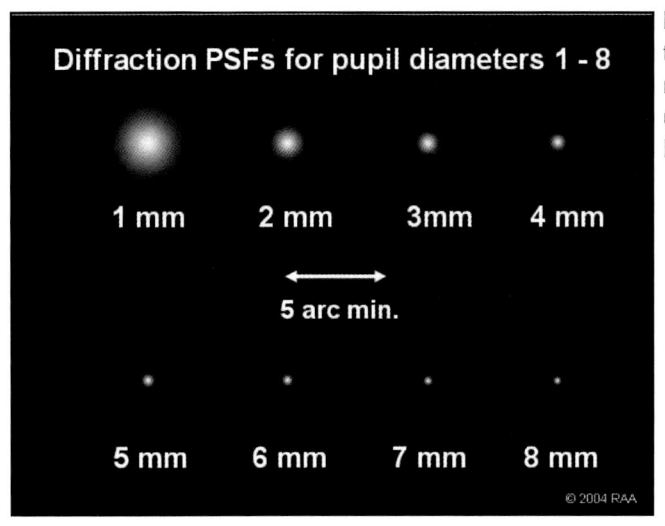

Figure 2-3. Diffraction limited (eyes with no wavefront error) two-dimensional PSFs for eight different pupil diameters ranging in diameter from 1 to 8 mm. PSFs were generated using Visual Optics Laboratory (v 6.72 Sarver and Associates, Inc). (Courtesy of R.A. Applegate, OD, PhD.)

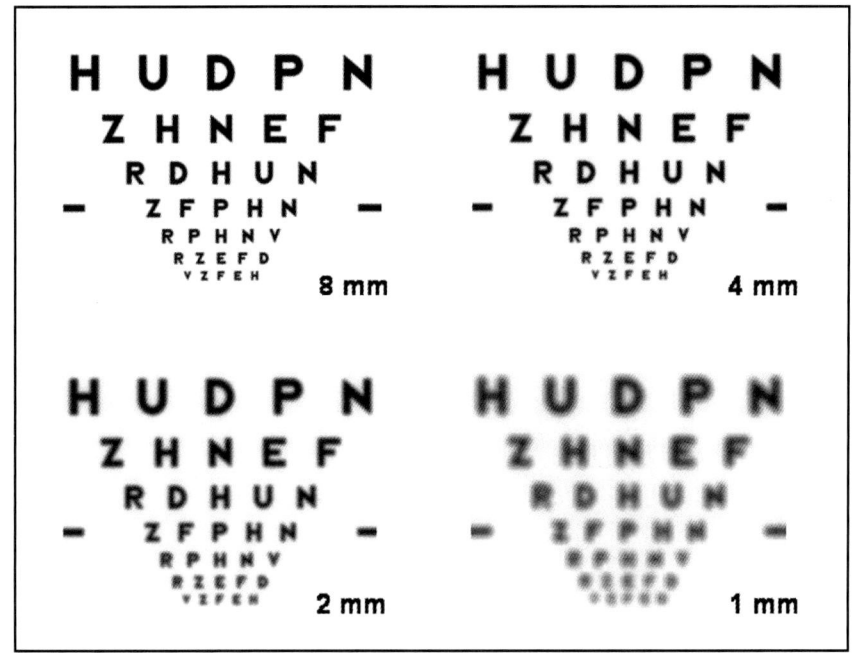

Figure 2-4. Simulated retinal images of an aberration-free eye (no wavefront error) viewing a logMAR chart though four different pupil diameters ranging from 1 to 8 mm. Notice that in an eye with no wavefront error, retinal image quality is best when the pupil is the largest. The single bar on each figure represents the 6/6 line. Chart generation and simulations were generated using Visual Optics Laboratory (v 6.72 Sarver and Associates, Inc). (Courtesy of R.A. Applegate, OD, PhD.)

* Diffraction effects increase as pupil size decreases, making the quality of the retinal image poorer and poorer as pupil size decreases.

Wavefront Error

All eyes have optical aberrations (wavefront error) that cannot be corrected with a sphero-cylindrical correction. Wavefront error that can be corrected with a sphero-cylindrical correction are typically referred to as the low-order wavefront error or low-order aberrations. Low-order aberrations in the uncorrected ammetropic eye account for the vast majority of the eye's wavefront error. Wavefront errors that cannot be corrected with sphero-cylindrical corrections are collectively referred to as higher-order aberrations. In the past, higher-order aberrations have been referred to as irregular astigmatism. Now, however, individual components of the irregular astigmatism can be identified (eg, coma, spherical aberration, secondary astigmatism), as well as their relative magnitudes. Furthermore, knowing the wavefront error of the eye provides fundamental information for the design and construction of corrections intended to minimize the adverse affects of both the low- and high-order aberrations of the eye.

To understand wavefront error, it is helpful to change our thinking from rays of light to waves of light. Once it is understood what a wave of light is, we can then define wavefront error. In Figure 2-5, light from a distant source forms parallel rays as it approaches an optical system symbolized by the simple positive lens. These rays can be easily converted to wavefronts by connecting small perpendicular line segments on each ray at the same elapsed time from when light left the point source (same phase). After refraction by a perfect optical system, the rays will come to a diffraction-limited focus forming an Airy disk. As with the incoming rays, small line

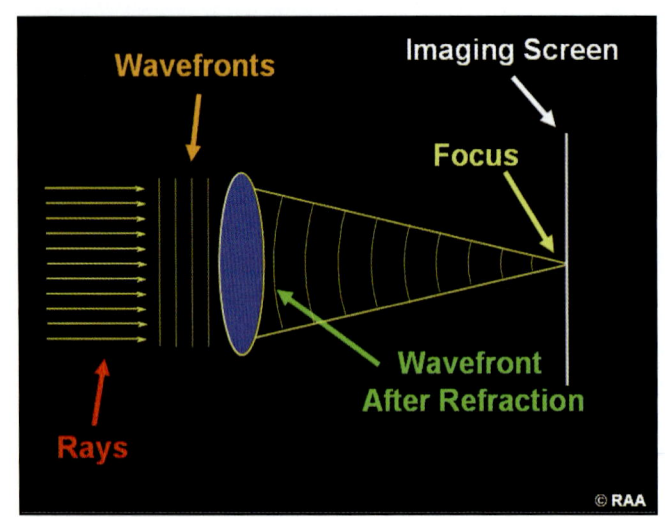

Figure 2-5. Converting rays of light to wavefronts. See text for explanation. (Courtesy of R.A. Applegate, OD, PhD.)

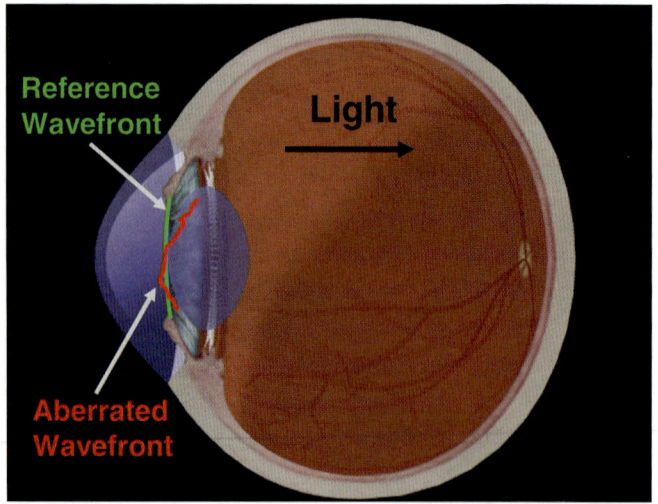

Figure 2-6. Wavefront error is the difference between the reference wavefront (green) and actual wavefront (red) point by point within the pupil. Eye simulation generated using Visual Optics Laboratory Light (v 1.31 Sarver and Associates, Inc). (Courtesy of R.A. Applegate, OD, PhD.)

segments can be drawn perpendicular to the refracted rays at the same elapsed time from when light left the point source. Connecting the infinite number of small perpendiculars will form spherical wavefronts whose radii get progressively smaller as the diffraction-limited focus is approached.

Now, if we define what we consider to be a perfect wavefront, we can in turn define wavefront error. For light entering the eye headed for the retina, the ideal wavefront for a perfectly focused distance point source is spherical having a center of curvature at the retina (Figure 2-6). This ideal wavefront serves as a reference representing the shape of the wavefront that forms an ideal image of a distant point source on the retina. Typically, the eye's optics will distort the incoming wavefront. After refraction, the distorted wavefront (represented in red) enters image space through the exit pupil of the eye.

For light entering the eye, the difference between the reference wavefront (green) and the actual wavefront (red) point by point across the extent of the exit pupil defines the wavefront error of the eye. By convention, the wavefront error at the center of the pupil zero.

Wavefront Error Fitting Functions and Maps

In order to describe the wavefront error in a manner that gives insight as to the type and magnitude of the errors, wavefront error is generally fit with a fitting function. The Optical Society of America recommended fitting function for describing ocular aberrations is the Zernike expansion.[9] These recommendations have been refined to form the ANSI standards for fitting the wavefront error of the eye (Z80.28). The second through fourth radial orders of the Zernike expansion are displayed in Figure 2-7.

The reader is referred to the OSA recommended standard[9] and the ANSI Z80.28 standard for details such as the **proper method for comparing right and left eyes**, and the reference

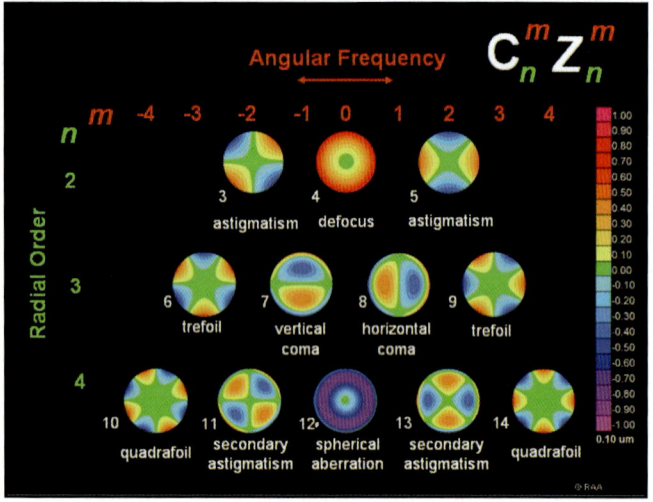

Figure 2-7. The second through fourth radial orders of the Zernike expansion illustrating the recommended double index system (green and red numbers), the recommended single index system (white numbers), one of the recommended color scales, and the common names of the aberrations. (Courtesy of R.A. Applegate, OD, PhD.)

coordinate system.

Wavefront error maps can either plot the actual measured values or the fitted values. Typically, they plot the fitted values with the low-order aberrations attributable to the sphero-cylindrical correction set to zero. Removing the low-order aberrations from the map and displaying them as a standard sphero-cylindrical correction prevents the low-order aberrations from masking the presence of higher-order aberrations (Figure 2-8) in the displayed map.

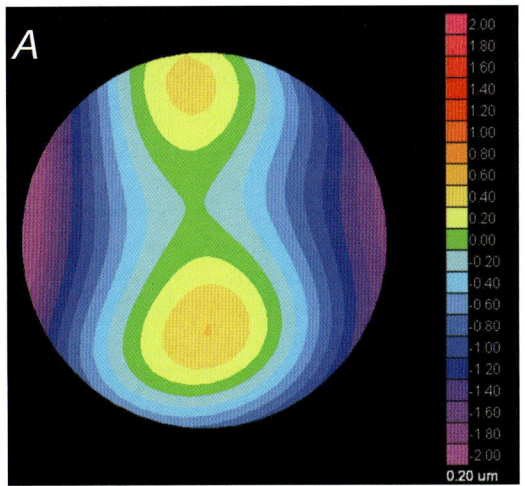

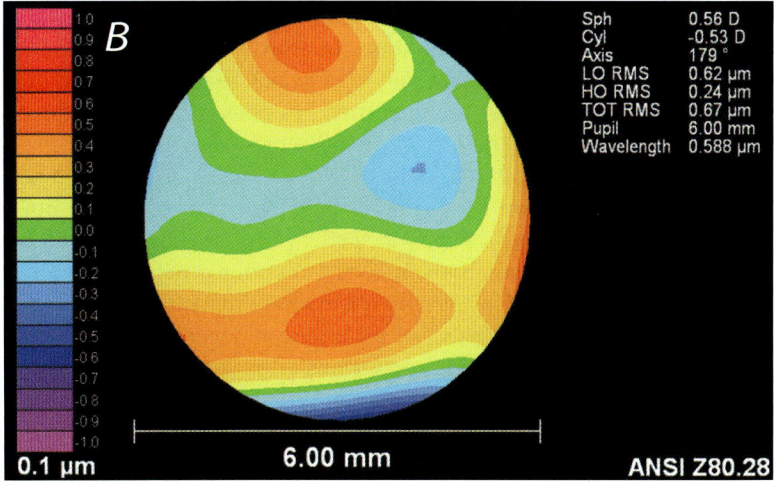

Figure 2-8. (A) A wavefront error map over a 6-mm pupil for a subject with a modest sphero-cylindrical refractive error (+0.56 -0.53 x 179). Notice the scale is twice as big as panel (B), which plots only the higher-order wavefront error and numerically displays the low-order aberrations in the typical sphere, cylinder, and axis format. The total high-order aberration in typical normal 20-to 40-year-old eye over a 6-mm pupil is ~0.3 µm. This eye has 0.24 µm of high-order aberrations (HO) and the total low-order aberrations (LO) are more that 2 times higher (0.62 µm) even though the sphero-cylindrical correction is a modest +0.56 -0.53 x 179. Wavefront error maps were generated using Visual Optics Laboratory (v 6.72 Sarver and Associates, Inc). (Courtesy of R.A. Applegate, OD, PhD.)

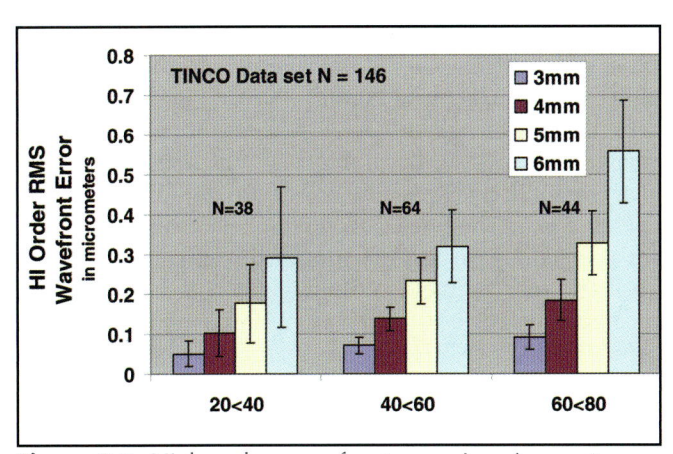

Figure 2-9. High-order wavefront error in micrometers as a function of age and pupil size. Data is from the Texas Investigation of Normal and Cataract Optics funded by the National Eye Institute grant EY 08520 entitled *Aberrations in Normal and Clinical Populations* to RAA. (Courtesy of R.A. Applegate, OD, PhD.)

Figure 2-10. A comparison of a diffraction-limited eye (no wavefront error) and the PSF of a typical normal eye wearing a sphero-cylindrical correction. Below 3 mm, diffraction effects dominate the normal eye's PSF, and the perfect eye and real eye have very similar PSFs. Above 3 mm, wavefront error dominates. (Courtesy of R.A. Applegate, OD, PhD.)

Wavefront Error, Age, Pupil Size, and Acuity

Higher-order wavefront error varies as a function of pupil size and age as can be seen in Figures 2-9 and 2-10.

Wavefront error degrades retinal image quality and cannot increase retinal image quality over the diffraction-limited case. The fact that wave aberrations decrease image quality is easily viewed by comparing perfect diffraction limited PSFs to those of a patient with their spherical and cylindrical error corrected as a function of pupil size (see Figure 2-10). In Figure 2-10, notice that for pupil sizes less than 3 mm, diffraction dominates (it is hard or impossible to tell the diffraction limited PSFs from the patient's PSFs). At 3 mm, the point spread for the diffraction limited and typical normal eye produce PSFs that are nearly equivalent. Above 3 mm, the normal eye PSF becomes worse than the diffraction limited case.

Wavefront error also varies as a function of accommodation. The major change is in the spherical aberration term, which shifts increasingly in the negative direction as level of accommodation increases. Although the change in aberration structure due to accommodation is real and significant, it is unlikely the benefits of a wavefront-guided correction will be negated by the change in aberration structure induced by accommodation.[10] Perhaps more importantly, not all aberrations impact visual performance equally.[11-13] In general, aberrations near the center of the Zernike tree affect visual performance more than aberrations near the edge for any given magnitude of wavefront error. Furthermore, combining the right mix of various aberrations can provide better or worse acuity than the individual aberrations themselves. For example, defocus and spherical aberration when mixed in ideal proportions provides better acuity than either of these subcomponents by themselves.[14] Consequently, RMS wavefront error is not the best metric of potential visual performance. Researchers are working on a variety of single value metrics of retinal image quality based on wavefront error that are more predictive of visual performance than RMS error.[15,16] These new metrics are much better correlated with measures of visual acuity (in particular, mesopic low contrast acuity) than RMS error.[2]

For many clinical eyes (eg, keratoconics), it is important to correct the higher-order aberrations. For the normal eye, the gains obtained by correcting higher-order aberrations are primarily for large pupil sizes and diminish as the pupil size gets smaller. In other words, decreasing the aberrations of the eye will increase the pupil diameter at which aberrations become the primary degrader of retinal image.

Clinical implications of wavefront error include the following:
* The adverse effects on retinal image quality of wave aberrations in the normal healthy eye increase with pupil diameter.
* Retinal image quality in the normal healthy eye has the highest fidelity for pupil diameters around 3 mm.
* Wavefront error decreases retinal image quality compared to the diffraction limited case.
* Wavefront errors attributable to different Zernike modes are independent mathematically; however, in terms of visual performance, Zernike modes interact. When compared to the visual impact of individual modes, these interactions can reduce visual performance, increase visual performance, or have little impact on visual performance.
* The effects of diffraction and increased depth of focus cause most eyes to see the same for pupil diameters <2 mm.
* Correlations between visual performance and wavefront aberrations must be made for the same pupil size.

Whole Eye vs Corneal Wavefront Error

The optics of the healthy eye are primarily defined by the corneal and crystalline lens optics, the relative placement of the crystalline lens with respect to the cornea, and axial length. The cornea/air interface experiences the largest optical index change of all the optical components of the eye. Combining this fact with the fact that the radius of curvature of the corneal first surface is the order of 7 to 8 mm makes the corneal first surface the most powerful refracting surface in the eye accounting for nearly three-quarters of its refracting power. Despite this important fact, corneal topography alone cannot be used to determine the sphero-cylindrical refractive errors of the eye. Nonetheless, corneal topography can be used to calculate the shape of the corneal first surface. Assuming an optical index for the cornea allows for the calculation of corneal first surface wavefront error with respect to a reference wavefront of interest. This technique is particularly powerful in eyes with abnormal corneal first surface optics in that it helps to identify the site of the major optical defects. Whole-eye aberrometry measures the optical errors of the whole-eye, it does not by itself identify the origin of the errors. By subtracting the wavefront errors of the corneal first surface from the whole eye wavefront error, a good estimate of the aberrations attributable to the internal optics (primarily the crystalline lens and corneal back surface) can be made.[17-19] It is important to emphasize that in order to estimate the optical errors of the internal optics, care must be taken to align the corneal first surface wavefront error and whole eye wavefront error to the same reference point (eg, the center of the pupil when fixating a object point on the optical axis of the measuring device—the line of sight). I remain amazed that corneal topography and wavefront sensing are not commonly combined into one device aligned to the same reference axis. The reasons to combine the two instruments are compelling particularly for corneal refractive surgery. The rationale is simple and straight forward. The difference between corneal topography before and after surgery defines the surgically induced correcting lens. The difference between the surgically induced lens and the planned ablation lens defines the error in the procedure.

The Modulation Transfer Function

The optics of the eye filters the retinal image. Filtering means some of the information contained in the object is not transferred to the image. Filtering is seen in the PSF by the fact that each point is not imaged to a perfect point. Although filtering can be seen in the PSF, it is difficult to quantify what information has been lost. The manner in which any given optical system (eg, the eye) filters spatial information is easily visualized in the modulation transfer function (MTF). The MTF defines how much contrast as a function of spatial frequency is transferred by the optical system to the image plane (Figures 2-11 and 2-12).

In Figure 2-12, it is easy to see that a diffraction-limited 1-mm pupil filters more spatial information (the curve goes to 0 at a lower spatial frequency and transfers a lesser contrast for any given spatial frequency) than a diffraction-limited 3-mm pupil or a 5-mm pupil, etc.

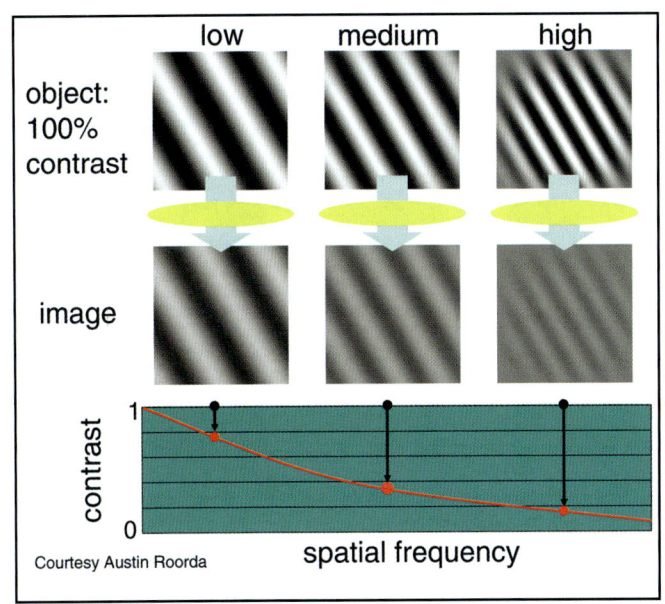

Figure 2-11. Schematic representation of the meaning of the MTF. The MTF reveals how much contrast is lost at each spatial frequency as a result of being imaged through the optical system of interest. Across the top of this schematic representation are three spatial frequencies increasing in spatial frequency from left to right each having 100% contrast. As each is imaged through the optics of interest, contrast is lost as illustrated in the row labeled "image." The MTF is a plot of the resulting image contrast as a function of spatial frequency (graph at bottom of the figure). One hundred percent of the contrast is transmitted to the image plane if the object contrast is 1 and 0% of the contrast is transmitted to the image if the contrast is 0. (Courtesy of R.A. Applegate, OD, PhD.)

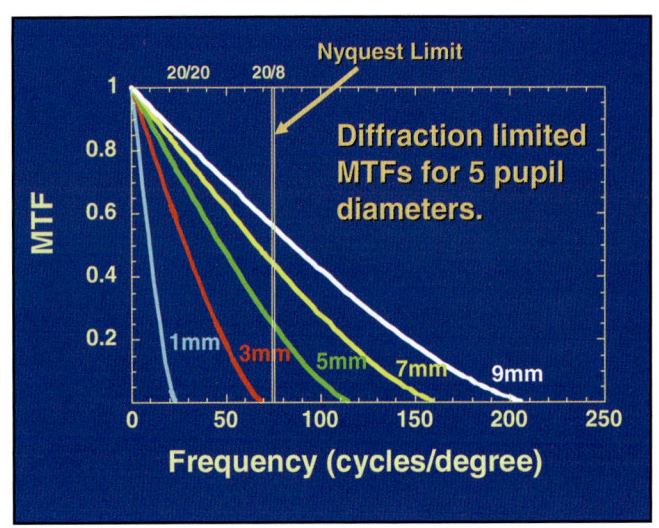

Figure 2-12. In an aberration-free eye, the MTF varies as a function of pupil diameter. Plotted here are the diffraction limited (no aberration) MTFs for five different pupil diameters. (Courtesy of R.A. Applegate, OD, PhD.)

In Figures 2-11 and 2-12, the MTFs are plotted for one orientation of the sinusoidal gratings. In well aligned rotationally symmetric optical systems (a system that has rotational symmetry with respect to their optical properties such as a simple positive of negative lens), plotting the MTF for one orientation is generally sufficient. However, for nonrotationally symmetric optical systems such as the eye, it is not sufficient to measure the aberrations in one orientation. Instead, it is necessary to know the modulation transfer for all orientations of the grating. In Figure 2-13, the two-dimensional MTF over a 6-mm pupil is graphed showing a typical normal eye with a sphero-cylindrical correction (left) and a diffraction limited eye (no aberrations). Notice that the transmitted contrast varies with grating orientation in the real eye, and that even when the eye is corrected for sphero-cylindrical errors, the higher-order aberrations are reducing the transmitted contrast compared to the diffraction-limited eye. The reduction is due to the fact that the higher-order aberrations of the eye are not correctable with a sphero-cylindrical correction. A goal in corneal refractive surgery is designing ideal corrections to maximize the area on the two-dimensional MTF by balancing both the low- and high-order aberrations of the eye to create a retinal image that renders the best visual percept.

The two-dimensional MTF of an eye can be calculated from the wavefront error measured with an aberrometer in a matter of milliseconds.

Neural Limits

The very center of the fovea, the foveola, has the highest density of photoreceptors and highest spatial resolution. In the foveola, cone photoreceptors are between 2 to 2.5 µm in diameter. An individual cone photoreceptor responds to light falling on it in a graded manner. Therefore, it does not differentiate image detail. For example, if a letter E is imaged totally within a single photoreceptor, the visual system cannot differentiate the E from a period. In order to differentiate the E from a period, the letter E must be large enough such that each component of the letter E is stimulating a different photo receptor. Said differently, the Nyquist Sampling Theorem must be respected. The Nyquist Sampling Theorem states: the maximum spatial frequency that can be detected is equal to half of the sampling frequency. For the case of the letter E, each white gap and dark bar can be no smaller than a photoreceptor (Figure 2-14).

Given the dimensions of the eye and the diameter of the foveolar cones of approximately 2 to 2.5 µm, the Nyquist sampling limit in terms of Snellen acuity is between 20/8 and 20/10. Consistent with the Nyquist sampling theorem, Austin Roorda (at the School of Optometry, University of California, Berkeley) using his adaptive optics confocal laser scanning ophthalmoscope with stimulus generator to minimize the aberrations of his own eye was able to recognize targets to 20/8 (personal communication).

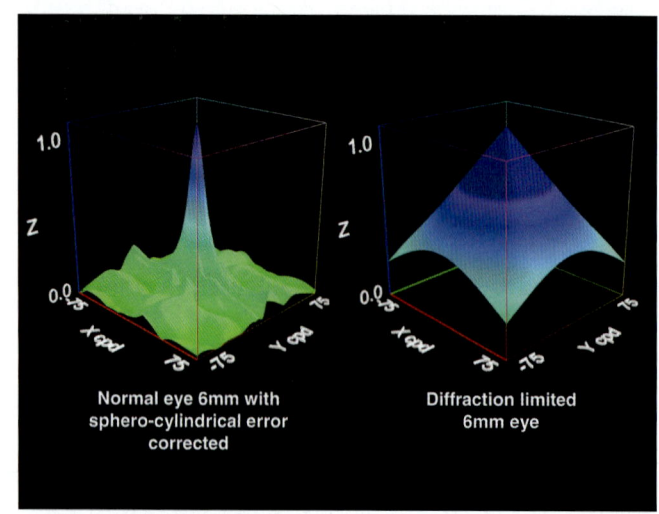

Figure 2-13. Two-dimensional MTFs. Left: A typical normal 6-mm eye with the sphero-cylindrical errors of the eye corrected by setting the second radial order of the Zernike polynomial to zero. For comparison, on the right is the two-dimensional MTF of an aberration-free 6-mm eye. Notice that there is a lot of room for the normal eye to be improved with corrections designed to minimize higher-order aberrations. The Snellen equivalent for 60 cycles/degree (cpd) is 20/10. These two-dimensional MTFs were generated using Visual Optics Laboratory (v 6.72 Sarver and Associates, Inc). (Courtesy of R.A. Applegate, OD, PhD.)

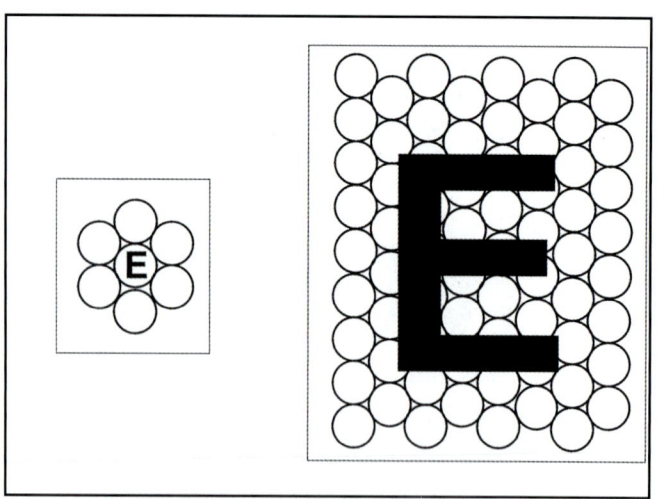

Figure 2-14. Each circle represents the cross-section of a cone photoreceptor in the foveola. Left panel: A letter E is imaged within a single photo-receptor. Given that an individual photoreceptor responds with a graded response depending on the number of photons captured, the letter E cannot be differentiated from a period. Right panel: According to the Nyquist sampling theorem, to be differentiated as a letter E, each white gap and dark stroke can be no smaller than a photoreceptor. (Courtesy of R.A. Applegate, OD, PhD.)

Aliasing and Other Possible Adverse Consequences of Decreasing Higher-Order Aberrations

Correctly recognizing an object (eg, a letter E) is a different task than detecting the presence of an object. In the case of aliasing, targets smaller than the resolution limit defined by the Nyquist sampling theorem can be detected in aliased form (the perception does not look like the actual object). For example, a bar grating with a spatial frequency smaller than the Nyquist sampling limit (smaller than the photoreceptors sampling the grating) can be seen as an aliased image (Figure 2-15 right panel) due to undersampling.[20] Diffraction effects prevent the normal eye from seeing spatial frequencies smaller than the photoreceptor diameter for pupil diameters less than 3 mm. For larger pupils, higher-order aberrations prevent the normal eye from seeing spatial frequencies smaller than the photoreceptor diameter.

As wavefront corrections continue to improve, will aliasing be a problem for the visual system? For a variety of reasons it is highly unlikely that we will decrease ocular aberrations in a normal healthy eye by more than a factor of 2 or 3. Even if we decrease high-order aberrations by a factor of four and perfectly corrected the low-order aberrations of sphere and cylinder, the contrast at 75 cycles/degree and above is still low compared to diffraction limited case (Figure 2-16) and is unlikely to handicap vision for a variety of reasons:

* For pupil sizes less than 3 mm, diffraction effects prevent spatial frequencies that cause foveal aliasing from being passed.
* For moderate size pupils (3 to 5) in near aberration-free eyes, the contrast for spatial frequencies >70 cycles/degree are unlikely to be high enough to make aliasing a problem.
* For larger pupils, it is unlikely that ocular aberrations can be decreased to the point that aliasing will be a problem.
* Even if reduced, experiences in peripheral indicate that gains in contrast outweigh the adverse effects of aliasing.

What may be a handicap in having the aberrations reduced by a factor of 4 is a loss in depth of field, particularly when the pupil is large. The "right" collection of higher-order aberrations (yet to be clearly defined) increases the depth of field at the expense of contrast. The fact that some eyes readily adapt and prefer multifocal designs indicate that the loss in contrast may not outweigh a presbyopic patient's satisfaction in being able to see both distance and near relatively well. On the other hand, we will need to carefully balance patient needs with public safety. It has been shown in driving simulators that a loss of contrast in distance vision decreases reaction time, increasing the probability of an accident.[21]

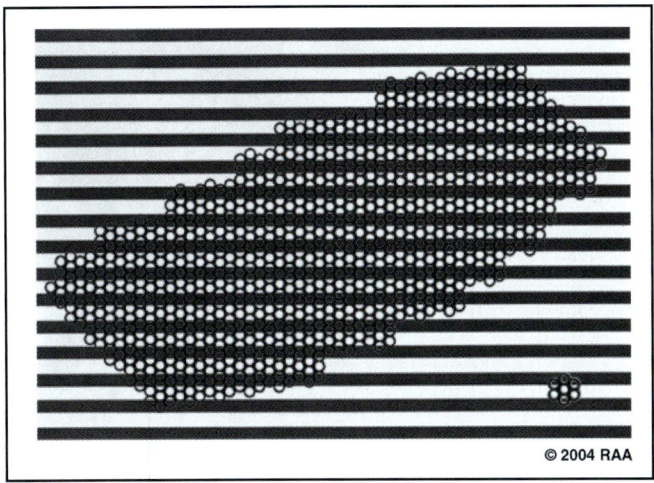

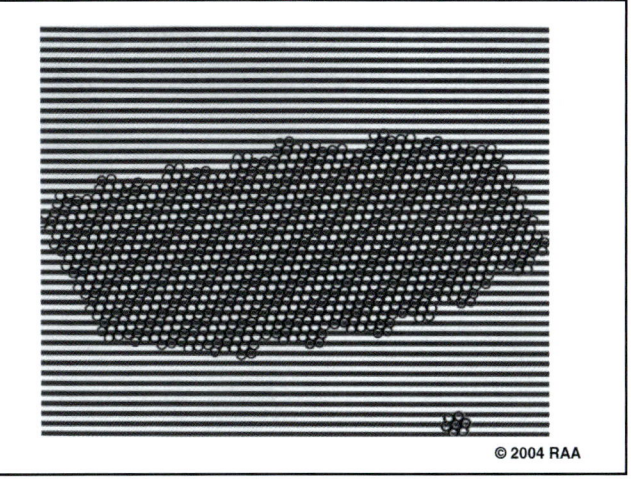

Figure 2-15. Aliasing. If the spatial detail of an object is greater than the Nyquist sampling limit (bar grating left panel) imposed by the photoreceptor mosaic (represented by the small circles), then the spatial detail can be correctly detected. However, if the spatial detail of an object is smaller than the Nyquist sampling limit (bar grating right panel) imposed by the photoreceptor mosaic, then an aliased percept is formed (diagonal bars) having a lower spatial frequency than the actual object. (Courtesy of R.A. Applegate, OD, PhD.)

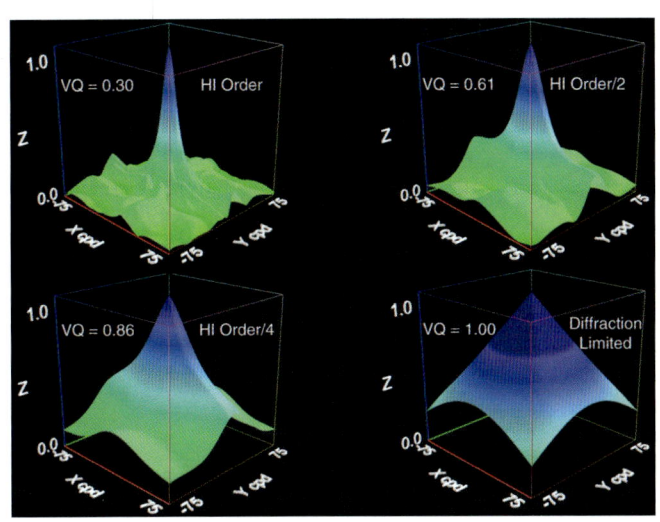

Figure 2-16. Two-dimensional modulation transfer functions for a typical normal eye through a 6-mm pupil. Upper left with sphero-cylindrical error corrected; Upper right, with sphero-cylindrical error corrected and higher-order aberrations reduced term by term by half their initial amount; lower left, with sphero-cylindrical error corrected and higher-order aberrations reduced term by term by three-quarters their initial amount; lower right, an diffraction-limited 6-mm eye. (Courtesy of R.A. Applegate, OD, PhD.)

Goals for Wavefront Corrections of the Eye

In the late 90s, I advocated that refractive surgery would come of age when it routinely corrected the sphero-cylindrical errors of the eye to less than 0.25 D without changing the presurgical higher-order wavefront error. That is, leave the higher-order aberrations as is and only correct the sphero-cylindrical error. Work by Artal et al, reinforces this initial goal with the finding that simply rotating the existing higher-order aberration structure of an eye (no change in magnitude) reduces visual performance.[22,23] Despite this finding in 2002, I revised my initial goal for refractive surgery to include reducing higher-order aberrations in eyes with large amounts (greater than the average eye) of higher-order aberrations. The argument is simple. The gains in retinal image contrast in a normal eye with greater than normal higher-order aberrations out-weigh the risks of altering the structure of the higher-order aberrations so long as the aberrations are lowered and not increased. Just as we adapt to an astigmatic correction, we will adapt to new aberration structures rather quickly. Similarly, in eyes with unusually low higher-order aberrations care should be taken not to increase aberrations, for these individuals are more likely to be dissatisfied. The reason is simple. The effect on visual performance of a relatively small increase in higher-order aberrations of an eye with above normal higher-order aberrations is most likely to be small. The same increase in aberrations will have a greater impact on an otherwise normal eye with unusually low higher-order aberrations.

Summary

It is useful for a refractive surgeon to know the following:
* High contrast acuity is relatively insensitive to minor variations in higher-order aberrations.
* Mesopic low contrast acuity is much more sensitive to small variations in the higher-order aberrations than photopic high contrast acuity.
* Retinal image quality is determined principally by diffraction, aberrations, scatter, and chromatic aberration. The effects of diffraction and aberrations are pupil size dependent.

- Given the aging population, scatter will become an increasingly important parameter defining visual performance.
- It is more informative to display high-order wavefront error maps separately from those that include both the lower and higher-order wavefront error.
- In the normal eye, diffraction dominates retinal image quality for pupil sizes <3 and wavefront error dominates retinal image quality for pupil sizes >3.
- Wavefront error varies as a function of pupil size, age, and level of accommodation.
- Not all wavefront error is equal in its affects on visual performance.
- RMS wavefront error—while the most commonly used single value metric of optical quality—is not the best metric for predicting visual performance.
- Corneal topography can be used to describe the optical aberrations of the corneal first surface and is particularly useful in highly aberrated eyes.
- The two-dimensional MTF describes how the eye's optics filter the spatial content of objects.
- The diameter of the foveolar cones limit visual resolution to somewhere between 20/8 and 20/10.
- Aliasing is unlikely to significantly alter the benefits of minimizing the eye's higher-order aberrations.
- The goal of refractive corrections in the typical normal eye or an eye with abnormally low amounts of higher-order aberrations should be to reduce the sphero-cylindrical error to less than 0.25 D without altering the eye's higher-order aberrations.
- The goal of refractive corrections in otherwise normal eyes with atypically large amount of higher-order aberration should be to reduce the sphero-cylindrical error to less than 0.25 D and reduce the eye's higher-order aberrations to normal levels.
- The previous two goals are mostly likely best achieved by using a state-of-the-art wavefront guided correction particularly as the systems continue to evolve.

This work is supported in part by: NIH/NEI grant EYR01-008520 to RAA, NIH/NEI CORE grant NIH/NEI EY07551, the Borish Endowment, the Visual Optics Institute, and the College of Optometry, at the University of Houston.

Acknowledgements: I wish to acknowledge my Colleagues and friends in Optometry and Ophthalmology, Jason Marsack for reading and commenting on the chapter, and the many patients that have served as subjects over the years. It is this group of people along with the loving support of my wife Rachel and my children Aaron, Ryan, Camille, and Olivia that make my work enjoyable and rewarding.

Disclosures: In the interest of full disclosure, I consult for Sarver and Associates, Inc and have consulted for Alcon.

References

1. Schneck ME, Haegerstrom-Portnoy G, Lott LA, Brabyn JA, Gildengorin G. Low contrast vision function predicts subsequent acuity loss in an aged population: the SKI study. *Vision Res.* 2004;44:2317-2325.
2. Applegate R, Marsack J, Thibos L. Metrics of retinal image quality predict visual performance in eyes with 20/17 or better visual acuity. *Optom Vis Sci.* In press.
3. Donnelly WJ III, Applegate RA. Using Shack-Hartmann images to evaluate nuclear cataract. *Invest Ophth Vis Sci.* 2003;44,Abstract 223.
4. Donnelly WJ III, Pesudovs K, Marsack JD, Sarver EJ, Applegate RA. Quantifying scatter in Shack-Hartmann images to evaluate nuclear cataract. *J Refract Surg.* 2004; 20:S515-S521.
5. van den Berg TJ, IJspeert JK, de Waard PW. Dependence of intraocular straylight on pigmentation and light transmission through the ocular wall. *Vision Res.* 1991;31:1361-1367.
6. van den Berg TJ, Hagenouw MP, Coppens JE. The ciliary corona: physical model and simulation of the fine needles radiating from point light sources. *Invest Ophthalmol Vis Sci.* 2005;46:2627-2632.
7. Guell JL, Pujol J, Arjona M, Diaz-Douton F, Artal P. Optical Quality Analysis System; Instrument for objective clinical evaluation of ocular optical quality. *J Cataract Refract Surg.* 2004;30:1598-1599.
8. Sommerfeld, A. Zur mathematischen theorie der Beugun-serscheinenungen. *Nachr Kgl Acad Wiss Gottingen.* 1894;4:338-342.
9. Guirao A, Gonzalez C, Redondo M, et al. Average optical performance of the human eye as a function of age in a normal population. *Invest Ophthalmol Vis Sci.* 1999;40:203-213.
10. Cheng H, Barnett JK, Vilupuru AS, et al. A population study on changes in wave aberrations with accommodation. *J Vis.* 2004;4:272-280.
11. Applegate RA, Ballentine C, Gross H, Sarver EJ, Sarver CA. Visual acuity as a function of Zernike mode and level of root mean square error. *Optom Vis Sci.* 2003; 80:97-105.
12. Applegate RA, Sarver EJ, Khemsara V. Are all aberrations equal? *J Refract Surg.* 2002;18:S556-562.
13. Marsack JD, Pesudovs K, Donnelly WJ III, et al. Prediction of visual acuity with combinations of wavefront aberration metrics. *Invest Ophth Vis Sci.* 2004;45: Abstract 2768.
14. Applegate RA, Marsack JD, Ramos R, Sarver EJ. Interaction between aberrations to improve or reduce visual performance. *J Cataract Refract Surg.* 2003;29:1487-1495.
15. Thibos LN, Hong X, Bradley A, Applegate RA. Accuracy and precision of objective refraction from wavefront aberrations. *J Vis.* 2004;4:329-351.
16. Chen L, Singer B, Guirao A, Porter J, Williams DR. Image metrics for predicting subjective image quality. *Optom Vis Sci.* 2005; 82:358-369.
17. Artal P, Guirao A. Contributions of the cornea and the lens to the aberrations of the human eye. *Opt Lett.* 1998;23:1713-1715.
18. Artal P, Berrio E, Guirao A, Piers P. Contribution of the cornea and internal surfaces to the change of ocular aberrations with age. *J Opt Soc Am A Opt Image Sci Vis.* 2002;19:137-143.
19. Artal P, Guirao A, Berrio E, Williams DR. Compensation of corneal aberrations by the internal optics in the human eye. *J Vis.* 2001;1:1-8.
20. Wang YZ, Bradley A, Thibos LN. Aliased frequencies enable the discrimination of compound gratings in peripheral vision. *Vision Res.* 1997;37:283-290.
21. Personal communication. Steve C. Schallhorn.
22. Elliott DB, Yang KC, Whitaker D. Visual acuity changes throughout adulthood in normal, healthy eyes: seeing beyond 6/6. *Optom Vis Sci.* 1995;72:186-191.
23. Artal P, Chen L, Fernandez EJ, Singer B, Manzanera S, Williams DR. Adaptive optics for vision: the eye's adaptation to point spread function. *J Refract Surg.* 2003;19:S585-587.

CHAPTER 3

Clinical Application of Differential Wavefront Aberrometry

Phil Buscemi, OD; Harkaran S. Bains

Synopsis

The NIDEK OPD-Scan (Gamagori, Japan) is a combination unit that provides information on topography, wavefront, autorefraction, keratometry, and pupillometry. Measuring over 8000 data points, the optical path difference scanning system (OPD-Scan) utilizes dynamic spatial skiascopy and placido disk topography to measure normal to extremely aberrated eyes. This compact unit plots 13 different maps to provide information on the corneal shape, wavefront, internal aberrations, and visual quality of the eye.

This diagnostic platform is employed for a variety of uses including patient screening, preoperative evaluation, and follow-up care. The OPD can determine the source of visual blur, and qualify and quantify the components of "irregular astigmatism." Among other uses, the OPD-Scan can be used for determining the effect of corneal and intraocular procedures, following the wavefront and refractive progression of a cataract, CL fitting, or the effect of pharmacological constriction of the pupil. Part of the Node Advanced Vision Excimer Laser Platform (NAVEX), the OPD-Scan is also widely used for customized ablation of primary and highly aberrated eyes.

The NIDEK OPD-Scan simultaneously performs all measurement in one sitting without moving the patient, ensuring the data from the various modalities are aligned and registered with respect to each other. This facilitates the correlation of corneal contribution to the wavefront aberrations of the eye and the internal contribution to wavefront.

The OPD-Scan uses a unique measurement principle, based on retinoscopy called "spatial dynamic skiascopy" to determine the wavefront aberrations of the eye. The fundamental differences between retinoscopy and dynamic skiascopy include the use of infrared light instead of visible light and the measurement of time lag for photodetector simulation instead of lenses to determine the refractive power of 1440 data points within the physiologically dilated pupil. The raw data is plotted in refractive power maps and converted to conventional wavefront maps and graphs. The OPD-Scan employs placido disk technology to plot corneal topography.

Unique to the OPD-Scan is the presentation of wavefront data in terms of refractive diopters and the ability to directly distinguish front corneal surface aberration from lenticular and back corneal surface aberrations.

The addition of a software package called the OPD-Station allows simulation of visual acuity charts and the effect on visual quality due to the refractive and wavefront status of the eye. The automated screening program, the corneal navigator, for screening corneal pathologies such as keratoconus and pellucid marginal degeneration and abnormal corneas further enhances the clinical utility.

OPD-Scan and OPD-Station

The OPD-Scan is a combination aberrometer and topographer that uses the principle of spatial dynamic skiascopy to measure the aberrations of the eye and placido disk topography to measure the corneal shape. This unit uses over 8000 data points to plot the aberrations of the eye and the corneal topography. In addition to aberrometry and topography, the OPD-Scan provides autorefractometry, keratometry, and pupillometry functions integrated into one unit, allowing accurate data registration between the different exam types. Due to this integration of functions, the OPD-Scan is currently being employed for surgical planning and preoperative and postoperative evaluations for a variety of refractive and intraocular procedures. A separate workstation termed the OPD-Station allows further application such as visual quality

Figure 3-1. Measurement principle of the NIDEK OPD-Scan.

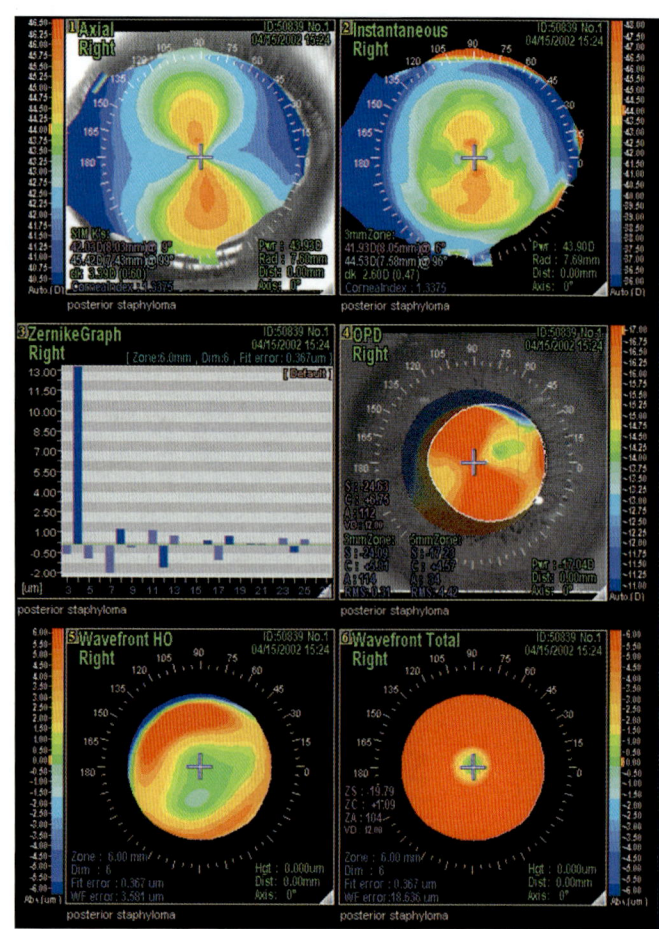

Figure 3-2. Patient with axial myopia, corneal astigmatism, and posterior staphyloma with an OPD refraction of -24.63+ 6.75 x 112. RMS value of 4.42 D indicates high irregular astigmatism and higher-order wavefront error of 3.581 µm indicates reduced optical quality.

simulation and provides clinically-useful maps that plot the refractive effect higher-order aberration in diopters.

ABERROMETRY MEASURING PRINCIPLE

The aberrometry measuring method consists of an infrared light-emitting diode housed within a chopper wheel with slit apertures. The receiving system consists of a photodetector array that converts the time differences of stimulation into dioptric power maps that correlate the refractive error in a two-dimensional map at the entrance pupil. The projection and receiving systems are optically conjugate. The dioptric power maps or refractive maps are displayed as "OPD maps" from which traditional Zernike based maps, out to the eighth order, can be derived. The aberrometry principle is termed spatial dynamic skiascopy. Plotting 1440 points, the projecting optical system scans at a constant speed in a single direction on the pupil center. The receiving optical system includes an aperture and photo diode array that detects the light reflected by the retina. The aperture is optically positioned in front of the retina for myopes or behind the retina in the case of hyperopia and on the retina in the case of emmetropia.

Figure 3-1 illustrates the measuring principle for aberrometry. By correlating the time differences with refractive errors, the refractive error at each position on the cornea (photo diode position) with respect to the corneal center can be derived. One complete scan on the retina obtains the distribution of refractive powers for all meridians within 0.4 seconds; by rotating the measurement system 360 degrees, the distribution of refractive powers through 360-degree meridians is obtained. An eyetracker with x, y, z autofocus maintains the eye in the correct position during measurement. The advantage of this method is that it allows the widest range measurement for aberrometers. Unlike traditional position-based aberrometers, the NIDEK OPD-Scan does not suffer from an inability to detect spot array pattern correctly on a CCD image plane that results in a narrow measurable range for Hartmann-Shack, Tscherning, and Tracey aberrometers. Additionally, in moderate and highly aberrated eyes, many of the traditional aberrometers cannot provide measurements or provide inaccurate measurements due to crossover of data points. The NIDEK OPD-Scan has a measurable range of refractive errors from -20.0 D to +22.0 D, with astigmatism measurement up to ± 12.0 D. Hence, the OPD-Scan can reliably measure highly myopic or astigmatic eyes, keratoconus, and excessively irregular eyes (Figure 3-2).

TOPOGRAPHY MEASURING PRINCIPLE

For the corneal topography, a placido disk principle is employed. The corneal topography is plotted using an arc step method that calculates the slope of the corneal surface

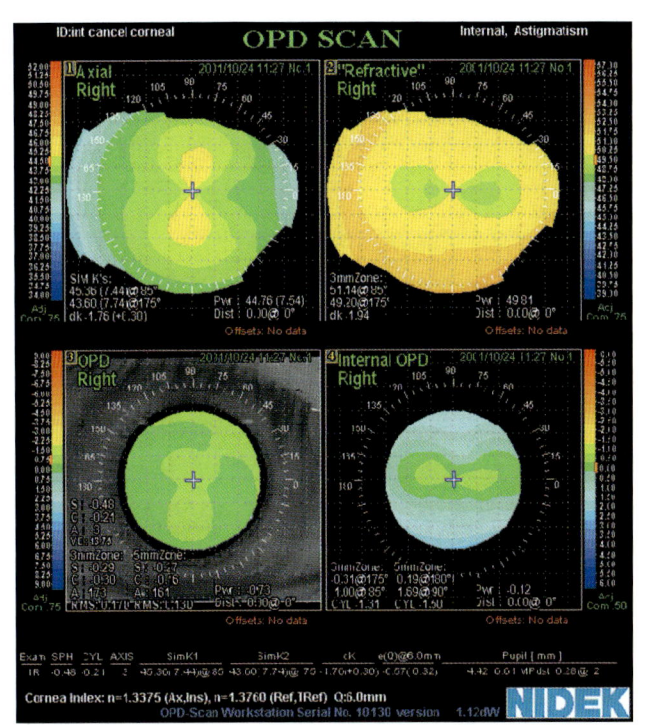

Figure 3-3. Compensation of corneal astigmatism (axial map) by the internal aberrations of the eye (internal OPD map). OPD-Scan refraction -0.48 -0.21 x 3. Corneal cylinder -1.76 D, internal cylinder -1.5 D. Note the OPD map shows homogenous refractive power distribution that is near emmetropic, yet corneal maps and internal OPD maps both show bow-tie patterns of astigmatism.

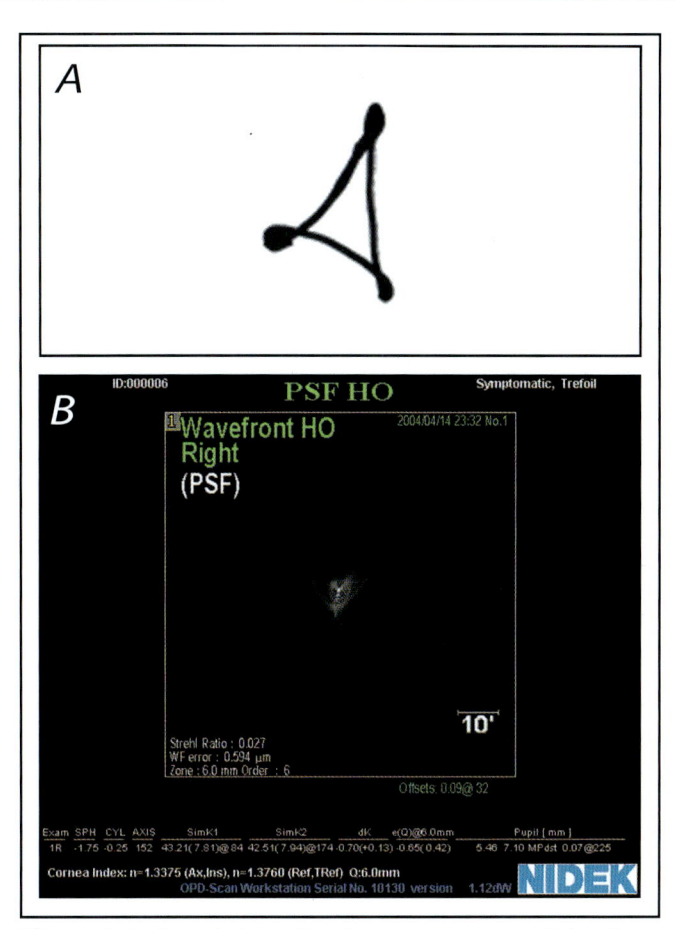

Figure 3-4. Correlation of patient symptoms and the simulated point spread function of a symptomatic post-LASIK patient.

at each placido ring edge and elevation. Corneal shape indices such as eccentricity (e), asphericity (Q), and keratometry values are provided. Corneal topography maps presented via this method are axial, instantaneous, refractive, and three-dimensional elevation maps.

CLINICAL APPLICATIONS

Clinically, the OPD-Scan provides standard corneal topography and wavefront information. The wavefront data plots wavefront total maps, higher-order maps, and Zernike graphs cataloging the aberration profile along with the associated wavefront error values. Higher-order wavefront error values between 0.3 and 0.5 µm are considered normal. Additionally, the Strehl ratio is provided, which serves as a metric of the optical quality of the eye (0.04 is considered normal).

The integration of the corneal topographer (CT) and wavefront analyzer (WF) components into one unit enables the direct evaluation and diagnosis of corneal and internal aberrations of the eye. The measured data is registered on the same; hence, the simultaneous measurement of corneal topography and wavefront allows point-by-point analysis of regions of interest, if required. The OPD-SCAN is the only unit available that plots the internal aberrations of the eye, separating corneal front surface aberrations (tear film interface with air) from the internal aberrations of the eye that can arise from the back corneal surface or the lens (Figure 3-3).

Up to 12 different topography and aberrometry maps can be separately displayed on the OPD-Scan. Unique to the OPD-scan are refractive diopter maps termed "Internal OPD" and "OPD" maps. The "OPD" map presents the spatially resolved refractive and aberrometric status of the entire optical path of the eye. As shown in Figure 3-3, there is -1.75 D of corneal astigmatism present; however, the OPD-Scan refraction shows very little cylinder. The Internal OPD map shows -1.5 D of cylinder that is compensating of the corneal cylinder.

The point spread function simulates the distortion of a point of source of light due the aberrations of the eye. The point spread function can be simulated for the total wavefront profile, the higher-order profile and the effects of the individual types of aberrations such as coma or trefoil. This can be useful in the subjective confirmation of patient symptoms and as a patient teaching tool to simulate the effects of the aberrations and explain them in simple terms (Figures 3-4). An ideal screening tool for the wavefront based treatment, custom intraocular lenses, laser ablation, or contact lenses versus conventional treatments are the OPD higher-order maps (OPD HO) and modulation transfer function graphs (MTF).

Traditional wavefront HO maps plotted in microns provide little clinical utility. The OPD HO map plots the effect of all the higher-order aberrations of the eye in diopters.

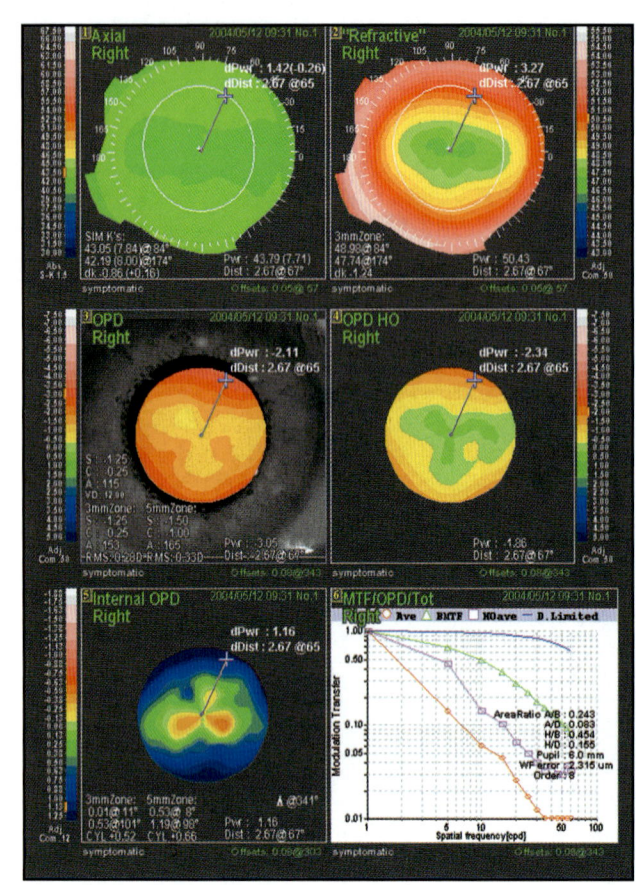

Figure 3-5. OPD-Station analysis of a symptomatic post-LASIK patient.

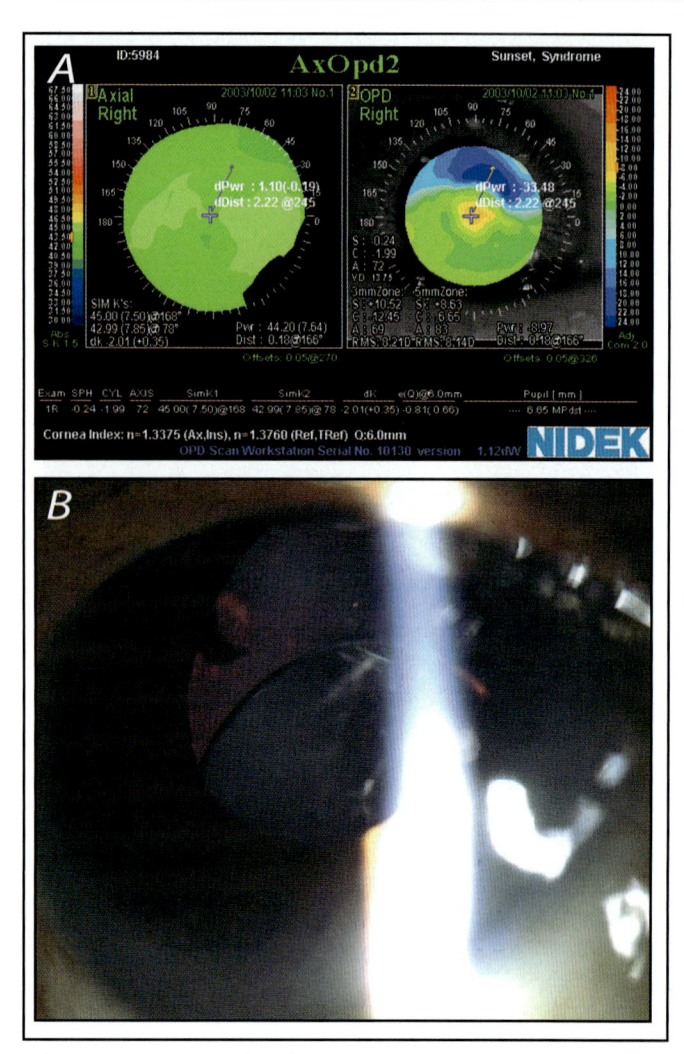

Figure 3-6. Example of OPD-Scan measurement of an eye with sunset syndrome with a 33.0-D refractive gradient across the open pupil and a 3-mm OPD refraction of +10.52 -12.45 x 69.

Effectively, this map presents what is remaining after sphere and cylinder (the lower-order aberrations) are removed. The MTF graph plots the visual performance of the eye. The various curves denote the best human MTF (green), diffraction limited MTF (dark blue), the effect on visual performance once the sphere and cylinder are removed (red), and the effect of correcting the higher-order aberrations of the eye (pink). As a rule of thumb, the larger the area under the curves, the better the visual performance of the eye. The OPD internal map displays the refractive status of eye due to the internal aberrations of the eye by subtracting the effects of the corneal front surface from the total aberrometry. This map allows one to determine if the source of the aberrations is corneal, internal, or a combination. This can be a critical factor in the clinical outcome of refractive surgery. Figure 3-5 plots OPD-Station analysis for a symptomatic post-LASIK patient. The OPD map shows induced spherical aberration and trefoil as shown by the trilobed pattern centrally. These aberrations combine to form a refractive gradient of -2.11 D across the pupil. Once the lower-order aberration is removed, the OPD HO maps shows that the higher-order aberrations are causing a larger refractive gradient, which is unmasked as sphere and cylinder is removed. Hence, it is clinically intuitive to surmise that this patient requires a custom ablation treatment to reduce the complaints of glare. This observation is further reinforced by the MTF graph, which shows a larger area under the pink curve (visual performance with higher-order aberration corrected) compared to the red curve (visual performance with just lower-order aberration corrected).

For intraocular surgery, the internal OPD map allows the determination of the centration of the IOL and the optical effect of the surgery (Figures 3-6A and B). The OPD and internal OPD map shows hallmark patterns for various IOL associated complications. Figures 3-6A and B show the characteristic OPD map for sunset syndrome showing hyperopic crescent superiorly with a larger myopic areas below with a 33.0-D difference in refraction. Figure 3-7 shows the characteristic pattern for a tilted IOL showing myopic and hyperopic areas bisecting the pupil but with significantly reduced refractive gradient compared to that shown in Figures 3-6A and B.

For refractive surgery procedures, there are various indices that allow the determination of the corneal vertex, the pupil center, and the photopic and mesopic pupil centers (Figure 3-8). Preoperatively, this information provides vital information on the centering of the treatment; postopera-

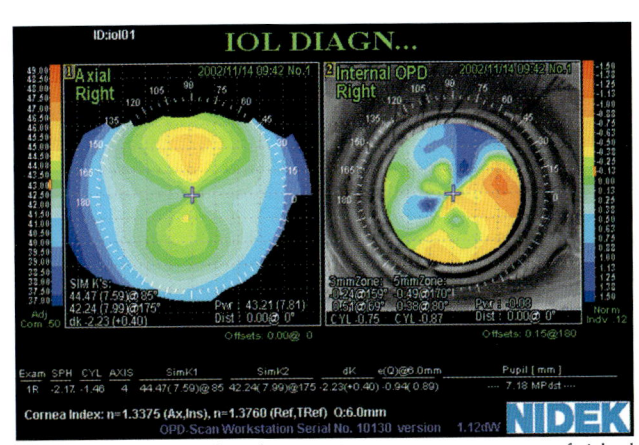

Figure 3-7. Example of OPD-Scan measurement of titled IOL. Notice the hyperopic and myopic areas bisecting the pupil on the Internal OPD map.

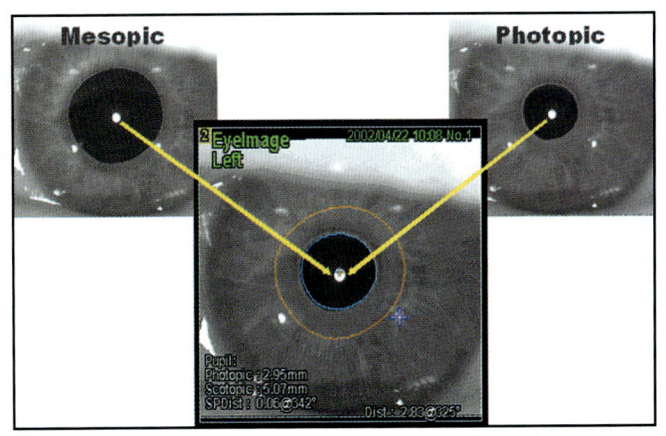

Figure 3-8. Pupillometry and alignment of Purkinje images on corneal topography and aberrometry (mesopic pupil) that allows correct centering procedure.

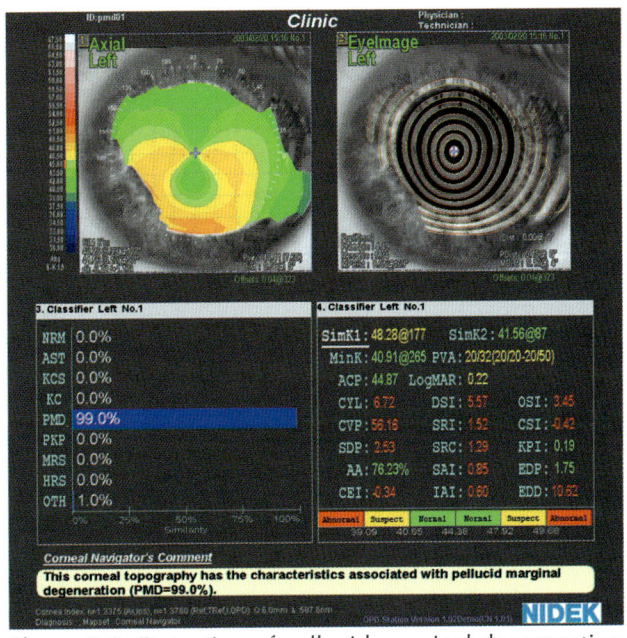

Figure 3-9. Detection of pellucid marginal degeneration (PMD) with corneal navigator function of the NIDEK OPD-Scan.

tively, these indices can be used to determine the centration of the procedure. Additionally infrared pupillometry allows accurate determination of the scotopic pupil size.

Screening for corneal pathology is fundamental to prevent surgery on corneas with progressive corneal dystrophies such as pellucid marginal degeneration or keratoconus. The OPD-Station contains an automated corneal topography screening device that classifies corneal topography into nine different classifications of normal vs abnormal, keratoconus, keratoconus suspect, and pellucid marginal degeneration. Forme fruste keratoconus is only detectable by corneal topography; hence, such screening algorithm will aid the clinician in diagnosis of abnormal corneas. Figure 3-9 shows an example of a pellucid marginal degeneration showing the percent likelihood that this is PMD and the color coded values that are largely red denoting abnormal values. Since undiagnosed pellucid marginal degeneration has been the etiology of postsurgical ectasia, this is an especially important clinical tool.

In summary, the NIDEK OPD-Scan presents multiple clinical diagnosis and management functions that allow the user to prescreen, diagnose, follow-up, and address complications due to intraocular and refractive surgery.

CHAPTER 4

Understanding Wavefront: Microns vs Diopters

Stephen D. Klyce, PhD

The eye's low-order aberrations of defocus and astigmatism are conveniently corrected in spectacles with sphere and cylinder. "However, interface shape irregularities—particularly those at the corneal surface—can create higher order (HO) aberrations that in turn cause symptomatic blur and ghosting. The effects of these aberrations can range from a minor annoyance to being functionally debilitating. For example, these HO aberrations are often the source of reduced acuity in corneal transplant patients. Even normal eyes, however, exhibit a certain amount of HO aberrations; some are not clinically significant and others may even be beneficial to vision. For example, Schallhorn (personal communication) has found that a small amount of vertical coma correlated with better uncorrected visual acuity among US Navy Top Gun pilots. While the object of individualized laser refractive surgery is to eliminate all aberrations, doing so may not provide optimal visual function. Yet, clinical trials have shown that customization of laser corrective procedures does lead to improved outcomes when compared to standard treatments that correct only sphere and cylinder. Further study is necessary to determine the optimum final wavefront pattern that would provide the best functional vision.

The corneal surface generally contributes the bulk of ocular HO aberrations due to the high refractive index gradient between air and the tears. Lenticular defects associated with aging, leading to changes in shape and eventual cataract formation, can produce aberrations as well. Therefore, the use of a wavefront sensor to measure the optical characteristics of an entire eye should provide the best data for the correction of that eye's total aberrations. Combining data from the wavefront sensor and the corneal topographer provides the most useful information possible to the clinician, both for diagnostics and for refractive surgery.

Wavefront Basics

The wavefront sensor measures the distortion of a lightwave that is altered by the optics of the eye. A plane wave of monochromatic light will be curved by the positive power of the cornea and lens (Figure 4-1). A mismatch between this combined power and the axial length of the eye produces ametropia or focus errors. Shape irregularities in the cornea and lens cause distortion and aberrations in the wavefront. Note that wavefront sensors do not measure light scatter (from stromal haze, scarring, or cataracts), chromatic aberrations, or diffraction phenomena, although wavefront sensor measurements can be degraded, or even rendered useless, by these factors. Clinically, though, light scatter is often the only property of consequence; if there is sufficient corneal or lenticular light scatter to obscure the retina, wavefront sensors generally will not provide useful data.

An easy way to understand aberrations is to realize they are caused by differences in the travel time and path lengths of parallel rays entering the pupil and projecting toward the retina. As light enters the eye from the air, its speed is retarded according to the optical density of the material along its path to the retina (index of refraction). The arrival time is also retarded by an increase in the distance of travel. These two factors, density and dimensional variations, can be measured with a wavefront sensor, which will be described below. The measurement data can be expressed as either a refractive error in diopters (D) or a distortion in microns (μm). The data can be used as well to calculate the point spread function, which is the image of a distant point of light that is formed on the retina, and these data are subsequently used to assess image quality of an individual eye. As shown in Figure 4-1, optical data are referenced to different planes in the eye. Corneal

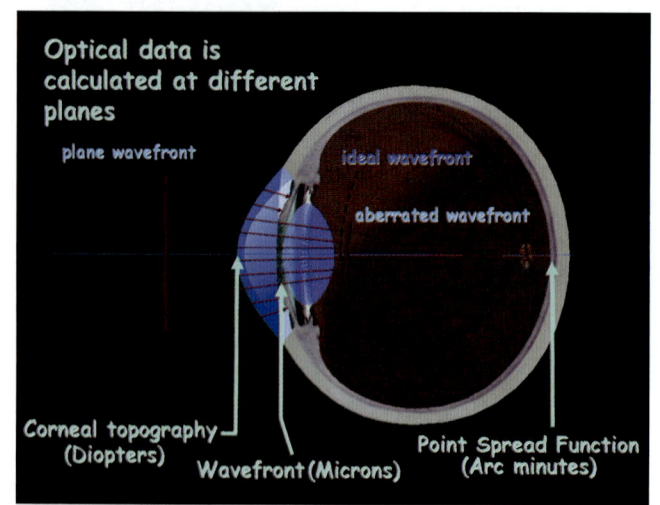

Figure 4-1. A wavefront of light changes shape (is aberrated) by the optics of the eye. An eye with perfect optics would focus a point of light at infinity onto the retina as an Airy disk pattern. One can observe the optical properties of the eye with corneal topography analysis, which is expressed in diopters at the corneal plane; as a wavefront expressed (most often) in microns at the pupil plane or in diopters at the corneal plane (less frequent); and as a point spread function in minutes of arc at the retinal plane.

topography has the corneal plane as its reference. Wavefront data generally, but not always, is referenced to the pupil plane. It will be seen that expression of wavefront data in units and reference planes that are different from those used in corneal topography are the main factors that prevent efficient clinical use of wavefront data.

The measurement of wavefront must also consider the role of the pupil in the formation of images, as this aperture affects the depth of field as well as the extent of the corneal and lenticular landscape in use. A decrease in pupil size increases the depth of field, but more importantly, a small pupil constrains light to the better, central optics of the eye. The latter comes into play with refractive surgeries that leave the cornea with a small optical zone. For this reason, it is important to consider what pupil size is being used when analyzing wavefront data; analyzing a 3-mm diameter of wavefront data to simulate daytime vision can show good optical characteristics, but analyzing the same data out to a 6-mm pupil to simulate night vision can reveal significant aberrations. The effect of pupil diameter on wavefront data will be illustrated.

One last, important observation about wavefront analysis: one can analyze the wavefront produced by the whole eye or from any single part of the optical path. This means that one can construct a wavefront pattern derived from corneal topography and subtract these data from the total wavefront of the eye to determine how much of the eye's aberrations arise from the cornea and how much stem from the rest of the eye. This feature can be used diagnostically.

Wavefront Sensors

With the recognized potential for newer generation tracking and scanning excimer lasers to go beyond the "simple" correction of sphere and cylinder, industry responded with the introduction of wavefront measurement systems based upon several different principles. The Shack-Hartmann approach is probably the most widely adopted and uses the observation of a laser ray projected onto the retina and viewed through a 12-by-12 or greater grid of micro-lenses. Each lens observes the retinal ray image at a unique angular location within the pupil so that distortions in the eye's optics are measured on a pointwise basis. The strength of this approach is that all positions within the pupil can be measured simultaneously to avoid potential movement artifact. The weakness is that generally only a few hundred points can be measured within the pupil, placing a limit on spatial resolution. It is noted that sensors have been developed with up to 3000 elements within a circular aperture, but at this spatial density, even minor HO aberrations can confuse the accurate location of the array of point images.

A second method used to measure wavefronts from the eye is the Tscherning method. Here, a specific pattern, usually a grid, is projected onto the retina and the resulting distortions in its shape are related to the aberrations of the eye. The Tracey ray tracing system belongs to this class of wavefront sensor, although the pattern it projects occurs in a serial pointwise fashion. The advantage of this device is that the pattern is totally programmable, and therefore, the spatial resolution can be increased or decreased to suit the application. However, there is a trade off. The higher the spatial density and number of points projected, the longer the time necessary for measurement, and movement artifact can intrude upon accuracy before very high spatial resolution can be achieved over the whole measured area.

A third method used to measure wavefront is that of refractometry. The Emory spatially resolved refractometer relies on subjective patient response and takes the longest time for measurement of any of the wavefront devices. The NIDEK OPD-Scan uses a similar principle—dynamic skiascopy—to measure the refraction of the eye through the pupil over 1440 points. This device has the highest usable spatial resolution of all the available instruments and has an added bonus in that it includes the measurement of corneal topography, allowing nearly simultaneous wavefront and corneal topography measurement. As a consequence, wavefront and corneal topography can be more closely aligned with each other and the eye during surgery to improve the accuracy of customized corneal treatments. In addition, near simultaneous capture of ocular wavefront and corneal topography permits calculation of the internal optics of the eye. A potential shortcoming of the OPD-Scan is that the wavefront measurement requires up to 400 mSec compared to the CCD camera acquisition time of 33 mSec for Shack-Hartmann devices and corneal topography systems, including that of the OPD-Scan. However, movement artifact does not seem to manifest itself as a problem in the OPD-Scan measurements.

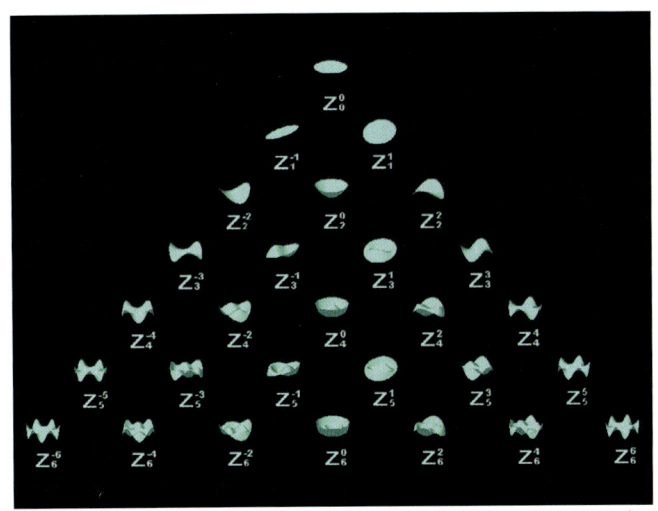

Figure 4-2. Zernike pyramid of wavefront models up to the sixth order; this set of often used in clinical trials of customized ablations. Different mathematical combinations of these modes are used to fit wavefronts. The indexing uses superscripts to denote the angular frequency, and subscripts to denote the radial order. Commonly named terms include Z00 = piston, Z1-1 = tip, Z11 = tilt, Z2-2,2 = astigmatism, Z20 = defocus, Z3-1,1 = coma, Z3-3,3 = trefoil, Z40 = spherical aberration.

Wavefront Data Analysis

In the past, methods were developed to describe the optical distortions in microscope and telescope optical components. These techniques were thought to be appropriate to describe the aberrations of the eye and have, therefore, been adopted for use in wavefront measurements. At least three related analytic techniques have been used to extract optical characteristics from three-dimensional wavefront structures or surfaces. These include the Taylor Series, Zernike polynomial series, and the Seidel series. In 1999, the Optical Society of America formed the Vision Science and Its Applications (VSIA) Taskforce on Standards for the Reporting of the Optical Aberrations of the Eye to examine issues arising from the fledgling field of ocular wavefront measurement. The group proposed a refinement of the Zernike method for the description of ocular aberrations. With the Zernike method, individual coefficients can be used to measure separate optical aberrations including defocus, cylinder, prism, spherical aberration, coma, trefoil, and other HO terms (Figure 4-2). Generally, all of the Zernike terms above first order (excludes so-called piston, tip, and tilt) are included to calculate the total wavefront aberrations. HO aberrations typically include all of the Zernike terms above second order (excluding piston, tip, tilt, defocus, and astigmatism). Hence, the HO aberrations intentionally exclude optical defects of the eye that can be corrected with standard spectacle optics and should reveal what might be corrected with more elaborate means (customized corrections).

Since the Zernike method, like the other methods, is a potentially infinite polynomial series, it was argued that it could be used to fit any degree of ocular wavefront distortion simply by increasing the number of terms used. However, there are caveats in the blanket use of the Zernike polynomials in clinical applications, including diagnostics and refractive surgical corrections. Zernike terms are based on terms that exhibit radial symmetry, which is to say that they can accurately model surfaces, such as telescope mirrors, that are intended to be rotationally symmetric. Normal corneas exhibit a good degree of radial symmetry, but irregular corneas, such as transplants and those with keratoconus, produce enough nonrotationally symmetric irregularity that the Zernike approach is not ideal. As ordinarily used, the sixth order Zernike polynomial smooths wavefront data and as such does not faithfully capture all of the aberrations responsible for diminished vision in highly aberrated eyes.[1-3] Furthermore, as more Zernike orders are added to improve the accuracy of fit to aberrated wavefronts, a limit is reached beyond which the fitting procedure becomes unstable and inaccurate.[4] As a result, the performance of laser custom ablation in aberrated eyes, based on Zernike models, can be suboptimal, and because of this, other strategies, such as Fourier Series analysis, are being applied.

Nevertheless, Zernike decomposition of wavefront structure remains a powerful tool with which to measure the contribution of the HO aberrations to visual function. The measurement unit traditionally chosen to describe the shape of a wavefront has been the micron. This unit provides a pointwise measure of the amount light is advanced or retarded with reference to a plane that is usually the pupil. The integrated or total amount of distortion from a reference surface is measured with the root mean square (RMS), a commonly used engineering method for reporting signal distortion. Microns are directly useful for guiding laser ablation, as the amount of material removed in an area is expressed in this fashion. However, for diagnostics, wavefront data cast in diopters is more easily compared to standard topography. The duality of wavefront presentation is the central theme of this chapter and is covered in detail below.

As noted above, Fourier analysis is another approach to analyzing wavefront data. There are two basic ways to use the Fourier method. Fourier Series analysis can be used as a three-dimensional surface fitting routine to model wavefront data. As such, it can do so more accurately than the Zernike method for use in customized laser sculpting.[4] A second method is the direct Fourier transform, which can be used to model complex data exactly, and this is often used in image analysis. In understanding the consequence of different aberrations on visual performance, the Fourier transform is used to show how a point source of light should appear on the retina. This is illustrated with the point spread function (PSF) (Figure 4-3). The Fourier transform can also be used to demonstrate how certain wavefront aberrations affect visual acuity by calculating their impact through the mathematical convolution of the PSF with common images such as a visual acuity chart shown in Figure 4-4. Camp, and coworkers[5] provided one of the first demonstrations of this capability a decade before wavefront sensors made their appearance in clinical use. Such presentation forms should become useful

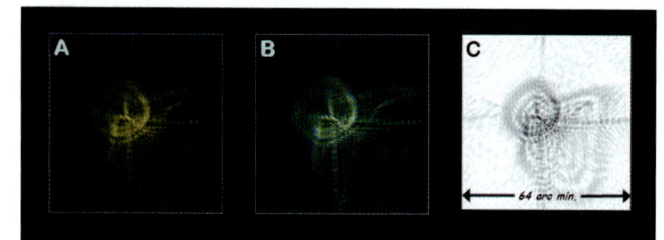

Figure 4-3. Example of a PSF from a large (7 mm) pupil, myopic refractive surgery with a small optical zone. The major features in this PSF include starburst, halo, and ghosting; these are often included in the night vision complaints reported by symptomatic patients after refractive surgery. The lower intensity components of these PSFs have been emphasized mathematically for visualization—the dimmer pixels would not be sensed. (A) Polychromatic PSF created with white light and using the photopic response function of the retinal cone receptors. (B) Polychromatic PSF created with white light and using the mesopic response function of the retinal rod receptors. (C) Black and white inverse image of (A), an alternative presentation format.

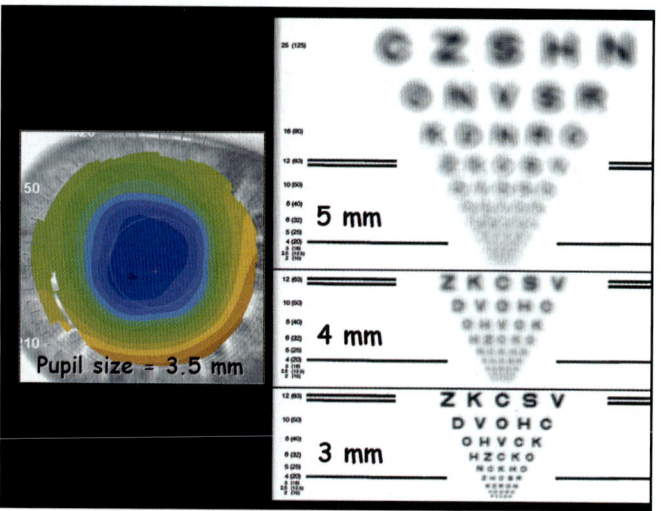

Figure 4-4. The corneal topography of a very aspheric LASIK correction for myopia. The photopic pupil diameter for this eye was 3.5 mm measured topographically. The PSF was calculated from the HO aberrations in the topography data and convolved with a National Eye Institute Snellen eye chart for simulated pupil sizes of 3, 4, and 5 mm. Note the progressive loss of acuity as well as a decrease in contrast owing to the blur created in this multifocal topography. Compensation for the Stiles-Crawford effect was applied to avoid an overestimate of the loss of Snellen lines at the larger pupil sizes.

clinical adjuncts to evaluate the quality of vision in individual eyes and the effect of specific refractive corrections thereupon.

Clinical Applications

There are two basic uses of wavefront data: diagnostics and customized refractive correction—both surgical (keratorefractive) and nonsurgical (contact lenses, intracorneal lenses, and intraocular lenses). In order to be used by devices such as lasers for sculpting lens shapes, the wavefront data must be expressed in micron units of distance that relate to the amount of material that needs to be removed at each location on the corneal or lens surface to achieve the desired refractive result. For diagnostic use, the wavefront data should be expressed in diopters—units of refractive power that would allow direct comparison of wavefront data with corneal topography data. In this way, it is possible to determine the source of any aberrations measured. In simple terms, units of microns are needed for machining lenses, while units of diopters are needed for diagnostics.

The Micron Scale for Wavefront Display

One of the biggest challenges facing the integration of wavefront measurements in clinical practice was the presentation format. The format chosen did not seem comparable to corneal topography displays despite the fact that ordinarily, most of the aberrations in an aberrated eye arise from the corneal surface. What had been learned from the development of corneal topography scales used in color-coded contour maps[6-8] needed to be applied to the display of micron wavefront data: 1) a scale contour interval needed to be chosen to be just adequate to perceive clinically significant features; 2) a range needed to be establish that would encompass the bulk of aberrations seen clinically; and 3) a color palette needed to be chosen from a contrasting color set so that aberrations would stand out. A final feature that was thought to be essential for a meaningful micron wavefront scale was the use of a progressive color scheme that would be consistent with the colors used in topography: an area of cornea that was lower in power than normal and presented with a blue color, would correspond to an area in a wavefront that was also cool in color. An example of the use of this scale, developed by Smolek and Klyce,[9] is shown in Figure 4-5. Studies showed that with wavefront data the bulk of the HO aberrations are included in the range of -6.5 to 6.5 μm and clinically significant aberrations become evident using an interval of 0.5 μm. With this scale, maps of ocular wavefront errors decomposed with the Zernike polynomials clearly reveal abnormalities while masking variations among normal eyes with excellent visual acuity.

It is important to point out again that the extent of the data that is collected and the aperture through which it is analyzed are of paramount importance. Wavefront sensors often have a limited diameter over which they can reliably collect data, generally up to 6 mm through the dilated pupil. Clearly, if a patient has 7- or 8-mm pupils at night, the average wavefront sensor will not be able to carry its analysis to the margin of the pupil. Since the optics of the eye degrade progressively with the diameter of the pupil, most wavefront sensors will

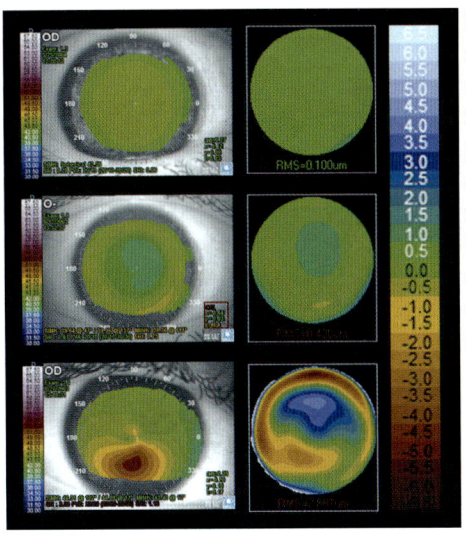

Figure 4-5. Axial power corneal topography maps in units of diopters are shown in the left-hand column, while wavefront maps of these topographies in units of microns are shown in the right-hand column. The scale to the right is the Smolek/Klyce wavefront scale in microns; it's range is -6.5 to 6.5 μm in 0.5 μm steps. Note the correspondence between the topographies presenting optical properties at the corneal plane and the wavefront data, which present the same corneal data fitted with the Zernike method at the pupil plane. Displayed in this fashion, there is a correspondent similarity that makes interpretation and comparison clinically useful. The top cornea is a normal spherical cornea, the center cornea has had LASIK for myopia, and the bottom cornea has clinical keratoconus topography.

not be able to provide accurate estimates for vision beyond their normal scope. However, since the corneal surface is normally responsible for most of the HO aberrations in the eye and since topographers generally capture data out to 9 mm and beyond, it seems reasonable to use corneal topography data to assess quality of vision after corneal surgery. It is noted that this assumption can be tested using the NIDEK OPD-Scan internal aberrations display described below. The effect of pupil size on optical aberrations is shown in Figure 4-4, as previously noted.

Zernike decomposition can be a useful adjunct for the clinician to understand the quality of vision and the cause of visual complaints, particular in surgical corneas. Using Zernike decomposition, one can dissect out specific aberration types (eg, spherical aberration and coma), in order to see how these contribute to vision in specific cases. Examples of a Zernike decomposition display are shown in Figures 4-6A through 6C. Combined with the micron color scale described above, these show the contributions of each of the major HO aberrations on vision quantitatively, as well as graphically. In addition, they are constructed so as to indicate aberrations that are outside the range found in normal, unoperated corneas. The micron wavefront data shown in the figures arises from corneal topography data rather than from ocular wavefront sensors and, therefore, has a high spatial resolution and can be used to assess aberrations over any simulated pupillary aperture up to the diameter of the area analyzed by the corneal topographer.

Diopter Scale for Wavefront Display

As noted above, expressing wavefront errors in microns may not be as useful for diagnostics as the more clinically familiar units of power expressed in diopters. The NIDEK OPD-Scan is unique among the wavefront sensors in that it directly measures the refractive status of the eye in diopters, and the data are referenced to the corneal plane. This provides an important opportunity for clinical use; the wavefront sensor data provide a corneal plane refraction map of the eye over the entrance pupil, while the Placido topography provides corneal plane power map data of the corneal surface. Normally, the axial power map is used diagnostically in the clinic, but corneal topography can be expressed as refractive power using Snell's Law and in units of diopters. Hence, the corneal refractive power topography map data can be registered with and subtracted from the OPD whole eye wavefront refraction map. The result is a dataset that can be used to map the internal aberrations of the eye (Figures 4-7 and 4-8). This is a powerful tool that allows the clinician to detect instances where aberrations arise from within the eye. One can expect that aberrations arising from conditions such as lenticonus and significant intraocular lens decentration and tilt should be detectable with this strategy.

Summary and Conclusions

It is clear that wavefront analysis is here to stay. While the Zernike polynomial approximation is useful for describing the lower-order aberrations, studies have shown that this method lacks the precision necessary to capture the fine, often random irregularities in the corneal surface. Either the raw wavefront data or another method with greater fidelity, such as Fourier Series analysis, must be used in the planning of customized laser refractive surgery. Corneal topography is also here to stay and needs to be coupled mathematically to wavefront data for the best representation of the eye's aberrations. Improving the spatial density or number of measurement points taken by an aberrometer from within the pupil will improve the visual results after laser sculpting.

As with the interpretation of corneal topography, wavefront maps need to be presented using scales and units that are appropriate for the particular application. Laser sculpting needs data to be expressed in microns, while clinicians need a diopter scale to appreciate the relative contributions of the corneal surface and internal optics of the eye. For both

Figure 4-6. Zernike HO decomposition display as implemented on the NIDEK Magellan corneal topographer (NIDEK, srl, Padua, Italy). (A) Analysis of a slightly astigmatic (0.75 D), un-operated cornea. The corneal topography is shown in the upper left panel using the axial map with the Universal Standard Scale. This is fit with the Zernike polynomials with an adjustable radial order (here eighth order) and over a defined pupillary diameter (here 4.0 mm). The lower-order Zernike terms, including the tip, tilt, and cylinder, are not included in the HO display. Hence, in this cornea, otherwise normal except for the small amount of cylinder, there are no significant HO aberrations. Spherical aberration, coma, trefoil, the remaining HO aberrations (irregular), as well as the total HO aberrations show no features in the color-coded aberration maps. Further, the RMS values below each Zernike element are green, meaning that each of these is within ±2 standard deviations from the average of normals for this pupil size and Zernike order. The residuals map is included so that the user can evaluate the goodness of fit of the Zernike method to an individual corneal topography. PSFs are also plotted below each decomposition display. These can be selected to display photopic, mesopic, or monochrome representations as shown in Figure 4-3. In addition, one can select the eye chart mode to display their aberrated form as in Figure 4-3. The enhance PSF feature can be selected to boost the intensity of the parts of the PSF that are generally below the sensory threshold for visualization purposes. (B) This is a contact lens patient who is experiencing warpage. A high-riding contact lens has produced a furrow across the lower part of the visual field. This can cause spectacle blur, which the display clearly indicates will have its optical origins predominately in vertical coma and some irregular HO aberrations. Note that the RMS values of all the aberrations are red, which means they are all more than 3 standard deviations distant from the average measured in normals. (C) A keratoconus corneal exhibiting a good deal of spherical aberration, coma, and irregular HO aberrations. One can also see in this display a significant amount of residual aberrations that are not fit well with the eighth order Zernike fit employed. In the corneal topography map, the pupil outlines are displayed. This is the approximate area that was analyzed in this calculation.

applications, a strict adherence to the use of display scales with a fixed range and fixed contour interval is necessary so that only detail of visual consequence can be appreciated. The micron scale for expressing wavefront presented in this chapter should help the clinician relate traditional wavefront data to the diopter maps that are the standard for presenting corneal topography.

The wavefront maps measured with the NIDEK OPD-Scan are expressed directly in units of diopters at the corneal plane. Because the device incorporates a standard Placido corneal topographer that captures corneal and ocular data along the same axis and in rapid succession, these two data sets are comparable and can be subtracted to provide information about the internal aberrations of an eye. This has far-reaching implications to extend our knowledge regarding the optics of intraocular lenses *in situ*.

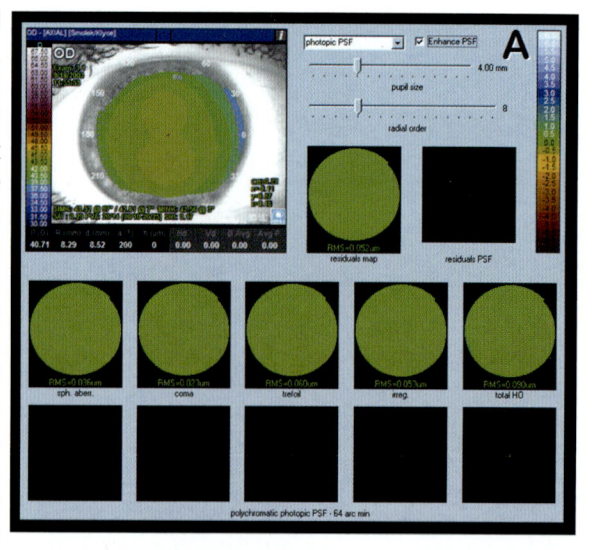

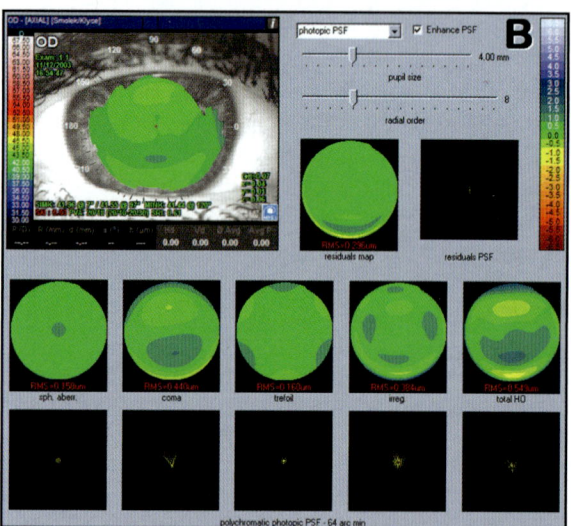

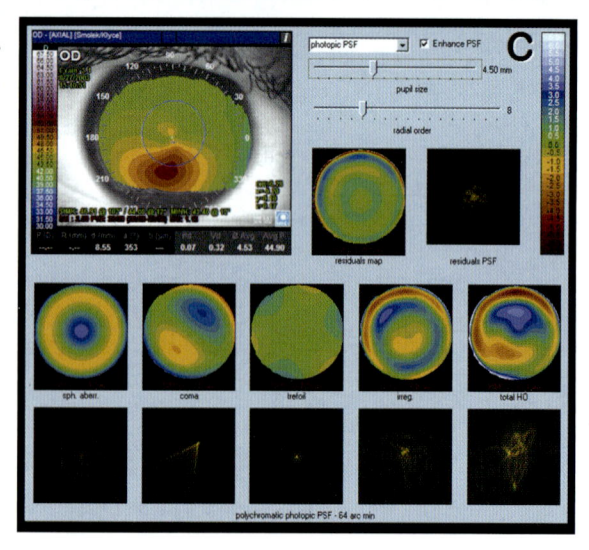

Acknowledgments

This work was supported in part by US Public Health Service grants EY03311 from the National Eye Institute, National Institutes of Health, Bethesda, MD.

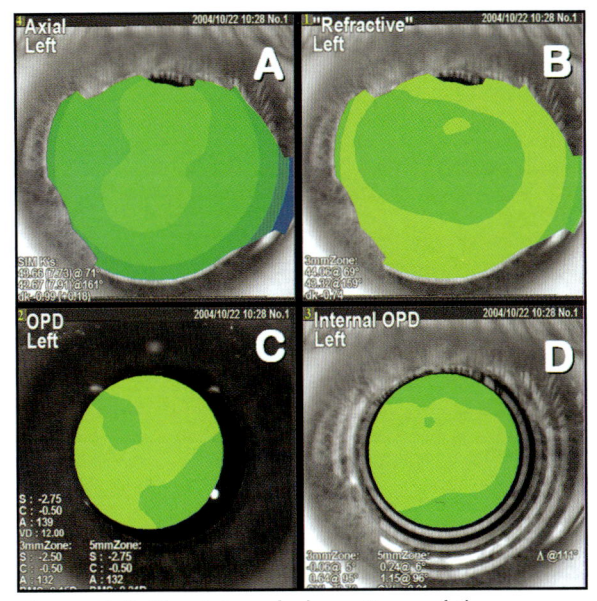

Figure 4-7. The internal aberrations of the eye can be assessed with the NIDEK OPD-Scan. This is a normal eye with all data expressed in the standard 1.5 D contour interval using the same color palette. (A) The OPD-Scan corneal topographer component produces an axial power map. (B) The same data are used to calculate a "refractive" power map which should match the way in which the wavefront sensor data is expressed. (C) The ocular refraction map is measured in diopters using the principle of skiascopy. (D) Compensating for any tilt differences, the "Internal OPD" map is calculated by subtracting the corneal aberrations from the whole eye aberrations: D = C - B. In this eye, there are few aberrations anywhere.

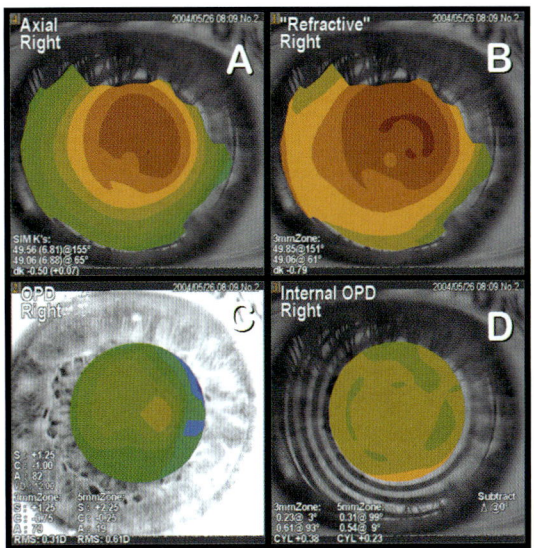

Figure 4-8. The internal aberrations of the eye can be assessed with the NIDEK OPD-Scan. This is a cornea after LASIK for hyperopia. (A) Axial power map. (B) "Refractive" power map. (C) Refraction map. (D) "Internal OPD" map: D = C - B. In this eye, essentially all of the significant aberrations arise from the corneal topography.

Dr. Klyce has been a consultant to NIDEK, Inc, Gamagori, Japan.

References

1. Smolek MK, Klyce SD. Zernike polynomials are inadequate to represent HO aberrations in the eye. *Invest Ophthalmol Vis Sci.* 2003;44:4676-4681.
2. Klyce SD, Karon MD, Smolek MK. Advantages and disadvantages of the zernike expansion for representing wave aberration of the normal and aberrated eye. *J Refractive Surg.* 2004;20:S537-S541.
3. Smolek MK, Klyce SD. Goodness-of-prediction of zernike polynomial fitting to corneal surfaces. *J Cataract Refract Surg.* 2005;31:2350-5.
4. Alchagirov A, Klyce SD, Smolek MK, Karon, MD. Comparison of accuracy of zernike polynomials and fourier series in corneal surface representation. ARVO Abstract #851, Association for Research in Vision and Ophthalmology, Fort Lauderdale, Fa, May 1-5, 2005. [for text, see http://www.arvo.org]
5. Camp JJ, Maguire LJ, Cameron BM, Robb RA. A computer model for the evaluation of the effect of corneal topography on optical performance. *Am J Ophthalmol.* 1990;109(4):379-386.
6. Maguire LJ, Singer DE, Klyce SD. Graphic presentation of computer-analyzed keratoscope photographs. *Arch Ophthalmol.* 1987;105:223-230.
7. Wilson SE, Klyce SD, Husseini ZM. Standardized color-coded maps for corneal topography. *Ophthalmology.* 1993;100:1723-1727.
8. Smolek MK, Klyce SD, Hovis JK: The universal standard scale: proposed improvements to the ANSI standard corneal topography map. *Ophthalmology.* 2002;109:361-369.
9. Smolek MK, Klyce SD: Standard absolute scales for corneal wavefront error maps. ARVO Abstract #2565, Association for Research in Vision and Ophthalmology, Fort Lauderdale, Florida, May 2-5, 2003.

Patient Selection for Surface Ablation

Paolo Vinciguerra, MD; Luca Maestroni, MD

Examining Candidate Patients for Refractive Surgery

INTRODUCTION

Refractive surgery is a valuable tool for improving the quality of life of individuals affected by myopia, astigmatism, hypermetropia, and presbyopia, but it is important to remember that it is rarely an obligatory solution. Thus, we recommend being extremely selective in choosing patients for this procedure and attempt to clarify not only the themes pertaining to the localized or systemic disorders, but also above all the psychological and motivational aspects at the time of the preoperation examination.

This is the only way to be able to determine whether photorefractive treatment is the most appropriate solution or whether it might be preferable (for both patient and surgeon) to recommend other types of corrective measures.

CASE HISTORY

Naturally, this is first aspect of the ophthalmic examination and, as mentioned, has special importance with respect to the norm.

FAMILY HISTORY

First of all, the family history must be investigated in order to ascertain any potential disorder that may be latent, or which might manifest themselves in later life. Metabolic disorders such as diabetes and immune or collagen-related disorders, which might alter the bodies repair responses (see below), are particularly relevant.

In relation to the eyes, it is important to ascertain any familial keratoconus; glaucoma; degenerative retinal disorders such as retinitis pigmentosa, hereditary maculopathies, and Stickler's syndrome; zonular changes; or alterations of the vitreous body associated with collagen-related disorders. Each of the disorders may constitute a contraindication to the operation.

MEDICAL HISTORY

A patient's medical history, besides determining their general state of health, must identify any previous or current disorders that might prejudice the operation's good outcome.

General State of Health

This should be examined carefully; any behavioral and, above all, dietary habits should be investigated so as to identify any potentially hazardous situations. First of all, any recent and sudden changes in body weight should be clarified. Unsuitable diets may deplenish the body of those substances (eg, vitamins, amino acids, oligoelements) constituting the substrates for cellular metabolic processes and cause delayed re-epithelialization, poor epithelial adhesion to the newly formed Bowman's capsule, and recurrent epithelial erosions, aggravated by a qualitative and quantitative deficiency of the lachrymal film and altered stromal inflammatory response. Vitamin complexes are fundamentally important for tissue regeneration, and some in particular play a specific role in the eye. Vitamin A plays an essential role in epithelial metabolism; deficiencies lead to serious alterations of mucosa, which in the eye, manifest themselves as xerophthalmia and keratomalacia. It is not without reason that topical preparations are used in the treatment of various disorders of the eye surface. Aside from the above, their crucial role in the synthesis of retinal photopigments should be remembered. The B-complex vitamins play an important role in epithelial turnover and in neuromuscular transmission. Their deficiency can lead to alterations in the corneal and conjunctival epithelial surface. Vitamin D can cause changes in the eye, not only due to deficiency but also due to excessive haematic levels, which can result in scleral, conjunctival, and corneal calcium accumulation (band shaped keratopathy). Essential amino acid deficiencies may lead to delayed epithelialization and corneal melting. The investigation must also take account of any particularly physically demanding sporting activities, which may lead to analogous problems in individuals certainly not affected by any of the above disorders. In relation to cigarette smoke, there is no scientific evidence of potentially negative effects on immediate or long-term postoperative recovery following refractive surgery, even if exposure to the conjunctival mucosa and the corneal surface immediately following photoablation. However, if the patient is treated with contact lenses, there may be increased risk of inflammation and infection if exposed to smoke. It is recommended to avoid exposure to smoke, at least until epithelial repair is complete. Alcohol consumption in moderate quantities does not appear to have any influence on this type of surgery, even if there is no scientific evidence.

Refractive surgery should not be considered for pregnant or nursing patients for a number of reasons. First of all, the hormonal changes occurring during such periods may induce alterations in the production of the lachrymal film. This essentially causes problems in terms of repair and the mechanisms for nourishment and defence against infection in the outer corneal layers, considering also that photoablation is, in itself, a cause of hypolacrimia. Furthermore, it is believed that during pregnancy there may be refractive fluctuations that may alter the correct measurement of refractive deficiencies, and in the final analysis, invalidate the precision of the treatment. In addition, pregnancy has been identified as a potential cause of regression following refractive surgery.[1] It is then necessary to consider the consumption of the medications (eg, antibiotics, NSAIDs, cortisones) that are necessary following treatment and to which the baby would also be exposed, as the teratogenic or toxic potential of which is not always known. Hence, it is undoubtedly best to postpone the operation until after weaning.

Metabolic Disorders

Given the high prevalence of affectations, it is very important to verify their presence, also in the family history (see the previous paragraph). Foremost among such disorders is, without doubt, diabetes mellitus, which notoriously delays the tissue repair response and promotes the onset of infections. Even though no cases of postoperative complications following refractive surgery have ever been published, it is known to all vitreoretinal surgeons that re-epithelialization following vitrectomy, where the corneal epithelium frequently undergoes such alterations in transparency as to require removal in order to allow good visibility, may be very slow and problematic. The authors of this chapter have had to deal with a case of PTK in a diabetic patient that required a full 25 days to re-epithelialize. Besides the aforementioned risk of an altered wound-healing response, diabetic patients should be evaluated during the preoperational stages for refractive surgery with particular care for other reasons. First of all, fluctuations in glycemia frequently cause changes in the hydration state of the lens which, in the final analysis, result in changes in refraction; hence, during the preoperative stage, it may be difficult to determine refraction with any degree of precision and if by any chance successful, this may change following surgery. Hence, potential refractive instability constitutes a further contraindication to surgery. The aforementioned alterations in lens metabolism frequently lead to precocious opacification of the organ,[2-4] whereby this problem, aggravated by the fact that the calculation of the intraocular lens for implantation is made significantly more difficult and imprecise by previous corneal surgery, must also be evaluated. It need hardly be mentioned how diabetic retinopathy must make even the most tenacious surgeon (or patient) cautious. It is highly inadvisable to propose such surgery in patients with poorly compensated diabetes or affected by one or more of the numerous complications typical of the disorder. If the compensation situation is good and long lasting, with no organ damage or any signs of diabetic retinopathy, it is very important to assess the quality of the adhesion of the corneal epithelium to the Bowman's membrane. First of all, any epithelium appearing to show localized or widespread milkiness is an indicator of altered localized metabolism and it would be advised to not continue with refractive surgery. Verification of adhesion may be performed by observing blinking (there should be no slippage of the epithelium on the underlying layers) or with a cotton wad placed in contact with the cornea, which will highlight any surface alterations. In essence, diabetic patients must be exhaustively evaluated, both generally (metabolic compensation, organ damage, duration of the disorder) and locally, paying particular attention to the quality and adhesion of the corneal epithelium. To avoid any potential reparative problems of the eye surface, some authors recommend performing the operation using the LASIK technique. Less common, but worthy of equally careful assessment, is the presence of any other metabolic problem (liver or kidney failure, anorexia, etc) that may impede correct epithelial regeneration or interfere with the stromal reaction.

Endocrine System Disorders

Aside from glandular disorders, which are without doubt important and incompatible with refractive surgery but which rarely come to the attention of the refractive surgeon (disorders affecting the pituitary, adrenal, hypothalamus etc), thyroid disorders are of particular interest due to their relative high occurrence and the frequency with which they affect the eye. There are essentially two causes to recommend against performing refractive surgery. First, immunological disorders affecting the thyroid may constitute one of the complications of systemic collagenopathy and, hence, be associated with or lead to Sjögren's syndrome or altered collagen repair response typical of such disorders. Second, thyroid-associated ophthalmopathy may lead to varying degrees of lagophthalmos but may be sufficient to prejudice lachrymal film dynamics. Given that one of the first indications of thyroid-associated ophthalmopathy is retraction of the upper eyelid, evaluation of the dynamics of blinking assumes great importance. The parameters to be verified include complete closure of the eyelid and the position of the upper eyelid with respect to the pupillary margin, which under photopic conditions must remain at least 2 mm apart.

Immunological and Collagen Disorders

A case of anomalous wound healing following photorefractive keratectomy, sufficiently serious as to require perforating keratoplasty, has been reported in the literature.[5] Subsequent investigation showed the patient was recognized as being affected by systemic lupus erythematosus. The immune-related collagenopathies are a group of disorders with overlapping clinical symptoms, often affecting the eye, frequently requiring chronic treatments that are potentially harmful for the apparatus of the eye. With regard to the ophthalmologist, the most frightening manifestations leading to photorefractive surgery not being recommended are the tendency to form keloids or unpredictable wound-healing, and the frequency of severe Sjögren's syndrome. Furthermore, it is known that among the factors that might promote the onset of or re-exacerbation of lupus erythematosus is the exposure to particular wavelengths of light. Although not supported by any scientific data, exposure to excimer lasers might be harmful in such patients. Prolonged treatments to which the patient is frequently imposed, and which also have potential effects on the visual apparatus, must be considered. Of the most frequently used drugs, chloroquine may deposit on the retina causing a maculopathy or in the cornea; corticosteroids, especially in high doses, may cause cataracts and/or glaucoma; and immunosuppressant drugs may promote postoperative infections.

Keloid Formation

With wound healing anomalies, photorefractive surgery is not advised given the delicate role of the modulation of the repair response in order to guarantee maintaining corneal transparency and uniformity. In such cases, some surgeons believe the LASIK technique to be applicable.

Neurological Disorders

The refractive surgeon frequently encounters patients undergoing treatment for epilepsy, who otherwise enjoy good health and request photorefractive surgery. In such cases, the doubts are manifold since it is known that an epileptic attack can be brought on by lights or high intensity flashes and, hence, potentially by laser radiation. In this regard, advice from a neurologist is undoubtedly essential, even though from personal experience it may be difficult to obtain any guarantees. Frequently, however, a simple adjustment of the therapy prior to the procedure can allow the operation to go ahead in complete safety. For this reason, it would not seem prudent to undertake a procedure that may need to be immediately interrupted due to an attack with all the consequences this would involve, whereby the full cooperation of the specialists following the patient from the neurological viewpoint is imperative. Neurological disorders resulting in alterations of the dynamics of the eyelids, such as acute myasthenia (Wilk's syndrome), should also be considered at the preoperative stage.

Infectious Diseases

Numerous disorders with infective aetiologies, besides compromising the patient's general condition, may lead to such alterations in the eye as to recommend great prudence when planning refractive treatments. Leaving aside rare or acute disorders, there are numerous clinical conditions that may come to the attention of the refractive surgeon. Due to its increasing frequency in recent years, tuberculosis should undoubtedly be given careful consideration mainly for two reasons: the potential reactivation of a pulmonary focus following steroid therapy (even if the typical steroids do not seem to have such an effect) and the involvement of the eyes in an active infection. For the cornea, the manifestations described include interstitial or ulcerative keratitis and the formation of phlyctenules, but practically any area of the eye may be involved.[6] In essence, a previous history of tuberculosis does not constitute an absolute contraindication to refractive surgery but must demand prudence, and it would be wise to ascertain accurately that the disease truly is dormant. Analogous evaluations should be made for syphilis even though this infection may be effectively treated using appropriate therapies. A case history of a primary infection that has been diagnosed and adequately cured does not constitute a contraindication. In our opinion, patients who have exhibited more advanced stages of the disease (secondary or worse still, tertiary), aside from the numerous systemic and ophthalmological complaints that may manifest themselves, should in any case be excluded from this type of surgery since there is insufficient guarantee of postsurgical compliance. Acquired immunodeficiency syndrome or being positive for the HIV virus constitutes an absolute contraindication even if the treatments currently available allow prolonged maintenance of excellent general health. Herpes infections should be discussed particularly thoroughly; a positive history of eye infection (keratoconjunctivitis, ulcers) of sure herpetic nature, must involve great prudence given that exposure to ultraviolet radiation may cause a dendritic ulcer. The phenomenon has been studied in PTK on herpetic leukomas,[7] and a case of herpes infection flaring up 2 weeks after PTK, which later progressed into a corneal perforation,[8] is described in the literature. However, there is no consensus of opinion in relation to the above point given that other studies show that the rate of herpes reactivation is equal in patients exposed to excimer laser as to those not exposed[9] and that in any case, the phenomenon is generally observed some months after the operation.[7] Furthermore, the role of topical steroids, which might completely or partially be responsible for herpes reactivation, is not entirely clear. Some authors propose a 2-week preventive treatment with oral acyclovir.[5]

Musculoskeletal Apparatus

Certain disorders of the musculoskeletal apparatus may be associated with eye disorders, given that certain collagen types are common to bone, muscle, and eye structures. Marfan's syndrome is a rare hereditary disorder (occurrence 1/15,000), which is almost invariably associated with axial myopia, whereby it is not so infrequent that patients affected by slight, undiagnosed forms (the pathology has very variable expressivity) come to the ophthalmologists attention seeking correction for their refractive defect. Refractive surgery is absolutely not advised for various reasons. Due to the frequency of pathologies affecting the zonular apparatus (from simple phacodonesis to ectopia lentis), the uveal layer (iridodonesis, incomplete development of the angle structures and the ciliary body), and the retina (frequent retinal detachment), and even if there are no known anomalies of the corneal collagen, it is not possible to precisely predict the biomechanical response of the eye structures to refractive surgery. Since patients affected by Marfan's syndrome have rather typical habitus and facies (elevated stature, arachnodactyly, long arms, kyphoscoliosis, sunken chest, capsule-ligament laxity), it is important to perform a more thorough investigation in all myopic patients exhibiting some or all of the aforementioned signs in addition to researching the eye related manifestations of the disorder with particular care. Since, in the vast majority of cases, transmission is autosomal dominant, it may be useful to perform a thorough familial investigation in all suspect cases. Even more difficult to diagnose is Stickler's syndrome, an autosomal dominantly transmitted hereditary collagenopathy with variable penetration, characterized by altered levels of type-II collagen. The systemic signs in this disorder (pineal dysplasia, laxity of the ligaments, enlarged knees, wrists, and also the heavy facial bones, epicanthus, dental anomalies) may not appear obvious. The eye-related signs may be manifold and range from axial myopia, to subcapsular cataract, to premature opacification of the lens nucleus. The distinctive sign is vitreal syneresis and the observation of an optically empty vitreous body. The retinal anomalies, which frequently lead to giant and/or multiple bilateral ruptures, are frequent and very serious. If the above is added to the previously discussed points regarding the unpredictability of the mechanical responses in collagen alterations, it is easily understood how such cases should be carefully identified and not be treated by means of refractive surgery.

Skin

Among the numerous dermatological disorders that might involve the eye, atopic dermatitis merits particular attention. Aside from the most obvious clinical manifestations involving the eyelids (trichiasis, entropion, thickening, and scab formation on the eyelid margin), conjunctiva (papillary conjunctivitis, scar formation, and retraction), lens (subcapsular cataract), and cornea (ulcers, epithelial erosions, corneal neovascolarisation), it should be remembered that in individuals affected by this disorder, there is an estimated predominance of keratoconus of approximately 25%.[10] Hence, atopic dermatitis does not constitute an absolute contraindication to refractive surgery even if it is in clinical remission. Particular attention should be paid to the identification of any keratoconus even if there have been no eye complications to advise against it.

Allergies

This is an extremely widespread problem. Pollen allergies are seasonal in nature, so if the eye is affected particularly violently, it is highly recommended to plan the refractive surgery for an appropriate time. Among the most significant drug allergies are antibiotics, and in this case, an antibiotic should be selected from a different class to the one that is not tolerated.

One-Eyed Patients With an Eye Prosthesis in the Adelphous Eye

As already mentioned, refractive surgery is a procedure burdened by somewhat rare risks; therefore, we recommend avoiding it in functionally or anatomically one-eyed patients, as the impact on the patient's life would be particularly devastating if complications develop. Furthermore, in prosthetized patients, it is necessary to consider that the anatomical condition of the eviscerated or enucleate bulb and the presence of the prosthesis itself (which is always a foreign body) promote infections, making any surgical procedure in the healthy eye even more hazardous.

PHARMACOLOGICAL HISTORY

The consumption of any drugs must be carefully evaluated. First, the consumption of a drug may reveal a previously undetected disorder. Secondly, in order to verify that the drug intended for administration does not interact with any others normally taken, so as to be able, if possible, to modify the eye-specific or systemic treatment. Finally, numerous systemic drugs may potentially have effects on the eye.

In refractive surgery, the most important interactions relate to medications that may induce dry eye and those that might cause midriasis. Dry eye is a recognized cause of delayed re-epithelialization[10] and haze[11] following PRK. There are a large number of drugs associated with dry eye; the class most frequently encountered by the surgeon, given the generally young age of refractive surgery patients, is that of oral contraceptives,[11] which should be suspended for a few months before and after the surgical procedure (the authors suggest 1 month prior and up to 2 to 3 months following surgery). Isotretinoin,[12] a dermatological drug used to treat acne, is frequently associated with dry eye. Further, numerous cardiocirculatory drugs have an effect on lachrymal film production, foremost beta-blockers (even when administered topically) but also other less commonly used antihypertensive acting molecules including Clonidine, Reserpine, Prazosin, and Methyldopa. In relation to the gastrointestinal system, certain antispastic drugs should be mentioned, including Methocarbamol, Cyclobenzaprine, and above all, Methoclopramide, given their widespread use. Certain decongestants, such as ephedrine and pseudoephedrine, have a certain decree of significance since they may be used chronically. Even corticosteroids, taken chronically, may cause dry eye.[10] Lastly, we mention the benzodiazapines, which are widely used and which patients frequently neglect to mention. For the purposes of completeness, we can add to this list the tricyclic antidepressives and certain drugs used for the treatment of Parkinson's disease (eg, Biperidene, Procyclidine), even though, obviously, surgery in patients affected by such serious disorders appears unlikely.

Cases involving iatrogenic midriasis should be evaluated carefully since this can result in errors in measuring the refractive defect, and because it may result in giving rise to halos, particularly if dealing with a high refractive defect, or corneal thickness insufficient for the creation of a wide optical zone.

Besides the drugs used in the acute stages of cardiovascular disease (Adrenaline, Atropine, etc), antihistamines and antimuscarinic bronchodilators (Ipratropium, Oxytropium) must be taken into consideration due to their high frequency of use.

Patients taking such substances cyclically or chronically must be evaluated carefully, and a pupillometry must naturally be performed to predict and evaluate any postoperative problems.

EMPLOYMENT HISTORY

The refractive surgery candidate's job has numerous important aspects that might have an influence on the choice of whether or not to operate and on which technique to adopt. First of all, certain jobs involve specific visual needs and, consequently, the patient may have expectations which are unrealistic or which are impossible to guarantee. Similarly, refractive surgery may be requested in order to obtain the necessary requirements to participate in competitions or to perform specific tasks (eg, air force pilots).

In such cases, the patient's requirements and expectations should be discussed carefully, since what would normally be considered by both patient and surgeon as a good result (eg, a 1.0 D residue from a defect of 10.0 D) might instead be seen as unsuccessful; hence, it is always best to attempt to understand what the patient expects and to always be rather cautious with regard to professions requiring a high standard of visual performance.

Generally, from a professional viewpoint, jobs can be distinguished as those predominantly requiring near vision (eg, VT operators, microscope operators, editors, students) and jobs predominantly requiring distance vision (eg, drivers, representatives). Such distinctions are mainly important for determining the refractive target. Given that the lasers currently on the market are not absolutely precise, it is possible to select (taking account of the patient's age) whether to "aim" at a target of 0 with slight hypermetropia or 0 with slight myopia, depending on which of the two, slight myopia or hypermetropia, might be more advantageous for the patient.

Another important subject is work-related exposure to substances or environmental conditions that might compromise the good outcome of the operation. Patients need to be advised that in the postoperative period, all environments that might be infectious or polluted with harmful substances (fumes, chemical agents, dusts) should be avoided. Therefore, it may be appropriate to abstain from professions inevitably avoiding exposure to such environmental conditions.

The risk of eye infections is certainly present until re-epithelialization has occurred, but even following epithelial repair and though increased pathogen susceptibility has not been demonstrated, it is certain that any infections may have very serious consequences.

Polluting environments may also lead to epithelial alterations and/or induce stromal inflammation, so they should be avoided during the postoperative period. It is very difficult to establish general rules, and since it is impossible for the surgeon to evaluate each situation in detail, it is important to inform the patients and make them responsible for their behavior.

On the other hand, the potentially harmful effects of certain wavelengths of light, which might affect the cornea, lens, and retina, is much more certain. Corneal lesions due to ultraviolet radiation depend on wavelength and intensity.[14,15] Wavelengths that can damage the cornea range from 260 to 290 nm, but fortunately, such wavelengths are curbed by the stratospheric ozone layer, whereby they rarely reach ground level. Therefore, light damage occurs only with prolonged exposure such as that which takes place with snow, which reflects a high percentage of ultraviolet radiation.[17]

The most frequent cause of corneal lesions is exposure to artificial light sources, such as tanning or germicidal lamps and electric arc welders. At a wavelength of 270 nm, an energy intensity of even 0.005 mJ/cm^2 produces damage, while wavelengths of 300 and 310 nm, respectively, require intensities of 0.01 and 10.5 mJ/cm^2.[6] The clinical manifestation is a widespread punctate superficial keratitis appearing approximately 8 to 12 hours following exposure. Chronic exposure leads to the formation of corneal vacuoles and appears to be associated with the onset of pterygium.[18,19]

The consequences of exposure to ultraviolet radiation following refractive surgery are entirely different and potentially much more serious; it is known that following PRK, there may be activation of stromal keratocytes with consequent deposition of anomalous newly-formed stromal tissue, resulting in stromal opacification (haze). The problem is evidently very widespread and potentially hazardous; therefore, it is essential to discuss with the patient during the preoperative stage and ascertain that the risks have been understood and that they are willing and ready to avoid hazardous work-related exposure or ultraviolet environments for at least 3 months following the operation.

There is no direct correlation between lens disorders and refractive surgery, but opacification of the organ certainly prejudices the result of the refractive surgery, making further surgery necessary, so it is best to thoroughly evaluate exposure to potentially cataractogenic agents. Some studies have shown a correlation between UV-A and UV-B type radiation with cataract formation, predominantly cortical, due to the formation of free radicals that interfere with the bodies metabolic processes.[20-22]

Infrared radiation is also considered to be a cause of cataract; for some time, the cataracts affecting glass-blowers has been considered a work-related disorder due to infrared exposure.[23] This type of work-related risk potentially affects many professional categories, and must be given due regard by suggesting particular prudence in patients considered to be particularly at risk, so as to avoid having to deal with unsatisfactory results and a second operation for cataracts.

Objective Examination

With candidates for refractive surgery, the ophthalmic examination must be as complete as possible and must evaluate anatomical or functional conditions that normally have no clinical significance but which might influence postoperative recovery. Furthermore, it is fundamentally important to precisely document each detail and discuss them with the patient. The normal slit-lamp examination should be supplemented with instrumental examinations, indispensable for detecting subclinical eye disorders and for the correct planning of the ablation.

Eye Motility

Without considering tropias, muscular paralysis, nystagmus, and other serious alterations whose treatment lies out of our scope during the planning stage, it is important to consider whether surgery may unbalance any phoria, causing the patient to suffer transient or permanent diplopia (double vision). Therefore, any refractive procedure must always be preceded by a thorough study of eye motility. The postoperative situation is well simulated by contact lenses, so if the patient has never used them, it is certainly useful in dubious cases to perform tests with complete correction of the refractive defect by application of contact lenses.

Sometimes, photorefractive surgery may, on the contrary, try to resolve the accommodative component of a strabismus. Again, in this case, it is best to thoroughly evaluate every factor underlying the aforementioned strabismus during the preliminary stage, because frequently the accommodative factor is not unique, which may be disappointing in relation to correcting eye alignment following refractive surgery. Undoubtedly, in any case, it is recommended to perform an orthoptic examination in order to precisely document every parameter influencing motility and to detect any dysfunctions that may have escaped the ophthalmologist.

Eye Adnexa

The conjunctiva, eyelids, and glandular apparatus should be carefully explored since corneal reparation may be seriously compromised by even slight anomalies in each of the above mentioned regions. The eyelids must not show any anomalies such as lagophthalmos, ptosis, reduced blinking, entropion, ectropion, or trichiasis, which may compromise correct lachrymal film distribution or cause mechanical lesions to the corneal epithelium. Analogously, the presence of proptosis of any kind must be identified and considered carefully.

Any disorders involving the palpebral glands (chalazions, meibomitis, styes) or blepharitis must be treated in advance, due to the potential bacterial super-infection and because such conditions cause alterations to the lachrymal film. There must not be any signs of acute or chronic inflammation in the conjunctival area, indicating bacterial or viral infections or allergic reactivity. Any condition of this type should be treated in advance.

Lachrymal Film

This merits special consideration since it is essential for correct epithelial repair. Certain signs detected by slit-lamp examination are useful for its qualitative and quantitative evaluation. Any imbalances in the constituents, with predominance of the lipoprotein component, may be indicated by the presence of mucous aggregates or filaments spread around or localized in the inner canthus. Various parameters can quantify an adequate presence, or otherwise, of the lachrymal film; the lachrymal meniscus must have a height of approximately 0.3 mm, the film break-up time (BUT) must be greater than 10 seconds.[24] A reduction of the lachrymal meniscus, a reduced BUT and any signs of punctate keratitis, are considered signs of dry eye. The Schirmer type I, II, and III tear production tests and the Jones test are also useful.

Further clarification and evaluation of the dynamics of the lachrymal film may be obtained using dedicated instruments, such as the tearscope (Keeler), or by means of keratoscopy. Having identified a lachrymal deficiency, the decision of whether or not to proceed with the refractive surgery depends largely on the extent of the aforementioned deficiency, by any correlation with recent use of contact lenses. In this case, a prolonged postponement may improve the situation if there is concomitant presence of other problems of the eye surface or other areas. It is important to take into account any potential complications (delayed re-epithelialization, epithelial softening, increased susceptibility to infection) and to proceed with caution. In such cases, some authors suggest resorting to an intrastromal procedure (LASIK).

Cornea

This is the organ on which the photoablation is performed; thereby, it seems unnecessary to underline the importance of a thorough examination. The slit-lamp is used to verify the integrity of each of the overlying layers.

The corneal epithelium must not have any interruptions or areas of sufferance that may reflect a lachrymal deficiency or an infectious or dystrophic disorder. An epithelium with a milky appearance is an indicator of altered metabolism or dystrophy.

Good adhesion between the epithelium and the Bowman's membrane is also important, even if adhesion of the epithelium to newly formed Bowman's lamina following surface photoablation is generally firmer. Adhesion may be verified rather simply by observing blinking (which must not show any slippage of the epithelium on the underlying layers) or with a cotton wad placed in contact with the cornea, which will highlight any surface alterations.

The stroma must not show any alterations, in terms of transparency and uniformity, an unequivocal sign of a progressive or full-blown disorder. Aside from the acute infective pathologies that are so obvious as to leave no doubt in terms of diagnosis, stromal opacity can occur rather more frequently as a result of foreign bodies, previous infections, or dystrophic disorders. In such cases, it is necessary to first consider the extent, location, and nature of the stromal opacities; for example, a small leukoma from a peripheral foreign body will not have any influence on the refractive procedure, as opposed to widespread opacity affecting the optical zone. This should absolutely not be treated by means of a photorefractive procedure but possibly by means of a phototherapeutic intervention (see Chapter 30).

Slit-lamp examination is also very useful in determining corneal thickness and allows the identification of any localized areas of thinning, which must be evaluated with particular suspicion and investigated more thoroughly by means of appropriate instrumental examinations. Even localized thickening is clearly identifiable and is usually accompanied by altered stromal transparency due to the depositing of newly formed collagen, while widespread thickening is an indicator of stromal imbibition due to an endothelial deficiency or due to a marked increase in intraocular pressure.

The thickness of the different corneal components (stroma and epithelium) must be analyzed carefully; in the case of stromal thinning, the epithelium tends to fill the trough formed due to stromal tissue deficiency, restoring normal or almost normal thickness. Where surgical ablation is planned, it is necessary to thoroughly evaluate what remains once the epithelium is removed in order not to find oneself in the unpleasant situation of having to suspend the operation due to lack of tissue or worse.

It is possible to evaluate the presence of guttae in the entire endothelium-Descemet's membrane complex, as the presence of which would mean advising against photorefractive surgery, even if it appears that laser ablation does not induce any loss of endothelial cells.

LENS

The organ's transparency is a fundamental condition. In the case of cataract, it should be evaluated whether an operation on the lens might be more appropriate even in light of the possibility for implanting multifocal or accommodative lenses to compensate for the loss of physiological accommodation. Naturally, everything depends on the degree and the evolutive potential of the cataract.

A similar situation applies to somewhat older patients with no lens opacity that desire to undergo refractive surgery. Given the poor/absent residual accommodative capacity, and the likelihood of the future development of cataracts, then the alternative lensectomy also seems valid here. In refractive surgery patients, it is still difficult to calculate the intraocular lens (IOL), therefore, it is very useful to be provident and perform a biometry prior to the operation.

EYE PRESSURE AND GLAUCOMA

A diagnosis of glaucoma is clearly incompatible with refractive surgery for various reasons. First of all, the cortisone treatment that is frequently necessary in the postoperative stage may imbalance tone; furthermore, given that any drug may be toxic for the corneal epithelium, this might involve the suspension of the antiglaucomatous therapy for a lengthy period of time. There might be serious problems in the follow-up for the disease since eye pressure measurements are altered by changes in corneal curvature and thickness, and even if this problem will soon be resolved by the advent of new equipment not influenced by such factors (eg, the Pascal tonometer). It should also be considered that any deterioration of the disorder not linked to the refractive surgery might be seen by the patient as being due to the operation with obvious unpleasant contentions or possible legal ramifications.

The attitude to take in the case of ocular hypertony without perimetral alterations of the optic nerve or nerve fibres is rather more controversial. Obviously, the degree of hypertony is determinant, it should not be forgotten that tonometric data is related to corneal thickness and curvature. The glaucoma risk factors, such as age, family history, myopia, and ethnic origin, should then be taken into consideration. In dubious cases, a tonometric curve may be useful, and in any case, it is always appropriate to be extreme cautious.

RETINA AND VITREOUS BODY

Among the potential complications of laser photoablation, one worthy of mention is vitreoretinal disorder in that the relationships between refractive surgery and retinal rupture/detachment have always been rather controversial. Photorefractive techniques have historically been used to treat myopia, and it is well known how the myopic population is frequently affected by vitreal and peripheral retinal degenerations, predisposing the patient to the formation of retinal perforations and ruptures and, lastly, retinal detachment.

Two factors have been analyzed as potential joint causes of retinal rupture and detachment in photorefractive surgery:
* Excimer laser-generated shock waves.
* The compression and decompression action of the suction ring on the base of the vitreous.

In relation to the direct action of the laser on the retina and on the vitreous base, there have been various hypotheses, but there is no scientific evidence of a potentially pathogenic mechanism at that level. Instead, the suction ring (where used) is considered with greater suspicion, in that this tool firstly generates a strong increase in intraocular pressure (over 60 mm/Hg), followed by a rapid decompression, returning the eye to normal pressure levels. This action gives rise to a process opposite to that operated by a surgical cerclage, which is aimed at releasing the retina from vitreal traction.

In the case of suction rings, since the eye is a closed system whereby the product of pressure by volume is a constant, increased pressure leads to a reduction in volume and vice versa, with the result of generating traction at the base of the vitreous due to the shape which the eye transiently assumes. Also, the position where such rings act is crucial, as larger sized rings position themselves precisely at the pars plana, where the compression and release mechanism described is potentially more hazardous.

Notwithstanding the above points, in thousands of operations performed using the LASIK or PRK technique with the aid of suction, there has been no appreciable increase in the incidence of retinal rupture or detachment. Isolated cases of extensive retinal rupture in strict temporal correlation with suction, which seem to have occurred in widespread regmatogenic degenerations not previously treated by laser barrage are described in the literature.

It would certainly be worthwhile to conduct a scientific evaluation of the incidence of retinal detachment in surgical patients and controls, and determine whether or not a suction ring was used in those having surgery. However, the relative rarity of retinal problems, the presence or absence of predisposing lesions, the extent of any myopia, the time interval between surgery, and the complications that arise make such an undertaking infeasible.

Since it is not possible to completely exclude a potentially pathogenic role for refractive surgery on the periphery of the retina and on the vitreous, particularly if the use of suction rings is envisaged, it is essential that the surgeon adopts a very prudent attitude. The vitreoretinal area must be examined very thoroughly, and any predisposing lesions must be treated by laser in advance.

In the case of being faced with a retina with widespread degeneration, a tendency to rupture, multiple perforations, or that may be considered a high regmatogenous risk, it is necessary to forgo any refractive surgery at least prior to having performed effective prophylactic laser treatment and having protracted the retinal follow-up.

Maculopathies of various degrees are encountered rather frequently in myopic individuals. There does not appear to be any correlation between refractive surgery and the formation or progression of neovascular membranes or areas of chorioretinal atrophy; nonetheless, it does not seem appropriate to operate on serious forms, which are atrophic or proliferative, or showing any evolutive potential.

VISUAL ACUITY AND REFRACTION

The determination of visual acuity and refraction is crucially important when dealing with refractive surgery because correct measurement is a fundamental requirement for good correction of the ametropies, and measuring a patient's visual acuity allows evaluation of the functional potential of the organ and the identification of any deficiencies that may or may not be difficult to detect any other way (and which should be investigated further).

Diagnosis and measurement of ametropies may be performed various ways, and each specialist frequently relies more on their experience rather than standardised techniques. Notwithstanding the above, in our opinion, it is important to follow certain "rules" that allow the absolute precision necessary for planning surgery, which are sometimes neglected if the aim of the examination is the prescription of an eyeglass.

First of all, it is important to have a period of time where the use of contact lenses is suspended given the potential (and frequent) mechanical effect on curvature and on the corneal epithelium, which might have a significant influence on refractive parameters.

It is impossible to indicate a sufficiently long period of suspension that can guarantee the complete restoration of corneal curvature because the deformation (the warpage visible to the corneal topograph) depends on manifold factors, such as the type of lens (soft or semirigid), since when and for how long it has been used, the support, the mobility, etc. However, it is best if prior to measuring the refraction, the lens is not applied for at least 4 days.

Nonetheless, variations in the spherical and/or cylindrical component of the ametropia in patients who, for reasons of age and case history, should be stable are always rechecked following a longer suspension period in order to ascertain whether the change observed is not due to a particularly persistent reversible corneal deformation. Naturally, in such cases, corneal topography is usually decisive (see below).

Having eliminated this factor, or reduced it as much as possible, the first step in the refractive examination is measuring the previous correction; it is necessary to measure both the glasses for distance and close-up and any contact lenses.

If possible, it is useful to also measure the parameters relating to old prescriptions, to be able to monitor the progress of the ametropia over time and more certainly establish whether facing a stable or progressive situation.

Classically, the methods for measuring refractive defects are distinguished as either objective or subjective.

OBJECTIVE METHODS

Keratometry

This determines the curvature, expressed in diopters, of the two main corneal meridians. It may be measured using a Javal ophthalmometer, automatic keratometers, or by corneal topography. It provides an undoubtedly reliable indication of the astigmatism of the anterior corneal surface, but only at the point where it is determined, and does not give any indications on the status of the other dioptric media, whereby its potential use in refractive surgery is undoubtedly limited.

Autorefractometry

The autorefractometer is now routinely used as the first approach. There are many on the market, with varying levels of precision, and they usually provide a good starting indication. Without discussing at length which instruments may be more or less reliable, it may be useful to specify certain aspects. Firstly, various studies in the literature indicate that the error margins for all the instruments analyzed are not in the least negligible.[25-27] The same reproducibility of the examination is frequently rather low; hence, it is always appropriate to repeat a number of acquisitions (at least 3) so as to reduce the error margins. In other words, this is an undoubtedly useful examination, providing good indications and speeding up the ophthalmologists work, but which is not critically transformed into an eye lens, or worse still, into a surgical plan and constitutes a data value to be compared with others (corneal topography, aberrometry, subjective refraction) from which it may be comfortably refuted.

Skiascopy

This allows the evaluation of the refractive power of each meridian and constitutes an irreplaceable tool for uncooperative patients. Nevertheless, in expert hands, it is a very useful method and very close to reality; it does not allow the level of precision necessary for refractive surgery whereby, like autorefractometry, it may be used as an indication to be verified using other instruments.

Aberrometry and Corneal Topography

These will be discussed more extensively elsewhere but constitute important means of refractive diagnostics. Topography is extremely useful in identifying the astigmatic component of ametropia and precisely determines the axis and the extent of the cylinder, which is particularly useful above all in high levels of myopia where the cylinder is frequently underestimated. Aberrometry allows understanding of the variation of the refractive defect with varying pupillary diameter (it is usually shown at pupillary diameters of 3 and 5 mm).

The subjective methods for measuring ametropies are those requiring responses from the patient and constitute the most important data to be followed both for the prescription of lenses and for planning refractive surgery.

Since the examination is reliable and does not generate confusion in either the patient or the examiner, it is appropriately executed using standardised methods and instruments. The patient should be in a condition to provide simple answers and not generic impressions. The ophthalmologist should be fast, clear, and decisive in proposing the alternatives. Finally, one or more objective refractometry examinations should be performed beforehand. The clinician should start with the lenses that are as close to the natural lens as possible and perform the examination quickly to avoid any loss of concentration from the patient due to tiredness.

Since the patient's participation includes comparing the effect of two optical corrections, it is important that these are proposed in rapid sequence. For this reason, use of a phoropter is undoubtedly preferable, which also allows greater precision in measuring the axis and power of the astigmatic component and excludes the optical aberrations induced by overlapping several lenses in the test spectacles (not always perfectly in axis with one another).

Various methods may be used effectively to verify or to "refine" the correction (eg, fogging test, crossed cylinders, dichromatic test, astigmatic quadrants), and undoubtedly, the more accurate the measurement, verified using various methods, the more precise it will be.

It is fundamentally important that the refraction is determined in cycloplegia. Cycloplegia is the paralysis of the ciliary muscle performed by instilling anticholinergic substances into the conjunctival sac.

The hypermetropia is compensated by accommodation that may be more or less complete, depending on the extent of the defect and the patient's age; hence, it is obviously impossible to quantify it without eliminating said compensation. A hypermetropic candidate for refractive surgery must become accustomed to the complete correction of the ametropia and not only the expressed component. Hence, if the patient has been previously prescribed a correction for just the expressed component, the operation must be preceded by a period where the patient combats the complete correction, even at the cost of discomfort and a temporary loss of correct visual acuity, in order to simulate the postsurgical situation and allow the ciliary muscle to accommodate.

In myopia, the cycloplegia assumes even greater importance for a number of reasons; first of all, some myopic individuals tend paradoxically to accommodate, whereby the extent of the refractive defect may be overestimated. Secondly, it happens rather frequently, more in younger patients, that a hypercorrection is prescribed, which is easily detected by an examination in cycloplegia. In essence, in myopic individuals, the lens, either spontaneously or due to an erroneous prescription, is not always in the most functional refractive state for the reduction of the myopia, and this explains the significance of the cycloplegia in such cases.

Specifically in the case of refractive surgery, it is necessary to consider the effects of an erroneous measurement of ametropia from not having performed complete cycloplegia. This includes, in the case of hypermetropia, undercorrection of the defect and, in the case of myopia, hypercorrection of the defect. Between these two evils, undercorrection of a hypermetropic patient is certainly more acceptable (as opposed to making a myopic patient hypermetropic) because, in the first case, the reduction of the defect will always result in a benefit. This benefit could even be complete for some time if the patient is young enough. In the second case, the new refractive situation will be unsatisfactory for the patient, who will certainly complain of loss of near visual acuity and, in the worst-case scenario, even distance visual acuity. Hence, it is well understood why the previous affirmation, in relation to the utmost importance of cycloplegia in myopic patients, is in no way exaggerated.

In relation to the methods of execution and the evaluation of the results obtained with respect to noncycloplegic refraction, it is first necessary to take into account the eye drops used; 0.5% or 1% atropine has a slow and very prolonged action over time, whereby it is not in fact used. Cyclopentolate has a more rapid, relatively short-lived action and efficacy similar to that of atropine. For complete blockage, two instillations a few minutes apart are generally performed. Maximum effect lasts from 20 minutes to 1 hour following application. Tropicamide has the undoubted advantage of a reduced duration of action and is instilled 3 to 4 times for complete cycloplegia but is less effective compared to cyclopentolate.

Cycloplegia must be absolute in hypermetropic patients, where the accommodation is strong and may be particularly enduring, while in myopic patients, a milder action may be sufficient given that the extent of the accommodative phenomenon does not normally exceed 1.0 D.

The evaluation of the refraction obtained depends on the level of completeness of accommodative block given that complete cycloplegia interferes with the basal accommodative tone; the lens, even in an emmetropic patient fixing on infinity, has a certain amount of accommodation, defined as the basal accommodative tone. In ametropic individuals, the basal accommodative tone does not depend on the refractive defect and is, hence, not corrected by glasses or any other means, including refractive surgery.

Cycloplegic substances relax the accommodation more than that which occurs in the maximally physiologically relaxed state; for this reason, normally about 1.0 to 1.25 D are subtracted from the value obtained if the cycloplegic substance used is atropine, 0.50 to 0.75 D if 1% cyclopentolate or tropicamide is used.

Visual Acuity

From a purely medical viewpoint, the determination of this parameter is of rather minor importance with respect to refraction; indeed, for the purposes of the operation, it is essential to know the exact amount of the ametropia; it is somewhat less useful to know whether, with optimal correction, the patient can see 20/30 or 20/20.

Since, unfortunately, medical litigation is increasing rapidly, the refractive surgeon can on no account omit measuring visual acuity and must precisely document primarily those conditions where optimal visual acuity is less than that commonly considered to be normal. In cases to the contrary, they might be accused of causing a reduction in visual acuity for which they are blameless.

For similar reasons, it is best to always document incorrect visual acuity even when, such as in the presence of high ametropia, it may appear absurd or even probing.

It is important that measurement takes place under standardised conditions, with well-illuminated optotypes and an equal number of letters on each line. The visual acuity to be attributed to the patient is that corresponding to the smallest correctly read line.

Instrumental Examinations

Besides a thorough clinical examination, nowadays, the refractive surgeon cannot ignore the valuable contribution provided by even more sophisticated dedicated instruments that allow analyzing morphology, the thickness of corneal curvature (the wavefront) of the aberrometry, indispensable until just a short time ago.

KERATOSCOPY

Keratoscopy is based on the reflection of luminous rings projected from a dedicated apparatus (keratoscope). Correct data acquisition is fundamental for achieving a reliable examination.

Great attention must be paid to the correct positioning of the head as well as ensuring that the patient focuses on the luminous sight, that the lachrymal film is well laminated, and that the rings are in focus.

In relation to the keratoscope, a frontal position is certainly the most comfortable but not the best for acquisition. Indeed, it would be better to turn the head so that the patient fixes on the luminous ring while drawing away the eye being examined, then move to the left while analyzing the right eye and towards the right while analyzing the left eye. This way, the shadow of the nose is reduced, and the slight lowering of the upper eyelid due to convergence is eliminated, thus increasing the range of the area covered by the rings. With deep-set eyes, it would be expedient to increase the thickness of the instrument's forehead rest; the resulting hyperdistention of the head reduces the shadow cast over the cornea from the frontal bone and allows more extensive exploration of the upper sectors.

Keratoscopy provides morphological information; hence, each evaluation must be performed based on the appearance of the corneal rings. The regularity and the continuity of keratoscope rings are indicators of good surface quality at each point; the lachrymal film and corneal epithelium give good reflection, ensuring the specularity of the cornea. Such characteristics are only compromised in the most evident stages of altered curvature with corneal ectasy; a descemetocele with focal opacification, hypercurvature to such an extent as to alter the lamination of the lachrymal film or the formation of a leukoma at the apex of the cone, appear as irregular and/or broken rings. Data processing in such cases is unreliable, if even possible, and the keratoscopic image is the only one capable of providing accurate information.

A regular reflection can only be produced by a surface with a constant radius of curvature. In a normal cornea, the rings appear concentric, well delineated, and defined. Irregularities indicate an abrupt variation in curvature.

Contrast is an important parameter in keratoscopic evaluation. This is generated by perfect corneal transparency; any reduction in contrast reflects a reduction in corneal transparency.

The topographic map is calculated based on the distance between the rings; this detail is very important in keratoscopic evaluation. Closer rings indicate a greater curvature of the surface undergoing analysis. On the contrary, widely spaced rings are indicative of a flat surface. Analysis of the overall curvature is just as important as localized variations. Often in the initial stages of keratoconus, it is difficult to observe keratoscopic distortions because the slight localized narrowing of the rings, an indicator of increased curvature of the anterior corneal surface, may go undetected, especially by an inexperienced or distracted observer.

The distance between the rings becomes fundamental in the evaluation of corneal leukomas of whatever origin. As mentioned previously, topographic extrapolation in such cases is frequently unreliable given the irregularity and the incompleteness of the rings, and it may not be simple to understand whether corneal opacity is raised or depressed. Simple evaluation of the behavior of the rings will show whether opacity is raised (converging rings in the vicinity of leukomatous formations), level, or depressed (divergent rings in the vicinity of lesions).

Variations in the distance between rings from the center to the periphery provides an estimate of corneal eccentricity. In a prolate cornea (more curved at the center, flatter at the margin), the distance between rings increases moving from the periphery to the center; in an oblate cornea (flatter at the center, more curved at the margin), the rings are closer at the periphery than at the center. Abrupt changes in curvature imply a significant increase in eccentricity and account for any associated deficiency of vision.

Evaluation of the keratoscopic examination may indicate processing errors in the evaluation of hypercurved surfaces. When two rings are very close, the software may ignore one, considering the subsequent ring directly.

The map calculation will be effected by this, and curvature will be underestimated, resulting in a cornea that appears more "normal" than it is in reality.

As mentioned previously, the keratoscope projects luminous concentric rings, hence the reflected rings must also be round. In the case of corneal astigmatism, the cornea has an oval and not spherical conformation; consequently, it reflects ovals, not rings. Depending on the characteristics of the astigmatism (with or against the rule, regular or irregular, large or small hourglass), there will be compression of the rings on one meridian with respect to the other, and focal or diffuse variations will be observed.

Another important aspect to be considered in a keratoscopic reading is the symmetry of the rings. Complete symmetry over the entire field examined is observed in emmetropic individuals or those affected by spherical refractive errors (myopia or hypermetropia); the rings appear round and concentric. Linear symmetry is typical in individuals affected by congenital regular astigmatism; the rings appear oval, and there is only perfect symmetry along the two main meridians.

The symmetry of the rings, whether complete or linear, is of fundamental importance because it indicates the possibility for correcting any refractive errors using lenses. Complete asymmetry is observed in abnormal corneas and compromises visual acuity and the possibility for complete correction of the refractive error with lenses. The rings may be irregular or even absent in some areas and show abrupt changes in the distances between one another.

Analysis of the complete examination will provide indications useful for recognizing congenital astigmatism. This is generally detected by regular rings closer on the more myopic (or less hypermetropic) meridian, giving a series of concentric ovals, irregular astigmatic in shape, where the asymmetry indicates a high variation in the curvature per unit of surface, and which may be a manifestation of a corneal disorder.

To assess how much a corneal alteration of whatever origin and extent influences a patient's visual acuity and quality of vision, it is essential to know the spatial relationship with the pupillary foramen. Generally, this rule especially applies to keratoconus, where the apex of the ectasy is frequently decentered and relatively slight astigmatism may be greatly incapacitating with respect to defects of greater extent, depending on their localization and the pupillary diameter of the individual in question.

Lachrymal Film

The colorimetric topographic corneal map, with whatever algorithm it is calculated, provides information on the curvature of the anterior corneal surface and the lachrymal film at any given time, but in the vast majority of cases, it does not indicate the cause giving rise to any anomalies and, above all, may frequently be misleading due to the presence of artifacts. Thus, keratoscopy constitutes an essential complement, since it allows proper analysis of the lachrymal film, which, as is well known, is indispensable for good reflection of the luminous mires and constitutes one of the major sources of artifacts. Keratoscopy is a dynamic examination and is, hence, an irreplaceable tool for evaluating lamination of the lachrymal film, a similarly dynamic process.

In many cases, the patient simply blinking is sufficient to establish whether a given alteration is due to lacking or poor lamination of the tear film, the presence of filaments, or mucous aggregates or secretions.

Anomalies of the corneal or conjunctival surfaces or disorders affecting the eyelids or tear ducts frequently compromise the lamination processes. In such cases, there is frequently supernatant accumulation in the lower sectors, which can distort the corneal curvature data shown by topography.

If there is any corneal hypercurvature, as in the case of keratoconus, the lachrymal film may level out the surface, making the curvature homogeneous and causing the pathology to go unrecognized or be underestimated. On the other hand, in the case where corneal tissue is lacking, the tear film may act as plaster, filling the defect, which may thus go unnoticed during processing.

A further advantage of keratoscopy is constituted by the possibility of a three-dimensional evaluation of the corneal surface and the lachrymal film, permitted by illumination of the keratoscope cone over multiple, even lateral, planes. This allows better evaluation of the area of defective lamination or stagnation, which have, among others, significant importance in giving rise to visual fluctuations.

The practice of acquiring keratoscopic and other images and then evaluating the computer results without knowing under what conditions they were surveyed and from which images they were calculated, should be prohibited. Alterations in the lachrymal film may give topographic patterns similar to keratoconus, whereby static evaluation of just the colorimetric map may give rise to gross diagnostic errors.

CORNEAL TOPOGRAPHY

This is computerized keratoscopy processing and constitutes the gold standard for measuring the curvature of the anterior corneal surface. In refractive patients, careful topographic analysis is indispensable for various reasons. First, topographic analysis is used for identifying corneal disorders such as keratoconus, which, in the initial stages, does not give rise to any clinical manifestations and is not identifiable any other way. In addition, nonprogressive localized hypercurvature such as forme fruste keratoconus may not be detected by means of simple objective slit-lamp examination but may lead to serious and irreversible alterations of corneal structure if they progress to corneal thinning for refractive purposes.

Progressive, or fruste, keratoconus represents the most obvious case where topography is of crucial importance, but all corneal disorders involving local or more widespread alteration of the curvature of the anterior surface may be identified and documented by means of this examination.

Even in nondisease conditions, corneal curvature represents an important preoperative parameter, above all in hypermetropies, where the possibility of obtaining good results depends on the curvature obtained. Indeed, if eccentricity becomes overaccentuated, a pattern similar to keratoconus is created with inevitable consequences for visual quality.

Another field where corneal topography has been shown to be irreplaceable is that of reversible corneal deformations brought on by contact lenses (warpage). A very high percentage of potential candidates for refractive surgery use them and show varying extents of warpage. Its presence may only be detected by means of corneal mapping, and at the risk of a bad outcome, all surgery should be suspended until the normal corneal profile is completely restored. Furthermore, warpage may frequently simulate a keratoconus, and differential diagnosis requires the prolonged suspension of using lenses and the subsequent repetition of the examination, which in the case of warpage will highlight the restored regularization of the corneal profile. This process may require some time, even up to 6 months.

Corneal topography may be calculated according to various mathematical formulae, known as algorithms. Until a few years ago, topographic reconstruction was performed exclusively using the axial algorithm. Today, it is accompanied by tangential, altimetric, and aberrometric analyses, which allow the attainment of superior information, undoubtedly more faithful to reality.

Indeed, it has been known for some time that due to the method of calculation, axial mapping involves a significant degree of approximation, which increases proportionally with the distance from the corneal apex and, for this reason, is considered poorly reliable outside the area of the central 3 mm.

Since many corneal disorders, including keratoconus, at least in the initial stages, may manifest themselves exclusively in paracentral or peripheral areas, the need to explore these areas more reliably and in further detail seems obvious.

The tangential algorithm calculates curvature based on the tangent to the anterior corneal surface in each point analyzed, whereby the analysis is not influenced by the distance from the center, and the map has good reliability even in peripheral areas. For this reason, it has become the gold standard for topographic analysis in numerous disorders, including keratoconus.

Tangential mapping, along with height mapping, provide information pertaining to corneal shape, while axial and aberrometric mapping evaluate the optical effect the cornea exerts on ocular diopter.

In order to best use the information provided, one should not be limited to a hasty glance at the map in the search for gross alterations such as a red stamp caused by an obvious keratoconus; instead, it is necessary to follow a precise analytical procedure.

As already underlined, topographic interpretation may not be left out from keratoscopic analysis; only the keratoscopic data can tell whether a particular alteration is due to the lachrymal film, to the erroneous processing of different anatomical parts (such as the eyelids or conjunctival surfaces), or a true corneal disorder and hence whether we are viewing a reliable map or an invention of the computer.

It would be appropriate for the acquisition of the images, a delicate and extremely important stage, to be entrusted to skilled operators, if not the ophthalmologist. That way, information would be obtained on the dynamics of the lachrymal film that would be lost with a single photogram. The first step in reading a map is evaluating the scale in which it is drawn.

The three colorimetric scale types available on all topographs are *absolute*, *normalized*, and *adjustable*.

With the *absolute* scale, each color corresponds to a fixed dioptric value, and the steps are further at the extremes of the scale and closer (1.5 D) between 35.0 and 51.0 D, which are the values most commonly encountered, while outside this interval, the chromatic variation is every 5.0 D. The *normalized* scale associates the darkest red with the most curved point and the most intense blue with the flattest point; the width of the steps depends on how much the "peak" rises over the "plane" (ie, the dioptric range between maximum and minimum curvature). The *adjustable* scale allows the operator to select the width of the dioptric interval necessary for the chromatic variation. The absolute scale is undoubtedly the most commonly used since it is much more reproducible and more readily interpreted. Furthermore, it allows good comparison of maps obtained at different times, even using different equipment. The adjustable map is useful for highlighting small dioptric variations that might be overlooked with larger intervals, but narrowing the chromatic interval increases the risk of overestimating each small variation in slope given the high color contrast generated. Furthermore, by selecting narrower "steps," above all with corneas having inhomogeneous curvature, there may be numerous unevaluated areas since they are off-scale, whereby better definition of detail is at the expense of the overall view.

The normalized scale has very variable resolution; it is comparable to the absolute scale if the corneal dioptric range is large and better if the slopes are not very steep; however, comparison with subsequent examinations is very difficult. Furthermore, very different corneas may take on very similar appearances.

It is generally always better to first analyze the absolute map, which rapidly provides a reliable overall view and is not subject to interpretational errors due to the colorimetric scale. To resolve and measure slight variations in curvature with greater precision, it may sometimes be useful to obtain an adjustable map.

Having processed the map, it is necessary to first evaluate whether processing is complete or whether there are any unprocessed areas in order to move on to careful analysis of the corneal profile, the homogeneity of curvature, the presence of any patterns associated with refractive defects, abrupt changes in slope, and any unprocessed areas.

A normal cornea has a prolate profile, one that is more curved at the center than at the edge. In the absolute scale, the central area will appear yellow or green and the color will gradually diminish until reaching the blue of the flatter edge. The progressiveness of the chromatic variation is an index of the homogeneity of the corneal surface and of the mildness of the variations in slope. Hence, evaluation of the tangential topograph allows a good estimate of corneal eccentricity.

The presence of different colors in adjacent areas should always be evaluated with extreme care (along with the non-processing of parts of the examination).

An area with a concentration of very different dioptric values is frequently an indicator of a corneal disorder, and when included within a pupillary field, gives rise to refractive defects that are difficult to correct, seriously affecting vision quality. In this sense, a useful compliment is provided by the indices calculated by the software, which express in numerical terms that which is expressed visually by topography. In the aforementioned case of an irregular corneal surface with abrupt changes in curvature, this is highlighted by a chromatically inhomogeneous map with correspondingly anomalous surface asymmetry index (SAI), coefficient of variation of corneal power (CVP), and standard deviation of corneal power (SDP) values.

The failure to process parts of the field under examination is frequently caused by corneal surface irregularities requiring careful assessment, first by means of keratoscopy.

Analysis of corneal morphology is very useful in defining refraction; for example, the identification of an astigmatic hourglass will provide valuable indications as to the extent, axis, and regularity of the refractive defect and on the most appropriate corrective method.

The evaluation of the pupil and its relationship with any alterations of the corneal surface is of fundamental importance.

It is obvious that a topographic irregularity of whatever origin will have an effect on visual acuity proportional to its closeness to the center of the pupil.

In keratoconus, the spatial relationship between the ectasia and the pupillary foramen has extreme clinical significance. The aberrations and the astigmatism generated by the conus, even when of relatively modest extent, can be very incapacitating, even more than greater dioptric defects, depending on their location and the pupillary diameter of the individual under examination.

In this sense, the recently marketed topographs allowing the execution of pupillometries and pupillographies have proved themselves extremely valuable.

Rather frequently, it is impossible to obtain good corrected visual acuity in patients with negative objectivity due to eye disorders; in such cases, the importance of a corneal topograph is frequently overlooked, since one of the greatest sources of optical aberrations and, hence, loss of visual acuity is precisely the cornea.

KERATOREFRACTIVE INDICES

Corneal morphology, on which optical characteristics depend, may be described by numerical indices and thus compared to a model cornea or a range of values defined as normal.

Each topograph calculates distinct indices, whereby differences may be encountered by using different equipment; nonetheless, they are very useful for summarily quantifying and analyzing a defined aspect of corneal optical quality.

Generally, the values for each cornea analyzed are compared with the mean values for a sample of normal corneas, and considered within the norm when included between +/- 2 SD, suspect when between ±3.0 SD, and altered when outside the aforementioned ranges.

The most commonly used indices include the following:

* *Sim-K* (simulated keratometry) and the keratometric value of the cornea under examination.

* *Astigmatism*: This is expressed as a function of the pupillary diameter; like corneal toricity, it is expressed in diopters of an area centered on the corneal vertex with a diameter equal to that of the pupil (normally, the most significant diameters used are 3 and 5 mm). It represents the extent and the axis of the regular astigmatic component of the cornea. A difference in axis or power between the two pupillary diameters indicates an irregular astigmatism that cannot be corrected by glasses.

* *Average pupillary power*: This is the mean axial curvature, expressed in diopters, of a diameter of 3 mm centered on the entry pupil, giving greater weight to the central corneal points. It represents the spherical equivalent of the aforementioned area. It is a useful parameter for describing mean curvature in very irregular corneas where, given the heterogeneity, simple morphological analysis is insufficient for understanding the true curvature.

* *Asphericity*: This is one of the parameters with greatest importance given that it describes the corneal profile and the difference in curvature between the center and the periphery. It indicates the degree to which the cornea is prolate or oblate. Corneal asphericity is determined by examining the asphericity of the conicoid most similar to the corneal segment of interest. It may be expressed

through four different indices, which are the shape factors p and SF, the eccentricity e, and the asphericity coefficient Q, which express exactly the same information and which are easily converted among one another by means of simple calculation formulae. In a prolate cornea, p varies from 0 to 1, while in an oblate cornea, it is greater than 1. $Q = p - 1$, hence a prolate ellipse ranges between -1 and 0, while an oblate surface is >0. If $e < 0$, this indicates an oblate surface; a normal cornea (prolate) has eccentricity values of around 0.5.

* *Spherical aberration*: The longitudinal spherical aberration (LSA) expressed in diopters within a corneal area of 4.5 mm. It expresses the difference between marginal and paraxial power.
* *Irregularity of curvature*: This is expressed (in diopters) as the standard deviation or mean square deviation of the instantaneous curvature with respect to the best-fit sphere (BFS).
* *Surface asymmetry index* (SAI): This is one of the first indices to have been introduced in corneal topography and represents the asymmetry of instantaneous curvature of the surfaces of the two hemimeridians opposing along each meridian. In the ideal cornea, it is equal to 0. In the case of asymmetry, the mean instantaneous curvature of the flatter hemisphere is colored blue, the most curved is red, and the SAI indicates the difference between the two.

ABERROMETRY

The increasingly widespread use of refractive surgery in recent years has created strong interest in comparisons of corneal surface optical quality. This has lead to the identification of many optical aberrations, potentially causing loss of visual acuity and poor quality of vision.

Optical aberrations are divided into various classes or orders; the prism constitutes the first order, and the traditional refractive defects (myopia, hypermetropia, and astigmatism) are the second order aberrations. The third order onwards relates to higher order aberrations, which cannot be corrected using lenses and may only be identified and measured using dedicated appliances, aberrometers.

But, what are optical aberrations? In the perfect eye, parallel light rays originating from infinity converge on a single point, the fovea centralis. If we consider the light rays reflected from the retina, the wavefront creating them will be planar and perpendicular to the aforementioned light rays. When considering ocular aberrations, reference is made to a planar wavefront produced by a nonaberrate eye; any deviation from this ideal profile constitutes an aberration and is measured by its distance from the aforementioned ideal surface (see Chapter 2).

Another important distinction is that between total aberrometry, which evaluates the aberrations produced by all ocular diopter constituents (lens, posterior corneal surface, vitreous body, etc), and corneal aberrometry, which analyzes the aberrations originating from the anterior corneal surface.

The software currently in use provide colored scale maps that, like in a geographical map, show how much a point is localized above or below "sea level," which is constituted by the ideal wavefront. The aberrometers are capable of calculating indices quantifying the total aberrations (RMS) and, furthermore, can break the overall aberrometry into its various components in order to show the effect of each aberration order on the calculated total.

In refractive surgery, aberrometry has various practical applications; firstly, the possibility to interface the diagnostic data with the operational part of the procedure (the laser) allows the attainment of customized ablation profiles that reduce high-order aberrations, both laser induced and pre-existing. In addition, the second order aberrations, the classical target of the ablative strategy, can be corrected with greater precision this way. Furthermore, the most sophisticated programs allow predicting of the effect that stromal subtraction will have on the corneal profile and on the wavefront. This allows for the planning of the operation with the double advantage of being able to visualize in advance and optimize the result (it is possible to simulate all the potential strategies, modifying those suggested by the software at will), saving tissue.

Resolving the corneal aberrometry from the total allows determination of the origins of the wavefront alterations and, hence, identification of that part that, not being generated by the cornea, cannot benefit from excimer laser correction. It is obvious that it would not be appropriate, for example, to modify the corneal profile in order to correct low- or high-order aberrations produced by anomalies of the lens. Hence, the optical aberrations, for which the indication is correction by excimer laser, are those of corneal origin.

Corneal aberrometric maps, despite providing entirely different data, frequently display a certain similarity to topographic maps. This is entirely understandable given that the anterior surface is the main source of corneal aberrations, whereby the characteristics, extent, and orientation must reflect the tangential topographic pattern.

HEIGHT TOMOGRAPHY AND THE RELATIONSHIP BETWEEN THICKNESS AND CURVATURE

The presence of reflection corneal topographs on the market for some years now means that ophthalmologists are used to considering the anterior corneal surface, which is the only parameter evaluated by this apparatus, as the sole source of information that may be interpreted erroneously as being more widespread than it is in reality.

Reflection topography solely evaluates the curvature of the anterior surface, and the data obtained is not used in any way to speculate upon corneal thickness or morphology. The availability of equipment capable of surveying the posterior corneal profile (Orbscan [Bausch & Lomb, Rochester, NY], Pentacam [Oculus, Lynnwood, Wash]) has clarified all this and provided a very valuable diagnostic aid.

Indeed, it has been known for some time that the corneal ectasy typical of keratoconus originates on the posterior surface, whereby such appliances are capable of observing much earlier stages of the disorder. In refractive surgery, this is vitally important for avoiding operations that, by thinning the cornea, might transform a fruste keratoconus into a progressive disorder or accelerate the progression of an already aggressive ectasy.

Besides this striking diagnostic implication, surveying the anterior and posterior surfaces allows the attainment of pachymetric topography and height tomography data. Pachymetric mapping is undoubtedly much more complete than the commonly used ultrasonic pachymetry, since the latter is acquired point by point and may miss areas of localized thinning. Furthermore, pachymetric topography is comparable with corneal topography and tomography in allowing measurement of the particular thickness of any given point of interest, something that is impossible with other types of pachymetric surveying.

Height tomography is also very useful in understanding corneal morphology; indeed, it permits establishing the relationships between curvature and anatomical structure. Initially, it takes significant effort to interpret height tomographs in that the subject of the analysis is not corneal surface curvature but rather its height with reference to a best fit sphere (BFS). For each point, the colorimetric scale will express a "hot" or "cold" color depending on the position above or below the aforementioned BFS.[28] For example, in an astigmatic cornea, the flattest and the most curved meridians appear inverted because the most curved meridian falls below the BFS and will be colored blue (while traditional maps indicate it as yellow or red). Such rudiments should be rigorously borne in mind, even more so when analyzing a cornea with abnormal morphology.

Corneal topography, being based on the principle of the reflection of Placido rings, is very much dependent on the integrity of the lachrymal film and the presence of any corneal alterations, whereby the data provided is not always a faithful description of the altered corneas. Furthermore, the maps are calculated by evaluating the distance of the rings from one another whereby points very close to one another are an indicator of a high degree of curvature, while further apart points are reflected by a flatter surface.[29-31]

Based on the above points, the importance of height tomography becomes clear, above all in profoundly altered corneas as a result of both previous surgery and an associated disorder.

Based on corneal topography alone, it is not possible to reconstruct the actual corneal morphology let alone estimate its residue, a fundamental factor in the selection of the correct therapeutic approach.

When analyzing a curvature map, it should always be borne in mind that the analysis of any given part of the cornea must include the surrounding areas and that the terms "flat" or "curved" are always in relation to the surrounding zones.

At this point, the height map becomes fundamentally important since it allows the determination of the position (raised or sunken) of each point on the cornea with respect to the BFS.[28,33]

In corneal topography, the presence of an overabundance of tissue causing an eversion (continuous red line) or a depression (dotted red line) on the corneal surface in both cases appears as blue areas in that they are both locally flattened.

Naturally, the situation relating to corneal thickness will be completely reversed. In the first case, there is abundant residual corneal thickness that will allow further corrective surgery (eg, PTK), if necessary. In the second case, there is thinning that will have to be considered when planning treatment.

It is easily understood how the data provided by this examination can profoundly influence therapeutic choice, such as residual corneal thickness, which is obviously a determining factor if considering phototherapeutic ablation.

Pachymetric mapping allows the determination of residual thickness and, hence, definition of the relationship between corneal curvature and thickness.

It provides additional information with respect to the height profile since, in the first case, the data provided are absolute, and secondly, they are relative to the BFS. Hence, even a peak in height on the anterior surface cannot coincide with increased thickness since this is in relation to the BFS and because, in any case, it is necessary to evaluate the corresponding posterior surface.

As mentioned previously, the thickness/surface ratio does not follow any predefined rules; a flat area may be thick (normal corneal margins, areas of stromal fibrosis) or thinned down (myopic photoablation optical zone, corneal ulcer), just as a curved area may be thin (keratoconus) or thick (corneal scarring).

The information obtained by pachymetric mapping is of fundamental importance but, for various reasons, should be examined carefully prior to accepting its validity.

First, the acquisition system leads to a great number of artefacts in and around the eyelids and a "shadow area" at the medial nasal and temporal periphery due to the incidence of scanning.

Furthermore, normal thickness is not necessarily caused by stromal tissue since it is well know how thinned areas (erosions, ulcers, etc) are frequently filled by epithelial lamina until level with the surrounding area, causing unpleasant surprises during surgery and having to make do with less usable substrate for ablation than was previously estimated. Therefore, it is always necessary to also perform a qualitative analysis either using a simple slit lamp or with the evermore numerous and reliable instruments coming onto the market (Schempflug camera, Confoscan, Artemis, Pentacam).

PUPILLOMETRY

This measures pupillary diameter under photopic and scotopic conditions, correlating the pupillary diameter with the topographic and aberrometric data. Given that the extent of ablation is directly proportional to the width of the optical zone and the width of the optical zone depends on maximum pupillary diameter, it seems obvious that this examination should be indispensable for correct planning of the surgery.

Endothelial Microscopy

This is used to determine the state of the endothelial cells in order to confirm that there are no lesions that would lead to recommendation against refractive surgery (even though the excimer laser cannot cause any alterations at that level).

Besides the cell count (a young patient should have a cell density of 2500 to 3000 cells/mm^2), it is important to consider whether there are any signs of polymegatism or pleomorphism, indicating increased size and irregular shape in the residual cells, to make up for any loss.

Informed Consent and Patient Interview

Informed consent is a legally required document that safeguards the patient from undergoing surgery against his or her will. This is the first point that should be clarified since signing the consent form is often interpreted by the patient as a document relieving the surgeon from responsibility in the event of any drawbacks or complications. The consent form must be as clear as possible; it should not be written in overly technical language and should be understandable for those unfamiliar with medical matters. It must provide detailed information on all the problems related to the surgery, including any potential complications. Nowadays, all surgeons use forms that have been written by specialist associations and approved by ethics committees.

It may be best to give patients the informed consent form upon completion of the first ophthalmic examination. This will allow them to read it thoroughly, discuss it with their families, and above all, be able to clarify any doubts with the surgeon during the examinations before the surgery.

The patient interview is an essential time for the surgeon to properly clarify what are the reasonable expectations, the postoperative procedures, the need to comply with pharmacological prescriptions exactly, the rules relating to hygiene and behavior, the recovery times, any potential complications associated with inappropriate conduct, and the possibility of remaining residual refractive defects (above all in high ametropia). Patients should also be encouraged to ask questions, particularly in relation to their understanding of the previously signed informed consent and to what they have been told verbally. Any misunderstanding could continue, even after surgery, and might lead to the patient being dissatisfied even with a result the surgeon has deemed satisfactory.

Bibliography

1. Sharif K. Regression of myopia induced by pregnancy after photorefractive keratectomy. *J Refract Surg*. 1997;13(5 suppl):S445-S446.
2. Liang JN, Chylack LT Jr. Spectroscopic study on the effects of nonenzymatic glycation in human α-cristallin. *IOVS*. 1987;28:790.
3. Lee JH, Shin DH, Lupovitch A, Shi DX. Glycation of lens proteins in senile cataract and diabetes mellitus. *Biochem Biophys Res Commun*. 1984;123:888.
4. Liang JN, Chylack LT Jr. Non-enzymatic glycosylation of human diabetic lenses. *Diabetologia*. 1986;29:225.
5. Seiler T, Holchbach A, Derse M, Jean B, Genth U. Complications of myopic photorefractive keratectomy with the excimer laser. *Ophthalmology*. 1994;101:153-160.
6. Helm CJ, Holland GN. Ocular tuberculosis. *Surv Ophthalmol*. 1993;38:229-256.
7. Vrbec MP, Durrie DS, Chase DS. Recurrence of herpes after excimer laser keratectomy (letter). *Am J Ophtahalmol*. 1992;114:96-97.
8. Bialasiewitcz AA, Schaudig U, Draeger J, Richard G, Knobel H. Descematocele after excimer laser phototherapeutic keratectomy in herpes simplex virus-induced keratitis; a clinico-pathologic correlation. *Klin Monatsbl Augenhilkd*. 1996;208:120-123.
9. Seiler T, McDonnel PJ. Excimer laser photorefractive keratectomy. *Surv Ophthalmol*. 1995;40:89-118.
10. Frierdlander MH. *Allergy and Immunology of the Eye*. San Francisco, Calif: Harper and Row; 1979.
11. Tervo T, Mustonen R, Tarkkanen A. Management of dry eye may reduce haze after excimer laser photorefractive keratectomy (letter). *Refractive Corneal Surg*. 1993;9:306.
12. Murube J. History of the dry eye. In: Lemp MA, ed. *The Dry Eye: A Comprehensive Guide*. New York, NY: Springer-Verlag; 1992:183-220.
13. Fraunfelder FT, La Braico JM, Meyer SM. Adverse ocular reactions possibly associated with isotretinoin. *Am J Ophtahalmol*. 1985;100:147-152.
14. Voerhoeff FH, Bell L, Walker CB. The pathological effects of radiant energy on the eye. An experimental investigation with a systemic review of literature. *Proc Am Acad Arts Sci*. 1916;51:630-818.
15. Cogan DG, Kinsey VE. Action spectrum of keratitis produced by ultraviolet radiation. *Arch Ophthalmol*. 1946;35:370-376.
16. Pitts DG, Tredici TJ. The effects of ultraviolet on the eye. *Am Ind Hyg Ass J*. 1971;32:235-246.
17. Miller D. *Clinical Light Damage to the Eye*. New York, NY: Springer-Verlag; 1987.
18. Norm MS. Spheroidal degeneration of cornea and conjunctiva. Prevalence among Eskimos in Greenland and Caucasians in Copenhagen. *Acta Ophthalmol*. 1978;56:551-562.
19. Cameron EE. *Pterygium Throughout the World*. Springfield, Ill: CC Thomas; 1965.
20. Brilliant LB, Grosset NC, Ram PT, et al. Association among cataract prevalence, sunlight hours and altitude. *Am J Epidemol*. 1983;118:2350-2364.
21. Taylor H. The environment and lens. *Br J Ophtahalmol*. 1980;64:303-310.
22. Taylor H, West SK, Rosenthal FS, et al. Effect of ultraviolet radiation on cataract formation. *N Engl J Med*. 1988;319:1429-1433.
23. Langley RK, Mortimer CB, Mcculloch C. The experimental induction of cataract by exposure to heat and light. *Arch Ophthalmol*. 1960;63:473-488.
24. Nelson JD. Diagnosis of keratoconjunctivitis sicca. *Int Ophthalmol Clin*. 1994;34:37-56.
25. Orr PR, Cramer L, Hawkins BS, Bressler N. Manifest refraction versus autorefraction for measuring best corrected visual acuity. *Invest Ophthalmol Visual Sci*. 1997;38(suppl):S978.
26. Salvesen S, Kohler M. Precision in automated refraction. *Acta Ophthalmol (Copenh)*. 1991;69(3):338-441.
27. Goss DA, Grosvenor T. Reliability of refraction, a literature review. *J Am Optom Assoc*. 1996;67(10):619-630.
28. McRae SM, Krueger RR, Applegate RA. *Customized Corneal Ablation: The Quest for Supervision*. Thorofare, NJ: SLACK Incorporated; 2001.
29. Vinciguerra P, et al. Atlante di topografia corneale ed Fogliazza. 1995.
30. Koch DD, Haft EH. Introduction to corneal topography. In: Sanders DR, Koch DD, eds. *An Atlas of Corneal Topography*. Thorofare, NJ: SLACK Incorporated; 1993.
31. Bogan SJ, Waring GO, Ibrahim O. Classification of normal corneal topography based on computer-assisted videokeratography. *Arch Ophthalmol*. 1990;108:945-949.

32. Sher NA, Bowers RA, Zabel RW, et al. Clinical use of the 193 nm excimer laser in the treatment of corneal scars. *Arch Ophthalmol.* 1991;109:491-498.

33. McRae SM, Krueger RR, Applegate RA. *Customized Corneal Ablation: The Quest for Supervision.* Thorofare, NJ: SLACK Incorporated; 2004.

CHAPTER 6

BIOMECHANICS OF SURFACE ABLATION AND LASIK

Jennifer R. Lewis, PhD; Cynthia J. Roberts, PhD

Macromechanics

BIOMECHANICAL MODEL OF CORNEAL RESPONSE TO LASER ABLATION

The biomechanical response of the cornea to laser ablation of tension-bearing lamellae in a circumferential pattern was first proposed in 1995.[1] Although corneal biomechanics had been previously studied and modeled extensively with respect to nonlaser refractive procedures, these concepts had not been previously applied to excimer laser ablation, predominantly due to the prevailing analytical approach to ablation profile design, which was based on the Munnerlyn formula.[2] This formula was the result of a geometric analysis and predicted the change in curvature of the central cornea as a function of the depth and width of the ablation zone. The fundamental assumptions were that both the pre- and postoperative shapes of the cornea were spherical and that the change in anterior surface shape was strictly geometric in nature. In other words, the cornea was modeled as a homogeneous structure, like a plastic lens, without consideration of the change in structure induced by the ablative procedure.[3-9] The Munnerlyn approach cannot distinguish between surface ablation and LASIK and would predict no difference in ablation profile design or outcome. Yet, these two approaches are biomechanically distinct, as will be discussed in this section. The associated healing response is also distinct and will be discussed in the Micromechanics section of this chapter.

With empirical modification from large-scale population analyses, the Munnerlyn formula was quite successful in improving visual outcomes, as measured by visual acuity and refraction in bright light environments. Even with adequate correction of sphere and cylinder, some patients still complained of glare and halos in low-light conditions, especially with large pupils. The introduction of wavefront sensors highlighted the limitations of the Munnerlyn approach as well as increased the understanding of visual complaints in the face of excellent visual acuity. Significantly increased higher-order (HO) aberrations were measured following laser refractive procedures, most prominently spherical aberration.[10-13] Aberration induction was less with wavefront customization, but not eliminated.[14-16] The biomechanical response of the cornea to a change in structure offers an explanation for variability of the second-order outcomes of sphere and cylinder as well as spherical aberration induction.[16]

A schematic illustration of the biomechanical response of the cornea to central ablation is given in Figure 6-1. Preoperatively, the cornea consists of layers of tension bearing lamellae, with crosslinking between layers preferentially distributed in the anterior-peripheral regions. With the removal of tension bearing lamellae in the center, the remaining peripheral segments relax, allowing the peripheral cornea to swell. Due to the interconnections between lamellar layers, the resultant force is transmitted to the underlying lamellar layers, causing the central cornea to flatten as the peripheral cornea thickens and steepens.[6-7] Therefore, any procedure which circumferentially severs corneal lamellae will generate central flattening and peripheral steepening, mediated by individual biomechanical properties, as well as the nature of the procedure itself. The biomechanical response enhances a myopic procedure, is in opposition to a hyperopic procedure, and generates unintended central flattening in phototherapeutic keratectomy (PTK).[7] There are two main biomechanical differences between surface ablation and LASIK: 1) a lamellar flap is created with LASIK, and 2) the region of ablated lamellae is placed deeper in the corneal stroma with LASIK. These differences are illustrated in Figure 6-2, and their impact will be discussed in detail in the following sections.

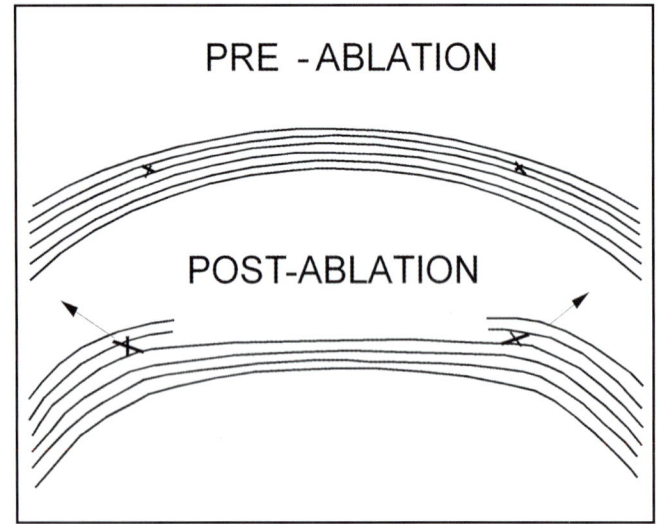

Figure 6-1. Schematic diagram of the proposed biomechanical response to laser ablation of tension bearing lamellae. The preoperative case is shown above, and the postoperative case is shown below. After ablation, the relaxed peripheral lamellar segments allow differential swelling which generates a force causing central flattening.

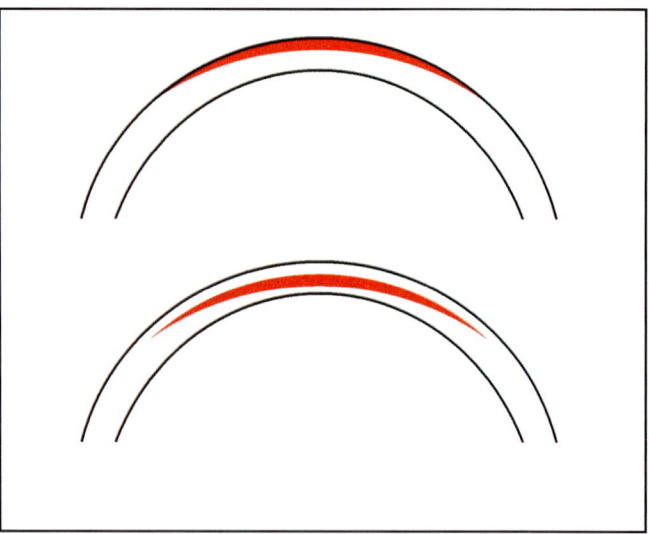

Figure 6-2. Illustration of an identical quantity of ablated tissue, both in a surface approach (top), as well as under a flap (bottom).

Table 6-1. Hyperopic Shift

Pt.	Preop Manifest Refraction (D)	Preop Sph Eq (D)	Operative Event	Postop Manifest Refraction (D)	Postop Sph Eq (D)	Postop Time
#1	-4.5 +0.5 x 30	-4.25	Buttonhole	-3.5	-3.5	1.5 mos
#2	+3 -0.25 x 15	+2.88	Buttonhole	+4.12 -1.5 x 30	+3.37	1.5 mos
#3	-8 +0.75 x 125	-7.625	Partial Flap	-8.25 +0.75 x 125	-7.875	3 wks
#4	-6.5 +0.25 x 90	-6.375	Partial Flap	-6.75 +0.5 x 90	-6.50	3 mos
#5	-2.75	-2.75	Free Cap	-2	-2	1 wk
#6	-2.25 +0.75 x 85	-1.875	Buttonhole	-1.25 +0.75 x 85	-0.875	3mos
#7	-10.75 -0.75 x 180	-11.125	Laser Failure	-10 -0.50 x 180	-10.25	4 mos

Avg (n=7)   -4.45 ± 4.50   -3.95 ± 4.63   (p <0.02)
Avg (n=5)   -3.42 ± 5.06   -2.65 ± 5.00   (p <0.001)
(excluding partial flaps)

BIOMECHANICS OF THE FLAP IN LASIK

When LASIK was initially conceived, the flap was assumed to be a neutral component of the procedure until early reports of anterior surface curvature alteration after the creation of a flap alone.[9,17-18] In a retrospective study of 7 subjects in whom a flap was created but no ablation was performed, a significant hyperopic shift was noted in those patients where the microkeratome passed the midline, with an average magnitude of 0.77 D.[17] In other words, the two partial flaps had no change in refraction. However, the patients with buttonholes, a free cap, and a flap after a laser failure all experienced a hyperopic shift, as shown in Table 6-1. Figure 6-3 represents a tangential difference map before and after the creation of flap, in which the laser subsequently failed and prevented ablation.[17] Multiple prospective studies have since been conducted to scientifically investigate the influence of the flap on LASIK outcomes.[19-22] In these studies, a flap was created and ablation was subsequently delayed by 2 to 3 months in order to evaluate the corneal response to the flap alone. All studies shared the common conclusion that the flap induces changes in either second-order aberrations, and/or HO aberrations. However, the nature of the change varied from study to study, depending on the technique used to create the flap, and the device used to evaluate the induced changes. Tran et al[22] reported only second-order aberrations after flap creation with a femtosecond laser and both second and HO aberrations after flap creation with a mechanical microkeratome. The hyperopic shift observed with both the femtosecond laser and the mechanical microkeratome is consistent with the biomechanical model presented. The HO aberrations observed with the mechanical microkeratome and not the femtosecond

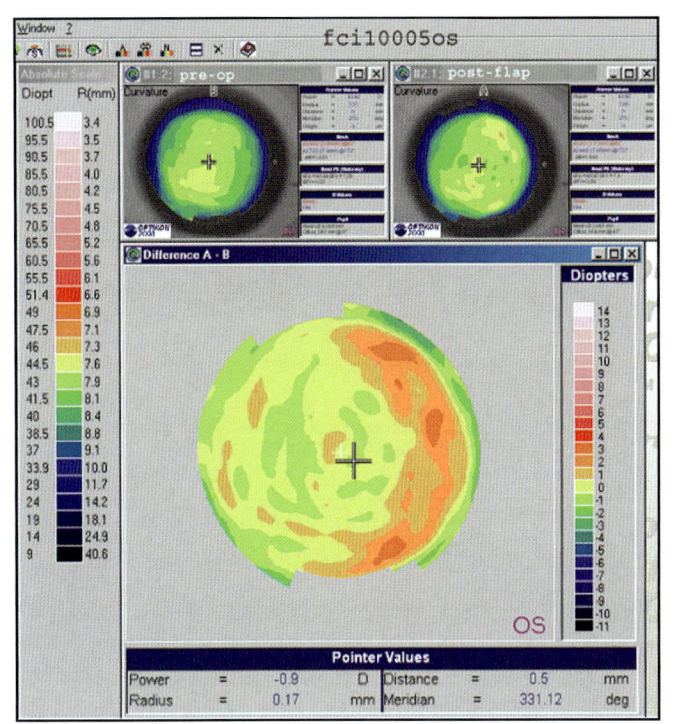

Figure 6-3. Preflap topography (upper left), postflap topography (upper right), and difference map demonstrating an increase in paracentral curvature after the creation of a lamellar flap with a mechanical microkeratome.[17]

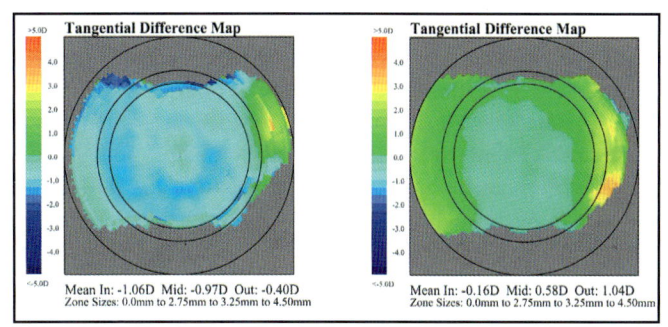

Figure 6-4. Average tangential curvature difference maps between 3 months postflap and preflap topographies. Left: Average (n=7) difference map from the group that had a flap created, but not lifted. Right: Average (n=10) difference map from the group that had a flap created, lifted, and replaced. Note the greater paracentral increase in curvature that corresponded to an increase in spherical aberration in the group where the flap was lifted.

laser is likely due to the more uniform flap thickness with the femtosecond laser. Potgeiter et al[21] reported that the magnitude of corneal response due to the flap was predicted by stromal bed thickness, flap diameter, and total corneal thickness. Thicker stromal beds and smaller flap diameters produced the greatest change in postflap topography. Flap thickness was not a significant predictor of response. This study suggests that the biomechanical response is driven strictly by the bed and not by the flap itself. In other words, two identical flaps would generate distinct responses if the underlying beds were of different thicknesses. MacRae et al[23] reported a significant difference in response between those flaps that were created but not lifted and those that were lifted and replaced. Figure 6-4 illustrates the difference between the shape change induced by the lift and the no-lift groups. This study suggests that flap manipulation plays an important role in flap response. In fact, in those flaps that were lifted, the spherical aberration induced by the flap alone was more than half of the total spherical aberration induced after the subsequent ablation, when compared to preop. Manipulation of the flap may lead to increased peripheral stromal swelling, according to the biomechanical model presented, magnifying the biomechanical response.

Once created, the flap offers little structural support to the cornea. Schmack et al[24] reported that a flap is 2.4% as strong centrally as an intact cornea and 28.1% as strong at the flap margins. Tensile strength was measured on postmortem eyes from donors who had a history of LASIK and compared to normal controls. The postmortem findings are consistent with clinical experience, in which a flap can be lifted 11 years after surgery. This work supports the conclusion that the mechanical strength of the cornea after LASIK lies predominantly in the residual stromal bed, which highlights a distinct structural difference between LASIK and surface ablation techniques.

STRUCTURAL COMPARISON OF LASIK AND SURFACE ABLATION

The apparent reduction in intraocular pressure (IOP) after refractive surgery has been reported by many investigators.[25-34] It has been assumed that the true pressure is not reduced, and the apparent reduction is an artifact of decreased corneal thickness after an ablative procedure. However, a theoretical analysis indicates that variation in corneal elasticity has a much greater impact on the error in Goldmann tonometry than thickness.[35] This is supported by clinical studies in which there was no correlation between thickness change and IOP reduction.[36-38] In addition, in the largest study reported,[34] the regression analysis of IOP change as a function of refractive change resulted in an R^2 of 0.009, which is associated with tremendous variability. The range of IOP change was approximately -15 mm Hg to +11 mm Hg over a range of refractive change from approximately 0 to 16.0 D in 8113 myopic procedures. All of these patients had reduced corneal thickness, but a substantial number had an *increase* in apparent IOP, which points to a mechanism other than thickness. In addition, the y-intercept of the regression was -1.36 mm Hg, which the authors predict would be the change in IOP due to structural alteration of the flap alone. An alternative explanation for the change in IOP after ablative surgery is a fundamental alteration in the biomechanical properties of the cornea due to a change in structure. It is then possible to compare surface ablation to LASIK in terms of apparent IOP reduction in order to investigate differences in biomechanical property modification between the two approaches. Sanchis Gemeno et al[27] reported a difference in the reduction of IOP between PRK and LASIK at 1 year postoperatively. Hjortdal et al[39] reported a long-term difference in apparent IOP reduction, comparing PRK to LASIK in two groups of patients who received similar myopic corrections. Despite the significant difference in apparent IOP reduction between LASIK and PRK, there was no significant difference in corneal thickness 36 months postoperatively. The LASIK group had a significantly greater reduction in apparent IOP than the PRK group, indicating a greater alteration in biomechanical properties after LASIK. This is likely due to both the creation of a lamellar flap, and the consequential placement of the ablated tissue region deeper in the cornea for the same correction (see Figure 6-2).

Corneal hysteresis is a new parameter that is a marker for the viscoelastic properties of the cornea. It is measured using a device called the Ocular Response Analyzer (Reichert, Buffalo, NY), which is an air puff tonometer that measures two applanation events.[40] The first occurs as the cornea is deflected inward, and the second occurs after the cornea reaches a state of concavity and then rebounds, reaching a second applanation before it recovers its original convex shape. Corneal Hysteresis is defined as the difference in the pressure between the first and second applanation events. If the pressure were the same at each applanation event, then the cornea would be a purely elastic material. The difference that occurs is representative of the viscoelastic properties of the cornea. Hysteresis is significantly reduced after LASIK,[40-41] indicating a fundamental change in biomechanical properties of the cornea. However, more research is needed.

IATROGENIC ECTASIA

Ectasia remains a rare, difficult to predict, yet very serious complication of refractive surgery. Literature reports relate predominately to iatrogenic ectasia as a complication of LASIK rather than PRK.[42-44] Several factors likely contribute to the difference in prevalence of ectasia following LASIK vs PRK. These include the lower residual stromal bed thickness in LASIK when compared to surface ablation for the same level of correction due to the need to ablate under a flap in LASIK. However, Vinciguerra et al[45] reported 5 years of long-term follow-up in ultrathin corneas without the occurrence of ectasia. In all of these cases, a PTK surface ablation was performed with an ablation zone width of 10 mm. The authors concluded that a wider ablation zone distributes the stress over the entire cornea and dramatically reduces the stress concentration produced by a thin central zone. From this study, it can be concluded that stromal bed thickness alone is insufficient to predict the occurrence of ectasia. Ectasia appears to be a multidimensional phenomenon related to both thickness and ablation zone width. In addition, an important factor that requires further investigation is that of biomechanical properties and their role in the development of ectasia. One hypothesis currently under investigation is that low hysteresis preoperatively may be a risk factor for the

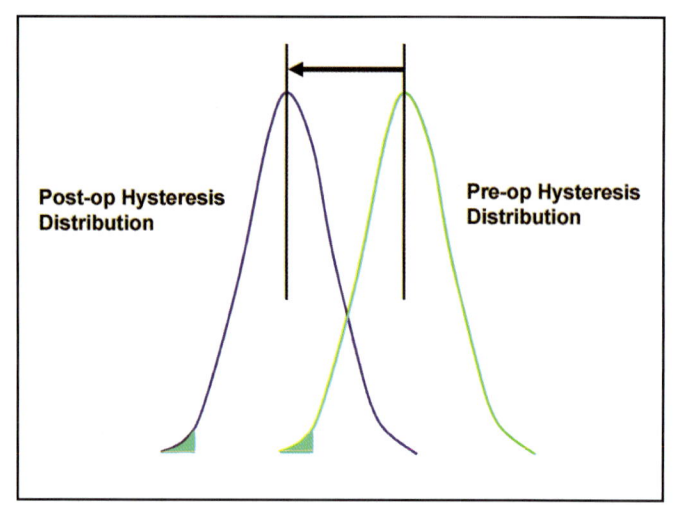

Figure 6-5. Illustration of the biomechanical properties hypothesis for iatrogenic ectasia. Corneal hysteresis is assumed to have a normal distribution preoperatively, shown on the right. After LASIK, the curve is shifted to significantly lower values.[41,46] Those individuals at the lower end of the bell curve (shaded) preoperatively are hypothesized to shift to a level of structural instability after LASIK.

development of ectasia, since it has been shown that both LASIK and LASEK cause a reduction in hysteresis postoperatively.[46] When this reduction is imposed on an already low hysteresis value, the cornea may become biomechanically unstable. This hypothesis is illustrated in Figure 6-5.

BIOMECHANICAL CUSTOMIZATION

An important question that emerges from the study of corneal biomechanics is whether the response can be manipulated to improve outcomes. Evidence has been reported that supports the concept that manipulation of response can be accomplished via ablation profile design, specifically by modifying the transition zone.[47-48] In a contralateral study in which one eye of 30 subjects was treated with a VISX S3 laser (Santa Clara, Calif) and one eye was treated with a Bausch & Lomb Technolas laser (Rochester, NY), the eye treated with the VISX laser had significantly greater spherical aberration induction than the eye treated with the Bausch & Lomb laser. All eyes had identical optical zone sizes of 6.5 mm. Therefore, the fundamental difference in the ablation profiles between lasers was the larger transition zone available with the Bausch & Lomb system. This is illustrated in Figure 6-6. The larger transition zone removed more of the peripheral lamellar segments (see Figure 6-1) that drive the biomechanical response, reducing the response and resulting in lower induction of spherical aberration. This study illustrates the importance of the transition zone, previously thought to be neutral, in influencing the induction of HO aberrations.

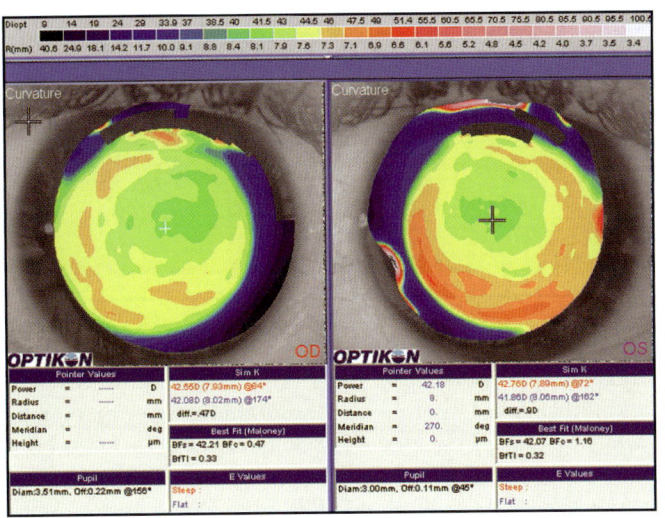

Figure 6-6. Contralateral postoperative tangential curvature maps from an individual treated with a different laser in each eye. Both eyes had a 6.5-mm optical zone. The map on the left (OD) had a transition zone out to 9 mm, while the map on the right (OS) had a blend zone to 8 mm. This smaller ablation zone resulted in a greater increase in paracentral curvature, corresponding to increased spherical aberration.[48]

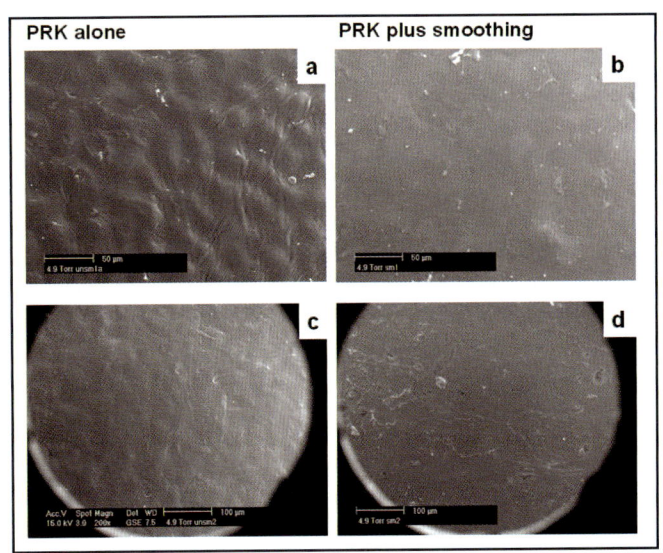

Figure 6-7. A & C: environmental scanning electron microscopy of two pair of human cadaver cornea following a -10.00 D PRK-ablation using a flying spot ArF excimer laser. B & D: matched-pair cornea received the same ablation and an additional therapeutic laser smoothing treatment with masking solution. After treatment, cornea were fixed in glutaraldehyde 2.5% for 3 hours and then stored in balanced salt solution at 4°C prior to imaging.

Micromechanics

Effect of Surface Irregularities After Photorefractive Keratectomy

Since the early testing and clinical trials of excimer laser PTK[49-52] and PRK,[2,53-56] millions of refractive procedures have been performed throughout the world with significant success to treat corneal irregularities and to correct refractive errors.[57] Identifiable complications such as haze and regression have been observed and quantified.[58-59] In vivo confocal imaging of stromal wound healing has been a useful tool to study these processes in living organisms;[60] however, the anatomical correlates and associated ultrastructural changes contributing to these complications are not well known. The observed complications do often correlate with specific treatment parameters and are thus often avoided clinically. However, once the mechanisms are identified, we may develop targeted therapies and enhance specific surgeries. Identifying targets to reduce these complications has lead researchers to examine the corneal ultrastructural and epithelial and stromal changes induced by surgery and healing. These changes may represent the ultra- and micromechanical response of the cornea, which correlate to changes in surface topography and corneal wavefront.

Stromal keratocyte differentiation is essential in maintaining corneal transparency after surgery and during healing. Keratocyte cell function including differentiation and proliferation may be altered by the stromal response to surface irregularities. Epithelial cell function following surface treatments respond to surface irregularities as regions of hyperplasia and the release of wound healing factors. Corneal healing response is regulated in part by these epithelial-stromal interactions and factors associated with the epithelial-stromal interface. Increased epithelial thickness typically results in regression observed 1 to 2 months postop. Comparing individual changes in corneal topography and ultrastructure in response to different treatment parameters, for example depth and optical zone, may lead to understanding the micromechanical response of the cornea to surgery. The purpose of this section is to examine the anatomical and biomechanical correlates associated with increased surface irregularities following deep ablations and gain insights into how these factors may relate to haze formation.

Imaging Ultrastructure Response and Corneal Surface Irregularities

Submicron-scale irregularities have been observed and quantified on excimer ablated polymethylmethacrylate and corneal tissue. Surface roughness does increase as a function of ablation depth as measured qualitatively by scanning electron microscopy (SEM)[61] and quantitatively by computerized laser interferometry[62] and atomic force microscopy.[63-64] Figure 6-7 is environmental scanning electron microscopy of 1-mm flying spot excimer ablated human cornea that have been fixed and imaged without critical point drying or metal coating, to illustrate the micron-scale surface features of the ablated corneal surface before and after smoothing.

Atomic force microscopy (AFM) has been a useful technique for visualizing surface nanotexture and measuring nanometer-scale surface features of cornea.[65-66] Structural information from AFM experiments can be obtained from corneas that have not been fixed, dehydrated, stained, or otherwise processed. An inherent problem with electron microscopic imaging of cornea, and most other biological tissue, is the need for tissue preparation (see Drawbacks of SEM). AFM can also detect many fine details that are not observed with SEM. Such details are likely masked by the deposited conductive metal layer or the dehydrated state required by the SEM preparation. AFM is, therefore, advantageous for studying natural cornea because it is nondestructive; it provides high three-dimensional spatial resolution without preparation effects; and it can be performed on fully hydrated specimens.

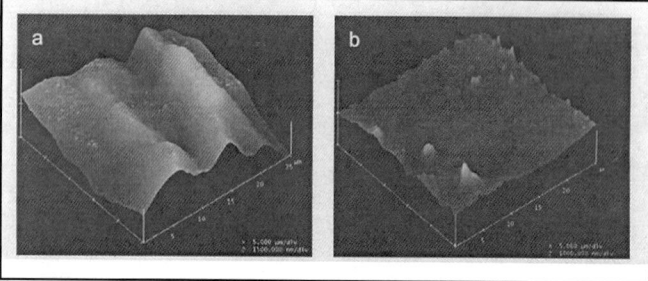

Figure 6-8. Atomic force microscopy of surface topography map of an ablated central corneal surface from a human cadaver eye following a -10.0 D PRK alone (a) and with additional phototherapeutic smoothing. (b) Specimens were imaged in balanced salt solution by low force contact-mode using silicon-nitride cantilevers with a nominal spring constant of 0.06 nm (NP20 from Digital Instruments, Santa Barbara, Calif).[63]

Drawbacks of SEM

It should be noted that analysis of intrinsic corneal surface roughness by SEM suffers drawbacks. These drawbacks include surface artifacts and contraction of the corneal tissue during fixation caused by chemical fixing with glutaraldehyde and osmium tetroxide as well as placement in a vacuum.[67] Small-angle x-ray scattering studies demonstrate that glutaraldehyde and ethanol treatments alter the intermolecular spacing of collagen fibrils in bovine cornea from 1.72 ± 0.06 nm to 1.81 ± 0.11 nm and 1.43 ± 0.04 nm, respectively, and do not alter the interfibrillar spacing. Critical point drying however dehydrates the cornea by decreasing the interfibrillar spacing from 63.8 ± 2.0 nm down to 54.0 ± 1.1 nm and intermolecular spacing from 1.72 ± 0.06 nm down to 1.43 ± 0.04 nm. For comparison, corneal collagen fibrils in humans have been measured by transmission electron microscopy (TEM) to be about 24 to 26 nm in diameter for fixed tissue; however, X-ray diffraction of physiologically hydrated cornea reveal larger fibril diameters of 31 nm for humans with a center-to-center collagen fibril spacing of 62 nm.[67-68] Fixation effects can be minimized by pair-controlled experiments.

AFM has advanced over the past decade to provide useful quantitative analysis with nanometer resolution of cornea and other hydrated biological substrates.[64,66,69-70] AFM of fixed, unablated human corneas revealed collagen fibril diameters ranging from 48 to 113 nm (mean 81.7 ± 19.9 nm) and beaded cross-bridges between adjacent, closely attached fibrils.[71] Mulitmode AFM has been performed on hydrated fixed and unfixed ablated human corneas that reveal micro- and nano-scale irregularities that vary with depth of ablation.[63] An increase in smoothness was measured on ablated corneal surfaces following a -10.0-D myopic ablation and phototherapeutic masking treatment.[63] Roughness values (mean RMS and Z range) were measured from 25-μm^2 regions across each surface of ablated corneas with and without phototherapeutic smoothing and demonstrate a decrease in roughness with smoothing similar to the images shown in Figure 6-8. The mean RMS of the two unsmoothed ablated human cornea were 612 ± 252 nm (n=18) and 479 ± 187 nm (n =24) and their paired-matched smoothed cornea were 102 ± 14 (n =5) and 147 ± 54 (n = 15). The Z range of the two unsmoothed human cornea were 3.611 ± 0.323 nm (n = 18) and 3.361 ± 0.930 nm (n = 24) and their paired-matched smoothed corneas were 1.177 ± 0.364 (n = 5) and 1.408 ± 0.503 nm (n = 15).

Optical profilometry and laser interferometry are effective noncontact methods to measure and characterize the surface roughness of material surfaces. Using these techniques, surface irregularities on ablated PMMA following 6-mm diameter PRK ablations (VISX 20/20) increased linearly with ablation depth from -1.0 to -15.0 D.[72] Each diopter increment resulted in an approximately 300 nm increased peak-to-valley measurement and 250 nm change in average roughness (Ra) per 10 μm of ablation. Therefore, a -15.0 D myopic ablation on a PMMA plate resulted in an average roughness of 6.5 μm, a root mean average height of 0.8 μm, and a peak-to-valley distance of 5 μm. Optical profilometry roughness data in Figure 6-9 were collected from curved PMMA lenses following an 8-mm diameter PTK by a 1-mm flying spot laser (LadarVision) from 0 to 80 μm deep. Analysis of the central ablation roughness shows a linear correlation between ablation depth and roughness.

To compare the ablation profile of corneal tissue and PMMA, computerized laser interferometric microscopy (Zygo Corporation, Middlefield, Conn) was used to measure average (Ra) and RMS roughness (root-mean-square deviation from the best fit surface relative to the reference surface) on five New Zealand white rabbit corneas and PMMA test blocks. Ablations were generated by a 5-mm diameter 80-μm deep argon fluoride broad beam therapeutic excimer laser system (VISX 20/20). The mean roughness values of the ablated corneas were significantly higher than the ablated PMMA. The mean Ra and RMS of the ablated corneas were 183.3 ± 20.6 nm and 240.1 ± 23.1 nm, and of the PMMA, 79.5 ± 23.0 nm and 96.5 ± 27.1 nm, respectively. The authors could not detect a significant difference between the central and peripheral areas of the ablation zone in either sample.[62]

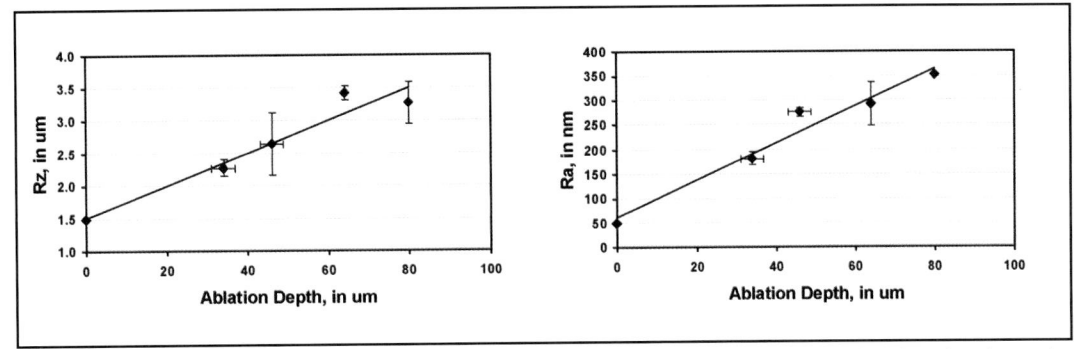

Figure 6-9. The mean surface roughness (Ra and Rz) of the central surface of ablated polymethylmethacrylate lenses was measured using optical profilometry (Veeco Instruments Inc.) with a 10x objective lens and tilt and curvature correction, and averaged across four 525x525 µm² areas for each measurement. Each lens received a central 8-mm diameter PTK flying spot treatment. Roughness increases linearly with depth of ablation (linear correlations for Rz, $R^2 = 0.96$ and for Ra, $R^2 = 0.93$), where Ra is the average roughness defined as the mean deviation from the best fit surface relative to the reference surface, and Rz is the average maximum height of the profile.

INCREASED SURFACE IRREGULARITIES AND LASER ABLATION

The appearance of haze is often more pronounced following deeper ablations observed in both LASIK and PRK. Surface roughness increases as a function of depth of laser ablation measured on acrylic plates as well as on porcine and human corneas. Furthermore, treatments that smooth corneal surface irregularities prior to healing reduce haze. Thus, a correlation between haze following deep (≥6.0 D) photorefractive keratectomy and surface roughness is likely. This association provides a mechanism to study corneal response to surface roughness and explore haze formation to surface irregularities during corneal remodeling and wound healing.

Subtle differences in videokeratographic outcomes suggest that laser modalities can improve visual outcome as a function of reduced surface microtopography. For example, a smaller beam flying spot provides better outcomes when compared to a broad beam.[73] Laser modality can also generate different degrees and profiles of roughness. Electron microscopy of porcine corneas and quantitative laser interferometry and Hommel-Werkel rugosimetry of ablated calibration plastic verify significant differences in surface irregularities generated by different clinical lasers. These differences were measured using myopic correcting ablations ≤9.0 D and a variety of lasers:[74] VISX S2 Smooth Scan (Santa Clara, Calif), NIDEK EC-5000 Autonomous Ladar Vision System (Gamagori, Japan), Bausch and Lomb Technolas (Rochester, NY),[75] VISX-Star, Coherent Schwind Keratom I/II, and Chiron Technolas Keracor 117C (Plano Scan).[76] SEM analysis of argon fluoride excimer ablated de-epithelialized porcine corneas shows fewer surface irregularities are generated at lower repetition rates, comparing 2 Hz versus 10 Hz (VISX 20/20). Corneas treated with a masking fluid, regardless of repetition rate, have the fewest irregularities.[77]

Corneal curvature may also affect the relative laser efficiency and surface roughness profile. If laser efficiency varied with curvature as a function of effective surface area, then laser-associated roughness would also vary.[78] However, such data has yet to be presented.

CORNEAL STRUCTURE, TRANSPARENCY, AND HAZE FOLLOWING PHOTOREFRACTIVE KERATECTOMY AND LASIK

Understanding how the cornea maintains its transparency and structural integrity during wound healing may be a key to understanding the effects of micro/nanotopography and changes in corneal ultrastructure. Corneal transparency is maintained by the regular fibril spacing that is regulated by the fibril diameter and the glycosaminoglycan chains of the proteoglycans keratan sulphate and dermatan sulphate. These fibrils are interspersed with quiescent keratocytes that vary in density throughout the stroma. Alterations in this spacing will affect transparency, either by hydration or composition, as well as activated keratocytes/fibroblasts whose morphology and nuclei increase reflectivity. Corneal keratocytes have been shown to contain water-soluble proteins called crystallins that render these quiescent cells transparent at visible wavelengths.[79] Further, the interwoven structure of the stromal collagen fibers[80] and resistance to swelling in the anterior one-third likely[81] contribute to a depth-dependent corneal biomechanical response.

Meek and colleagues have used transmission electron microscopy and x-ray scattering to detect differences in fibril ultrastructure across species and found that corneal collagen fibrils in humans typically measure about 24 to 26 nm in diameter in dehydrated, fixed tissue—and 31-nm diameter in physiologically hydrated tissue with a collagen fibril average center-to-center spacing of 62 nm.[82] Stromal regrowth after photoablation involves alterations in the collagen and proteoglycan matrix, similar to that observed in penetrating corneal scars. It has been proposed that the ultrastructural abnormalities in the newly deposited collagen may be a direct source of haze; however, Connon and colleagues[83] contend that this disorganized layer is too thin to affect corneal transparency, a concept that is supported by *ex vivo* confocal studies of post-LASIK human cadaver eyes.[84]

Connon and Meek[85] analyzed the scar tissue in rabbit corneas after 12 months and observed that collagen remodelling in the corneal scar tissue may continue for >1 year. After 12 months, the proteoglycan filaments in the scar were normal in size and number, whereas the collagen fibrils within the scar were still disorganized as evidenced by collagen interweaving and a lack of lamellar structure. Increased cellular reflectivity from stromal cells during wound healing is also observed by *in vivo* confocal microscopy and likely contribute to the observed haze.[86] Furthermore, the time scale of the haze formation is on the order of months from the initial surgery, suggesting a long-term response possibly involving multiple interactions and events that change during wound healing, possibly biomechanical in nature.

Loss of corneal transparency is typically explained by a combination of factors including 1) swelling or edema caused by abnormal water content, 2) scar tissue or fibrosis associated with abnormal collagen fiber diameter, spacing, and orientation, and 3) abnormal accumulation of macromolecules including proteins, glycosaminoglycans, and lipids. As mentioned, abnormal cellular-based reflections from multiple layers of stromal keratocytes and multiple structures (keratocyte nuclei, cell-body, and cell-processes) have been proposed to contribute to corneal haze.[87] The distinctions between reflective structures may require confocal microscopic examination to be discerned and further studies may provide insight into alternative mechanisms to address haze.

A comparison of eyes with complicated haze following PRK and LASIK revealed differences between early and late onset haze based on differences in epithelial structure measured by corneal permeability to fluorescein.[88] Corneal permeability to fluorescein increased following both PRK (2 to 8 weeks) and LASIK (4 to 6 weeks). Deeper ablations showed higher corneal fluorescein permeability for longer periods. In eyes with haze, an increased permeability to fluorescein was observed in the eyes with early postoperative haze onset (1 to 2 months), and a decreased permeability was observed in eyes with late postoperative haze onset (after 3 months). These permeability differences between haze groups suggest different mechanisms and anatomical correlates for early and late onset haze formation after PRK.

Surface Irregularities and Cell-Matrix and Cell-Cell Interactions

The mechanisms regulated by corneal cell-matrix and cell-cell interactions are multivariant and complicate corneal wound healing.[89] Following ablation, migrating corneal epithelial cells directly encounter the ablated stromal surface in the first days of wound healing during re-epithelialization.

A clinical study of corneal topography maps following PRK correlated increased epithelial migration rates to a reduction in ablation-related corneal surface irregularities.[90] Re-epithelialization may, therefore, be delayed or altered by irregularities in the substrate and contribute to haze formation and prolong wound healing, likely contributing to haze formation based on observed differences between LASIK and PRK.

In the ablated cornea, epithelial cells migrate directly over the corneal stroma by depositing fibronectin to serve as a temporary matrix for epithelial cell-ECM adhesion through integrins. The aggregation of actin stress fibers and associated intracellular proteins at focal contacts contribute to the spreading and migration of these epithelial cells. *In vitro* studies have shown that expression of ECM receptors is upregulated such that wounded corneal epithelial cells attach preferentially to collagen type I, type IV, or to laminin-1. The ultrastructure of the extracellular matrix underlying the anterior corneal epithelium of unablated, healthy human corneas has been characterized by Murphy and colleagues using scanning electron microscopy and atomic force microscopy.[91] This basement membrane has a very complex topography of fibrils intermingled with pores on the scale of 50 to 150 nm. Comparing the three techniques, TEM, SEM, and AFM, average feature heights were measured to be 149 ± 60 nm, 191 ± 72 nm, and 147 ± 73 nm, respectively. The microtopography of this surface may affect epithelial cell membrane structure and function. Amniotic membrane carriers for epithelial cell transplantation have a composition and topography that likely suits epithelial cell proliferation and integrity.[92-93]

In vitro studies support epithelial cell matrix-dependent behavior and biomechanical response to micro- and nano-texture. Culture studies have demonstrated a response of corneal epithelial cells as well as keratocyte cells to variations in nanotopography. Human corneal epithelial cells were cultured on nanofabricated textured surfaces with features similar to native basement membrane and altered cell behavior was observed. Nanoscale topography also modulated corneal epithelial cell-substratum adhesion.[94] Human corneal epithelial cells cultured on substrates with uniform grooves and ridges with pitches between 400 and 4000 nm aligned and elongated with the grooves as measured by their focal adhesions and associated stress fibers. Cell adhesion was greatest on the 400-nm pitch, the lowest limit tested. The small GTP-binding proteins that control cytoskeletal dynamics and cell behaviors in corneal epithelial cells were also regulated by nanotopography in culture. Rho protein, associated with stress fiber formation, is upregulated on nanoscale topography, whereas Rac protein, associated with lamellapodia formation, and Cdc42 protein, associated with filopodia formation, are down regulated (Christopher Murphy, personal communication). Thus, cell behavior can be modulated by nanoscale topographic cues and may play an important role in corneal wound healing following surface ablation.

Human corneal fibroblasts cultured on similar nanopatterned surfaces of grooves and ridges aligned more strongly than epithelial cells.[95-96] For example, on patterns with pitches of 800 nm and larger approximately 70% of the keratocytes (compared to 35% of epithelial cells) were aligned. On 70-nm-wide ridges with 400-nm pitch, keratocyte alignment dropped to 45% whereas epithelial cell alignment was constant. Focal adhesions and stress fibers aligned along the topographies; however, oblique orientations were also observed. Nanoscale patterns resulted in fewer stress fibers or focal adhesions than cells cultured on microscale patterns or on untextured substrates.

Corneal epithelial cell adhesion to porous polymers has also been studied in the study of corneal onlays, which provides insight into corneal cell-surface texture interactions. *In vitro* model systems have been used to examine the effect of polymer surface topography (pore sizes 0.1 to 3.0 μm diameter) vs nonporous surfaces on epithelial attachment and proliferation.[97] On these porous surfaces, corneal epithelial cells responded to a balance between the size of the pores and the amount of polymer surface between the pores. Basement membrane and hemidesmosome assembly was continuous and regular on 0.1-μm porous surfaces and limited to the polymer on 0.4- to 2.0-μm pores yet absent on smooth or 3.0 μm-porous polycarbonate surfaces.[98] Furthermore, 0.1- to 0.8-μm diameter porous surfaces supported superior stratification and protein deposition than porous or smooth surfaces ≥1.0 μm. Cytoplasmic processes tended to penetrate the 2.0- to 3.0-μm pore surfaces.[99] These results demonstrate that surface microtopography including porosity can significantly influence epithelial adhesion and stratification.

MICRO-/NANOMECHANICAL RESPONSE TO SURFACE IRREGULARITIES?

Numerous studies have shown evidence of epithelial hyperplasia and keratocyte activation following surface treatments. The degree of hyperplasia increases slightly with depth of ablation. TEM studies of primate corneas from 1.5 to 18 months after -1.5 and -3.0 D myopic corrective ablations revealed a thicker epithelium above the central treated area that was greater in the -3.0 D case. The number of activated keratocytes beneath the treated zone also increased, peaking at 4 months, then decreasing. Other studies have revealed fewer hemidesmosomes in the epithelium overlying the post-PRK treatment zone that may affect corneal function.[100] It has also been observed that initial epithelial attachment may correlate with corneal haze following PRK, such that patients with seemingly tighter epithelial attachment had a lower tendency to develop corneal haze.[101]

It is unclear how the wound-healing cornea, whose remodelling can continue for 1 to 3 years, responds during remodelling to the initial microtexture of the ablated surface. Ultrastructural variations throughout the cornea have been observed in the centers of postmortem LASIK corneas presumably resulting from interface irregularities in the presence of a flap.[84] *Ex vivo* confocal microscopy and histopathology identified slight changes in the corneal ultrastructure that have previously received little attention since they are invisible to clinical slit-lamp detection and do not seem to significantly affect corneal transparency. Both corneal epithelial and keratocyte cells are likely involved in these changes. The epithelium responds to biological and possibly longer-term biomechanical wound repair processes in the center of LASIK corneas. Focal areas of thickened epithelium are shown to result from basal epithelial cell hypertrophic modifications, and these cells tend to reside over low points on the corneal surface, therefore, filling in surface irregularities. Random undulations in Bowman's layer over the flap surface are also observed and are presumed to result from a lack of compatibility between the flap and the laser stromal bed. Structural variations in surface smoothness may, therefore, alter epithelial structure *in vivo*.

Local and regional changes in microstructure and tension would affect adherent cells such as epithelial and keratocytes that rely on their cell-matrix contacts to function. The stromal keratocyte cells function in wound healing by contributing to the maintenance of corneal ultrastructure and expression of keratan sulphate proteoglycans. Jester and Ho-Chang[102] have demonstrated the modulation of cultured rabbit corneal keratocyte phenotype by growth factors and cytokines that are released during stromal wound healing. These keratocyte phenotypes, in turn, control contractility (expression of α-smooth muscle actin) and extracellular matrix contraction in culture (marked by decreased keratan sulphate expression coupled with increased dermatan sulphate expression). In the absence of factors the keratocyte phenotype was non-contractile; however, application of TGFβ$_1$ induced myofibroblast differentiation with prominent focal adhesions and fibronectin assembly, α-smooth muscle actin expression, and significantly greater matrix contraction. Interestingly, IGF-I and IL-1α increased keratocyte proliferation but did not alter keratocyte phenotype nor induce matrix contraction. FGF$_2$ and PDGF induced fibroblast differentiation evidenced by focal adhesions and fibronectin assembly and significant extracellular matrix contraction. Therefore, release of specific factors in response to any remodelling of the irregular substratum could, therefore, affect the contractile response of the local keratocytes and induce a so-called "micromechanical response."

It should be noted that the haze associated with deep ablations is typically performed clinically on highly myopic corneas whose intrinsic ultrastructure and biological response may vary from other cornea. The impact of residual bed thickness, volume of tissue removed, and zone diameter may further alter the structural and biological response to confound the effect due to the surface irregularities alone. The challenge of developing an accurate biomechanical wound healing model will be to correlate differences in local ultrastructure to global biomechanical response.

CLINICAL REDUCTION OF HAZE AND SURFACE IRREGULARITIES

Wound healing can vary from subject to subject, and subepithelial haze can be categorized into different classifications including early (1 to 2 months postop) and late (>3 months) onset haze. These distinctions may support alternative mechanisms of haze formation. The grade and location of haze within the stroma will depend on many parameters including ablation depth. The haze effect is more pronounced following deep PRK and decreased but not absent following deep LASIK ablations. The risk of complicating haze generally limits myopic PRK corrections to depths of -6.0 D or less. The minimum residual bed thickness requirement also limits LASIK depths more than PRK; therefore, enabling deep PRK ablations without haze would improve the range of refractive treatments.

The development and duration of corneal haze increases proportionally with increasing stromal ablation depth.[86] In a rabbit PTK model to compare manual epithelial debridement vs transepithelial ablation, increased haze or backscattering of light, correlated with stromal photoablation depth but was unrelated to the depth of initial keratocyte loss. The increased haze appeared to be related to an increase in keratocyte density and reflectivity of migratory fibroblasts and transformation to myofibroblast phenotype.

Although the biomechanisms leading to haze are not well understood, they are likely multivariant. Effective methods to alter corneal wound response and reduce haze have been explored. Some effective methods include intraoperative mitomycin C application,[103-107] phototherapeutic masking solution smoothing treatments,[108-111] Epi-LASIK,[112] and plasminogen-activator inhibitor tear drops.[113-114] Epi-LASIK maintains the epithelial basement membrane and tight junctions, similar to a LASIK flap, and likely minimizes the release of factors into the stroma and consequently reduces the inflammatory haze response. Mitomycin C also reduces haze, however toxic to corneal keratocytes, and has been shown to remain toxic for 3 months after PRK in rabbits.[115] Clinical application of a masking-solution smoothing technique has been shown to reduce the prevalence of haze in human corneas following PRK.[108,116]

Vinciguerra and colleagues have demonstrated a correlation between such smoothing treatments to reduce posttreatment surface irregularities, decreased corneal haze, and improved spectacle-corrected visual acuity.[109] Analysis of epithelial wound healing rates following surface ablation also led to the hypothesis that surface irregularities decrease epithelial migration rates following PTK treatment.[90] Hastened re-epithelialization would likely diminish the impact of diffusive cellular factors such as epithelial-derived TGFβ by reducing their release and effective levels. A decrease of such factors would likewise impact the duration and degree of subepithelial haze.[117-118]

In an effort to understand the effect of smoothing on surface roughness, SEM comparison of the adjunct smoothing effect of therapeutic keratectomy using masking fluids on PRK ablated porcine corneas revealed a more marked effect at higher dioptric ablations (from -6.0 to -15.0 D spherical ablations).[119] Therapeutic smoothing using viscous 0.25% sodium hyaluronate masking solution on porcine corneas following -10.0 D spherical ablations with a 6-mm diameter and 3-mm transition zone (Technolas Keracor 217A Planoscan and NIDEK EC-5000) had a similar response.[120]

Clinically, Vinciguerra and colleagues have observed benefits based on optical and functional outcomes resulting from decreasing surface and intersurface irregularities following PRK using laser smoothing techniques.[109] Serrao and colleagues[116] completed a bilateral clinical study to compare the effect of smoothing on visual outcome, haze, and radial epithelial migration. Unilateral eyes of 20 subjects with manifest spherical equivalent -2.0 to -9.0 D received spherical PRK alone, and the contralateral eye received PRK with additional smoothing. Between 20 and 40 hours after surgery, the average velocity of radial epithelial migration was approximately 30% faster with smoothing. At 3 months, smoothing coincided with a slight hyperopic shift, however, resulted in an improved visual outcome and diminished regression and haze. In a related clinical study, postoperative smoothing after PRK for myopic corrections up to -6.5 D had more regular topographic indices (or decreased surface irregularity) and more predictable mean spherical equivalent refractions throughout follow-up up to 1 year than PRK alone.

In conclusion, surface irregularities may play a mechanistic role in wound healing following surface ablations and may induce a micromechanical response.

References

1. Dupps WJ, Roberts C, Schoessler JP. Peripheral lamellar relaxation: a mechanism of induced corneal flattening in PTK and PRK? *Invest Ophthalmol Vis Sci*. 1995;36(suppl 4):S708.
2. Munnerlyn CR, Koons SJ, Marshall J. Photorefractive keratectomy: a technique for laser refractive surgery. *J Cataract Refract Surg*. 1988;14:46-52.
3. Dupps WJ, Roberts C, Schoessler JP. Geometric bias in PTK ablation profiles and associated keratometric changes in human globes. *Invest Ophthalmol Vis Sci*. 1996;37(suppl 3):S57.
4. Dupps WJ. Chemomechanical modification of the corneal response to photokeratectomy. PhD Thesis. Ohio State University; 1998.
5. Dupps WJ, Roberts C. Suppression of the acute biomechanical response to excimer laser keratectomy. *Invest Ophthalmol Vis Sci*. 1999;40(Suppl 4):S110.
6. Dupps WJ, Roberts C. Peripheral stromal thickening and ablation pattern as predictors of acute corneal flattening in photokeratectomy. *J Refract Surg*. 2001;17:658-669.
7. Roberts C, Dupps, WJ. Corneal biomechanics and their role in corneal ablative procedures. In: MacRae SM, Krueger RR, Applegate RA (eds). *Customized Corneal Ablation: Quest for Super Vision*. Thorofare, NJ: SLACK Incorporated; 2001:109-132.
8. Roberts C. The impact of corneal biomechanics on outcomes in laser refractive surgery. In: Burrato L, Brint S, eds. *Custom LASIK: Surgical Techniques and Complications*, 2003;14(4):489-491.
9. Roberts C. The cornea is not a piece of plastic. *J Refract Surg*. 2000;16:407-413.
10. Oliver KM, Hemenger RP, Corbett MC, et al. Corneal optical aberrations induced by photorefractive keratectomy. *J Refract Surg*. 1997;13(3):246-54.
11. Miller JM, Anwaruddin R, Straub J, Schwiegerling J. Higher-order aberrations in normal, dilated, intraocular lens, and laser in situ keratomileusis corneas. *J Refract Surg*. 2002;18(5):S579-S83.
12. Moreno-Barriuso E, Lloves JM, Marcos S, et al. Ocular aberrations before and after myopic corneal refractive surgery: LASIK-induced changes measured with laser ray tracing. *Invest Ophthalmol Vis Sci*. 2001;42(6):1396-403.
13. Llorente L, Marcos S, Barbero S, Merayo-Lloves J. How total and corneal aberrations change with standard LASIK surgery for hyperopia. *Invest Ophthalmol Vis Sci*. 2002;43:U474-U.

14. Nagy ZZ, Palagy-Deak I, Kelemen E, Kovacs A. Wavefront-guided photorefractive keratectomy for myopia and myopic astigmatism. *J Refract Surg.* 2002;18:S615-S619.
15. Nuijts RMMA, Nabar VA, Hament WJ, Eggink FAGJ. Wavefront-guided versus standard laser in situ keratomileusis to correct low to moderate myopia. *J Cataract Refract Surg.* 2002;28:1907-1913.
16. Roberts C. Future callenges to aberration-free ablative procedures. *J Refract Surg.* 2000;16:S623-S629.
17. Lembach, RG, Roberts C, Carones F. The refractive effect of the flap in laser in situ keratomileusis. *Invest Ophthalmol Visual Sci.* 2001;42(suppl 4):3235.
18. Roberts C, Castellano D, Mahmoud AM. Intra-operative flap topography during laser in situ keratomileusis. *Invest Ophthalmo Vis Sci.* 2001;42(suppl 4):3894.
19. Pallikaris IG, Kymionis GD, Panagopoulou SI, et al. Induced optical aberrations following formaiton of a laser in situ keratomileusis flap. *J Cataract Refract Surg.* 2002;28:1737-1741.
20. Porter J, MacRae S, Yoon G, Roberts C, Cox IG, Williams DR. Separate effects of the microkeratome incision and laser ablation on the eye's wave aberration. *Am J Ophthalmol.* 2003;136(2):327-337.
21. Potgieter FJ, Roberts C, Cox IG, et al. Prediction of flap response. *J Cataract Refract Surg.* 2005;31:106-114.
22. Tran DB, Sarayba MA, Bor Z, et al. Randomized prospective clinical study comparing induced aberrations with IntraLase and Hansatome flap creation in fellow eyes. Potential impact on wavefront-guided laser in situ keratomileusis. *J Cataract Refract Surg.* 2005;31:97-105.
23. Cox I, MacRae S, Porter J, et al. What causes the increase in higher-order aberrations after LASIK? The cut, the flap manipulation and/or the ablation? *Association for Research in Vision and Ophthalmology.* 2004:211.
24. Schmack I, Dawson DG, McCarey BE, et al. Cohesive tensile strength of human LASIK wounds with histologic, ultrastructural, and clinical correlations. *J Refract Surg.* 2005;21:433-445.
25. Faucher A, Gregoire J, Blondeau, P. Accuracy of Goldmann tonometry after refractive surgery. *J Cataract Refract Surg.* 1997; 23:832-838.
26. Chatterjee A, Shah S, Bessant DA, et al. Reduction in intraocular pressure after excimer laser photorefractive keratectomy. Correlation with pretreatment myopia. *Ophthalmology.* 1997;104:355-359.
27. Sanchis Gimeno, JA, Alonso Munoz L, Aguilar Valenzuela L, et al. Influence of refraction on tonometric readings after photorefractive keratectomy and laser in situ keratomileusis. *Cornea.* 200X;19:512-516.
28. Garzozi HJ, Chung HS, Lang Y, et al. Intraocular pressure and photorefractive keratectomy: a comparison of three different tonometers. *Cornea.* 2001;20:33-36.
29. Fournier, AV, Podtetenev M, Lemire J, et al. Intraocular pressure change measured by Goldmann tonometry after laser in situ keratomileusis. *J Cataract Refract Surg.* 1998;24:905-910.
30. Zadok D, Tran DB, Twa M., et al. Pneumotonometry versus Goldmann tonometry after laser in situ keratomileusis for myopia. *J Cataract Refract Surg.* 1999;25:1344-1348.
31. Park HJ, Uhm KB, Hong C. Reduction in intraocular pressure after laser in situ keratomileusis. *J Cataract Refract Surg.* 2001;27:303-309.
32. El Danasoury MA, El Maghraby A, Coorpender SJ. Change in intraocular pressure in myopic eyes measured with contact and non-contact tonometers after laser in situ keratomileusis. *J Cataract Refract Surg.* 2001;17:97-104.
33. Alonso-Munoz L, Lleo-Perez A., Rahhal MS, Sanchis-Gimeno JA. Assessment of applanation tonometry after hyperopic laser in situ keratomileusis. *Cornea.* 2002;21:156-160.
34. Chang DH, Stulting RD. Change in intraocular pressure measurements after LASIK: the effect of the refractive correction and the lamellar flap. *Ophthalmology.* 2005;112:1009-1016.
35. Liu J, Roberts C. Influence of corneal biomechanical properties on intraocular pressure measurement: quantitative analysis. *J Cataract Refract Surg.* 2005;31(1):146-155.
36. Mardelli PG, Piebenga LW, Whitacre MN, Siegmund KD. The effect of excimer laser photorefractive keratectomy on intraocular pressure measurements using the Goldmann applanation tonometer. *Ophthalmology.* 1997;104:945-948, discussion 949.
37. Emara B, Probst LE, Tingey DP, et al. Correlation of intraocular pressure and central corneal thickness in normal myopic eyes and after laser in situ keratomileusis. *J Cataract Refract Surg.* 1998;24:1320-1325.
38. Feltgen N, Leifert D, Funk J. Correlation between central corneal thickness, applanation tonometry, and direct intracameral IOP readings. *Br J Ophthalmol.* 2001;85:85-87.
39. Hjortdal JO, Moller-PedersenT, Ivarsen A, Ehlers N. Corneal power, thickness, and stiffness: results of a prospective randomized controlled trial of PRK and LASIK for myopia. *J Cataract Refract Surg.* 2005;31:21-29.
40. Luce DA. Determining *in vivo* biomechanical properties of the cornea with an ocular response analyzer. *J Cataract Refract Surg.* 2005;31:156-162.
41. Pepose J, Qazi M, Roberts C. Relationship between corneal hysteresis, intraocular pressure and flap dimensions in LASIK patients. *Association for Research in Vision and Ophthalmolog.* 2005;4853/B56
42. Pallikaris IG, Kymionis GD, Astyrakakis NI. Corneal ectasia induced by laser in situ keratomileusis. *J Cataract Refract Surg.* 2001;27:1796-1802.
43. Randleman JB, Russell B, Ward MA, et al. Risk factors and prognosis for corneal ectasia after LASIK. *Ophthalmology.* 2003;110:267-275.
44. Twa MD, Nichols JJ, Joslin CE, et al. Characteristics of corneal ectasia after LASIK for myopia. *Cornea.* 2004;23:447-457.
45. Vinciguerra P, Torres Munoz MI, Camesasca FI, Grizzi F, Roberts C. Long-term follow-up of ultrathin corneas after surface retreatment with phototherapeutic keratectomy. *J Cataract Refract Surg.* 2005;31: 82-87
46. Pan X, Liu J, Roberts C, et al. Comparing LASIK and LASEK: indications of biomechanical response. *Association for Research in Vision and Ophthalmology.* 2005; 2728/B281.
47. Vinciguerra P, Camesasca FI, Torres IM. Transition zone design and smoothing in custom laser-assisted subepithelial keratectomy. *J Cataract Refract Surg.* 2005;31:39-47.
48. Twa M, Lembach R, Bullimore M, Roberts C. A prospective randomized clinical trial of laser in-situ keratomileusis using two different lasers. *Am J Ophthalmol.* 2005;140:173-183.
49. Trokel SL, Srinivasan R, Braren B. Excimer laser surgery of the cornea. *Am J Ophthalmol.* 1983;96:710-715.
50. Puliafito CA, Steinert RF, Deutsch TF et al. Excimer laser ablation of the cornea and lens: experimental studies. *Ophthalmology.* 1985;92:741-748.
51. Bowers RA, Sher NA, Gothard TW, et al. The clinical use of the 193-nm excimer laser in the treatment of corneal scars. *Invest Ophthalmol Vis Sci.* 1991;32(Suppl):720.
52. Serdarevic O, Darrell RW, Krueger RR, Trokel SL. Excimer laser therapy for experimental *candida* keratitis. *Am J Ophthalmol.* 1985;99:534-538.
53. L'Esperance FA Jr, Warner JW, Telfair WB, Yoder PR, Martin CA. Excimer laser instrumentation and technique for human corneal surgery. *Arch Ophtlamol.* 1986;107:131-139.
54. Taylor DM, L'Esperance, FA Jr, Del Pero RA, et al. Human excimer laser lamellar keratectomy: a clinical study. *Ophthalmology.* 1989; 96:654-664.
55. Gartry DS, Muir MGK, Marshall J. Excimer laser photorefractive keratectomy: 18-month Follow-up. *Ophthalmology.* 1992;99:1209-1219.
56. Pallikaris IG, Siganos DS. Excimer laser in situ keratomileusis and photorefractive keratectomy for correction of high myopia. *J Refract Corneal Surg.* 1994;10:610-617.
57. Rajan MS, Jaycock P, O'Brart, Hamberg-Nystrom H, Marshall J. A long-term study of photorefractive keratectomy: 12 year follow-up. *Ophthalmology.* 2004;111:1813-1824.
58. Jain S, Khoury JM, Chamon W, Azar DT. Corneal light scattering after laser in situ keratomileusis and photorefractive keratectomy. *Am J Ophthalmol.* 1995;120:532-534.
59. Maldonado MJ, Arnau V, Navea A, Martinez-Costa R, Mico FM, Cisneros AL, Menezo JL. Direct objective quantification of corneal haze after excimer laser photorefractive keratectomy for high myopia. *Ophthalmology.* 1996;103(11):1970-1978.

60. Moller-Pedersen T, Cavanaugh HD, Petroll WM, Jester JV. Stromal wound healing explains refractive instability and haze development after photorefractive keratectomy: a 1-year confocal microscopic study. *Ophthalmology.* 2000;107:1235-1245.
61. Taylor SM, Fields CR, Barker FM, Sanzo J. Effect of depth upon the smoothness of excimer laser corneal ablation. *Optom Vis Sci.* 1994;71:104-108.
62. Liang FQ, Geasey SD, del Cerro M, Aquavella JV. A new procedure for evaluating smoothness of corneal surface following 193-nanometer excimer laser ablation. *Refract Corneal Surg.* 1992;8(6):459-465.
63. Lewis JR, Agarwal G, Roberts C. Atomic Force Microscopy Investigations of Corneal Tissue after Photoablative Treatment. *Biophysical Journal.* 2004;2468.
64. Nogradi A, Hopp B, Revesz K, Szabo G, Bor Z, Kolozsvari L. Atomic force microscopic study of the human cornea following excimer laser keratectomy. *Exp Eye Res.* 2000;70: 363-368.
65. Fullwood NJ, Hammiche A, Pollock HM, Hourston DJ, Song M. Atomic force microscopy of the cornea and sclera. *Curr Eye Res.* 1995; 14:529-535.
66. Lydataki S, Lesniewska E, Tsilimbaris MK, et al. Observation of the posterior endothelial surface of the rabbit cornea using atomic force microscopy. *Cornea.* 2003,22:651-664.
67. Fullwood NJ, Meek KM. A synchrotron x-ray study of the changes occurring in the corneal stroma during processing for electron microscopy. *J Microscopy.* 1993;169(1):53-60.
68. Meek KM, Quantock AJ. The use of x-ray scattering techniques to determine corneal ultrastructure. *Progr Retin Eye Res.* 2001;20(1):95-137.
69. Tsilimbaris MK, Lesniewska E, Lydataki S, et al. The use of atomic force microscopy for the observation of corneal epithelium surface. *Invest Ophthalmol Vis Sci.* 2000;41:680-686.
70. Ushiki T, Hitomi J, Umemoto T, et al. Imaging of living cultured cells of an epithelial nature by atomic force microscopy. *Arch Histol Cytol.* 1999;62:47-55.
71. Meller D, Peters K, Meller K. Human cornea and sclera studied by atomic force microscopy. *Cell Tissue Res.* 1997;288(1):111-118.
72. O'Donnell CB, Kemner J, O'Donnell FE. Surface roughness in PMMA is linearly related to the amount of excimer laser ablation. *J Refract Surg.* 1996a;12:171-174.
73. Fiore T, Carones F, Brancato R. Broad beam vs flying spot excimer laser: refractive and videokeratographic outcomes of two different ablation profiles after photorefractive keratectomy. *J Refract Surg.* 2001;17:534-541.
74. O'Donnell CB, Kemner J, O'Donnell FE. Ablation smoothness as a function of excimer laser delivery system. *J Cataract Refract Surg* 1996b;22:682-685.
75. Thomas JW, Mitra S, Chuang AZ, Yee RW. Electron microscopy of smoothness of porcine corneas and acrylic plates with four brands of excimer laser. *J Refract Surg.* 2003;19:623-628.
76. Argento C, Valenzuela G, Huck H, et al. Smoothness of ablation on acrylic by four different excimer lasers, *J Refract Surg.* 2001;17:43-45.
77. Fasano AP, Moreira H, McDonnell PJ, Sinbawy A. Excimer laser smoothing of a reprodible model of anterior corneal surface irregularity. *Ophthalmology.* 1991;98:1782-1785.
78. Mrochen M, Seiler T. Influence of corneal curvature on calculation of ablation patterns used in photorefractive laser surgery. *J Refract Surg.* 2001;17(5): S584-587.
79. Jester JV, Moller-Pedersen T, Huang J, et al. The cellular basis of corneal transparency: evidence for 'corneal crystallins.' *J Cell Sci.* 1999;112(5):613-622.
80. Fullwood NJ, Meek KM. A synchrotron X-ray study of the changes occurring in the corneal stroma during processing for electron microscopy. *J Microscopy.* 1993;169(1):53-60.
81. Muller LJ, Pels E, Vrensen GFJM. The specific architecture of the anterior stroma accounts for maintenance of corneal curvature. *Br J Ophthalmol.* 2001;85:437-443.
82. Meek KM, Fullwood NJ. Corneal and scleral collagens—a microscopist's perspective. *Micron.* 2001;32:261-272.
83. Connon CJ, Marshall J, Patmore AL, Brahma A, Meek KM. Persistent haze and disorganization of anterior stromal collagen appear unrelated following phototherapeutic keratectomy. *J Refract Surg.* 2003;19:323-332.
84. Dawson DG, Holley GP, Geroski DH, et al. Ex vivo confocal microscopy of human LASIK corneas with histologic and ultrastructural correlation. *Ophthalmology.* 2005;112:634-644.
85. Connon CJ, Meek KM. The structure and swelling of corneal scar tissue in penetrating full-thickness wounds. *Cornea.* 2004;23:165-171.
86. Moller-Pedersen T, Cavanagh D, Petroll WM, Jester JV. Corneal haze development after PRK is regulated by volume of stromal tissue removal. *Cornea.* 1998;17(6):627-639.
87. Moller-Pedersen T. Keratocyte reflectivity and corneal haze. *Exp Eye Res.* 2004;78:553-560.
88. Polunin GS, Kourenkov VV, Makarov IA, Polunina EG. The corneal barrier function in myopic eyes after laser in situ keratomileusis and after photorefractive keratectomy in eyes with haze formation. *J Refract Surg.* 1999;15:S221-S224.
89. Suzuki K, Saito J, Yanai R, et al. Cell-matrix and cell-cell interactions during corneal epithelial wound healing. *Prog Ret Eye Res.* 2003; 22:113-133.
90. Serrao S, Lombardo M. One-year results of photorefractive keratectomy with and without surface smoothing using the Technolas 217C laser. *J Refract Surg.* 2004;20:444-449.
91. Abrams GA, Schaus SS, Goodman SL, Nealey PF, Murphy CJ. Nanoscale topography of the corneal epithelial basement membrane and descemet's membrane of the human. *Cornea.* 2000;19:57-64.
92. Koizumi N, Fullwood NJ, Bairaktaris G, Inatomi T, Kinoshita S, Quantock AJ. Cultivation of corneal epithelial cells on intact and denuded human amniotic membrane. *Invest Ophthalmol Vis Sci.* 2000;41:2506-2513.
93. Fukuda K, Chikama T, Nakamura M, Nishida T. Differential distribution of subchains of the basement membrane components type IV collagen and laminin among the amniotic membrane, cornea, and conjunctiva. *Cornea.* 1999;18(1):73-79.
94. Karuri NW, Liliensiek S, Teixeira AI, et al. Biological length scale topography enhances cell-substratum adhesion of human corneal epithelial cells. *J Cell Science.* 2004;117:3153-3164.
95. Teixeira AI, Nealey PF, Murphy CJ. Responses of human keratocytes to micro- and nanostructured substrates. *J Biomed Mater Res A.* 2004; 71(3):369-376.
96. Flemming RG, Murphy CJ, Abrams GA, Goodman SL, Nealey PF. Effects of synthetic micro- and nano-structured surfaces on cell behavior. *Biomaterials.* 1999;20:573-588.
97. Xie Y, Sproule T, Li Y, Powell H, Lannutti JJ, Kniss DA. Nanoscale modifications of PET polymer surfaces via oxygen-plasma discharge yield minimal changes in attachment and growth of mammalian epithelial and mesenchymal cells. *J Biomed Mater Res.* 2002;61:234-245.
98. Evans MD, Dalton BA, Steele JG. Persistent adhesion of epithelial tissue is sensitive to polymer topography. *J Biomed Mater Res.* 1999;46:485-493.
99. Dalton BA, Evans MD, McFarland GA, Steele JG. Modulation of corneal epithelial stratification by polymer surface topography. *J Biomed Mater Res.* 1999;45:384-394.
100. Beuerman RW, McDonald MB, Shofner S, et al. Quantitative histological studies of primate corneas after excimer laser photorefractive keratectomy. *Arch Ophthal.* 1994;112:1103-1110.
101. Lipshitz I, Fisher L, Lazar M, Loewenstein A. Epithelial cell adhesion and haze after photorefractive keratectomy. *J Refract Surg.* 1997;13: S451.
102. Jester JV, Ho-Chang J. Modulation of cultured corneal keratocyte phenotype by growth factors/cytokines control in vitro contractility and extracellular matrix contraction. *Exp Eye Res.* 2003;77(5):581-592.
103. Mirza MA, Qazi MA, Pepose JS. Treatment of dense subepithelial corneal haze after laser-assisted subepithelial keratectomy. *J Cataract Refract Surg.* 2004;30(3):709-714.
104. Carones F, Vigo L, Scandola E, Vacchini L. Evaluation of the prophylactic use of mitomycin-C to inhibit haze formation after photorefractive keratectomy. *J Cataract Refract Surg.* 2002;28:2088-2095.

105. Chalita MR, Roth AS, Krueger RR. Wavefront-guided surface ablation with prophylactic use of mitomycin C after a buttonhole laser in situ keratomileusis flap. *J Refract Surg.* 2004; 20(2):176-181.
106. Camellin M. Laser epithelial keratomileusis with mitomycin C: indications and limits. *J Refract Surg.* 2004;20(5):S693-698.
107. Gambato C, Ghirlando A, Moretto E, Busato F, Midena E. Mitomycin C modulation of corneal wound healing after photorefractive keratectomy in highly myopic eyes. *Ophthalmology.* 2005;112(2):208-218
108. Vinciguerra P, Azzolini M, Airaghi P, Radice P, De Molfetta V. Effect of decreasing surface and interface irregularities after photorefractive keratectomy and laser in situ keratomileusis on optical and functional outcomes. *J Refract Surg.* 1998a;14:S199-S203.
109. Vinciguerra P, Azzolini M, Airaghi P, Radice P, Sborgia M, De Molfetta V. A method for examining surface and interface irregularities after photorefractive keratectomy and laser in situ keratomileusis: predictor of optical and functional outcomes. *J Refract Surg.* 1998b;14:S204-S206.
110. Vigo L, Scandola E, Carones F. Scraping and mitomycin C to treat haze and regression after photorefractive keratectomy for myopia. *J Refract Surg.* 2003;19(4):449-454.
111. Kornmehl EW, Steinert RF, Puliafito CA. A comparative study of masking fluids for excimer laser phototherapeutic keratectomy. *Arch Ophthalmol.* 1991;109:860-863.
112. Pallikaris IG, Naoumidi II, Kalyvianaki MI, Katsanevaki VJ. Epi-LASIK: comparative histological evaluation of mechanical and alcohol-assisted epithelial separation. *J Cataract Refract Surg.* 2003;29:1496-1501.
113. Csutak A, Tozser J, Bekesi L, et al. Plasminogen activator activity in tears after excimer laser photorefractive keratectomy. *Invest Ophthalmol Vis Sci.* 2000;41:3743-3747.
114. Lohmann CP, Marshall J. Plasmin- and plasminogen-activator inhibitors after excimer laser photorefractive keratectomy: new concept in prevention of postoperative myopic regression and haze. *Refract Corneal Surg.* 1993;9(4):300-302.
115. Kim T, Pak JH, Lee SY, Tchah H. Mitomycin c-induced reduction of keratocytes and fibroblasts after photorefractive keratectomy. *Invest Ophthalmol Vis Sci.* 2004;45:2978-2984.
116. Serrao S, Lombardo M, Mondini F. Photorefractive keratectomy with and without smoothing: a bilateral study. *J Refract Surg.* 2003;19:58-64.
117. Wilson SE, Mohan RR, Hong J-W, et al. The wound healing response after laser in situ keratomileusis and photorefractive keratectomy. *Arch Ophthalmol.* 2001;119:889-896.
118. Wilson SE. Analysis of the keratocyte apoptosis, keratocyte proliferation, and myofibroblast transformation responses after photorefractive keratectomy and laser in situ keratomileusis. *Trans Am Ophthalmol Soc.* 2002;100:411-433.
119. Horgan SE, McLaughlin-Borlace L, Stevens JD, Munro PMG. Phototherapeutic smoothing as an adjunct to photorefractive keratectomy in porcine corneas. *J Refract Surg.* 1999;15:331-333.
120. Lombardo M, Serrao S. Smoothing of the ablated porcine anterior corneal surface using the Technolas Keracor 217C and NIDEK EC-5000 excimer lasers. *J Refract Surg.* 2004;20:450-453.

SECTION II

General Principles

CHAPTER 7

GENERAL PRINCIPLES IN SURFACE ABLATION

*Paolo Vinciguerra, MD; Fabrizio I. Camesasca, MD;
Maria Ingrid Torres Munoz, MD*

Surface Ablation: Predictability, Regularity, and Smoothing

Although the first clinical application of excimer laser refractive surgery dates back to Trokel in 1985, and its use and technology have tremendously expanded since then, it is well-known among refractive surgeons that final refractive results may still be quite different from those planned. Until recently, the unpredictability of the corneal stromal and epithelial reparatory response was considered the main culprit for this phenomenon. Irregularities of the ablated corneal surface have been proven to play an important role in enhancing collagen deposition and, therefore, variation from the planned refractive result. On the contrary, a smooth ablated surface induces less reparatory response, leading to a lower degree of haze formation and unpredictability of refractive result.[1-5]

In 1990, when we first began our studies on excimer laser ablation, with the Meditech laser, the ablation was obtained by inserting discs of progressively smaller diameter in a steel cylinder. Step height was 8 µm. When the 99-step mechanical diaphragm was introduced and the ablation step height was decreased to 5 µm, we noted a reduction in regression and haze. During those years, a regression of 2.0 to 3.0 D was commonly regarded as tolerable. Another major improvement was observed when excimer laser with ablation steps of 0.30 to 0.25 µm (ie, Summit and VISX models) became available. From then on, greater attention was devoted to ablation step height reduction.

In the 1990s, we noticed that haze always ensued, even after a PRK of just 3.0 D, occasionally with relevant regression even with prolonged steroid therapy. On the contrary, after PTK—at the time performed with methycellulose since no masking fluid was currently available—no haze was observed. A 100-µm ablation with PTK did not induce haze, while a 30-µm PRK did. The idea of somehow introducing this PTK advantage to PRK was born. The main difference we observed at the end of ablation was that the PTK surface was smooth, while the PRK surface was always rougher. Another detail could be noted: while preoperatively PTK patients with profoundly deformed surfaces had very poor vision, immediately after surgery, their vision improved considerably, even with correction. On the contrary, PRK patients had good BSCVA preoperatively, but postoperatively, 10 to 15 days were necessary to achieve good vision.

Moreover, while in PRK the ablation border always showed a marked change in curvature—high curvature gradient—PTK eyes showed topographically normal peripheral corneal curvatures.

Thus, in the early 1990s, we decided to introduce the PTK ablation pattern in the most frustrating cases, PRKs for high myopia, almost constantly associated with marked regression and haze. In these cases, the well-known possible hypercorrection-related hyperopic shift of PTK would have been an advantage to minimize the expected marked regression. We used methylcellulose, laminated in a thin layer and applied a 5-mm wide (the widest available diameter) 10-µm ablation. To our great surprise, patients had better immediate vision, and in the first month, hyperopic shift was less than usual; haze was still present but much less than usual, and refraction was much more stable. Since then, we have introduced and progressively improved smoothing in the final phase of refractive surgery.[3,4]

Besides microscopic reduction of irregularities, smoothing provides an important macroscopic aid in regularizing the border of the ablated cornea where it connects to normal, unoperated corneal curvature. Essentially, smoothing can be seen as a microtransition between the steps of the amphitheater-like multi-zone ablation pattern. Even with flying spot lasers, which in any case induce a curvature gradient between center and periphery of the ablation, smoothing makes the transition between zones of different dioptric power more progressive. Finally, we observed a more rapid re-epithelialization rate for eyes in which smoothing was performed, decreasing from 7 to 10 days to 3 to 5 days. This is easily understandable, since the epithelial cells did not have relevant micro-irregularities to fill after smoothing and were able to cover the stromal surface more rapidly.

A revolutionary approach to the problem of unpredictability has been introduced by Cynthia Roberts with the concept of corneal biomechanical response to laser ablation (see Chapter 6).[6] The concept is based on the anatomical lamellar structure of the corneal stroma and on its tensile strength: central severing of lamellae due to creation of a new refractive surface by excimer laser tissue removal causes elastic contraction of the remaining peripheral lamellae, with consequent corneal curvature variation. This consists in peripheral corneal increase in curvature and thickness and in central flattening, leading to refractive change just where the curvature was carefully modified to achieve a planned power.

A delicate point in the creation of a new surface with excimer laser ablation is the transition zone (TZ). In this portion of the ablation, the new central curvature must be connected with the unchanged peripheral corneal curvature. In both stromal and surface ablation, marked variation of curvature in this peripheral portion leads to a response which aims to reduce curvature variation but which may induce regression and restriction of the effective OZ. The smoothing technique presently adopted to remove corneal microirregularities of a size inferior to the spot size (0.89 mm) and to the height of ablation (0.25 µm), in state-of-the-art surface ablation, whether it is PRK, LASEK, or Epi-LASIK, is described in detail in Chapter 8.

Surface Ablation and Corneal Curvature Gradient

In this chapter, we deem it necessary to define the anatomical and functional concepts of ablation zone (AZ) and optical zone (OZ) size. AZ size is the diameter of the corneal area where the tissue has been ablated for optical purposes. In topography, it is closest to the instantaneous algorithm analysis, which defines the borders of the ablation and the so-called "red ring" (Figure 7-1). The "red ring" is the change of curvature between the treated and the untreated cornea and is visible only in the instantaneous (tangential) or elevation map. OZ size is the optical diameter of the zone of achieved correction calculated according to the Snellen formula. In topography, it is closest to the axial algorithm analysis that defines the refractive results of the ablation.

The history of excimer laser ablation for refractive surgery shows a progressive increase in the diameter of the OZ, from 3 mm with Summit lasers to the presently available 6 to 7 mm. In recent years, after recognition of the importance of

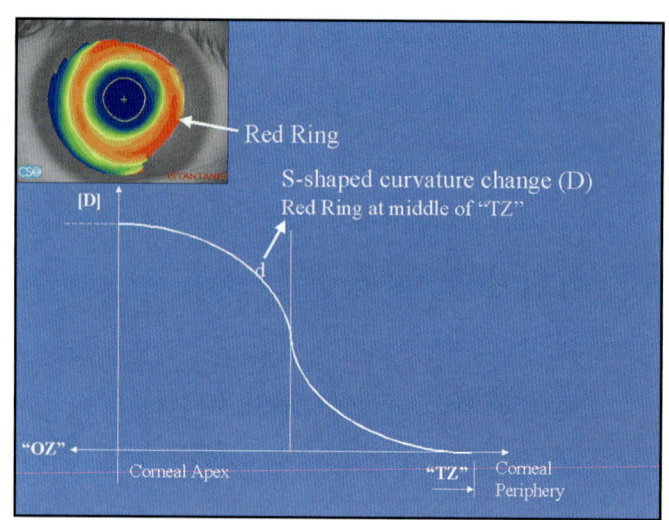

Figure 7-1. Topography and curve showing induced curvature change (D) from corneal center to periphery (corneal curvature gradient), conventional ablation. On topography, note the "red ring" in the middle of the transition zone (TZ).

the scotopic pupil diameter in the generation of visual disturbances at night after excimer laser refractive surgery, the ideal diameter of the OZ has been defined as corresponding to the maximal scotopic pupil diameter. Actually, despite the apparent soundness of this approach, even patients today may occasionally complain of night vision disturbances with halos and ghosting. The recent introduction of aberrometric analysis in refractive surgery has provided a useful insight into the problem. The importance of the corneal curvature gradient has been highlighted: a marked postoperative increase in corneal curvature from the center to the periphery (eg, 38.0 D at 6 mm and 55.0 D at 7 mm visible in tangential algorithm topography) may determine major vision disturbances (see Figure 7-1). This curvature variation is clearly highlighted by the "red ring" visible in tangential topographical maps as well as in aberrometric maps, indicating the presence of a markedly high spherical aberration (SA). High SA always generates a restriction of the functionally useful OZ, even when the set AZ is equal to the pupil diameter; thus, corneal curvature gradient and SA must be contained if a wide OZ is our target.

An ablation minimizing the corneal curvature gradient will induce less visual disturbances. Figure 7-2 shows a case in which the AZ was not very wide (5 mm), but the TZ has been increased to 10 mm. Such a choice provides several advantages, such as less tissue removal, less sensitivity to decentration, as well as to pupil diameter change. The above-mentioned goal of achieving the widest possible OZ is in apparent contrast with this relatively small OZ approach, but careful observation of the tangential map shows that the central cornea has a more constant and wider curvature. The topography map shows that the corneal curvature increase from center to periphery is limited and constant. These features correspond to a functionally wider OZ, with low SA values. The main conclusion is that the TZ has a relevant optical function.

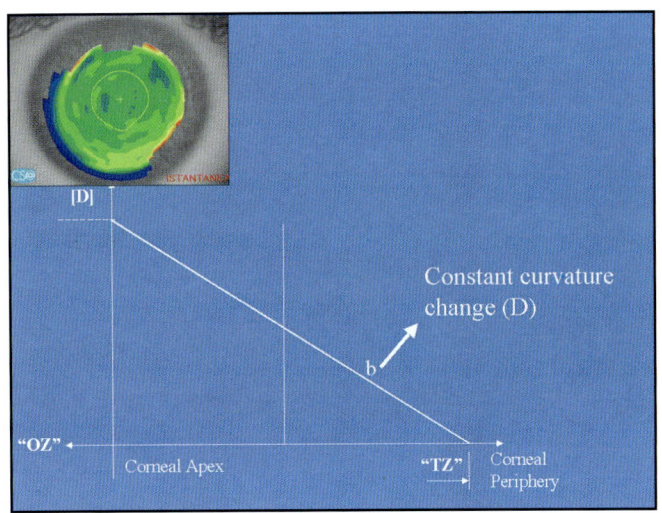

Figure 7-2. Topography and curve showing induced curvature change (Δ) from corneal center to periphery (corneal curvature gradient), ideal ablation. Note no "red ring" on topography.

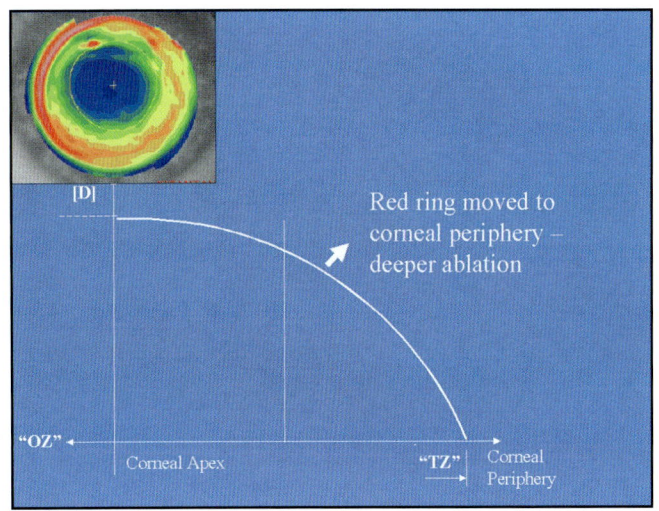

Figure 7-3. Topography and curve showing induced curvature change (Δ) from corneal center to periphery (corneal curvature gradient) in an ablation scheme aimed at widening the OZ and pushing the "red ring" as peripherally as possible. This scheme will ablate more deeply.

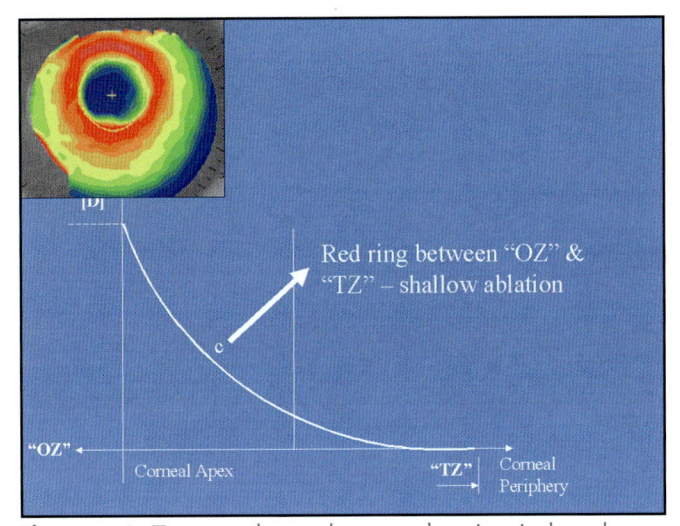

Figure 7-4. Topography and curve showing induced curvature change (D) from corneal center to periphery (corneal curvature gradient) in an ablation scheme aimed at restricting the OZ and pushing the "red ring" as centrally as possible. This scheme will save corneal tissue, requiring a shallow ablation.

Figures 7-3 and 7-4 show two opposite, extreme situations, in which the "red ring" has been pushed, respectively, as far peripherally as possible or as central as possible. These two extremes require profoundly different amounts of ablation, as well as induce different aberrations. A small OZ with red ring close to the center will require a limited ablation but will induce marked SA. A wide OZ with peripheral red ring will require use of much more tissue and will induce limited aberrations.

It must also be remembered that the center of the pupil often does not correspond with the corneal apex. Centering the ablation on the pupil or on the visual axis, as many current eye-tracking systems permit, implies that ablation-induced corneal tissue removal is nasally decentered, as this often happens if the pupil is decentered nasally. Usually, the ablation border induces a curvature variation visible in the tangential map as a red ring. With a decentered pupil and ablation, the nasal portion of this ring is located in the extreme corneal periphery, where the physiological curvature is low. Thus an ablation-induced 10.0-to 5.0-D change does not lead to a major increase in SA. On the contrary, the temporal portion of the ring will be located closer to the corneal apex in a region with higher corneal curvature, leading to a greater and optically more irritating change in the corneal curvature. The NIDEK Final Fit Software (Gamagori, Japan) that we use for custom ablations permits definition of the center-to-periphery corneal curvature variation. This provides a full range of possibilities from linear, gradual change in the curvature from center, to periphery, to total curvature variation concentrated in the extreme corneal periphery (see Figures 7-1 to 7-4).[7]

This opportunity is particularly useful in retreatments, providing the possibility of curvature change exactly where it is more useful, as is highlighted in Chapter 30. That is, when overcorrection has occurred during hyperopic ablation, the compensatory myopic ablation can be concentrated close to the corneal center, since this will lead to a consequent paracentral increase in curvature and widen the useful OZ. On the contrary, concentration of corneal curvature variation in the extreme periphery could be exceedingly useful when retreating undercorrected myopia to move SA as far as possible from the corneal center. The importance of SA in excimer laser refractive surgery is highlighted in Figures 7-5 and 7-6, showing corneal wavefront after a myopic ablation, with high corneal curvature gradient between corneal center and periphery. Note the marked SA and its resemblance in location with the "red ring" on instantaneous topography. If SA is subtracted from the wavefront, this shows substantial improvement.

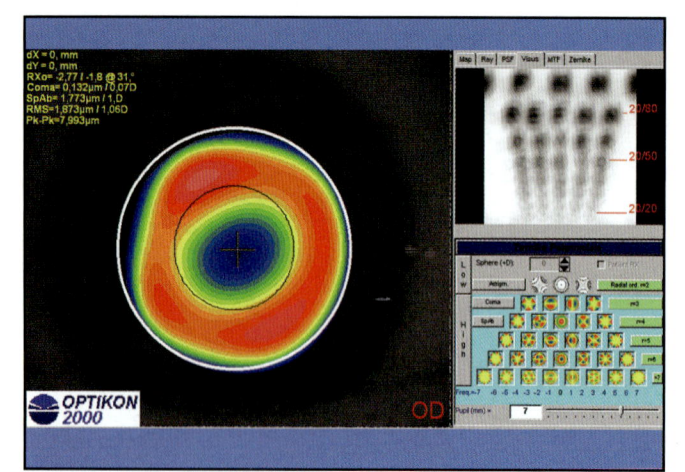

Figure 7-5. Importance of SA on corneal wavefront. Corneal wavefront after a myopic ablation, with high corneal curvature gradient between corneal center and periphery. Note the high SA, and its resemblance in location with the "red ring" on instantaneous topography.

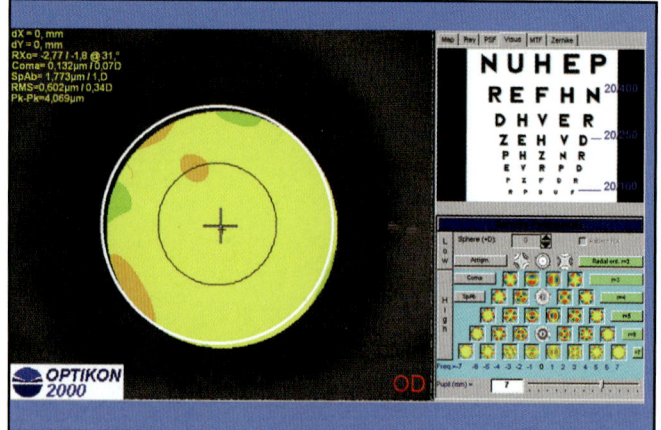

Figure 7-6. Same eye of Figure 7-5. SA has been subtracted from the wavefront (bottom left scheme, SA is deselected). Wavefront is substantially improved.

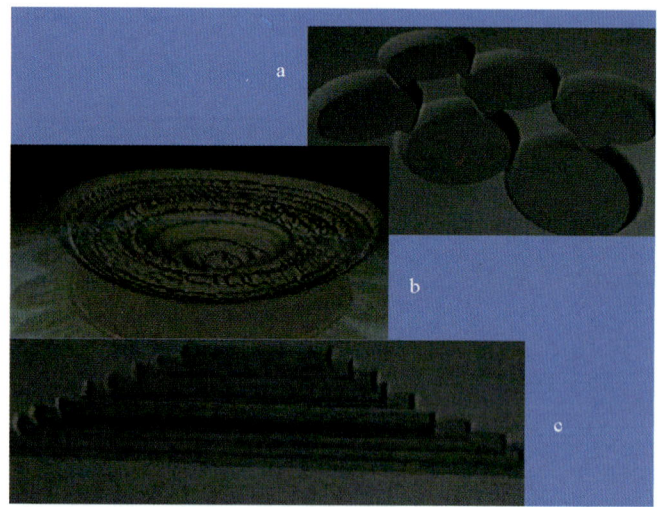

Figure 7-7. Surface irregularities generated by overlapping of different types of excimer laser ablations: (a) flying spot; (b) broad beam; (c) scanning slit.

Due to the ablation patterns of the different excimer lasers, as well as to the overlapping of the spots, any corneal ablation generates a surface with a certain number of micro-irregularities (Figure 7-7). Avoiding an increase in aberrations after refractive surgery is a difficult goal, and corneal irregularities induced by excimer ablation may cause aberrations, mostly relevant in scotopic conditions.[8] When high refractive defects are corrected, required ablations will be deep and will induce more irregularities, and it is assumed that the predictability of correction is inversely related to the level of refractive defect corrected. These irregularities may be macroscopic (ie, related to the centration and shape of ablation—rough or steep ablation margins—and induce mostly coma and SA) or microscopic, related to microirregularities of the ablated cornea, inducing high-order aberrations.

In surface ablation, the epithelium attempts to solve these macro-and microirregularities through several layers of epithelial cells and/or collagen deposition.[1,3,4,9] Collagen deposition may lead to postoperative haze. Marked variation of curvature in the peripheral portion of the ablation also leads to collagen deposition, a phenomenon that reduces this curvature variation but induces regression. These phenomena reduce the predictability of the imparted correction.

In LASIK, the corneal flap covers and thus solves the stromal microirregularities present after ablation. However, it may not be able to follow all the ablation-generated macroirregularities of the stromal bed, since this "blanket effect" may be reduced by markedly elevated stromal bed irregularity "peaks." Epithelial hyperplasia will then occur, with reduction of refractive predictability and regression. Large epithelial profile changes after LASIK have been demonstrated using a three-dimensional, very high-frequency digital ultrasound scanning system.[10] However, the simple LASIK flap creation changes the corneal wavefront (Figures 7-8 and 7-9) differently from creation of an epithelial flap, such as in LASEK and Epi-LASIK (Figure 7-10). It is our impression that marked variation of curvature in the peripheral portion of the ablation could thus lead to regression.

The observation of an increase in peripheral corneal steepness and thickness following central corneal flattening for myopic treatments prompted Cynthia Roberts to develop a theory on the influence of corneal biomechanical properties on refractive results after surface or stromal surgery.[6, 11]

This increase in steepness and thickness extends well beyond the ablated cornea and thus appears to be not entirely related to simple laser tissue subtraction. The biomechanical theory suggests that the central severing of elastic corneal lamellae following surface or stromal surgery may induce relaxation of the peripheral residual lamellae, with decompression of the extracellular matrix and an increase in curvature and thickness of peripheral stroma. This apparently results in tangential traction forces on the underlying lamellae, which in the central cornea, constitute the postoperative corneal surface, resulting in a central flattening not related

General Principles in Surface Ablation 79

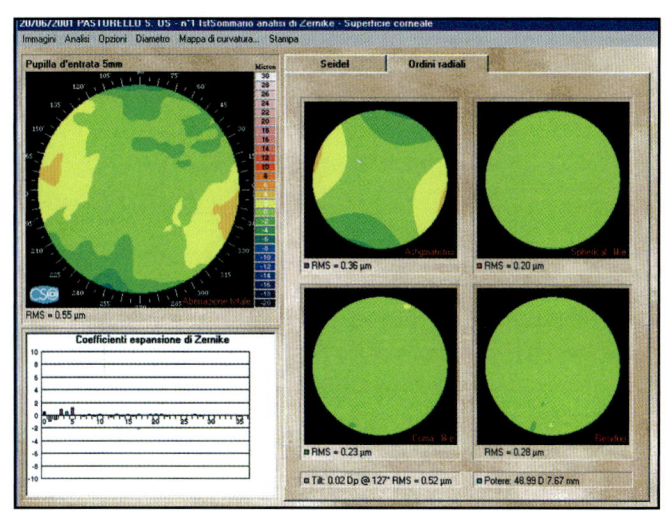

Figure 7-8. Intraoperative corneal wavefront before LASIK flap creation.

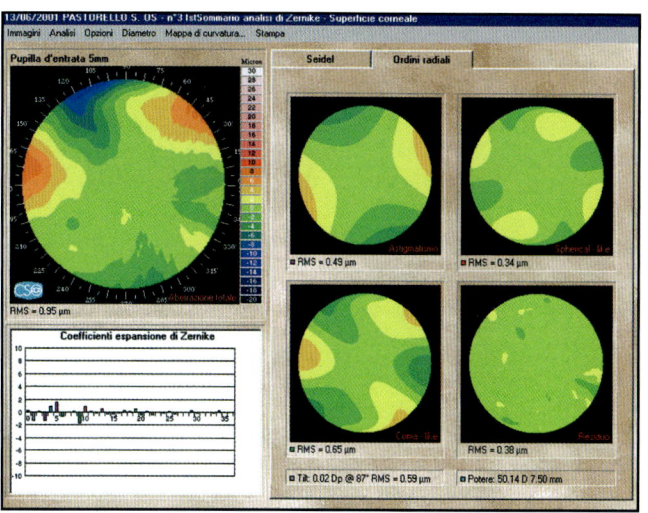

Figure 7-9. Intraoperative corneal wavefront after LASIK flap creation. High-order aberrations are induced.

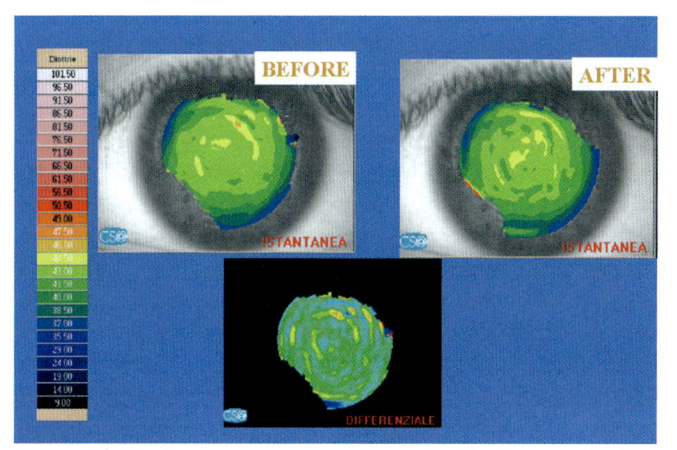

Figure 7-10. Instantaneous topography before and after creation of an epithelial flap with irrelevant induced corneal curvature changes.

to the ablation profile. This would lead to a hyperopic shift. Results will thus be increased in myopic treatments, while they will be decreased in hyperopic ones. This phenomenon will be more marked in LASIK, where the number of severed lamellae is tenfold that of PRK (see Chapter 6).[6]

In a previous study, we tried to overcome unpredictability connected with microirregularity and corneal biomechanics in several ways. Information on surface and total aberrometry provided in photopic, scotopic, and mesopic conditions by the NIDEK OPD integrated aberrometer, refractometer, topographer, and pupillometer, was integrated using the Final Fit software to provide a complete aberrometric optimization of the ablated corneal profile. The CATZ ablation pattern of the Final Fit imparts a refractive change in which all total OPD-detected ocular aberrations, and particularly SA, are optimized in the central 4.5 mm.[7,13] The curvature of the remaining cornea was then gradually modified in order to achieve a constant curvature gradient up to the external 10-mm margin of the ablation, at the same time maintaining the best possible reduction of ocular aberrations. The central 4.5-mm area of ablation must not be confused with an OZ. An advanced use of Final Fit was adopted for custom ablation in these cases. The segmental ablation for treatment of high-order components was applied first. This part of the treatment may change the axis and power of the cylinder, and thus at this point, the new axis and power of astigmatism were estimated. Finally, the resulting spherical component to be treated was calculated.

This surgical method adopted in this study offers several advantages. LASEK epithelial flap creation generated no biomechanical effect, as can be seen by the irrelevant curvature changes detected by comparing corneal topography pre- and postflap creation (Figure 7-10). The amount of tissue removed by the excimer ablation was limited, even with a wide final TZ diameter, and it was distributed all over most of the corneal surface, reducing the actual biomechanical effect. In LASIK, the actual induced biomechanical effect is hard to estimate, unless the ablative procedure is performed several days after flap creation once corneal curvature is stable. Moreover, in LASIK it may be hard to achieve a consistent flap thickness and diameter, and there may thus be a varying biomechanical effect.

In our LASEK cases, the final corneal curvature gradient was constant, as can be observed from an almost monochromatic postoperative topographic map on the axial algorithm, with an effective OZ much wider than the above-mentioned 4.5 mm, as well as a general containment of aberration increase (Figure 7-11). In routine myopic ablations, the sudden and marked variation in the corneal curvature gradient between central treated and peripheral untreated cornea is expressed topographically by a red ring visible on instantaneous algorithm, as well as by the aberrometric red ring of SA. With Final Fit, the corneal curvature gradient from center to periphery is reduced, and made more gradual. The gradient is positioned in the extreme periphery, beyond 9 mm, where the cornea is thicker and flatter. The topographical red ring will appear to be limited in width and diopter intensity, thus not actually red but in paler colors as well as being located very

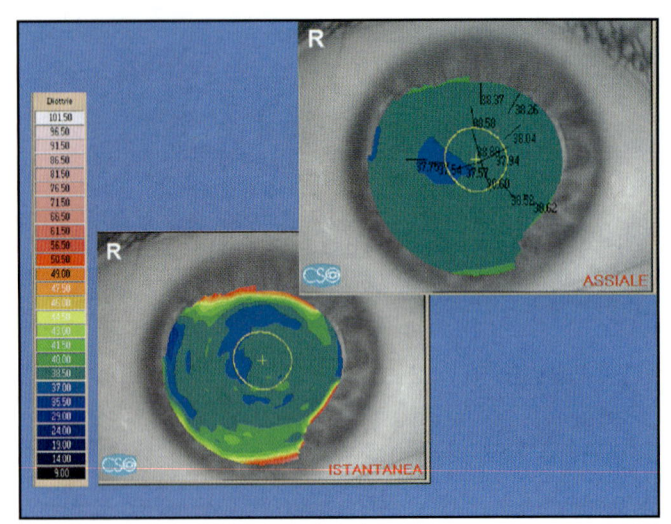

Figure 7-11. Corneal topography of a LASEK case, axial and instantaneous algorithm.

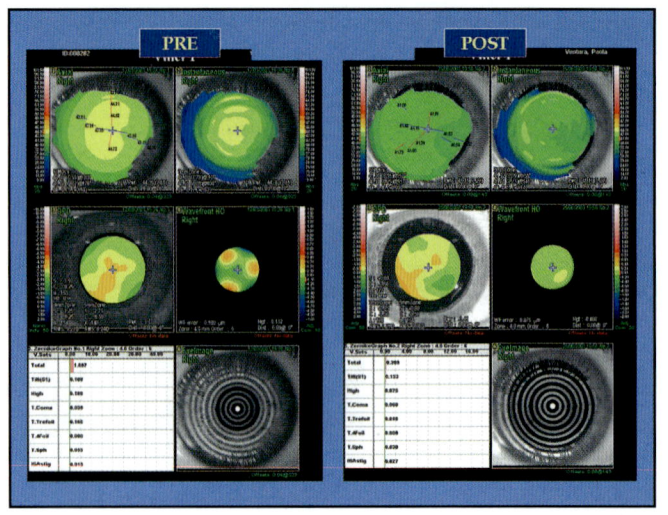

Figure 7-12. Pre- and postcustom ablation topography as well as aberrometry maps after custom ablation and smoothing.

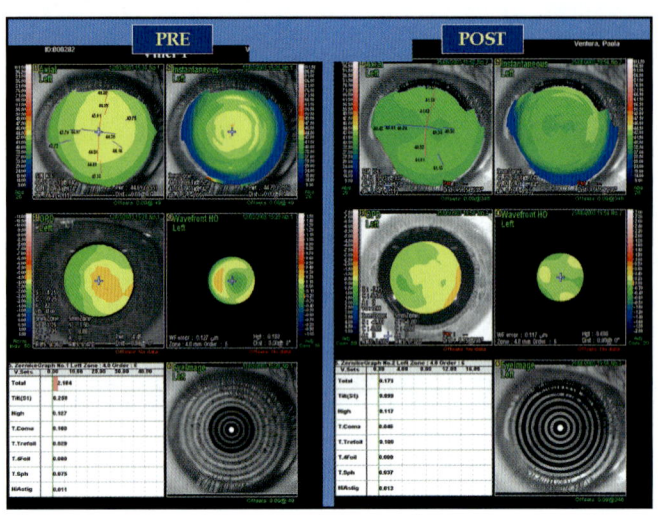

Figure 7-13. Another case of pre- and postcustom ablation topography, as well as aberrometry maps after custom ablation and smoothing.

peripherally. Furthermore, SA will be reduced, providing excellent vision quality even with dilated pupils. This strategy will make determination of pupil diameter less critical: at the corneal diameter corresponding to mesopic pupil—4 to 7 mm—the corneal curvature change will be constant with reduced aberrations for the incoming light.

In this study, surface aberrations were calculated up to the sixth order, when aberrations are usually considered only up to the fourth order. Surface aberrations at 1 year showed no substantial increase up to 5-mm pupils, but in the case of SA, they remained stable for 3-mm pupils and increased by 52.6% in value for 5-mm pupils.[12] Figures 7-12 and 7-13 show two such cases. These results were in accord with our previous studies.[14-17]

Conventional LASIK surgery increases total ocular aberrations.[8,18,19] To our knowledge, reports on wavefront-guided customized LASIK treatments on previously untreated eyes do not show change in postoperative higher-order aberrations in a predictable or reproducible fashion or show reduction of spherical-like aberrations or insignificant changes for dilated pupil after surgery.[20,21] In an interesting report, Yul et al compared the higher-order aberrations in 19 patients who underwent LASEK, without smoothing, using a conventional OZ in one eye and a larger zone with a blend zone in the fellow eye.[22] Refractive results at 3 months were comparable between the two groups. Higher-order aberrations increased at 1 and 3 months in both eyes compared with the preoperative situation. At 3 months, in the scotopic condition, higher-order aberrations after LASEK using a large OZ with blend zone ablation were smaller than those associated with conventional AZ treatment.

Concerning the ablation surface quality, in a previous study, one of the authors (PV) presented a method for examining surface and interface irregularities after refractive surgery, examining the quality of light transmitted through the cornea. This study showed a direct relationship between the immediate amount of postsurgical stromal surface irregularity and the 1-year haze and loss of one or more lines of visual acuity.[3,23,24] From this observation, a quest for better refractive surface regularization began, leading to the adoption of PTK-style smoothing as the final step of refractive laser surgery. In another study, we evaluated the results of smoothing on optical and functional outcomes.[4] Digitized retroillumination photography was used to grade the ablated surface (PRK eyes) or interface (LASIK eyes) according to a three-grade roughness scale. Eyes with grade 2 (mild) and 3 (severe) irregularity were randomized to PTK-style corneal smoothing or no smoothing. Eighteen months later, statistical evaluation of results showed less haze and better visual acuity in the eyes that received smoothing. Apparently, smoothing at the end of surgery provided a regular stromal bed for the corneal epithelium, reducing collagen deposition as well as haze formation with consequent possible reduction of imparted correction.[4] These results were confirmed by further PRK and LASEK studies.[17,25,26] Later on, Serrao et al. demonstrated that PRK plus smoothing lead to faster epithelial closure, better visual outcome, and less haze than simple PRK.[24,27]

The positive results of LASEK surgery reported in this study are comparable with those of other LASEK studies evaluating large numbers of eyes.[28-31] In particular, in the studies by Shahinian and Anderson, where LASEK was applied to highly myopic eyes, results appear to be similar, and no significant corneal haze was observed at the 1 year control.[29,30]

Conclusions

After the introduction of LASIK, surface refractive surgery has attracted less interest due to observed regression, haze, and postoperative pain. However, due to possible variations in flap size and thickness, the biomechanical factor at play in LASIK may render custom ablation less predictable as well as make containment of induction of aberrations less effective. The risk of late-onset postoperative corneal ectasia remains a rare but troublesome possibility.[33]

Surface refractive surgery remains an interesting option because it offers advantages such as a wider range of refractive correction and easier retreatments due to the contained stromal tissue ablation maintained. Apparently, the problem of regression can now to be solved by a different handling of the TZ and a better understanding of the biomechanical forces at play in the cornea. Creating a regular postoperative surface with smoothing can contain haze formation.

References

1. Huang D, Tang M, Shekhar R. Mathematical model of corneal surface smoothing after refractive surgery. *Am J Ophthalmol.* 2003;135:267-278.
2. Balestrazzi E, De Molfetta V, Spadea L, et al. Histological, immunohistochemical, and ultrastructural findings in humans corneas after photorefractive keratectomy. *J Refract Surg.* 1995;11:181-187.
3. Vinciguerra P, Azzolini M, Radice P, et al. A method for examining surface and interface irregularities after photorefractive keratectomy and laser in situ keratomileusis: predictor of optical and functional outcomes. *J Refract Surg.* 1998;14:S204-206.
4. Vinciguerra P, Azzolini M, Airaghi P, et al. Effect of decreasing surface and interface irregularities after photorefractive keratectomy and laser in situ keratomileusis on optical and functional outcomes. *J Refract Surg.* 1998;14:S199-S203.
5. Netto MV, Mohan RR, Sinha S, Sharma A, Wilson SE. Stromal haze, myofibroblasts, and surface irregularity after PRK. *Exp Eye Res.* 2005, 19 (on press).
6. Roberts C. Biomechanics of the cornea and wavefront-guided laser refractive surgery. *J Refract Surg.* 2002;18:S589-592.
7. Pop M, Bains HS. Clinical outcomes of CATz versus OPDCAT. *J Refract Surg.* 2005; 21:S636-639.
8. Oshika T, Klyce SD, Applegate AR, et al. Comparison of corneal wavefront aberrations after photorefractive keratectomy and laser in situ keratomileusis. *Am J Ophthalmol.* 1999; 127:1-7.
9. Netto MV, Wilson SE. Corneal wound healing relevance to wavefront-guided laser treatments. *Ophthalmol Clin North Am.* 2004;17(2):225-231.
10. Reinstein DZ, Silverman RH, Raevsky T, et al. Arc-scanning very high-frequency digital ultrasound for 3D pachymetric mapping of the corneal epithelium and stroma in laser in situ keratomileusis. *J Refract Surg.* 2000;16:414-430.
11. Qazi MA, Roberts CJ, Mahmoud AM, Pepose JS. Topographic and biomechanical differences between hyperopic and myopic laser in situ keratomileusis. *J Cataract Refract Surg.* 2005;31(1):48-60.
12. Vinciguerra P, Camesasca FI, Torres MI. One-year results of custom laser epithelial keratomileusis with the NIDEK system. *J Refract Surg.* 2004;20:S699-704.
13. Pieger S. Pearls, tips, and tricks for use of the NIDEK OPD-Scan and Final Fit software. *J Refract Surg.* 2004;20:S741-746.
14. Vinciguerra P, Camesasca FI, Urso R. Reduction of spherical aberration with the NIDEK NAVEX customized ablation system. *J Refract Surg.* 2003;19:S195-S201.
15. Vinciguerra P, Torres Munoz MI, Camesasca FI. Reduction of spherical aberration: Experimental model of photoablation. *J Refract Surg.* 2002;18:S366-370.
16. Vinciguerra P, Camesasca FI. Butterfly laser epithelial keratomileusis for myopia. *J Refract Surg.* 2002;18:S371-373.
17. Vinciguerra P, Camesasca FI, Randazzo A. One-year results of butterfly laser epithelial keratomileusis. *J Refract Surg.* 2003;19:S223-226.
18. Marcos S, Barbero S, Llorente L, Merayo-Lloves J. Optical response to LASIK surgery for myopia from total and corneal aberration measurements. *Invest Ophthalmol Vis Sci.* 2001;42:3349-3356.
19. Marcos S. Aberrations and visual performance following standard laser vision correction. *J Refract Surg.* 2001;17:S596-601.
20. Gimbel HV, Sofinski SJ, Mahler OS, et al. Primary multipoint (segmental) custom ablation. *J Refract Surg.* 2003;19:S202-208.
21. Sarkisian KA, Petrov AA. Clinical experience with the customized low spherical aberration ablation profile for myopia. *J Refract Surg.* 2002; 18:S352-356.
22. Yul SK, Bum LJ, Jaeyoung KJ, et al. Comparison of higher-order aberrations after LASEK with a 6.0 mm ablation zone and a 6.5 mm ablation zone with blend zone. *J Cataract Refract Surg.* 2004;30:653-657.
23. Vinciguerra P, Camesasca FI, Torres IM. Transition zone design and smoothing in custom laser assisted subepithelial keratectomy. *J Cataract Refract Surg.* 2005;31:39-47.
24. Serrao S, Lombardo M. Corneal epithelial healing after photorefractive keratectomy: analytical study. *J Cataract Refract Surg.* 2005;31:930-937.
25. Vinciguerra P, Torres I, Camesasca FI. Applications of confocal microscopy in refractive surgery. *J Refract Surg.* 2002;18:S378-381
26. Vinciguerra P, Camesasca FI. Treatment of hyperopia: a new ablation profile to reduce corneal eccentricity. *J Refract Surg.* 2002;18:S315-317
27. Serrao S, Lombardo M, Mondini F. Photorefractive keratectomy with and without smoothing: a bilateral study. *J Refract Surg.* 2003;19:58-64.
28. Autrata R, Rehurek J. Laser-assisted subepithelial keratectomy for myopia: two-year follow up. *J Cataract Refract Surg.* 2003;29:661-668.
29. Shahinian L Jr. Laser-assisted subepithelial keratectomy for low to high myopia and astigmatism. *J Cataract Refract Surg.* 2002;28:1334-1342.
30. Anderson NJ, Beran RF, Schneider TL. Epi-LASEK for the correction of myopia and myopic astigmatism. *J Cataract Refract Surg.* 2002; 28:1343-1347
31. Claringbold TV. Laser-assisted subepithelial keratectomy for the correction of myopia. *J Cataract Refract Surg.* 2002;28:18-22.
32. Dogru M, Katami C, Yamanaka A. Refractive changes after excimer laser phototherapeutic keratectomy. *J Cataract Refract Surg.* 2001;27:686-692.
33. Wang Z, Chen J, Yang B. Posterior corneal surface topographic changes after Laser In Situ Keratomileusis are related to residual corneal bed thickness. *Ophthalmology.* 1999;106:406-410.

CHAPTER 8

SMOOTHING IN EXCIMER REFRACTIVE SURGERY

Paolo Vinciguerra, MD; Fabrizio I. Camesasca, MD

The Quest for a Regular Ablated Surface

A cornerstone of refractive surgery is the concept that corneal regularity is more important than its transparency. This can be easily clarified with an example. A window pane is transparent and raindrops on it are also transparent; however, a window pane covered with raindrops, even if transparent, does not permit good vision quality because of its lack of uniformity. Sunglasses, on the contrary, are not totally transparent, yet they permit good vision quality because of their regularity.

Refractive surgery may lead to inconstant results. Anatomo-functional (visual acuity, postoperative refraction, haze) as well as comfort (contrast sensitivity, night halos, glare) problems may be responsible for unreliable results. Several factors can be related to these problems: the patient, the instruments used, the set parameters, and the postoperative treatment. Patient-related causes are mainly connected to the corneal reparative response elicited by excimer ablation. Healing may be more or less exuberant in relation to patient's age (the reaction in younger patients is greater) or to the presence of previously undetected systemic diseases (diabetes may hinder re-epithelialization, a tendency to develop hyperplastic scars may lead to corneal stromal tissue hyperplasia, etc). Adequate tearing is another important factor, mandatory for a proper epithelial distribution in a laminar pattern.

Different types of excimer lasers have a different influence on the final result according to their beams and ablation geometry. Each ablation pattern induces a moderate surface irregularity, resulting from the overlap of each laser spot. No currently available laser beam, even if regularly positioned in a side-to-side manner, is capable of perfectly filling a surface without leaving small, unexposed areas.

Irregularities are, in part, related to the features of the excimer ablating beam and to intraoperative eye motion. Ocular motion may induce steep margins in a multi-step ablation—when concentricity is lost—and irregularities due to more or less prolonged loss of fixation as well as small irregularities related to saccadic eye motions. Even today, with excellent eyetrackers available, a certain amount of irregularity is induced, and extreme smoothness of ablation remains a distant goal.

The ablating beam may induce focal irregularities when homogeneity is scarce. Broad beam lasers, using repeated circular ablations with progressively decreasing diameters induce amphitheater-like ablation with concentric steps. Scanning slit beam lasers produce parallel ablations creating a fenestrated pattern with steps that can be particularly magnified by sudden eye movements. Flying spot lasers act by randomized ablation with a diameter ranging from 0.8 to 2 mm and may induce a fine granular, "beaten metal" pattern of irregularities by partial overlapping of small circular spots (see Figure 7-7).

In LASIK eyes, suboptimal flap overlap leads to changes in the interface with an inferior optical result and increase of the normal inflammatory response. The biological result of this irregularity is an increase of the inflammatory response with higher probability of haze and regression. Different ablation diameters as well as the presence and size of transition zones may also influence the final result. In LASIK, the microkeratome plays a relevant role related to factors such as plate stability, speed and sharpness of the blade, as well as quality, quantity, and stability of suction.

Furthermore, an extremely important factor for successful photoablation is the creation of a regular corneal profile without sharp and abrupt changes in curvature. These irregular curvature changes may induce an excessive reparative response with increased deposition of collagen and, possibly, reduction of the desired refractive effect. It is a well-known fact that treating low-grade ametropias leads to more constant results, while regular corneal profiles are hard to attain when correcting high ametropias. This observation leads us to assume the presence of a small error at each ablation that, when repeated a number of times, induces a substantial total level of error.

Finally, postoperative treatment may influence the course of refraction and haze. Several studies have taken into account all these factors and verified their possible influence, unfortunately, without a completely convincing explanation of the above-mentioned lack of reliability of the results. The search for improved reliability is currently spurring the development and application of custom ablation.

Looking for possible answers, we devoted our attention to the quality of the ablation surface.[1] Following corneal disepithelialization, refractive surgeons can observe the regular surface of the Bowman membrane. It features a continuous, mirror-like surface without macro- and microirregularities. Theoretically, perfect ablation should recreate this regular surface, while inducing a different profile of curvature. Loss of transparency, sudden changes in curvature, and surface irregularities all diffract light rays and decrease vision quality.

Evaluation of the Ablated Surface

Prompted by these observations, we decided to study surface qualities that may lead to a better result both in the immediate postoperative period and intraoperatively. Initially, we examined corneal surfaces with slit lamp, a method that unfortunately highlights only major irregularities.

The use of digitalized retroillumination with the Scheimpflug camera provided us with a better understanding of the corneal surface and its properties.[1] The Scheimpflug camera is a photographic system that provides a global analysis of the ablation surface both superficially as well as at stromal interface level. Digitalized retroillumination is attained through illumination of the ocular fundus, and the red reflex is used to examine the cornea illuminated from inside the eye when dioptric media are transparent. Figure 8-1 shows a simplified scheme of digitalized retroillumination with the Scheimpflug camera. With this device, we can obtain a representation of the ablated surface highlighting not only corneal opacities but also surface irregularities and even intrastromal changes in transparency in a very detailed fashion. All these changes induce light diffraction caused by light passing through media with differing refraction indexes and deviated from its original linear direction. It is essential to point out that light diffraction takes place not only in the presence of opacities but also when small irregularities of the corneal surface, changes in cornea and lens thickness, sudden curvature changes of the anterior and posterior corneal surface, as well as lacunae and folds in the LASIK

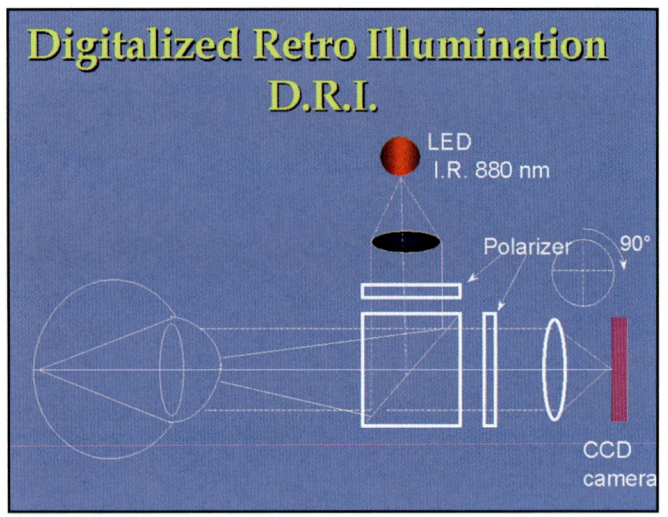

Figure 8-1. Simplified scheme of digitalized retroillumination with Scheimpflug camera.

flap interface are present. The Scheimpflug camera provides information on the quality of light transmission through the ocular media. Evaluation of severity, depth, light absorption, and, thus, density of the corneal surface can be obtained as well as stromal opacities and irregularities featuring different indexes of refraction with respect to normal cornea. Sudden and irregular changes in homogeneity of the refraction index of the cornea reduce the amount of light reaching the retina. The less lighted the corneal image is the less light that will be perceived by the patient. Thus, all the above-mentioned changes worsen the patient's vision. When observing a normal cornea with digitalized retroillumination and a dilated pupil, we will see an intensely lighted reflex indicating good transit of light through the cornea with no diffraction.

Scheimpflug camera examination allows identification of induced irregularity, influenced by the type of laser used. Whenever diffraction is present, the Scheimpflug reflex is weaker, proving that part of the light has not been transmitted to the retina. In these cases, the pupillary diameter will increase in the attempt to compensate diffraction by allowing more light into the eye. In this situation, the corneal profile situation becomes critical, because the aberration-reducing effect of a small pupil is absent.

On the contrary, when examining a patient immediately after refractive surgery, a fine irregularity is present with weaker light reflex, indicating the presence of diffraction. A weak light reflex means less light reaches the retina with reduced contrast sensitivity.

The Scheimpflug camera can also be applied in LASIK eyes for the evaluation of the flap interface. At this level, diffraction may occur because of incongruities of the two facing surfaces, flap, and stromal bed. These changes cannot be detected by topography and seldom by slit lamp examination.

We used the NIDEK NM 100 Scheimpflug camera (Gamagori, Japan) to evaluate corneal surface irregularities after refractive surgery.[1,2] We have thus been able to classify

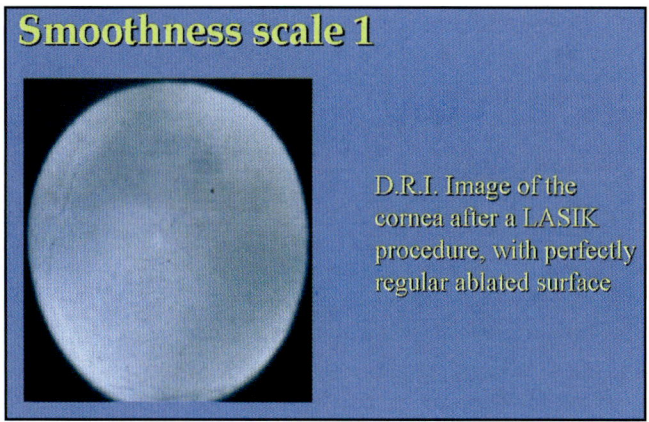

Figure 8-2. Grade 1, no irregularity. LASIK eye. Note smooth ablation surface, regular or with fine granularity, and no visible ablation border, no major irregularities.

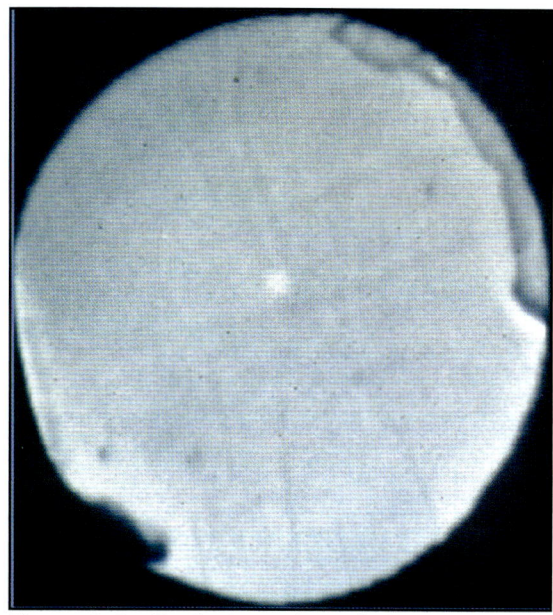

Figure 8-3. Grade 1, no irregularity. LASEK eye. Note border of epithelial flap.

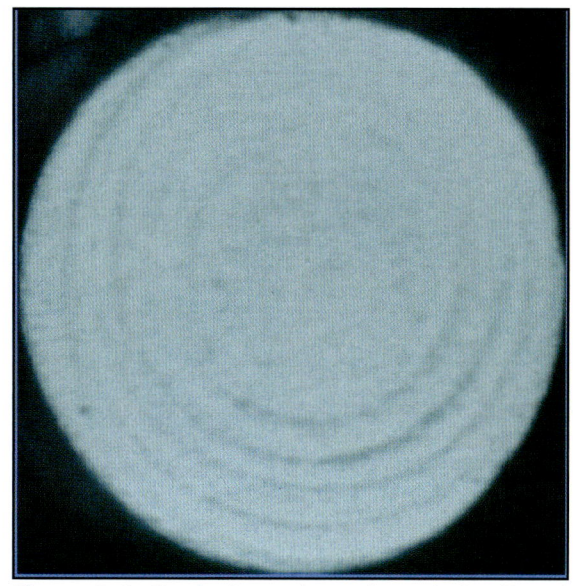

Figure 8-4. Grade 2, moderate irregularity. Broad beam laser.

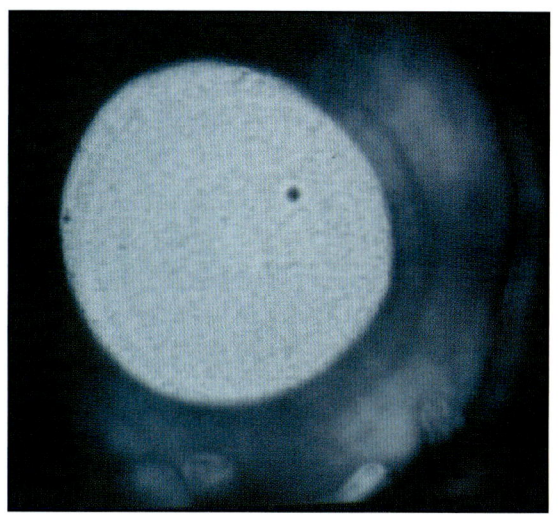

Figure 8-5. Grade 2, moderate irregularity. Flying spot laser. Irregularities are related to spot size.

these irregularities as follows:
- Micro-irregularities: Constantly generated during photoablation, due to saccadic eye motions, breathing, cardiac ocular pulse, and laser beam application modalities on the corneal surface even in the presence of an advanced eye tracking system.
- Macro-irregularities: Caused by sudden head or eye motions, incomplete cleaning of the stromal bed, or abnormalities in excimer laser operation as well as changes in the quality of the laser optical pathway.

A corneal surface irregularity scale may be established, and evaluated intraoperatively with the Scheimpflug camera immediately after photoablation, before contact lens application in PRK, epithelium repositioning in LASEK, or flap repositioning in LASIK. We have developed a scale with three different grades of severity:

1. *Grade 1.* No irregularity. Smooth ablation surface, regular or with fine granularity, with no visible ablation border, mostly concentric steps, and no major irregularities (Figure 8-2 and 8-3).

2. *Grade 2.* Moderate irregularities. Diffused or focal irregularities, ablation borders visible but not sharp, single steps sometimes decentered, and no flap interface folds (Figures 8-4 and 8-5).

3. *Grade 3.* Severe irregularities. Macroirregularities of ablation, relevant stromal islands inducing light diffraction, sharp ablation borders, decentered steps, and severe flap interface folds in LASIK. All these irregularities induce marked light diffraction, and show up in a very dark manner on Scheimpflug images. Therefore, they correspond to areas where the visual quality is markedly reduced (Figure 8-6).

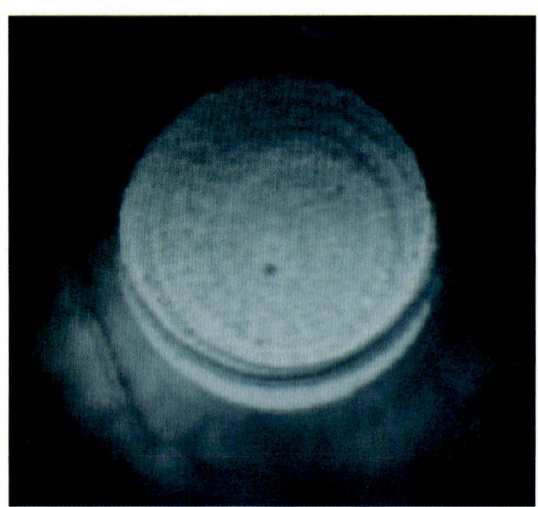

Figure 8-6. Grade 3, severe irregularity. Broad beam laser. Irregularities due to irregular centration.

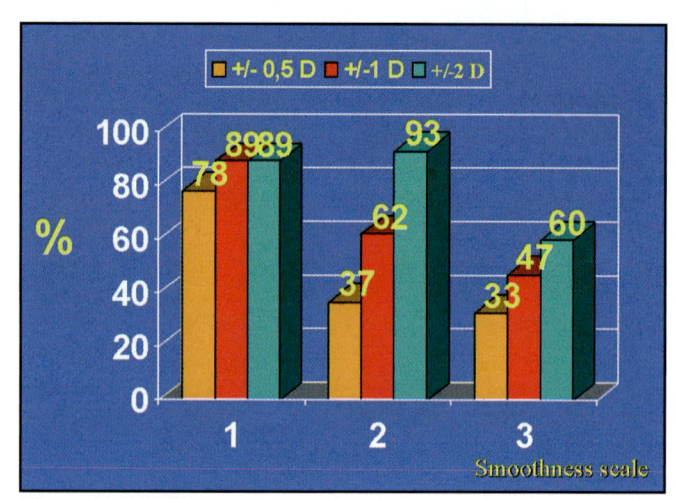

Figure 8-7. Difference from planned emmetropia among the three groups in LASEK eyes. Note how Group 1 eyes have higher percentages of eyes close to desired refraction.

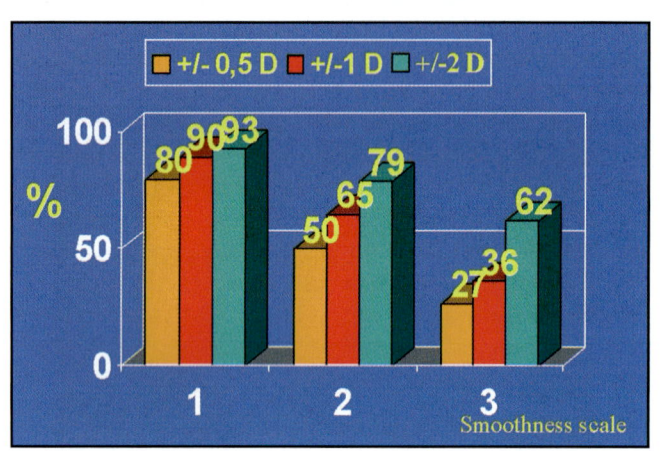

Figure 8-8. Difference from planned emmetropia at 12 months in LASIK eyes.

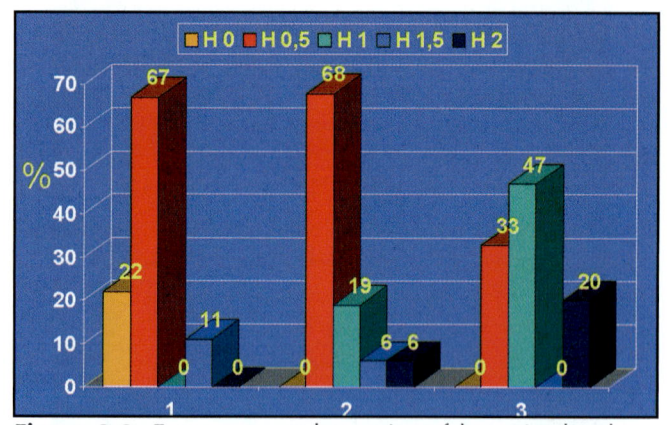

Figure 8-9. Frequency and severity of haze in the three groups of LASEK eyes, at 12 months.

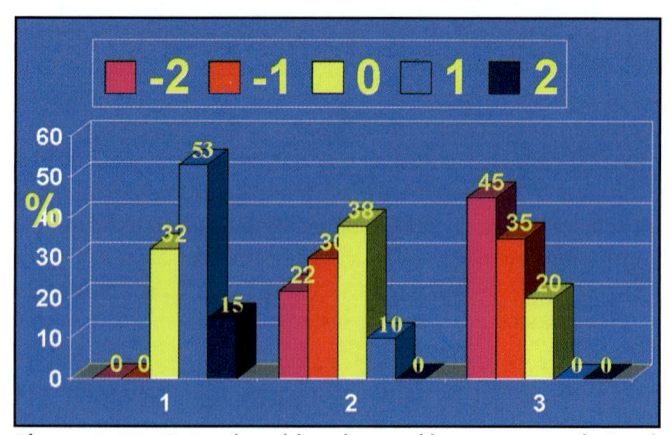

Figure 8-10. Gained and lost lines of best corrected visual acuity at 12 months, all cases.

CLINICAL STUDY - I

Using a Scheimpflug camera, we examined 80 eyes that had undergone LASEK (n = 40), or LASIK (n = 40), and divided them into three groups according to the above-mentioned scale of irregularity: Group 1 comprising eyes with no irregularity, Group 2 those with moderate irregularities, and Group 3 those with severe irregularities. At the end of follow-up, 12 months after surgery, spherical equivalent (SE) refraction was -0.23 ± 0.48 D in Group 1, -0.78 ± 0.8 D in Group 2, and -1.45 ± 0.92 D in Group 3. Figure 8-7 reports the difference from the planned emmetropia among the three groups in LASEK eyes and Figure 8-8 in LASIK eyes. Figure 8-9 reports the lower frequency of relevant haze observed in Group 1 LASEK eyes. Finally, Figure 8-10 shows the gained and lost lines of best-corrected visual acuity at 12 months in all cases. Group 1, including eye with no corneal irregularity, always fared better than the other two groups. This highlighted how corneal irregularities influenced precision of refractive result. A more regular surface stimulates a reparative process that may alter the refractive result to a lesser degree. More collagen deposition means reduction in the induced refractive effect, often in an unpredictable pattern. The end result is often a surface with unwanted refractive properties. The epithelium also plays a role, trying to provide a regular surface and filling gaps and irregularities. Furthermore, stimuli inducing collagen deposition may induce haze formation.

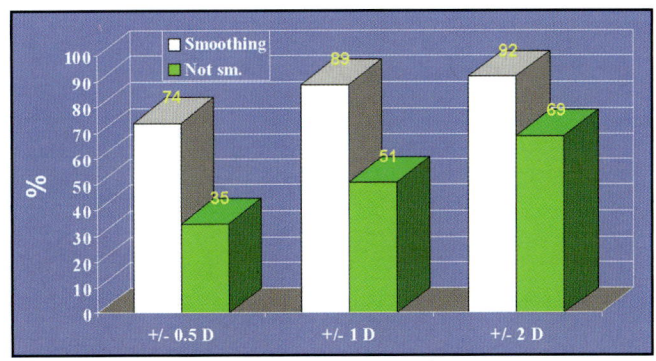

Figure 8-11. Smoothing after refractive correction. Comparison of refractive results in eyes with/without smoothing at 18-month follow-up examination. Percentages of eyes within ± 0.5, 1.0, and 2.0 D from planned emmetropia.

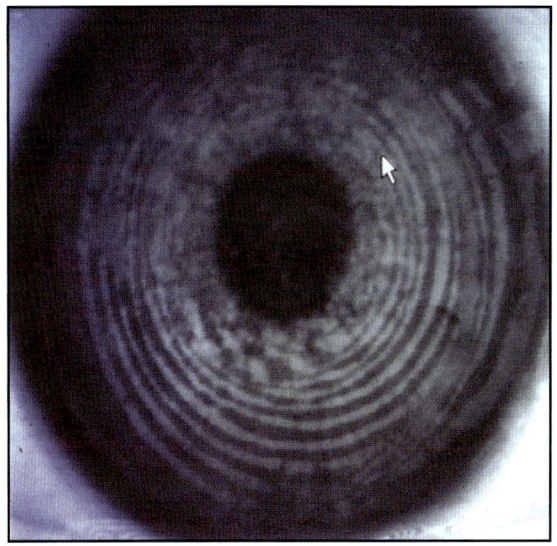

Figure 8-12. Group A eye, after refractive ablation and before smoothing.

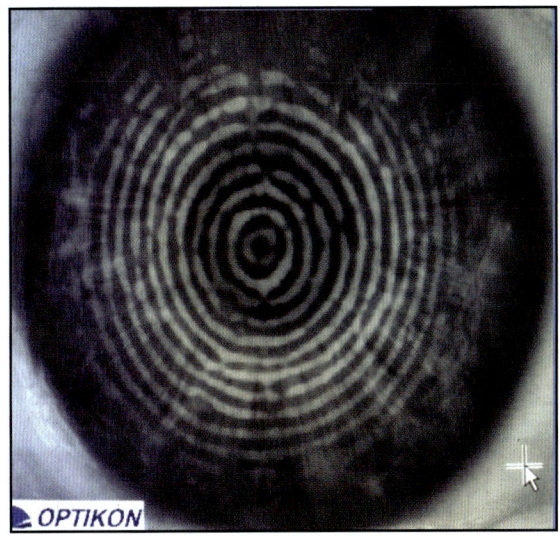

Figure 8-13. Same eye as Figure 8-12, during smoothing.

Smoothing of the Ablated Surface

Our idea of a smoothing treatment to increase postoperative regularity of the ablated surface originated a few years ago, performing phototherapeutic treatments for corneal dystrophies. After eliminating surface irregularities, we decided to correct ametropic defects too. When we did so, we observed a much higher refractive stability than in patients treated for the refractive defect only. Another interesting observation was that immediately after routine PRK, we could never perform satisfactory keratoscopy because the corneal surface did not reflect the Placido disc rings. This was not true of phototherapeutic ablations. Finally, these cases showed very limited haze, even if the treatment involved removal of more stromal tissue than normal refractive ablations. All these observations may be linked to the more regular surface we were obtaining in PTK by smoothing the corneal surface. Therefore, we looked for a way to obtain this surface quality in routine refractive treatments.

CLINICAL STUDY - II

We examined 225 LASEK eyes (Group A) and 76 LASIK eyes (Group B) prospectively with a Scheimpflug camera. Of these eyes, we classified 147 as having moderate (n = 80), or severe (n = 67), postoperative stromal irregularities. These eyes were randomized into two groups, Group A receiving a PTK-style smoothing with masking fluid after refractive ablation and Group B receiving the refraction ablation only. Mean preoperative refraction was -6.4 ± 3.2 D in Group A, -6.6 ± 3.1 D in Group B, and the two Groups were comparable for age and sex. After an 18-month follow-up period, Group A (smoothing) patients showed better refractive results (Figure 8-11) than Group B. Haze of 0.5 or less was present in 85% of Group A eyes and in 36% of Group B eyes. Figures 8-12, 18-3, and 8-14 show one eye before, during, and after smoothing.

Smoothing thus appeared as a technique that increased the optical properties of the treated surface by eliminating or reducing irregularities induced by refractive treatment. Its aim is to achieve a regular ablated surface (Grade 1 of the above mentioned scale). Severe irregularities are thus eliminated, if possible, and moderate irregularities reduced. Furthermore, ablation margins are smoothed, improving the anatomical connection between ablated and normal cornea (Figures 8-15 and 8-16). This last feature is decisive in PRK and LASEK to reduce the stimulus toward excessive scar tissue deposition with consequent regression and in LASIK to provide an interface without lacunae or folds. Reducing the high dioptric gradient (see Figure 8-15), a source of optical aberrations such as spherical aberration, improves the optical performance of the final corneal surface. The results of a recent study by Wilson demonstrate a relationship between the level of corneal haze formation after PRK and the level of stromal surface irregularity.[3] PTK-smoothing with methylcellulose was an effective method to reduce stromal surface irregularity and decreased both haze and associated myofi-

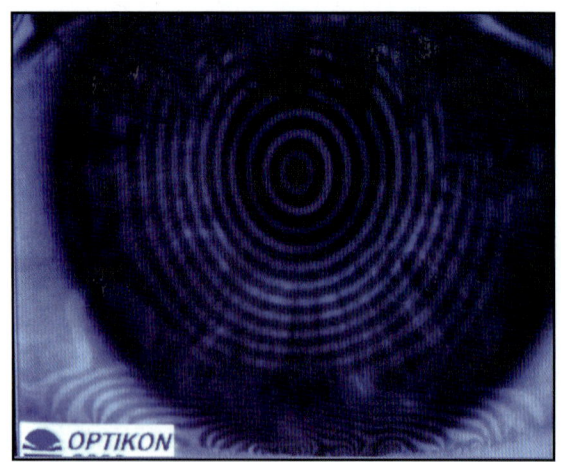

Figure 8-14. Same eye as Figures 8-12 and 8-13, at the end of smoothing.

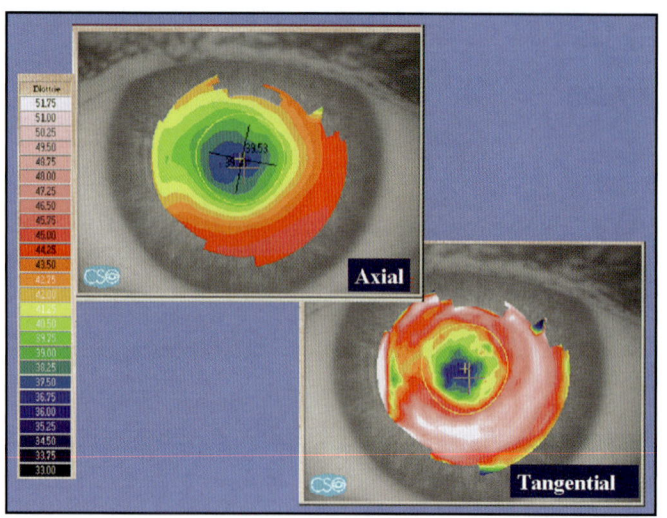

Figure 8-15. Postoperative topography of a LASEK eye treated with small ablation zone and no smoothing. The high dioptric gradient, indicated by the visible, thick red ring shows how anatomical continuity between treated and untreated corneas is profoundly altered.

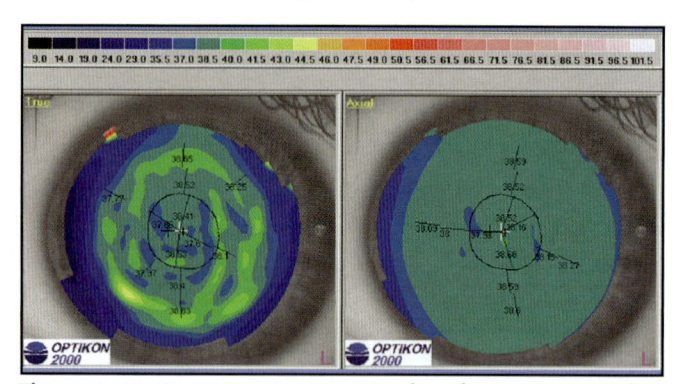

Figure 8-16. Postoperative topography of a LASEK eye after -7.0 D ablation, with wide ablation zone and smoothing. Note: 7 mm optical zone, low dioptric gradient, e = +0.2 (prolate cornea), and the almost monochromatic topography. The anatomical continuity between treated and untreated corneas is preserved.

broblast density. He conjectured that stromal surface irregularity after PRK for high myopia results in defective basement membrane regeneration and increased epithelium-derived TGFbeta signaling to the stroma that increases myofibroblast generation. Late apoptosis appears to have a role in the disappearance of myofibroblasts and haze over time.

Serrao has published several studies of stromal surface irregularity and haze after PRK, showing that PRK plus smoothing improves the visual results and diminishes regression and haze.[4-6]

Masking Fluid

Smoothing requires an appropriate masking fluid[7] with the following properties:

* Ablation rate similar to that of corneal rate. Ablation rate indicates the amount of material ablated at each laser pass. If the masking fluid has an ablation rate greater than that of the corneal stroma, stromal irregularities will be maintained, while a lower ablation rate will lead to undesired removal of parts of the stroma.
* Superficial tension equal to that of the corneal epithelium.
* Transparency.
* High bio-adhesiveness and low viscosity to be distributed in a thin regular film on the stromal bed.
* Shear rate similar to that of a viscoelastic substance. This permits lamination with a thickness related to the speed of the spatula passes, as described below.
* Non-Newtonian behavior with enough elasticity to permit a better absorption of the laser beam shock wave.
* Sterility with no impurities.
* High UV absorption.

Masking fluids commonly used in refractive surgery contain hyaluronic acid. Among these, we prefer those with short chains and low molecular weight.

Surgical Technique

The patient is informed about all the operative steps of surgical technique as well as the duration of treatment. A strong lid speculum should be used, such as the Castroviejo type for retinal surgery, to achieve a wide surgical field, proper cornea exposition, and allow rapid outflow of the fluids used intraoperatively without formation of pools.

After LASEK, before starting the smoothing process, it is recommended that the operative field be carefully washed with cooled BSS to eliminate all residues generated during ablation, as well as any surfactant.

Excessive corneal heating may induce stromal collagen chain changes. In order to limit corneal heating during smoothing, it is important to cool the cornea with chilled BSS

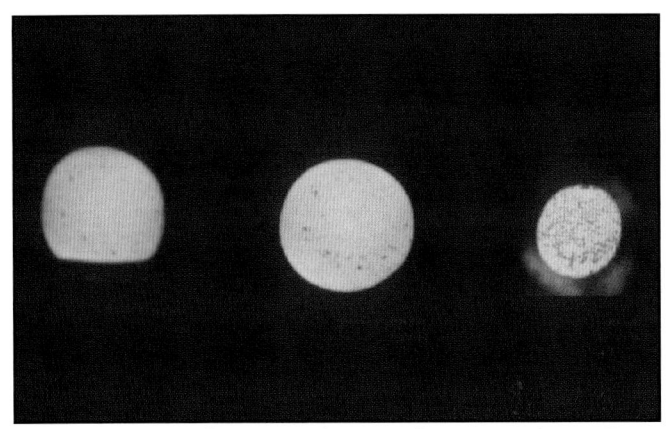

Figure 8-17. Grade 2 irregularities, flying spot laser. From right to left, progressive improvement of surface during smoothing.

or BSS ice cubes. Vinciguerra and Nizzola have developed special metallic cylinders that can be chilled separately and that limit tissue hydration, which are thus particularly useful in smoothing after LASIK.

After these preparatory maneuvers, smoothing is started with 1 to 2 drops of masking fluid on the center of the cornea. We use the Vinciguerra solution (hyaluronic acid 0.4%, Laservis, Chemedica, Munich, Germany), which features the same ablation rate as normal cornea and permits a regular ablation rate.[7-9] Masking fluid is carefully distributed with a special spatula (Buratto Spatula [ASICO, Westmont, Ill]). When a dry area appears, fluid is added and continuously redistributed with the special spatula. Never ablate on dry surfaces. Practice will provide the sufficient manual experience in continuous fluid redistribution to ensure that major irregularities emerge and are ablated. Fluid lamination can be performed with two methods: a fast, to-and-fro motion on the stromal surface permits a homogeneous lamination of the masking fluid. Conversely, a slow and unidirectional motion with final lifting of the spatula will induce thinning of the fluid. In the first phase of smoothing, when large irregularities may be present, lamination must be thin to allow the irregularity "peaks" to emerge and be selectively ablated while protecting the lower corneal areas ("valleys"). The surface will rapidly improve, as can be highlighted by intraoperative keratoscopy (Figure 8-17).

In the following phases, when only small residual irregularities remain, the masking fluid will follow their profile without highlighting peaks and valleys. It will now be useful to perform lamination while maintaining the fluid thicker to cover the entire stromal surface homogeneously. With a fluid that is thicker on valleys and thinner on residual peaks, ablation through the masking fluid will be performed mostly on the peaks. In fact, it must be remembered that excimer laser ablates even through the masking fluid. A precise determination of the best frequency of lamination can be achieved using fluorescein, which promptly shows dry areas, and by listening carefully to the changes in acoustic features of the corneal ablation process. Dry areas, often visible as umbilicate points on the surface of masking fluid disappear during smoothing, proving their nature as irregularities emerging from the masking fluid.

A neutral, PTK-style ablation is performed, with a diameter of at least 9 mm to avoid hyperopic shift. A low frequency ablation rate (ie, 10 Hz) is used to avoid corneal heating as well as preventing endothelial damage and postoperative stromal inflammation. The laser is set at maximum 30 μm ablation to obtain 8 μm of real ablation.

Smoothing in LASIK

When LASIK has been performed, generous preliminary washout of the operative field is contraindicated since it may induce flap hinge edema and hamper flap repositioning. A delicate factor during smoothing in LASIK eyes is the flap hinge, impeding a constant outflow of the excess masking fluid. This excess must be removed constantly with Merocel sponges to prevent a fluid meniscus, which could induce relevant refractive defects (astigmatism and hyperopia). During treatment, the flap must be adequately hydrated; otherwise, repositioning may be troublesome. Flap repositioning must be exact, stretching it if necessary to smooth folds or striae. The margins of the flap and of the stromal bed must be preserved to prevent epithelial ingrowth. If previous flap folds cannot be regularized, flap suturing may be indicated. A small flap (7.5 to 8 mm) may call for ablation of a very small corneal portion with consequent tissue removal in a limited stromal portion, a situation of localized flattening inducing hyperopia. Therefore, the risk of inducing hyperopia in such cases must be clearly explained to patients.[10]

PTK after LASIK is a procedure that must be limited in duration. Tissue hydration, induced by use of fluid, may become excessive and hamper precise flap repositioning. Flap irregularities will not be treated by PTK; they must be identified, and the patient must be informed of consequent limits in treatment results preoperatively

Considering all the above-mentioned facts, smoothing after LASIK is a procedure that should be approached only after adequate experience with smoothing in easier cases, such as in post-LASEK eyes.

Common Questions About Smoothing

* *Does smoothing influence final refraction?* The ablation induced by smoothing, if properly performed, does not hamper the final refractive result. The ablation diameter is important, because when it is inferior to 8 to 9 mm, it may induce hyperopia. An 8-μm ablation on 8 to 9 mm maintains the corneal curvature values without modifying the initial refraction.

* *Is the ablation frequency decisive?* We use 10 Hz ablation frequency since corneal heating may be induced by higher frequencies. However, corneal cooling before and after smoothing is always recommended.

* *Can smoothing be performed with a flying spot laser?* Yes, but in this case, the surgeon must verify that PTK-style ablation has an ultimately neutral ablation profile with no refractive effect.

* *If smoothing is so important, why it is not more commonly used?* Common doubts about smoothing include its reputation as a complex, refractively unpredictable, or useless technique. If the above-described technique is followed, smoothing is not a difficult technique. It is essential to set the laser appropriately, and approach the technique with caution and some intraoperative controls during initial cases (see Appendix A), to verify that smoothing does not negatively affect the corneal situation.

* *Can smoothing help me in retreatments?* Learning the smoothing technique improves the surgical tools that can be used in retreatments, specifically if intraoperative control techniques are mastered. Corneal irregularity is one of the most important factors in the unpredictable results associated with retreatments. Intraoperative topography is a mandatory exam to monitor treatment and the progression toward desired goals. This examination, in LASIK patients, must be performed directly on the stromal bed after the flap has been lifted, thus, only with instruments that can be used intraoperatively (such as the CSO [Florence, Italy] or the Keratron Scout [Optikon 2000, Rome, Italy]) with parts close to the ocular surface that can be sterilized. Contrary to smoothing after PRK, in LASIK, it is important to remember that when the flap is lifted, a topographical increase in curvature will always be present where the flap stromal bed meets the untreated cornea, indicating the cut margin on the stromal bed. Obviously, this curvature irregularity must not be treated, since it is essential for correct repositioning of the flap, and prevention of epithelial ingrowth.[4]

References

1. Vinciguerra P, Azzolini M, Radice P, Sborgia M, de Molfetta V. A method for examining surface and interface irregularities after photorefractive keratectomy and laser in situ keratomileusis: predictor of optical and functional outcomes. *J Refract Surg.* 1998;14:S204-206.
2. Vinciguerra P, Azzolini M, Airaghi P, Radice P, De Molfetta V. Effect of decreasing surface and interface irregularities after photorefractive keratectomy and laser in situ keratomileusis on optical and functional outcomes. *J Refract Surg.* 1998;14:S199-203.
3. Netto MV, Mohan RR, Sinha S, Sharma A, Dupps W, Wilson SE. Stromal haze, myofibroblasts, and surface irregularity after PRK. *Exp Eye Res.* 2005; (in press).
4. Lombardo M, De Santo MP, Lombardo G, Barberi R, Serrao S. Roughness of excimer laser ablated corneas with and without smoothing measured with atomic force microscopy. *J Refract Surg.* 2005; 21(5):469-475.
5. Serrao S, Lombardo M, Mondini F. Photorefractive keratectomy with and without smoothing: a bilateral study. *J Refract Surg.* 2003;19:58-64.
6. Serrao S, Lombardo M. Corneal epithelial healing after phorefractive keratectomy: analytical study. *J Cataract Refract Surg.* 2005;31:930-937.
7. Kornhehl EW, Steinert RF, Puliafito CA. A comparative study of masking fluids for excimer laser phototherapeutic keratectomy. *Arch Ophthalmol.* 1991;109: 860-863.
8. Vinciguerra P, Cro M, Giuffrida S, Airaghi P, De Molfetta V. A new strategy in excimer laser PTK: use of hyaluronic acid solution as masking fluid. *Inv Ophthalmol Vis Sci.* Annual Meeting Sarasota, FL, May 1-6, 1994.
9. Fasano AP, Moreira M, McDonnell PJ, Sinbawy A. Excimer laser smoothing of a reproducible model of anterior corneal surface irregularity. *Ophthalmology.* 1991;98:1782-1785.
10. Vinciguerra P, Prussiani A. Fotocheratectomia terapeutica (PTK). In: *Chirurgia Refrattiva: Principi e Tecniche.* Asti: Fabiano, 2000;439-462.

CHAPTER 9

EVALUATION AND DEVELOPMENT OF ABLATION PROFILES

Paolo Vinciguerra, MD; Fabrizio I. Camesasca, MD

Introduction

Correct calibration of the excimer laser is of great importance in achieving excellent visual results. Common and accepted calibration methods include ablation on paper and on PMMA, as well as use of fluency meter, voltage meter, and spot locator.[1,2] With the PMMA or paper tests, we can see the ablation power obtained; however, the profile and algorithm, the shape, and the quality of the ablation cannot be seen. In particular, we cannot evaluate ablation smoothness, optical gradient imparted, or evaluate the aberrometric behaviors of the ablated surface. Thus, the main limit of these calibration methods is that they are performed on a two-dimensional surface and, thus, do not show the effects of energy reduction due to the distribution on the curved corneal surface.

A New Method for Evaluation and Test of Ablation Profiles

We designed a three-dimensional PMMA hemisphere with a preset curvature of 43.0 D (Figure 9-1) to feature the dioptrical characteristics of a standard human eye and examine different ablation patterns in a setting closer to reality.[3] Due to its particular aspheric shape, aberrometric evaluation could be performed to show a normal wavefront. Different experimental ablation profiles performed with the NIDEK EC 5000 excimer laser were then evaluated. All profiles were examined with topography, wavefront, OPD, and keratoscopy. CSO topography (CSO, Firenze, Italy) and NIDEK OPD aberrometer (Gamagori, Japan) were used. Importantly, corneal topographers may detect differences in corneal curvature rays of 0.01 to 0.02 D and, in elevation maps, can show differences of 1 µm. Thus, on an ablation of 3.0 D, we can measure an error of 1/144 (0.020 D) when compared to the 1/12 error measurement of a lensmeter (0.25 D).

Calibration with the test hemisphere is safer and more accurate than with plastic. The test precision was 0.25 µm. Usually, a test with three-dimensional ablation areas with 6 mm of diameter created a 36-µm ablation, so that 1/144 of the ablation could be measured. In particular, we evaluated profiles for astigmatism, hyperopia (Figure 9-2), and myopia (Figure 9-3). Figure 9-3 shows seven different profiles for myopia obtained changing the focusing lens while maintaining unchanged ablation power and optical and transition zone diameters.

The hemisphere allowed successful and repeatable examination with topographer and aberrometer. Figures 9-4 and 9-5 show pre- and postoperative NIDEK OPD analysis with keratoscopy, axial and instantaneous topography maps, optical path deviation, and wavefront HO maps. Differential analysis was performed for topography and OPD maps. Stability of refractive treatment, as well as reproducibility, could also be assessed. Figure 9-6 shows the OPD analysis and map difference between two test ablations.

Surface regularity was studied in detail with the aid of keratoscopy. Figure 9-7 shows keratoscopy of a successful test with smooth ablation, while Figure 9-8 illustrates an ablation with dot defects, and Figure 9-9 a very rough surface.

Advantages of PMMA Hemisphere Test

This newly designed PMMA hemisphere represents a versatile tool that can be used both in the daily preparation routine and calibration for treatments, and in experimental evaluation of new profiles and algorithms. The evaluation may thus be performed for the first time in a three-dimensional manner.

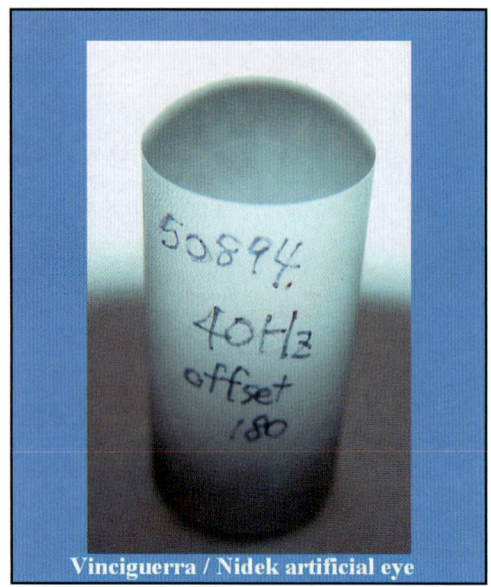

Figure 9-1. Experimental PMMA hemisphere with a preset curvature of 43.0 D.

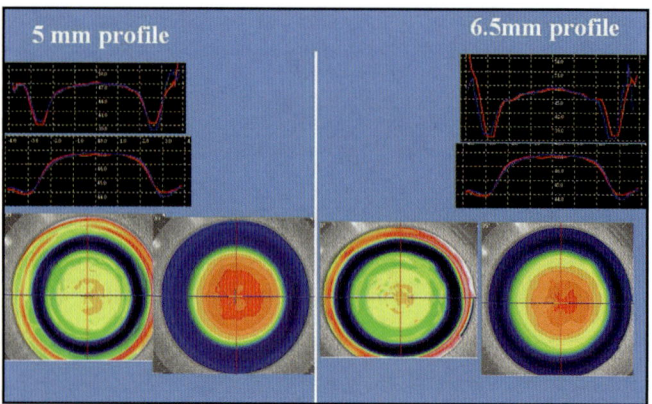

Figure 9-2. Comparison between two different experimental profiles for hyperopic correction.

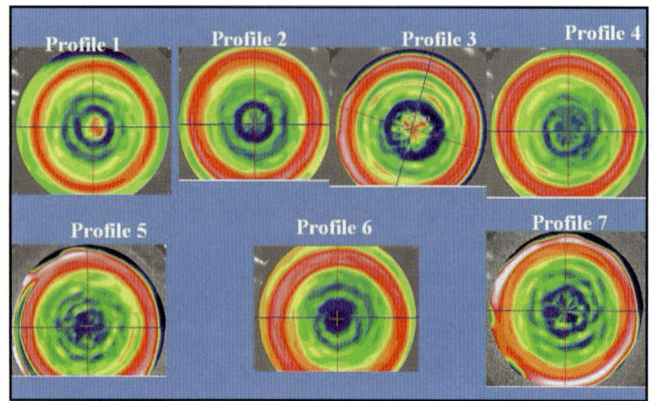

Figure 9-3. Seven different experimental profiles for myopia correction.

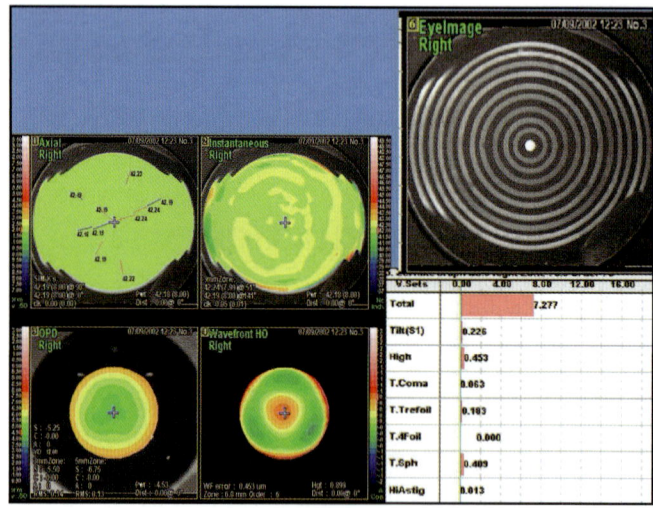

Figure 9-4. Preablation test hemisphere simulating a -5.0 D eye. NIDEK OPD analysis, with keratoscopy, axial and instantaneous topography maps, optical path deviation and wavefront HO maps.

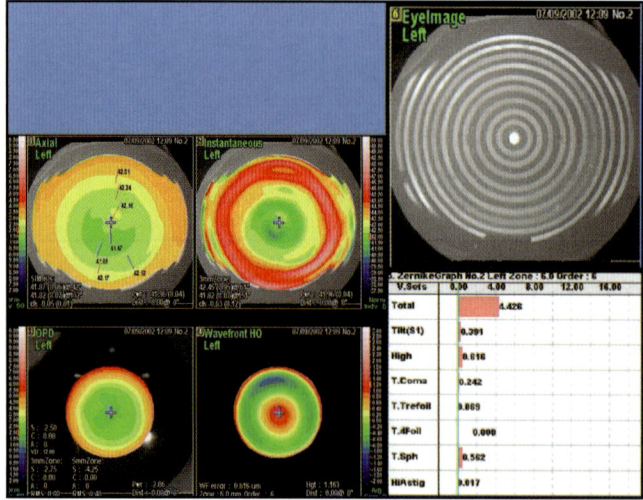

Figure 9-5. Test hemisphere after a -3.0 D treatment. Postoperative NIDEK OPD analysis, with keratoscopy, axial and instantaneous topography maps, optical path deviation and wavefront HO maps.

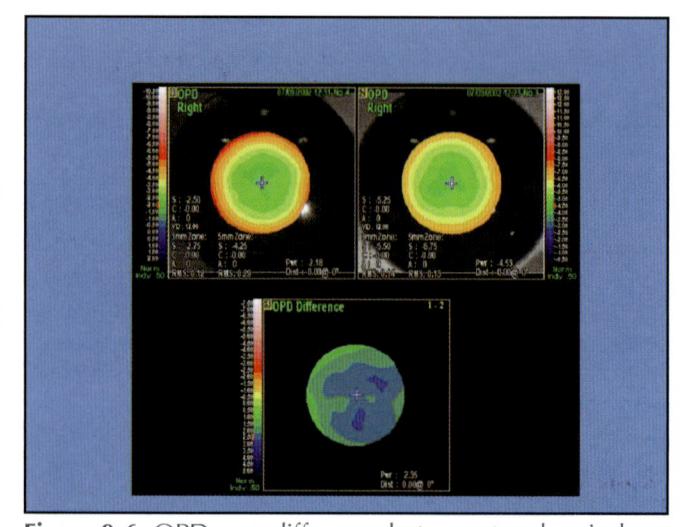

Figure 9-6. OPD map difference between two hemisphere tests

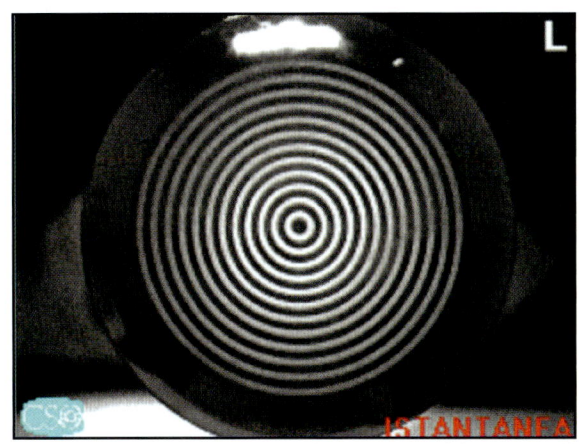

Figure 9-7. Keratoscopy of a successful test with smooth ablation.

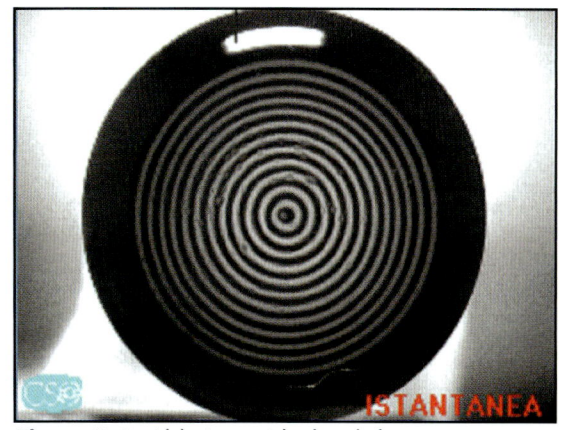

Figure 9-8. Ablation with dot defects.

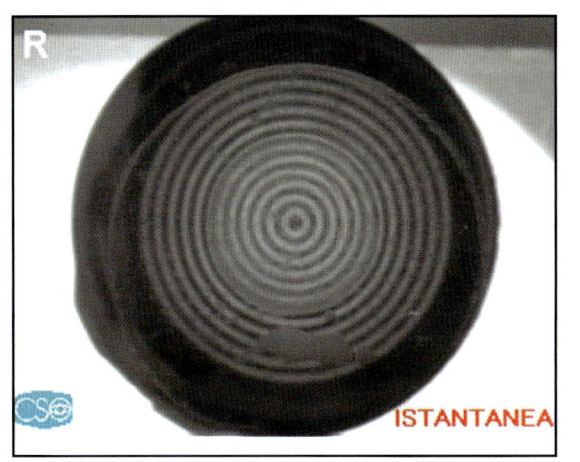

Figure 9-9. A very rough ablation surface.

Ablation on a spherical surface is closer to real ablation conditions in terms of progressive beam defocusing (ie, the beam focus on the apex is closer than in the periphery). Therefore, it is possible to detect laser ablation peripheral efficiency loss when applied on a curved surface.

The hemisphere is an easy tool for service technicians. A quality evaluation of the laser beam before any laser surgery can also be performed just like in a human eye. Ablation shape as well as centration may be examined. Any beam decentering with respect to the aiming beam can be easily detected, and as a result, laser treatment safety can be easily improved. Homogeneity and regularity of ablated surfaces can be evaluated, and the hemisphere may thus be used for analysis of defects in an excimer laser (eg, mirror defects). Experimental uses of this PMMA hemisphere include a preview of the surgical results obtainable with a new algorithm or profiles, enabling one to perform easy visual and instrumental evaluations and comparisons.

Ablation tests may be used to compare different lasers or ablation profiles. Using the customary plastic ablation plates, we can only measure ablation diameter and power, not asphericity (q value), the ablation profile, or the final corneal curvature gradient.

Conclusions

The test hemisphere introduces a common language among excimer laser developers, technicians and physicians. Its applications in everyday practice can include calibration and laser testing, monitoring results obtained with maintenance, as well as experimental purposes.

References

1. McDonald MB, Leach DH. Myopic photorefractive keratectomy: the U.S. experience. In: Thompson FB, McDonnell PJ. *Color Atlas/Text of Excimer Laser Surgery.* New York, NY: Igaku-Shoin; 1993:37-51.
2. Stein HA, Cheskes AT, Stein RM. *The Excimer. Fundamentals and Clinical Use.* Thorofare, NJ: SLACK Incorporated; 1997: 71-90.
3. Vinciguerra P, Camesasca FI, Torres Munoz MI. New test hemisphere for evaluation and development of ablation profiles. *J Refract Surg.* 2003; 19(2 Suppl):S260-264.

SECTION III

Surface Ablation

CHAPTER 10

TREATMENT OF MYOPIA

Fabrizio I. Camesasca, MD; Paolo Vinciguerra, MD;
Alessandro Randazzo, MD

Introduction

Myopia is the most common refractive defect in the world. Excimer laser refractive surgery has been challenging myopia since 1988 when the first excimer laser PRK for myopia on a normally sighted human eye was performed by McDonald and coworkers.[1]

Since then, the progress of surface ablation has been continuous and exciting. The introduction of LASIK, aimed at solving some of the less desirable problems and complications of PRK, such as postoperative pain, slow postoperative recovery of vision, haze, and regression, did not completely persuade the international ophthalmic community in abandoning surface ablation. Technological advancements, better knowledge of corneal reparation mechanisms, appropriate use of medications, the introduction of custom ablation, eye-tracking systems and new surface ablation techniques such as LASEK and Epi-LASIK, as well as the complexity of the rare but relevant complications associated with LASIK have maintained and strengthened the interest for surface ablation correction of myopia.[2]

Selection Criteria and Planning for Surface Myopic Ablation

The selection criteria listed in Chapter 5 must always be respected. The main guiding criterium is to pursue satisfactory final optical conditions. The upper limit in myopic ablation thus changes according to the preoperative corneal conditions (ie, corneal endothelium must be normal, without guttata or important reduction in cell counts).

Corneal thickness must always be taken into account, and a thicker than normal cornea (eg, 600 μm) will make the treatment safer and allow a wider ablation and transition zone (TZ) maintaining a safe residual thickness. A thin cornea or a wide pupil, requiring a wider ablation zone, will reduce the amount of diopters that can be ablated safely. Even when the corneal thickness is normal or high, though, we do not recommend treating more than 10.0 to 12.0 D of myopia because a deep ablation may induce a relevant scarring process with the risk of inducing haze or irregular central corneal surface. Use of Mytomicin C (see Chapter 29) is useful but may not be sufficient to control scarring for very high myopic ablations, and even if we could control scarring with consequent haze, surface irregularity, and regression efficiently, excessive ablation is not recommended for the following reasons:

1. Profound alteration of corneal biomechanical properties[3,4]
2. Lack of residual thickness for a retreatment
3. Reduced capacity to tolerate possible future corneal trauma or infection

All the criteria for identification of possible forme-fruste keratoconus must be respected (see Chapter 27 and Chapter 1). With the presently available knowledge and on the basis of our experience, we recommend leaving a final thickness of at least 300 μm. Nevertheless, as discussed in the Chapter 31 minimal residual thickness must not be considered as an exhaustive parameter. In our experience, a marked uniform reduction in thickness of the entire cornea is better than a thinning of lesser amount but concentrated all in the central cornea. The latter could more easily lead to ectasia.[4] Furthermore, a minimal myopic residual, of -0.50 to -0.75 D may be preferred if the patient's age is greater than 40 years and his working conditions require exhaustive use of near

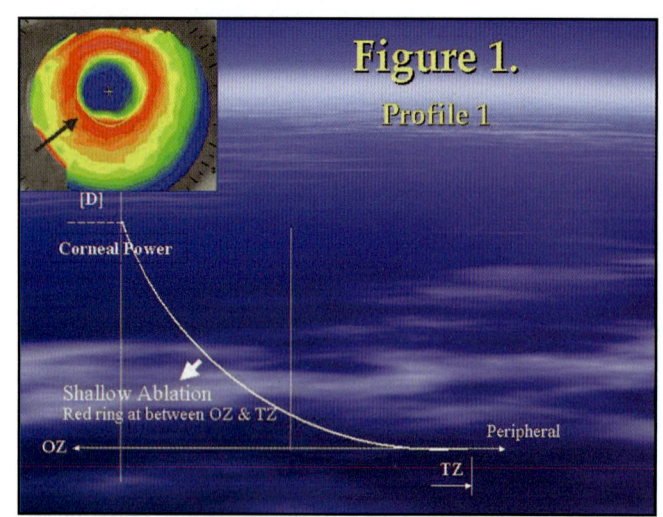

Figure 10-1. NIDEK Final Fit software allows visualization of simulated postoperative situation (target). Profile 1. This is a tissue-saving profile, but curvature change is all concentrated immediately after the optical zone (black arrow). Early types of excimer lasers adopted a similar profile.

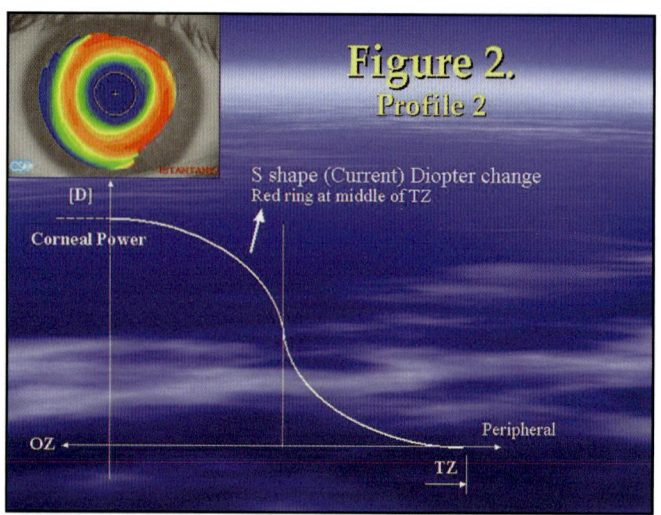

Figure 10-2. Profile 2. A similar profile is widely adopted by currently available lasers. Corneal curvature change is positioned in the middle of the transition zone. With this profile, tissue deposition elicited by this sharp corneal curvature change may influence the optical zone and lead to late regression, due to the proximity of the curvature change to the optical zone.

vision. Obviously, the final refractive goal must be carefully discussed preoperatively.

The most important step in planning a correction for myopia is the accurate definition of the refractive defect. We recommend determination of the defect first with the fogging technique and then after cycloplegia. Properly performed cycloplegia, with administration of cyclopentholate 1% eyedrops—we administer it three times every 20 minutes before performing refraction—will define the amount of sphere to be treated and avoid hyper- or hypocorrection.

A good knowledge of the used excimer laser and of its possible tendency to over- or undercorrect is also essential in planning the treatment. In our experience, a slight undercorrection, especially in patients over age 35, is preferable to overcorrection, even if the expectations of patients that request refractive surgery are always very high and need to be carefully tested with appropriate discussion of the procedure and its results. It has been shown that a scarce time dedicated to patients and a high volume practice are the major culprits for litigation.[5]

The Myopic Ablation Profile in Surface Ablation

A common myth in refractive surgery is that the ablation diameter set on the excimer laser will have a precise functional postoperative correspondence with the corneal zone featuring the desired uniform refractive features. Thus, that the postoperative topographic map will show a uniform curvature for the same preoperatively set diameter and the wavefront map a homogeneous wavefront error. This can be simplified stating that the ablation zone is considered to correspond precisely with the postoperative functionally useful optical zone (OZ).

Actually, as specified in the Chapter 7, features of the peripheral area of connection between ablated and nonablated cornea—the TZ—play an extremely important role in defining extension and properties of the so-called OZ. These properties may determine the final quality of vision.[6]

Another common myth is that a wider ablation zone will always provide a wider OZ. Again, if the TZ is not properly built, this may not happen. The corneal curvature gradient is the most important factor in defining the functional quality of a myopic ablation. The corneal curvature gradient defines the curvature change from the corneal center to the periphery.

Figures 10-1 to 10-4 present visualization of simulated postoperative situation based by NIDEK Final Fit (Gamagori, Japan) software based on OPD topographical acquisition. Final Fit allows seven different ablation profiles for myopia. Four typical profiles are described here, illustrating the possibilities for corneal curvature change distribution in relation to OZ and TZ, as well as the required amount of tissue ablation.

A very sharp curvature change will influence the functionally useful OZ, reducing its diameter. This statement can be easily understood when comparing instantaneous and axial topography views (Figures 10-5 and 10-6). A marked increase in curvature concentrated in a small corneal portion will increase spherical aberration. Light rays passing through this corneal portion will not contribute to retinal image; conversely, they will decrease its quality. An ablation creating a more gradual curvature gradient between center and periphery will create a more regular OZ, contain this increase in spherical aberration, and maintain it similarly to the physiological value aimed at balancing the spherical aberration of the lens. The peripheral portion of the cornea

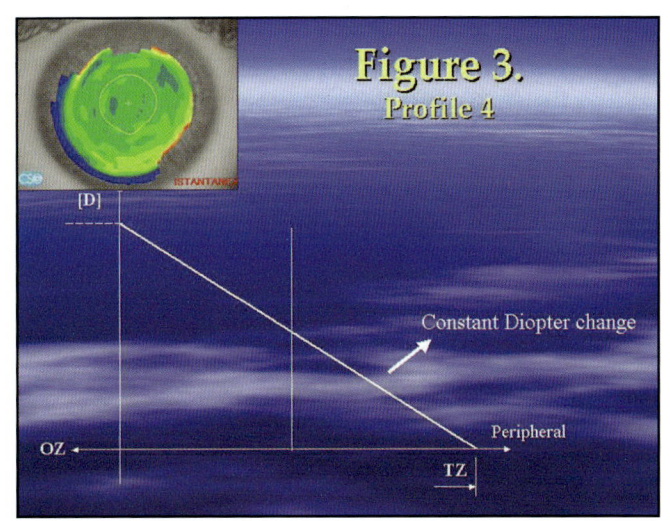

Figure 10-3. Profile 4. This profile provides constant curvature change from the end of the optical zone to the end of the transition zone.

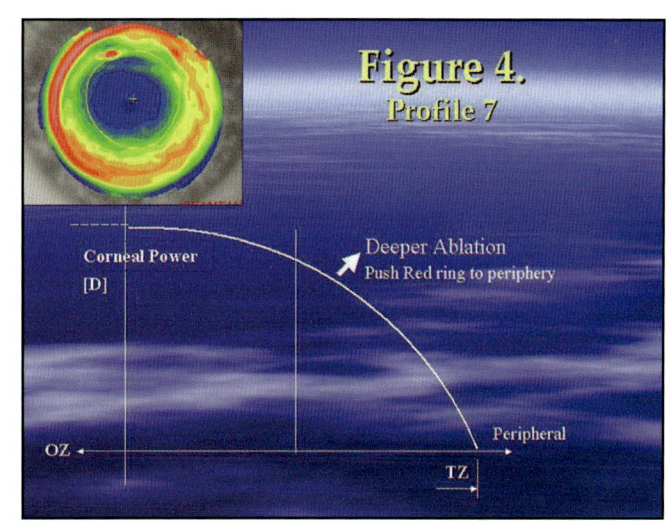

Figure 10-4. Profile 7. All profiles above no. 4 require more tissue removal, and concentrate corneal curvature center toward the end of the transition zone. Corneal curvature change is sharp because it is concentrated in a small area. A profile like this can be efficiently sued in corneas with a very flat periphery.

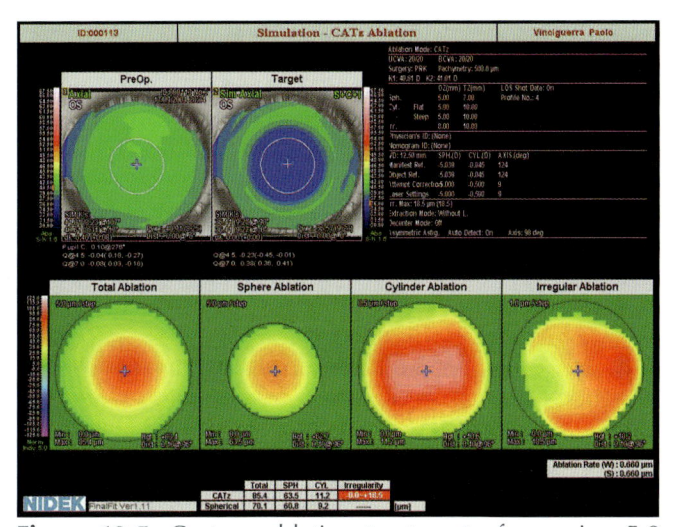

Figure 10-5. Custom ablation treatment of myopia, -5.0 D sph -0.50 (9) D cyl, axial algorithm. NIDEK Final Fit software, simulated postoperative situation. OZ is 5.0 mm, TZ is 7 mm, and ablation profile is no. 4. This view may induce the observer in thinking that the treatment will be appropriate, with a wide enough functional OZ (above right map). Ablation depth is 85 μm.

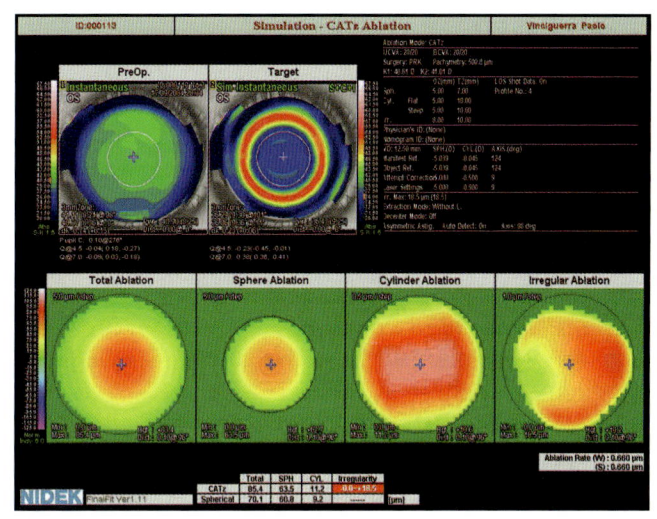

Figure 10-6. Same eye as in Figure 10-1, instantaneous algorithm, the target map shows a regular central cornea, but despite the 7-mm TZ, there is a marked change in curvature in the midperiphery, causing high spherical aberration and more chance of regression.

may thus contribute to the retinal image, and vision quality will be less sensitive to pupil size increase in scotopic conditions (Figures 10-7 and 10-8). It must be remarked that, presently, the attention of refractive surgeons is placed not only on obtaining a regular central curvature but increasingly on the optimization of asphericity factors (eg, q, e, p) in order to keep the corneal shape prolate as much as possible with preoperative-like curvature values.

However, another important topic must be remembered: even if the corneal curvature factors (ie, q) are maintained constant when the corneal curvature changes, so does spherical aberration. If for a q value of -0.025 and a mean corneal curvature of 43.0 D spherical aberration remains proximal to normal and compensates the lens spherical aberration, a similar q value and a corneal curvature of 32.0 D will be associated to a much different spherical aberration, thus impairing the physiological balance with the lens. In our opinion, for the future, it is more appropriate to consider spherical aberration as the most important parameter, since it autonomously encompasses changes in q when the corneal curvature varies, and it indicates more precisely how far the postoperative result may be from an optically acceptable situation.

The NIDEK Final Fit software helps the surgeon in understanding all these fine relationships, allowing simulation and modulation of final postoperative result according to different corneal shapes (Figures 10-5 through 10-12).

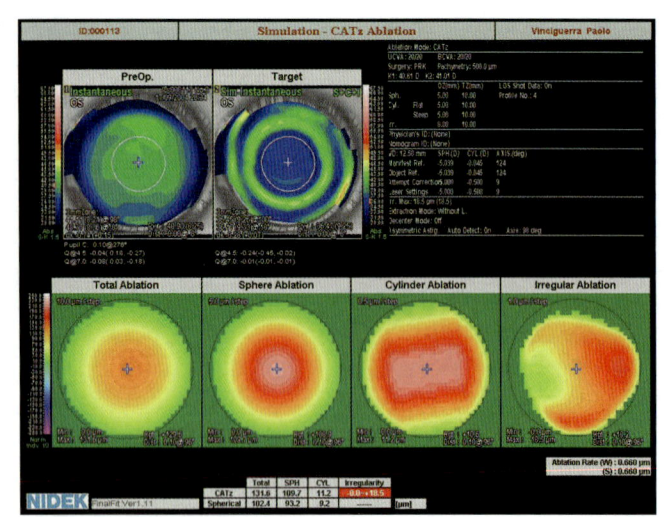

Figure 10-7. Same eye as in Figure 10-1, instantaneous algorithm. OZ is 5 mm, TZ has been increased to 10 mm. Widening the transition zone provides reduction of corneal curvature difference between center and periphery, with consequent reduction in spherical aberration. Ablation depth is 131 μm.

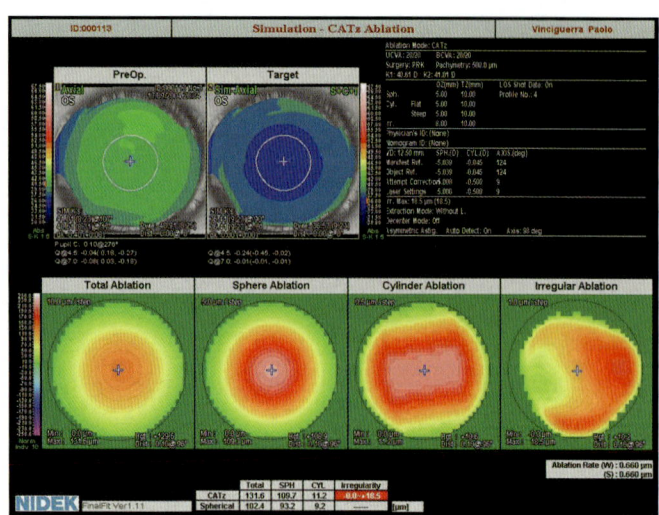

Figure 10-8. Same eye as in Figure 10-1, axial view of the strategy highlighted in Figure 10-3. Resulting functional OZ is extremely wide, with reduction of the corneal curvature gradient between center and periphery. High spherical aberration and perception of halos in mesopic conditions are prevented.

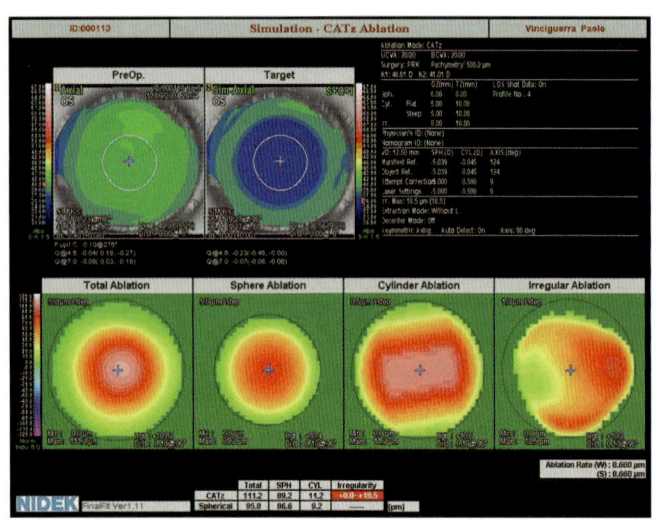

Figure 10-9. Same eye as in Figure 10-1, axial algorithm. OZ is 5 mm; TZ for sphere has been changed to 8 mm. Restricting the TZ to 8 mm provides tissue saving (111 μm). The resulting functional OZ is wide, even if less of that obtainable with a 10-mm TZ.

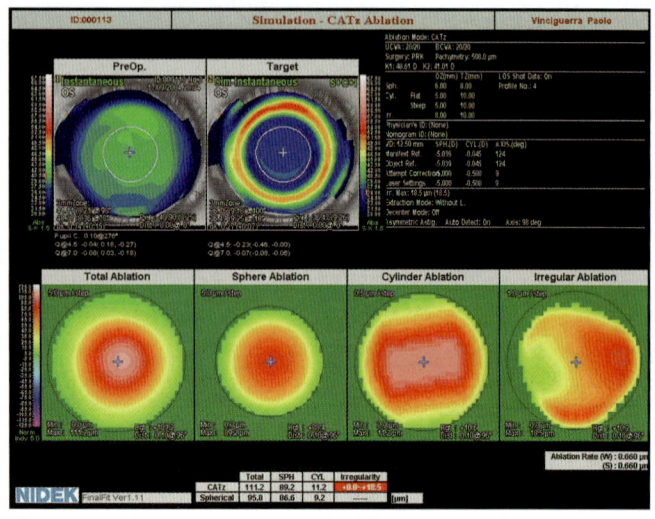

Figure 10-10. Same eye as in Figure 10-1, instantaneous algorithm. A marked red ring indicating high corneal curvature gradient and spherical aberration is present. A treatment with this strategy will have more chance of regression and halo perception in mesopic conditions.

Several other factors, in the myopic, as well as in the hyperopic and astigmatic ablation, also need to be taken into account. The pupil is important, and its diameter under scotopic conditions must be measured to provide a satisfactory OZ in eyes featuring wide scotopic pupil diameter. Location of the pupil is another important factor. Commonly, the pupil is decentered nasally with respect of the corneal apex, and since common eye-tracking systems center the ablation on the pupil and the physiological corneal shape is prolate with greater central curvature, the final TZ will be more gradual nasally (where the ablation involves the cornea up to the periphery) than temporally (where the ablation is applied on a more curved corneal portion and may not reach the corneal periphery).

Surgical Technique for Surface Myopic Ablation

The reliability and long-term stability of surface ablation for myopia has been demonstrated in several studies for a wide range of refractive powers and with different surgical techniques.[7-10] In the history of myopic correction, the

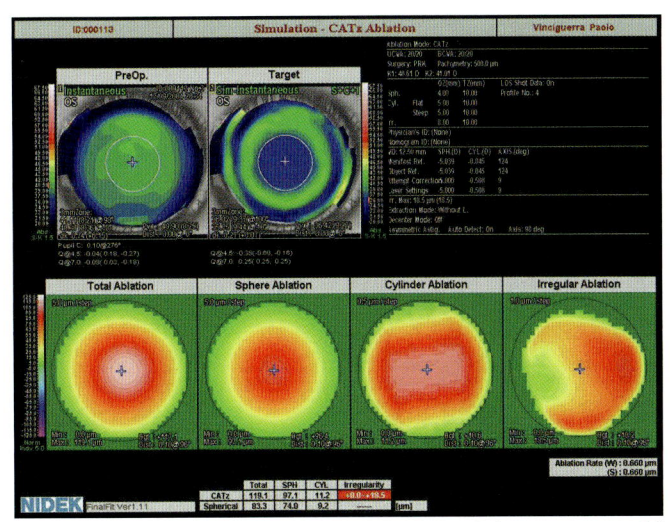

Figure 10-11. Same eye as Figure 10-1. If this case would have a thin cornea, with mandatory tissue saving, a possible strategy would be to reduce the OZ size. Here is shown the result of a treatment with a 4-mm OZ size, instantaneous algorithm. Ablation is of 119 μm.

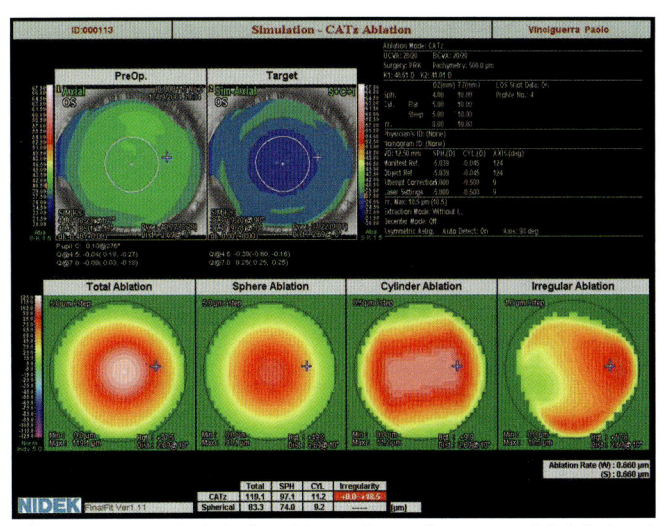

Figure 10-12. Axial algorithm view of strategy highlighted in Figure 10-7. Functional OZ has excellent width.

introduction of multiple ablation zones has been a milestone.[11] In a time when custom ablation was not available, this was a way to build a much more aspherical and, thus, physiological corneal profile than that is obtainable with a single ablation zone. Furthermore, the multiple ablation zone approach eliminated the sharp step of single zone ablation between treated and untreated cornea, providing a gradual "TZ" that reduced not only the extent of the reparative process but also regression and haze. Another advantage, more relevant when eye-tracking systems were not available, was that with a multiple zone ablation plan, possible tracking errors were minimized because the error would generally involve just a zone and, thus, a fraction of the planned ablated refraction. A third advantage was that the overlapping of these consecutive ablation zones reduced the intrinsic irregularity of the ablation pattern (see Chapter 8).

This ablation pattern, though, also had several limits. Often, it required a deeper ablation, especially when a wide ablation zone was preferred. Not all the available excimer lasers could easily perform this type of ablation and, as a result, the treatment could require longer times in order to set the desired zones.

The splitting of the refractive defect in different zones had to be carefully planned in order to create zones with identical or very similar power and to generate an identical corneal curvature gradient. Furthermore, the difference in diameter of the consecutive zones had to be constant in order to induce a similar scarring process throughout the ablated cornea.

Presently, custom ablation is our preferred technique for the correction of myopia.[12-15] Using the NIDEK Final Fit software with CATz option, we can identify easily if the minimal astigmatism often associated with myopia is true or determined by high-order aberrations that can be easily eliminated with the specific part of the ablation program (see Chapters 11 and 18). Smoothing is always performed at the end of surgery.

The NIDEK Final Fit software provides other opportunities for elaborating the final corneal profile, such as the correction of the total ocular wavefront (OPD option). The Final Fit OPD option utilizes the total ocular wavefront, evaluates it, and provides an ablation program that creates aspherical ablation zones and compensates all aberrations, including a possible lens astigmatism (Figures 10-13 through 10-16). Particular attention must be dedicated to the amount of preoperative corneal curvature; flat corneas require different strategy from more curved corneas (Figures 10-5 through 10-11, 10-17 through 10-24).

In our opinion, whenever a marked difference between corneal and total astigmatism is detected (ie, greater than -0.5 D), it is better to give up total astigmatism correction, and treat just the corneal portion. This is because the corneal astigmatism induced by total wavefront-based refractive surgery in order to compensate that of the lens will not have anymore this antagonist, particularly when the eventual removal of a cataractous lens is done at an advanced age. This situation may be optically disturbing, as it cannot be perfectly compensated with IOLs featuring a cylinder correction, and it might require further refractive surgery or be source of possible litigation.

Presently, the introduction of custom ablation and tracking systems has reduced the incidence of decentration—one of the most dreadful intraoperative complications in refractive surgery. After surgery, we always apply a protective contact lens and give a single administration of cyclopentholate 1% eyedrops, preservative-free steroid eyedrops, and fluoroquinolone eyedrops. The patient is then instructed to take fluoroquinolone eyedrops until complete re-epithelialization.

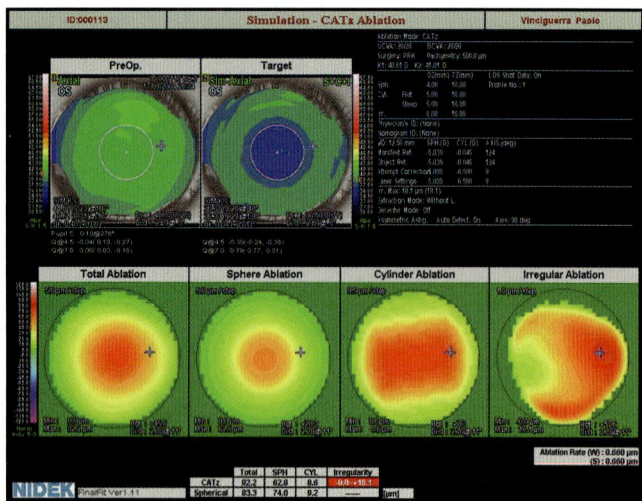

Figure 10-13. Axial algorithm view of strategy highlighted in Figure 10-7, with 4 mm OZ and 10 mm TZ. Ablation profile has been changed, from number 4 to number 1, moving the transition zone towards center of cornea, and thus restricting resulting functional OZ. This is a tissue-saving strategy: ablation depth is reduced to only 82 μm.

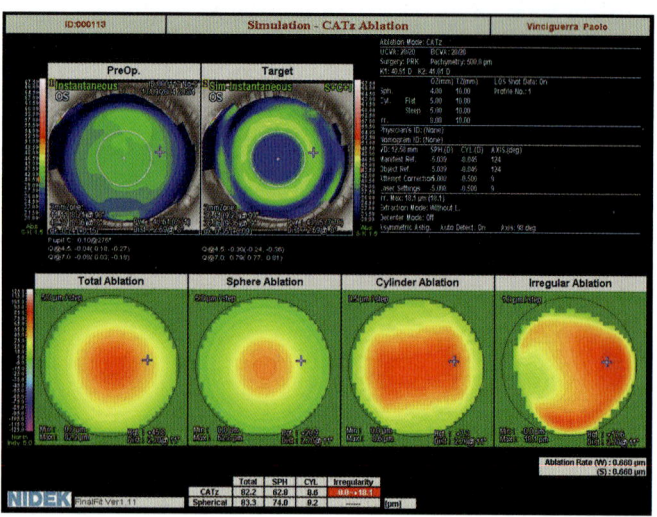

Figure 10-14. Same strategy as in Figure 10-9, instantaneous algorithm. The transition zone is close to the corneal center and the corneal curvature gradient remains elevated, even if not as much as in Figure 10-2.

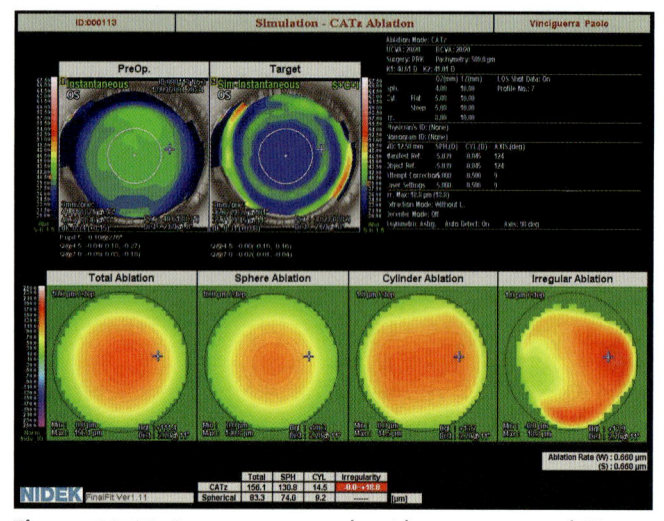

Figure 10-15. Instantaneous algorithm, strategy of Figure 10-7 (4 mm OZ), ablation profile number 7. The transition zone is more peripheral, the corneal curvature gradient is much reduced, and the ablation depth is of 156 μm. In the simulated postoperative instantaneous map, note the curvature gradient in extreme periphery. Such strategy is fit for low myopic powers.

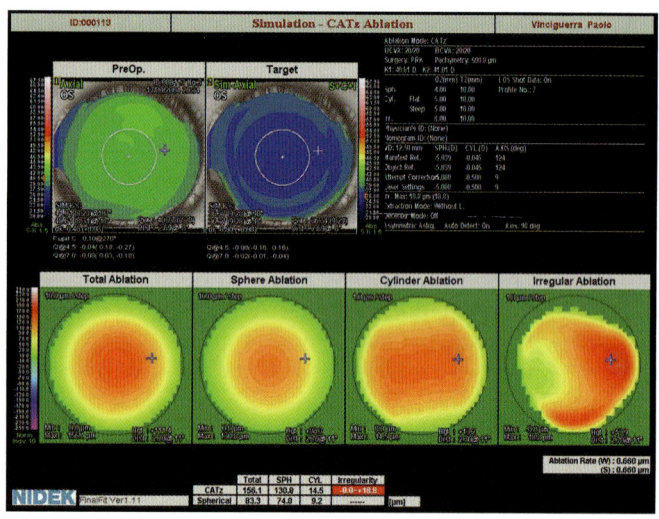

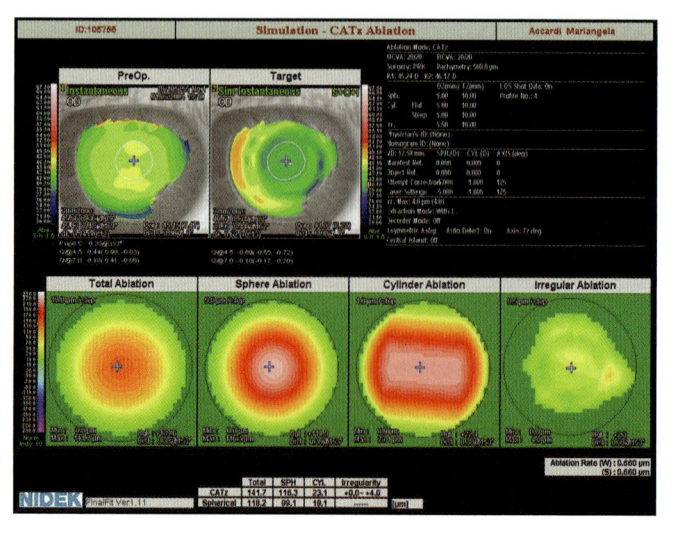

Figure 10-16. Same strategy as in Figure 10-11, axial algorithm. Functional OZ is extremely wide.

Figure 10-17. A case with a more curved cornea (mouse pointer 45.24 D, instantaneous map, upper left), -5.0 D sph -1.0 (175) D cyl, 5 mm OZ, 10 mm TZ, ablation profile number 4. Flattening the cornea becomes more critical, and more pronounced the resulting corneal curvature gradient. Ablation depth 141 μm.

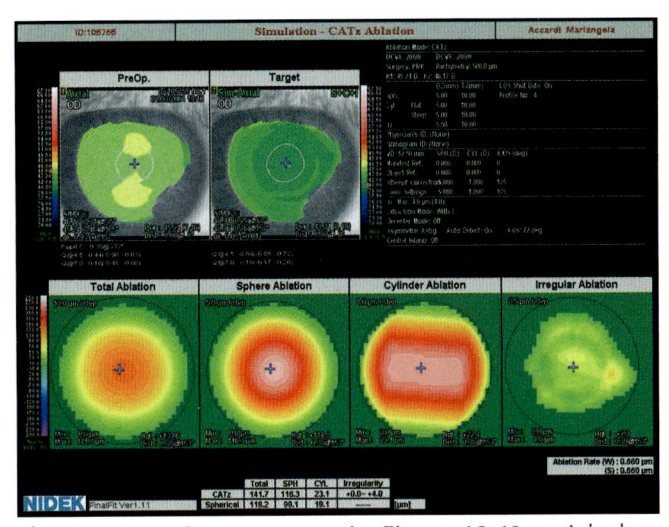

Figure 10-18. Same case as in Figure 10-13, axial algorithm. Functional OZ is very wide.

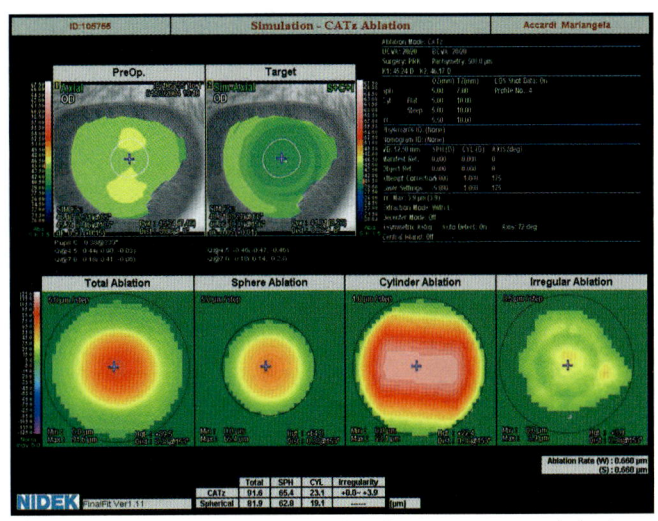

Figure 10-19. Same case as in Figure 10-13, axial algorithm, and ablation profile number 4, TZ is reduced to 7 mm. Ablation depth is reduced to 96 μm. Note how OZ is smaller than that in Figure 10-14.

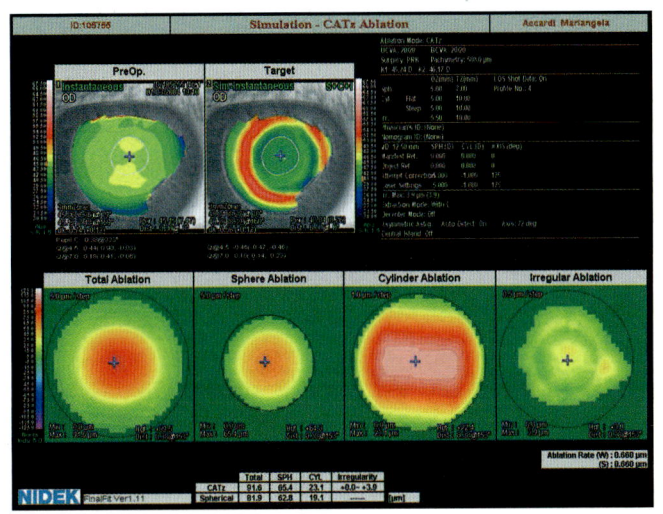

Figure 10-20. Same case as in Figure 10-13, strategy of Figure 10-15. Instantaneous algorithm, however, highlights marked corneal curvature gradient in the midperiphery. With such a high gradient, the risk of regression and halo perception is elevated.

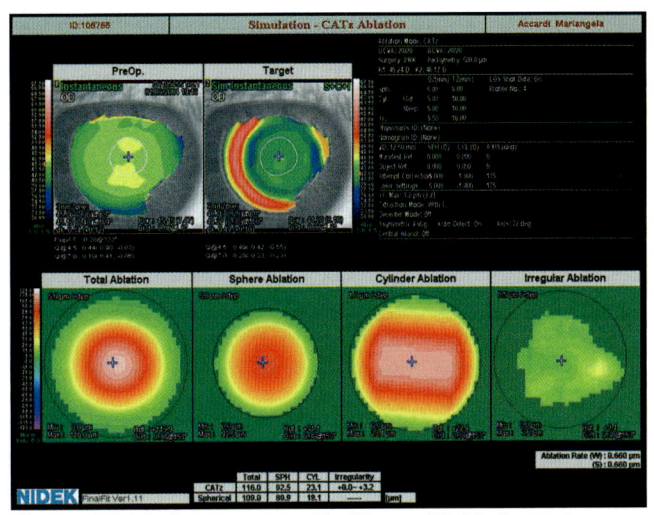

Figure 10-21. Same case as in Figure 10-13, instantaneous algorithm, ablation profile number 4. OZ has been widened to 6 mm, TZ restricted to 8 mm. Ablation depth has become 116 μm. The high corneal curvature gradient resulting from treating this highly curved cornea—visible as red ring—has been moved to the periphery.

Follow Up and Complications of Surface Myopic Ablation

Regardless of the technique (PRK, LASEK or Epi-LASIK), we carefully follow the patient during the postoperative period and remove the protective contact lens only when the epithelium is completely covering the corneal surface and appears stable. At that point, we change the therapy and prescribe fluorometholone eyedrops 3 times a day for 3 weeks, as well as preservative-free artificial tears several times a day (at least 6). The postoperative controls are routinely performed at months 1, 3, 6, and 12 with complete ophthalmologic examination and corneal topography. We do not administer a longer course of steroid because the surface regularity provided by smoothing—in our experience—greatly reduces the postoperative haze and regression (see Chapter 8).

The patient must be carefully instructed to report any stable reduction in vision beyond week 2 postoperatively, a period after which vision quality should improve constantly. Detection of residual refractive errors within the first months requires careful topographic examination. Detection of surface irregularity due to the epithelial closure line will be transitory. Central topographical irregularity may simulate regression with residual myopia or frankly the appearance of a central island. Paracentral topographical irregularity may cause astigmatism or hyperopia.

In these cases, we recommend that a soft disposable contact lens be applied constantly for up to 15 days. The pressure applied by the contact lens will regularize the epithelium

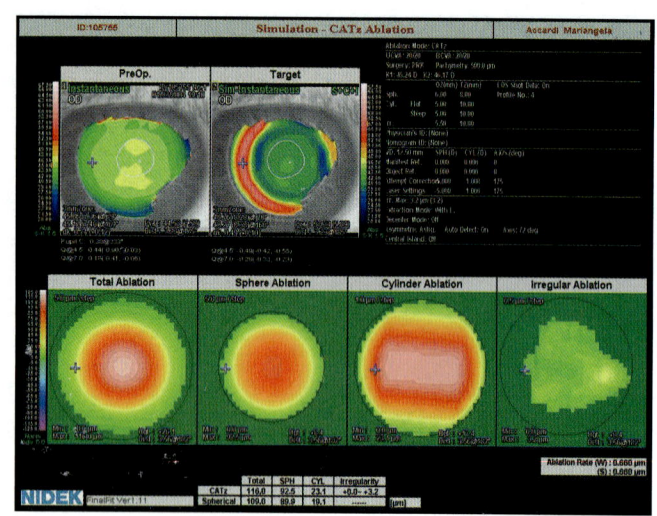

Figure 10-22. Same case as in Figure 10-17. If the mouse pointer is moved to the point where the corneal curvature gradient is higher, the value is of 57.33 D (instantaneous map, upper right).

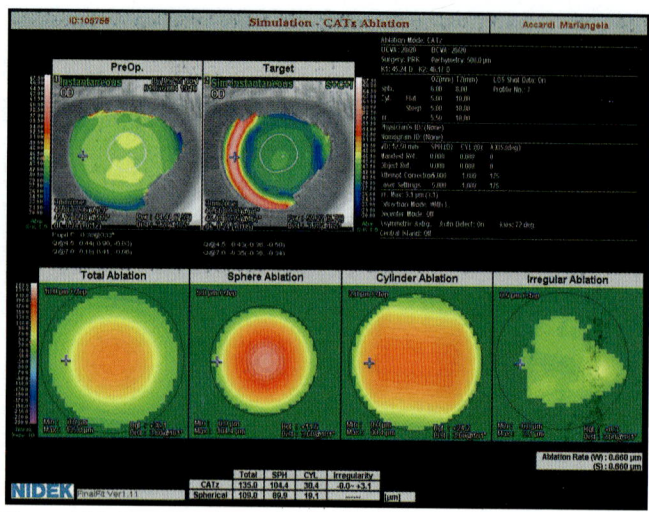

Figure 10-23. Same case as in Figure 10-13, instantaneous algorithm, 6 mm OZ, 8 mm TZ, ablation profile has been changed to number 7. Mouse pointer 59.22 D, instantaneous map, upper right. Ablation depth has become 135 µm. Compared with Figure 10-13, optical zone has been enlarged up to 6 mm. This requires deeper ablation. The high corneal curvature gradient resulting from treating this highly curved cornea has been moved as much as possible to the periphery.

and prevent possible excessive collagen deposition in areas where the epithelium is thicker. When detecting an undercorrection, the surgeon must proceed with caution to an accurate determination of visual acuity with fogging and, if in doubt, even cycloplegia. Patients with previous overcorrection and accommodative spasm may maintain this spasm for some time postoperatively, showing a false undercorrection. Differential topographical maps may be helpful in assessing the applied variation in curvature with the refractive map and axial algorithm providing information on the central change in curvature, the axial algorithm for the OZ extension, and the instantaneous for the whole corneal shape. Detection of frank undercorrection should be followed by a course of topical steroid (eg, desamethasone) eye drops for 1 to 2 weeks with successive monitoring of refraction and intraocular pressure, while keeping in mind the well-known underestimation of intraocular pressure after excimer refractive surgery. Generally speaking, this approach may be pursued, with progressively reduced possibilities of influencing refraction, until month 6 postoperatively.

Undercorrection associated with haze, as well as simple haze with reduction of visual acuity, must be likewise treated with courses of steroids. It has been demonstrated that haze associated with surface ablation regresses in the majority of cases with the course of time. We are especially pleased with the low haze frequency obtained applying smoothing after ablation (see Chapter 8). Sporadically and more often after treatment for high myopia (ie, above -6.0 D), we have observed cases of marked postoperative regression associated with haze and no apparent clinical cause, and treated them with repeated course of steroid eyedrops as mentioned above. We do not recommend retreatment before 1 year after the first surgery.

Treatment of overcorrection with courses of sodium diclofenac eyedrops has been mentioned sporadically, but to our knowledge, no adequate epidemiological report has been presented.

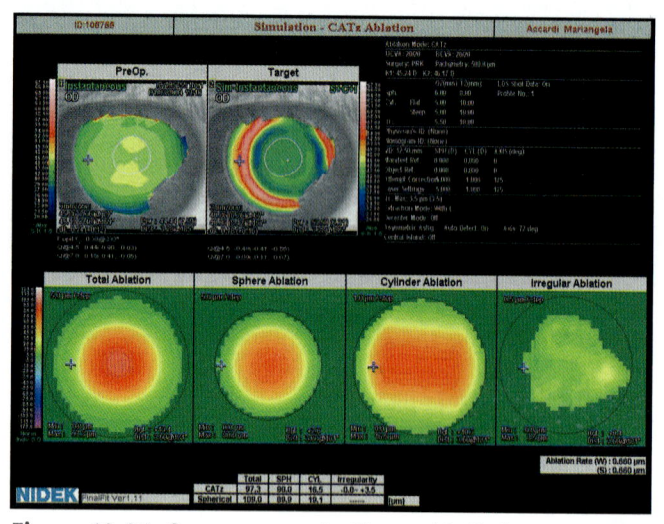

Figure 10-24. Same case as in Figure 10-13, instantaneous algorithm, 6 mm OZ, 8 mm TZ, ablation profile has been changed to number 1. Mouse pointer 53.5 D, instantaneous map, upper right. Ablation depth has been reduced down to 97 µm. The high corneal curvature gradient is now closer to the corneal center.

References

1. McDonald MB, Kaufman HE, Frantz JM, et al. Excimer laser ablation in a human eye. *Arch Ophthalmol.* 1989;107:641-2.
2. Roberts C. Biomechanics of the cornea and wavefront-guided laser refractive surgery. *J Refract Surg.* 2002;18:S589-92.
3. Vinciguerra P, Munoz MI, Camesasca FI, Grizzi F, Roberts C. Long-term follow-up of ultrathin corneas after surface retreatment with phototherapeutic keratectomy. *J Cataract Refract Surg.* 2005;31:82-7.

4. Piovella M, Camesasca FI, Fattori C. Excimer laser photorefractive keratectomy for high myopia. Four-year experience with a multiple zone technique. *Ophthalmology.* 1997;104:1554-1565.
5. Abbott RL, Ou RJ, Bird M. Medical malpractice predictors and risk factors for ophthalmologists performing LASIK and photorefractive keratectomy surgery. *Ophthalmology.* 2003;110: 2137-2146.
6. Nepomuceno RL, Boxer Wachler BS, Scruggs R. Functional OZ after myopic LASIK as a function of ablation diameter. *J Cataract Refract Surg.* 2005;31:379-384.
7. Vinciguerra P, Camesasca FI, Torres IM. Transition zone design and smoothing in custom laser-assisted subepithelial keratomileusis. *J Cataract Refract Surg.* 2005;31:39-47.
8. Vinciguerra P, Camesasca FI, Torres IM. One-year results of custom laser epithelial keratomileusis with the Nidek System. *J Cataract Refract Surg.* 2004;20:S699-704.
9. Mastropasqua L, Nubile M, Ciancaglini M, Toto L, Ballone E. Prospective randomized comparison of wavefront-guided and conventional phorefractive keratectomy for myopia with the meditec MEL 70 laser. *J Refract Surg.* 2004;20:422-431.
10. Twa MD, Nicholas JJ, Joslin CE, Kollbaum PS, et al. Characteristics of corneal ectasia after LASIK for myopia. *Cornea.* 2004;23:447-457.
11. Honda N, Hamada N, Amano S, Kaji Y, et al. Five-year follow-up of photorefractive keratectomy for myopia. *J Refract Surg.* 2004;20:116-120.
12. Pietila J, Makinen P, Pajari T, Suominen S, et al. Eight-year follow-up of photorefractive keratectomy for myopia. *J Refract Surg.* 2004;20:110-115.
13. Bilgihan K, Hondur A, Hasanreisoglu B. Laser subepithelial keratomileusis for myopia of -6 to -10 diopters with astigmatism with the MEL60 laser. *J Refract Surg.* 2004;20:121-126.
14. Rajan MS, Jaycock P, O'Brart D, Nystrom HH, Marshall J. A long-term study of photorefractive keratectomy: 12-year follow-up. *Ophthalmology.* 2004;111:1813-1824.
15. Nagy ZZ, Palagyi-Deak I, Kelemn E, Kovacs A. Wavefront-guided photorefractive keratectomy for myopia and myopic astigmatism. *J Refract Surg.* 2002;18:S615-619.

Treatment of Astigmatism

*Paolo Vinciguerra, MD; Fabrizio I. Camesasca, MD;
Guido Nizzola, MD; Daniel Epstein, MD, PhD*

Introduction

Treatment of astigmatism has been the second major challenge in the history of excimer laser refractive surgery. Regression, corneal haze, and functional symptoms secondary to optical aberrations are possible complications of astigmatism correction with excimer laser either using PRK, LASEK, or LASIK. The main cause of these complications lies in the high dioptric gradient induced by the commonly used ablation strategies in the transition area along the steepest topographical meridian (Figures 11-1 and 11-2).[1,2]

Understanding Astigmatism

A key point in the correction of astigmatism is comprehension of the corneal astigmatic profile. The true origin of astigmatism can be defined by proper use of several diagnostic methods, namely topography, aberrometry, and pachymetry.

A topography map will identify the location of astigmatism, whether it is with-the-rule, against-the-rule, or mixed; the symmetry of the astigmatic bow-tie pattern; and the degree of corneal curvature. Classic astigmatic corneal curvature (Figure 11-3) characteristically features a bow tie that is symmetric both in extension and in degree of curvature, with the steepest point of the upper segment showing the same curvature of the lower segment on an axial map. Figure 11-4 shows a summary of vision quality and Modulation Transfer Factor when astigmatism is present.

Correlation among axial, instantaneous, and elevation maps is particularly important in astigmatism. A classic, regularly astigmatic cornea will show an elevation map with a typical "bridge" pattern demonstrating the regularity of the astigmatic toroid (see Figure 11-3). An "island" pattern, on the contrary, may be indicative of an irregular astigmatism, and the cornea must be carefully evaluated by considering a pachymetric map. Pachymetry mapping can be presently performed with several instruments (eg, the Pentacam [OCULUS Optikgeräte GmbH, Wetzlar, Germany] and the Orbscan [Bausch & Lomb, Rochester, NY]).

As far as regular astigmatism is concerned, it is important to remember that a large or a small bow tie seen in axial topography is not directly related to the size of the corneal area involved in astigmatism. The size of the bow tie indicates the change in curvature, greater in the large bow tie, smaller in the small one. The radius of curvature changes rapidly from center to periphery in small bow ties (e values of more than 0.5), more gradually in large ones (e values of less than 0.5) (Figures 11-5 through 11-10).

The Astigmatic Ablation Profile in Surface Ablation

It is well known that regular astigmatism is characterized by the presence of two "main" orthogonal meridians: the steepest and the flattest meridians. In the past, two main strategies have been commonly adopted: ablation on one meridian only or split ablation on the two meridians of astigmatism and of axis and power. Treating all astigmatism on one meridian leads to marked corneal asymmetry, similar to the previous state of astigmatism; asymmetry is moved merely from the corneal center to the periphery. The corneal shape resulting from this correction is frequently oblate, much different from a physiological, normal, or an astigmatic prolate cornea (Figure 11-11). With even slight pupil dilatation (eg, up to 5 mm), eyes that received this type of treatment show an increase in aberrations, including spherical aberration, quadrafoil, and astigmatism.

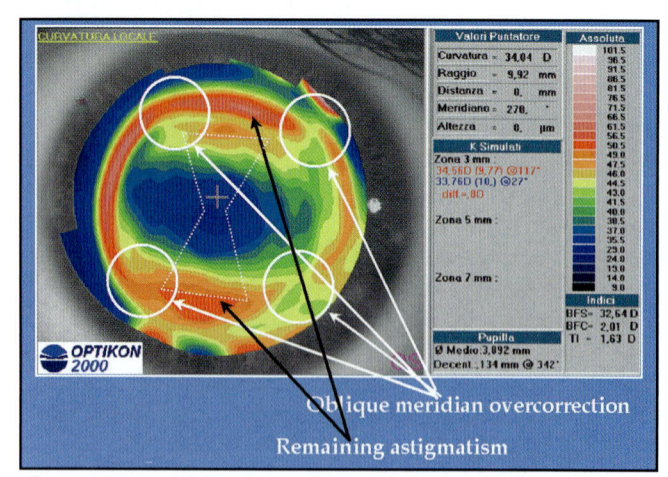

Figure 11-1. Oblique meridian hypercorrection. Treated: -7.25 D sphere -5.0 (173) D cylinder.

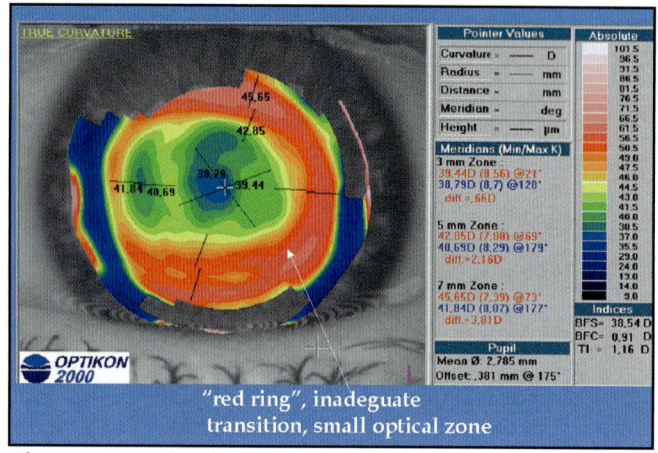

Figure 11-2. Inadequate preoperative transition on the steep meridian. Treated -6.0 D sphere -4.0 (5) D cylinder.

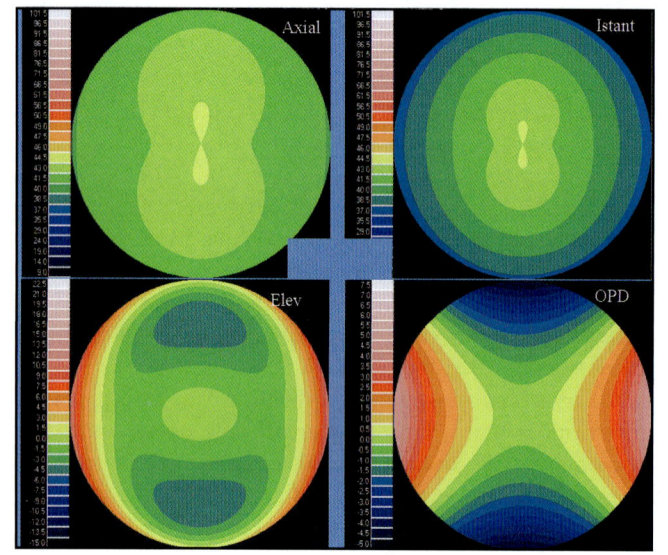

Figure 11-3. Topographical and OPD maps of classic astigmatic corneal curvature. The elevation map shows a typical "bridge" pattern.

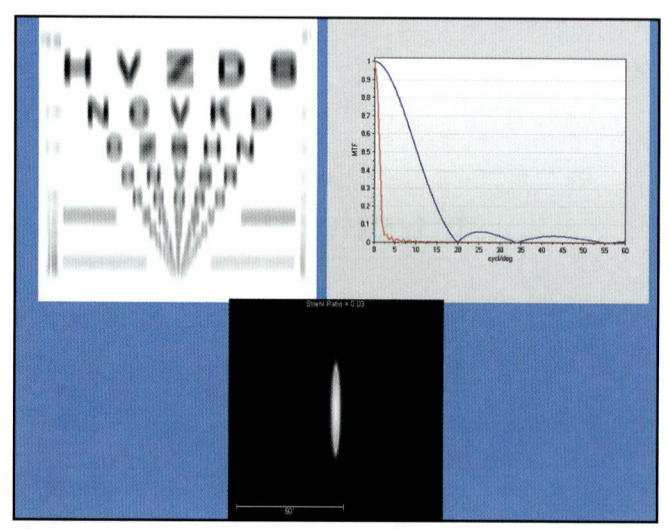

Figure 11-4. The same eye as in Figure 11-3, summary of vision quality and Modulation Transfer Factor.

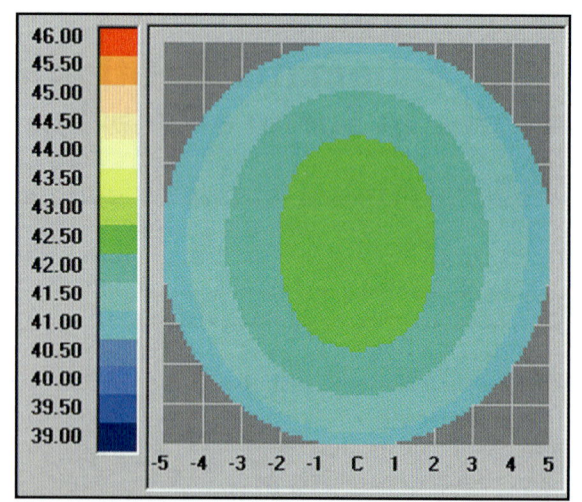

Figure 11-5. Low with-the-rule astigmatism (keratometry: 42.75/43.0 ax 180), medium eccentricity ($p = 0.8$) ($e = 0.45$)

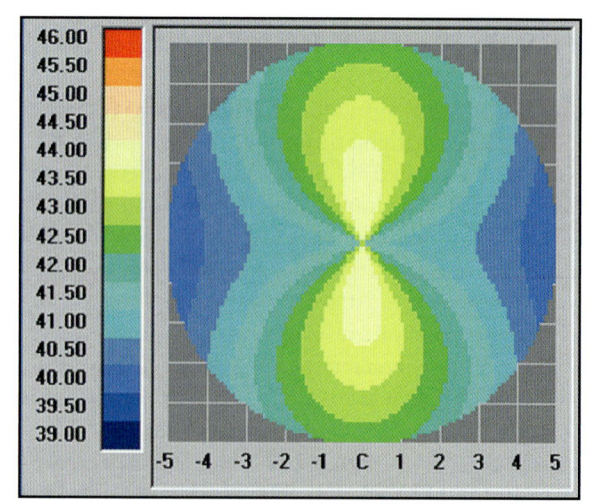

Figure 11-6. With-the-rule astigmatism 3.0 D (keratometry: 41.5/44.5 ax 180) medium eccentricity ($p = 0.8$) ($e = 0.45$).

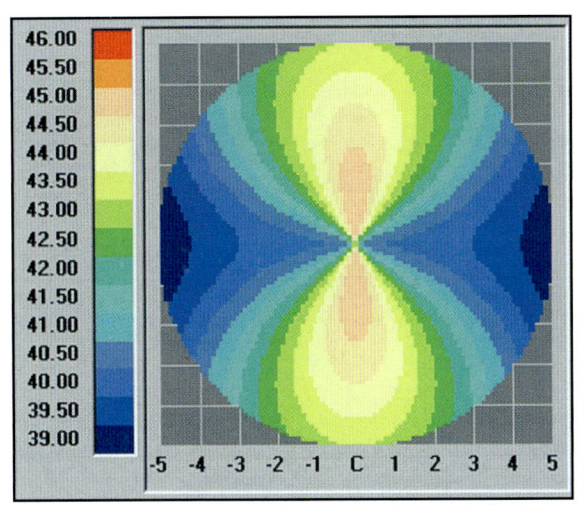

Figure 11-7. With-the-rule astigmatism 5.0 D (keratometry: 40.5/45.5 ax 180) and medium eccentricity (p = 0.8) (e = 0.45).

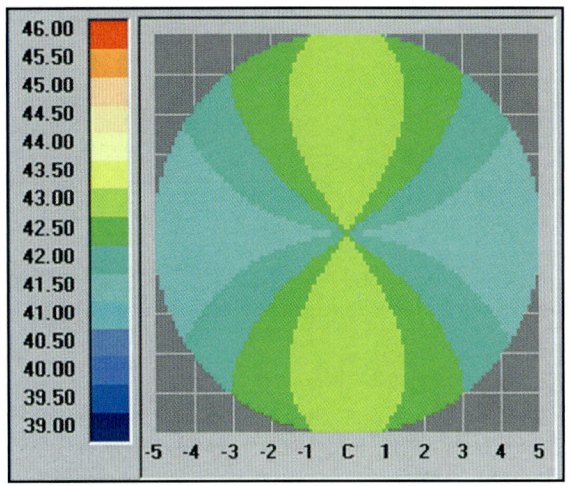

Figure 11-8. With-the-rule astigmatism 1.5 D (keratometry 42.0/43.5 ax 180) low eccentricity (e = 0.22) (p = 0.95).

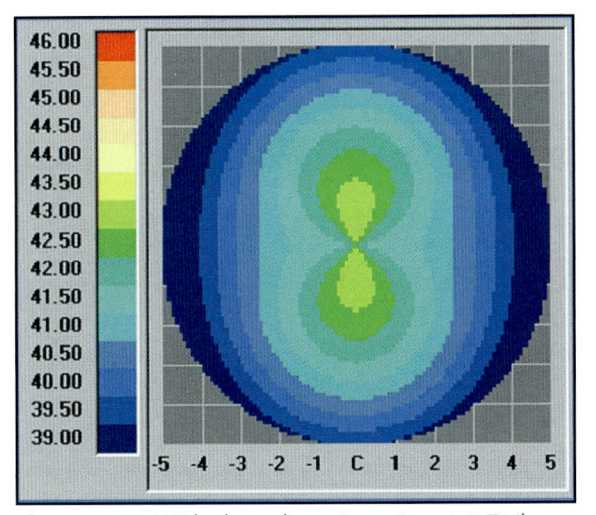

Figure 11-9. With-the-rule astigmatism 1.5 D (keratometry 42.0/43.5 ax 180) high eccentricity (e = 0.7) (p = 0.5).

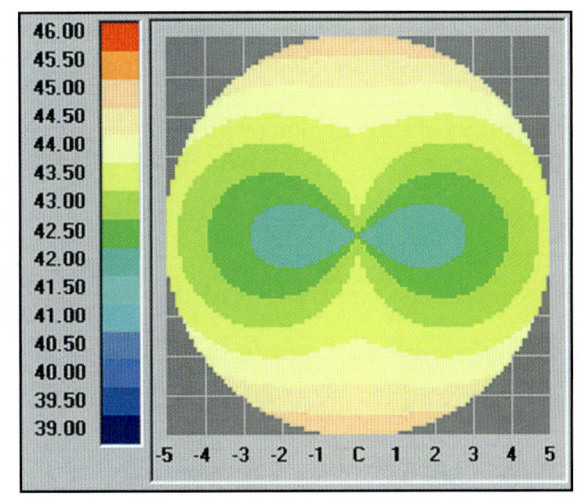

Figure 11-10. Against-the-rule astigmatism 1.5 D (keratometry 42.0/43.5 ax 180), oblate surface, negative eccentricity (e = -0.4) (p = 1.2).

Usually, precustom ablation techniques for the correction of myopic astigmatism were fairly satisfactory on the steepest meridian but generated overcorrection on oblique meridians, which have a lower dioptrical power. For example, if we treat for -5.0 D of cylindrical ablation with an optical zone (OZ) of 5 mm, we plan a 30-μm ablation on 126-degree axis. The actual ablation, however, is 40 μm with an overcorrection of 10 μm. A standard ablation appears to be adequate on the steepest meridian but, in fact, overcorrects the oblique ones, leading to a hyperopic shift. Overcorrection is spherical and about 20% with an irregular "four-leaf" astigmatism on the oblique meridians (Table 11-1, Figure 11-12).

Perfect ablation for myopic astigmatism should completely correct the steepest meridian, as well as the oblique ones in proportion to their curvatures. The flattest meridian should remain unchanged. A dioptrically progressive corneal shape is decisive in avoiding regression. Epithelial layering follows a superficial tension law.[3] When it meets irregular surfaces, corneal epithelium becomes thicker in order to fill gaps. A thicker epithelium induces formation of underlying scar tissue. Therefore, corneal irregularities are partially compensated by scar tissue deposition. Unfortunately, this mechanism leads to regression of a given correction.[4] Corneal scarring and epithelial thickening can also lead to midperipheral flattening. In order to avoid regression and visual acuity decrease, a regular and progressive change of corneal curvature is mandatory.

Epithelium hyperplasia covering corneal irregularities may lead to regression after LASIK, too.[5] The surgeon can eliminate regression by scraping the hyperplastic epithelium, but as weeks go by, the epithelium grows again, following the superficial tension law. Striae formation after LASIK represents another example of the importance of a regular corneal surface. After excimer ablation, striae occur when there is a high dioptric gradient between the OZ and the

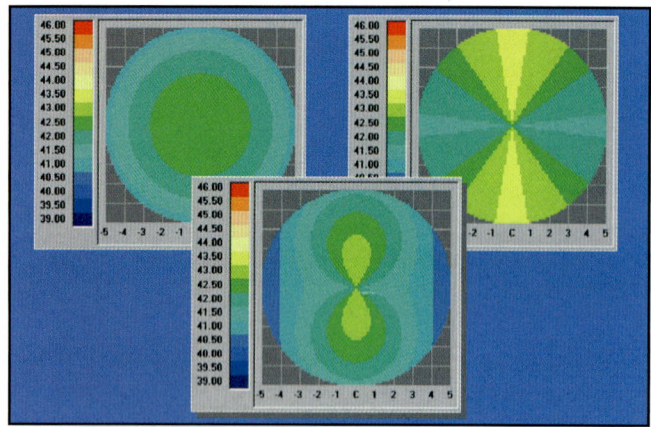

Figure 11-11. Top Left: aspheric, prolate, symmetric surface. Flattening of the cornea from center to periphery on any given meridian. At a given distance from the center, the curvature is the same on every meridian. Top Right: nonaspheric toric surface. The curvature along a single meridian remains the same at any given distance from the center. There is a change in curvature from one meridian to another. Bottom: aspheric toric surface. A combination of the two previously described curvatures. Classical bow tie shape in a normal cornea with a medium eccentricity.

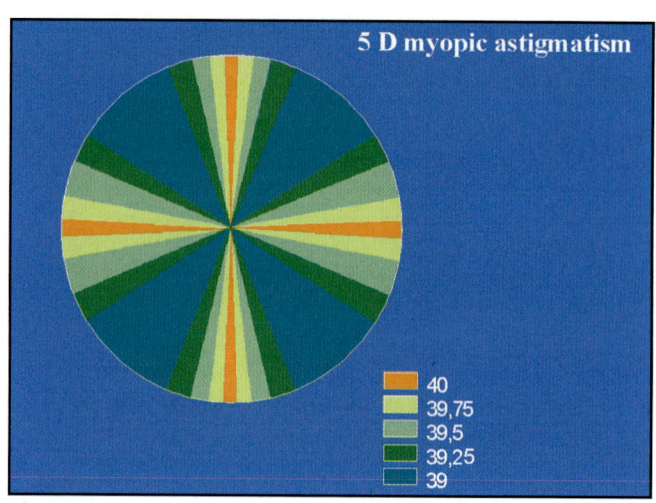

Figure 11-12. Five D myopic astigmatism. Irregular "four-leaved" astigmatism with overcorrection along the oblique meridians.

Table 11-1. Myopic Cylindrical Ablation

Axis	Theoretic Ablation (microns)	Real Ablation (microns)	Resulting Overcorrection (D)
90	50	50	0
108	40	47.5	+0.75
126	30	40	+1
144	20	29	+0.9
162	10	15.5	+0.55
180	0	0	0

peripheral "red ring" evidenced by topography.[6,7] Curvature variation from flat to steep cornea is substantial and reversed with respect to the physiological corneal curvature. The flap cannot lie evenly on this irregular stromal surface, and striae will occur.

Commonly, it is thought that a large ablation diameter (eg, 6.5 mm) is not associated with regression, while a small ablation diameter (eg, 4 mm) is. This is not completely true; by studying topographical maps, we have been able to see that, with large ablations too, there are changes to the ablation edge due to scar tissue formation, and/or epithelial hyperplasia. Changes take place at the edge of the ablation and far from the pupillary area, and thus the OZ remains uniform and patients are asymptomatic. On the contrary, in small ablations OZ edge modifications are within the pupillary area, thus the OZ becomes non-uniform with multifocality and optical aberration: patients note night halos, visual loss, and glare. Regression leads to a new myopic astigmatism on the steepest meridian (see Figure 11-1) and a positive spherical equivalent (SE) because of hypercorrection on the oblique meridian. Eventually, the refractive effect will be that of a mixed astigmatism, which is very difficult to retreat.

In recent years, emmetropia, as well as a regular corneal surface, has been pursued when correcting astigmatism. Correction of astigmatism on two meridians was introduced basically with two methods: the amount of correction split either evenly or unevenly between the two main meridians. Starting from the analysis of nomograms, which showed that a residual astigmatism was left on the untreated meridian, Chayet et al introduced an asymmetrical correction split onto the two astigmatism meridians.[3] He deserves much credit for his clever approach, though an asymmetrical correction retains the limits of creating an asymmetrical corneal surface with possible aberrations. In a thorough analysis of different available methods, Azar and Primack recommended correction on the hyperopic meridian only with the advantage of removing even less cornea than with any other technique.[8] However, in this case, treatment leads to corneal surface asymmetry also, even if on a different meridian, with possible induction of aberrations.

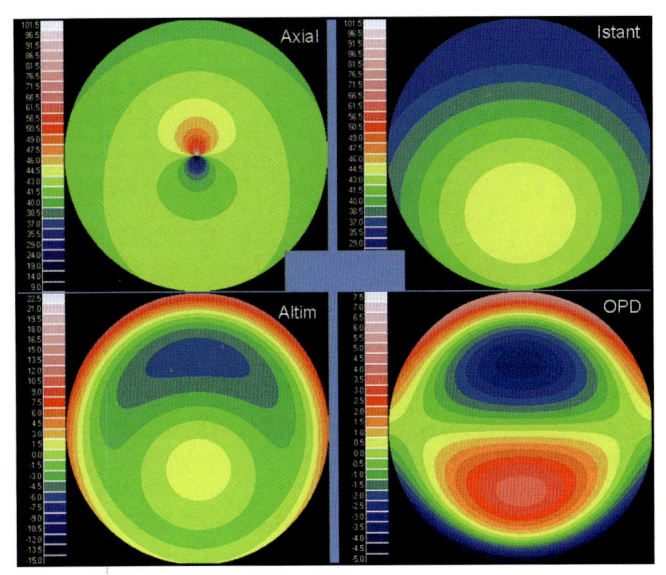

Figure 11-13. Topographical and OPD maps when coma is present.

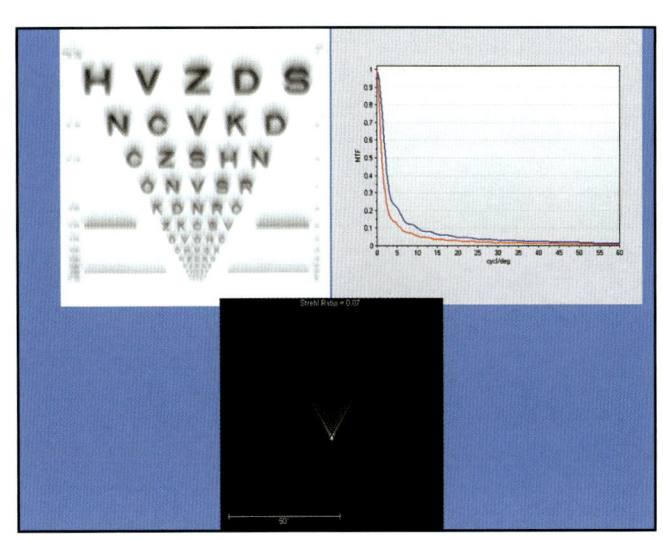

Figure 11-14. Visual function summary and Modulation Transfer Factor when coma is present.

We developed a technique for the correction of astigmatism with crossed cylinders, which, besides requiring limited tissue ablation, leaves the cornea prolate and symmetrical with a final shape closer to the normal prolate cornea, without inducing aberrations (eg, coma). Corneal regularity, previously almost an intuitive concept, can now be described as maintaining its eccentricity within physiological limits with a surface generating an aberration-free wavefront. Eccentricity indicates the corneal change in curvature from the center to the periphery and can be considered as a way to measure the shape of spherical aberration, not its effect on vision. When spherical aberration is high, the OZ diameter is very close to that of ablation zone (AZ). Containing spherical aberration within 1.0 to 2.0 D will provide an optical zone much wider than the AZ provided. When correcting astigmatism, the choice of the OZ diameter is usually related to the maximal pupil diameter.

Corneal Eccentricity

Our ideal postoperative target is a prolate cornea, maintaining corneal eccentricity. Eccentricity is the measure of corneal asphericity; therefore, it indicates the way the cornea changes from a flatter periphery to a more curved central portion. Normal eccentricity values (e values) range between +0.5 and +0.6 (normally prolate cornea: curved in the center, flat in the periphery).

Normal astigmatism correction on one meridian only leads to central corneal symmetry without changing the radius of curvature on the opposite meridian. Ablation on one meridian only changes corneal asphericity; a negative cylinder flattens the corneal center (oblate cornea), and a positive cylinder flattens the corneal periphery (excessively prolate cornea). Peripheral change in curvature is also important; the transition zone (TZ) concentrates it in a limited area with loss of physiological curvature creating a cornea that induces optical aberrations. Thus, if the two ablations are not symmetrical, the final result may be an asymmetrical cornea with high-order aberrations and poor visual quality. These aberrations negatively influence vision quality even at different pupil diameters, more than aberrations deriving from symmetrical changes (eg, coma), and the patients often complain of monocular double vision. Figures 11-13 and 11-14 show topographical maps, visual function summary, and modulation transfer factor when coma is present.

Cross-Cylinder Ablation Technique

Before the introduction of custom ablation, the cross-cylinder ablation technique was our method of choice for astigmatism.[5,9-11] The cornerstone of this treatment is the division of the cylinder power in two symmetric parts. Its main advantages are the preservation of the mean corneal radius of curvature, and therefore, of corneal eccentricity. Another advantage of this technique, as well as of other techniques (eg, positive cylinder), is a reduction in the quantity of ablated tissue. The cross-cylinder technique can be adopted with excimer lasers of recent generation that permit ablation both with negative and positive cylinders. The diameters of the ablation zone (AZ) and TZ must be symmetrical (eg,. 6.5 AZ with 1.0 TZ for a positive cylinder, and a 6.5 AZ and a 1.0 -9.5 TZ for the negative cylinder). In this way, the mean corneal curvature radius is unchanged, maintaining the physiological shape.

"Splitting" Technique

An "old-style" myopic excimer ablation with a single OZ and a small transition area increases the mid-peripheral curvature creating the typical topographic "red ring" (Figure 11-15). Instantaneous algorithm provides identification of the corneal curvature variation visible as a peripheral red ring. This is an oblate cornea. It is important to note how a 5-mm AZ treatment does not correspond to a real 5-mm OZ on the

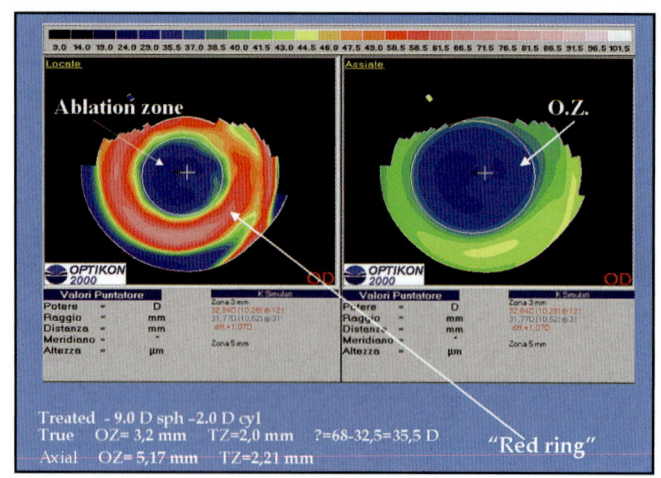

Figure 11-15. Presence of the "red ring" indicates a non-constant change in midperipheral curvature.

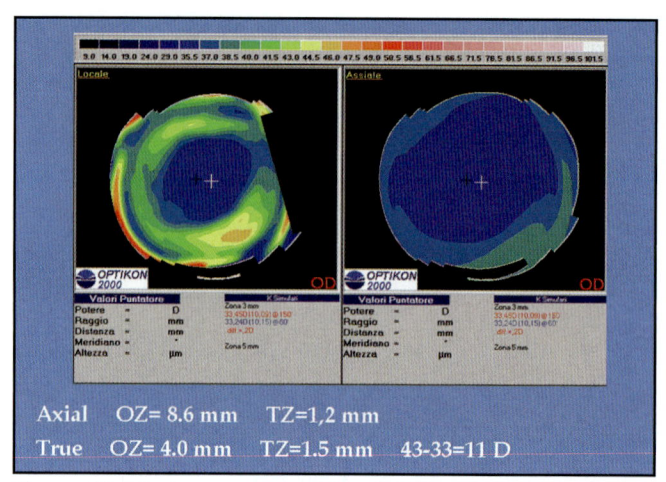

Figure 11-16. An eye treated for -9.0 D sph -2.0 D cyl (30). Hypercurvature in the midperiphery and "red ring" are prevented when the splitting technique is adopted.

topographic map and NIDEK OPD aberrometer wavefront map (Gamagori, Japan), because the true OZ edge, perceivable on instantaneous algorithm in corneal topography, is limited by the inner margin of the above-mentioned red ring. We usually obtain a different OZ than the programmed AZ. The instantaneous algorithm provides a reliable image of the actual AZ.

High myopia correction with small programmed ablation areas will lead to a red ring close to the pupillary area, so these patients will report night halos, loss of vision quality due to multifocality, and optical aberrations. In order to avoid this midperipheral hypercurvature, myopia correction requires the application of several OZs. This necessity to achieve a TZ with a more continuous-shape has led to development of solutions such as the multiple zone technique.[12] This technique requires a constant dioptric gradient for each OZ, not a constant ablation depth.

The "splitting technique" consists in dividing the entire spherical and cylindrical myopic ametropia into OZs that are dioptrically constant.[13] We program 7 or 8 OZs in high myopia. Every OZ corrects the same amount of spherical diopters as well as the same amount of cylindrical defect. The first OZ is the largest one, and the others are progressively smaller. There is a progressive dioptric gradient from the center to the periphery of the ablated area. We recommend remaining within a maximum of 3.0 D and a minimum of 0.50 D of correction for each OZ.

Such strategy finds an important application in LASIK in order to avoid striae and glare. Creation of hypercurvature in the midperiphery is, therefore, prevented (Figure 11-16). In a LASEK case, a homogeneously ablated area without red ring can be observed, and the axial map shows an enlargement of the ablated area (Figure 11-17).

Example 1

With the cross-cylinder technique, a mixed astigmatism of +2.0 sphere -4.0 (180) cylinder will be treated by ablating a +2.0 (90) cylinder zone and a -2.0 (180) cylinder zone because we must take the spherical equivalent (SE) into account.

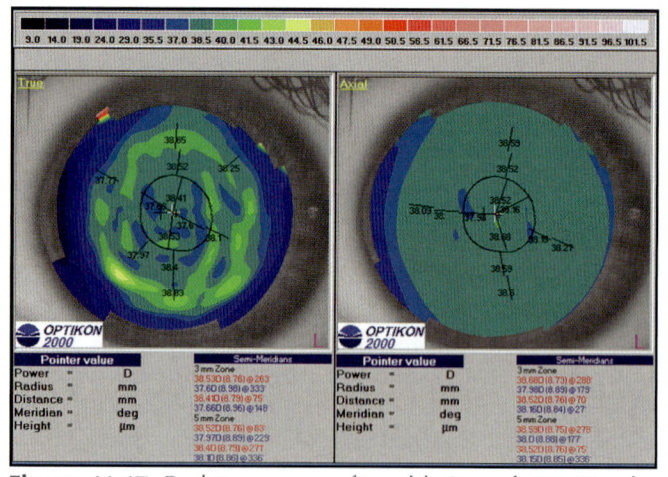

Figure 11-17. Prolate cornea after ablation of -7.0 D sph. Note that the postoperative optical zone is 11 mm. After ablation the cornea remains prolate.

* The SE of this defect is zero.
* According to the cross-cylinder formula, the amount of astigmatism must be regularly divided in two, half to be treated on the negative meridian and half on the positive meridian. Therefore, a -4.0 (180) cylinder is divided into two -2.0 (180) cylinder components, and one is transformed, taking the SE into account, into -2.0 sphere +2.0 (90) cylinder, while the other -2.0 (180) cylinder remains unchanged.
* The -2.0 sphere SE generated by converting the first half of the total cylinder nullifies the +2.0 sphere of the defect: the SE of the original defect, zero, is thus respected.
* The resulting refractive defect correction is, as quoted above, +2.0 (90) cylinder and -2.0 (180) cylinder. The mean radius of corneal curvature remains unchanged.

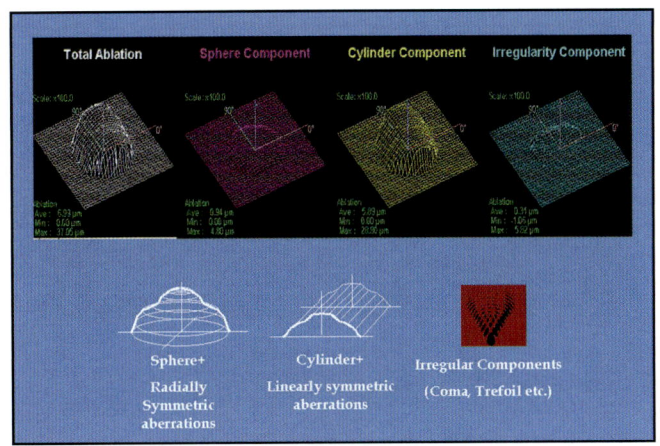

Figure 11-18. Final Fit ablation software with Custom Ablation Transition Zone software. Ablation includes a component for treatment of the spherical defect (radially symmetric aberrations), a toric component for treatment of the astigmatism (linearly symmetric aberrations), and a flying spot component for treatment of high-order aberrations (irregular components).

Example 2

+3.0 sphere -3.0 (80) cylinder.
* The SE of this defect is +1.5 sphere.
* The -3.0 (80) cylinder is divided into two -1.5 (80) cylinder components, and one is transformed, taking the SE into account, into a -1.5 sphere +1.5 (170) cylinder, while the other -1.5 (80) cylinder remains unchanged.
* The -1.5 sphere SE generated by converting the first half of the total cylinder plus the +3.0 sphere of the defect leads to a residual +1.5 sphere: the SE of the original defect, +1.5 sphere, is thus respected.
* The resulting refractive defect correction is +1.5 sphere +1.5 (170) cylinder and -1.5 (80) cylinder.

In summary, the multizone cross-cylinder method creates a progressive transition, with a low dioptric gradient, between the treated and untreated cornea. When an astigmatic defect is treated, this method maintains a postoperative physiologically prolate cornea. Advantages of the cross-cylinder technique as follows:
1. A physiologically prolate symmetric corneal shape
2. Less regression
3. Better visual quality
4. Tissue sparing by splitting part of cylinder ablation in periphery, especially useful in LASIK

The "splitting" technique leads to a spherical and more physiological corneal surface.

Custom Ablation

Until recently, the unpredictability of the corneal stromal and epithelial reparatory response was considered the main culprit for the well-known fact that final refractive results can still be quite different from those planned. Irregularities of the ablated corneal surface have been proven to play an important role in enhancing collagen deposition and therefore variation from the planned refractive result.[1-3]

On the contrary, a smooth ablated surface induces less reparatory response, leading to less haze formation and higher predictability of the refractive result.[14-17] We decided to introduce corneal smoothing in the final phase of refractive treatment after studies performed in 1998 (see Chapter 8).[16-17]

A revolutionary approach to the problem of unpredictability has been introduced by Cynthia Roberts with the concept of corneal biomechanical response to laser ablation.[18] The concept is based on the anatomical lamellar structure of the corneal stroma and on its tensile strength: central severing of lamellae due to creation of a new refractive surface by excimer laser tissue removal causes elastic contraction of the remaining peripheral lamellae with consequent corneal curvature variation. This results in peripheral corneal increase in curvature, thickness, and central flattening, leading to refractive change just where the curvature was carefully modified to achieve a planned power (see Chapter 6).

As mentioned previously, a delicate point in the creation of a new surface with excimer laser ablation is the TZ. In both stromal and surface ablation, marked variation of curvature in this peripheral portion leads to a response aimed to reduce curvature variation but may induce regression and restriction of the effective OZ.

We considered the above-mentioned concepts and the results of our previous studies and designed a surface corneal ablation strategy for custom LASEK and LASIK to increase predictability by reducing the biomechanical and reparative responses of the cornea.

We perform wavefront evaluation with the NIDEK OPD aberrometer, surgery with the LASEK technique, and ablation with the NIDEK EC 5000 excimer laser featuring 0.89 mm spot size, 130 mJ fluency rate, and 40 Hz rate. The ablation plan is elaborated the with the Final Fit ablation software featuring the Custom Ablation Transition Zone (CATZ) software (NIDEK) on the basis of the topographical and aberrometric data. Ablation includes an aspherical component for the treatment of spherical defect (radially symmetric aberrations), a toric component for the treatment of astigmatism (linearly symmetric aberrations), and a flying spot component for treatment of high-order aberrations (irregular components) (Figure 11-18). The TZ diameter is 10 mm.

After the ablation, we perform smoothing to remove corneal microirregularities of a size inferior to the spot size (0.89 mm) and to the height of ablation (0.25 μm), and to achieve a regular stromal bed as similar as possible to the physiological Bowman's layer. Smoothing is performed by applying a hyaluronic acid masking fluid (LASERVIS, Chemedica, Munich, Germany) and continuously distributing it over the corneal surface with a special spatula (Buratto's Spatula, ASICO, Westmont, Ill). The smoothing diameter is 10 mm, thus involving the entire corneal diameter and preventing a

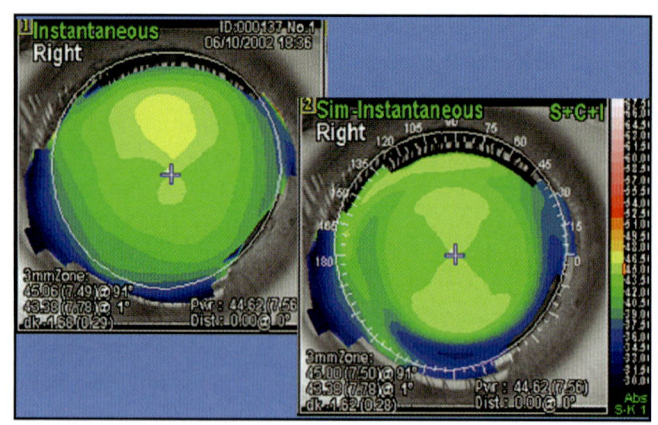

Figure 11-19. Left: preoperative instantaneous map, refraction -6.26 D sph -0.25 D cyl (1). Right: NIDEK Final Fit software target map shows that after simple high-order treatment (correction of high-order errors), the genuine cylinder power and axis can be unmasked. Even the most sophisticated custom ablation may result in residual wavefront errors.

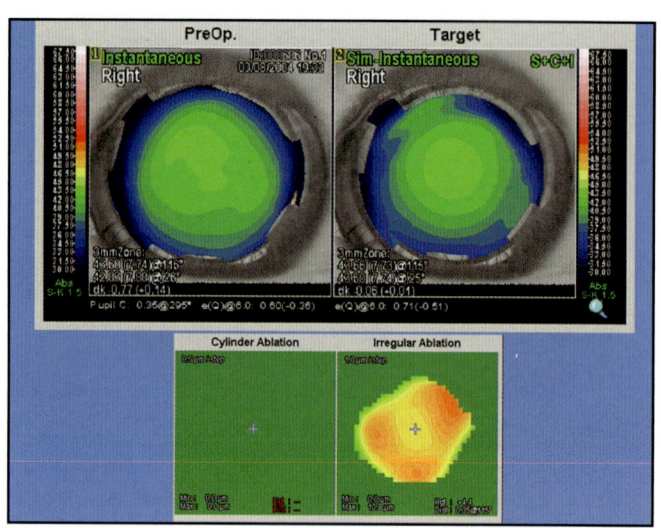

Figure 11-20. Left: preoperative instantaneous map. Right: NIDEK Final Fit software target map shows that after simple high order treatment (shown below), what looked like astigmatism was actually a combination of high-order aberrations. After those are treated actually no astigmatism is left.

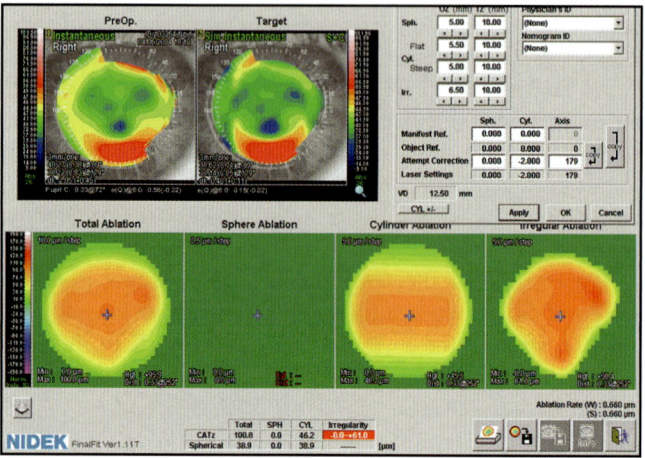

Figure 11-21. A retreatment case showing that after correction of -2.0 D cyl and high-order aberrations, a highly irregular surface is left (target instantaneous map, upper right).

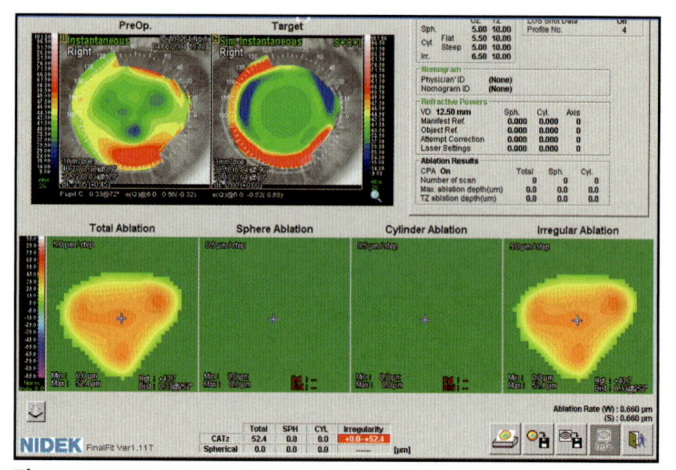

Figure 11-22. Same case as Figure 11-21: after simple treatment of high-order aberrations, a very regular corneal surface is obtained (target instantaneous map, upper right).

hyperopic shift. To avoid overheating the tissue, frequency is set at 10 Hz and the ablation at 30 µm. During the smoothing phase, the masking fluid is continuously added and evenly distributed with the spatula in order to maintain a thin layer of fluid and avoid the formation of dry areas. Because of the protective action of the masking fluid, the actual ablation imparted is almost 8 µm.[19,20]

Locating the True Cylinder Axis

Even the most sophisticated custom ablation treatment may lead to residual wavefront errors. We believe that an important factor in this process is related to the basic principle of custom ablation. High-order corneal surface aberrations, which are naturally irregular and asymmetric, influence the cylinder power and axis measured preoperatively. The correction of high-order aberrations may reveal the true cylinder power and axis, which can be quite different from the preoperative measurement (Figures 11-19 through 11-22). Avoiding increase in aberrations after refractive surgery is a difficult goal, and corneal irregularities induced by excimer ablation may cause aberrations.[21] Sometimes, what looks like pure astigmatism, perhaps irregular, is actually a combination of high-order aberrations. After those aberrations are treated, it may turn out that there is actually no astigmatism. Treatment of high-order errors may change the axis of the resulting, unmasked astigmatism. If this situation is not taken into account, several problems may occur: pseudo-decentration, residual astigmatism, induction of new high-order errors, or residual refractive error—all lead to poor vision. This happens in patients who, due to the information presently available on custom ablation, have high expectations on their final visual result.

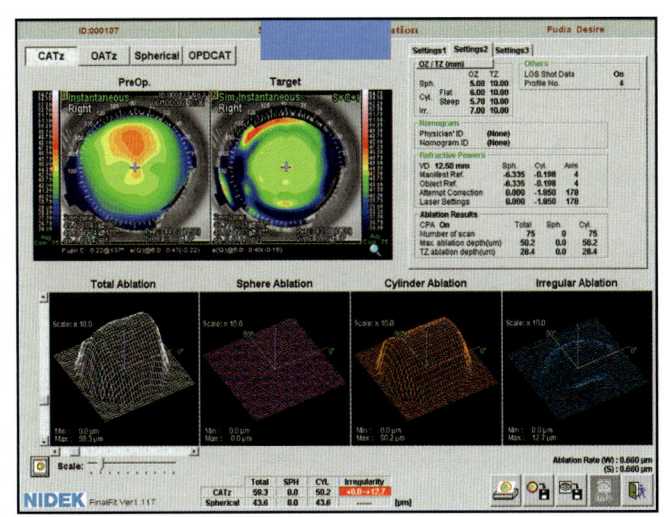

Figure 11-23. The CATZ ablation pattern of the Final Fit imparts a refractive change in which all total OPD-detected ocular aberrations, and particularly spherical aberration, are optimized in the central 4.5-mm.

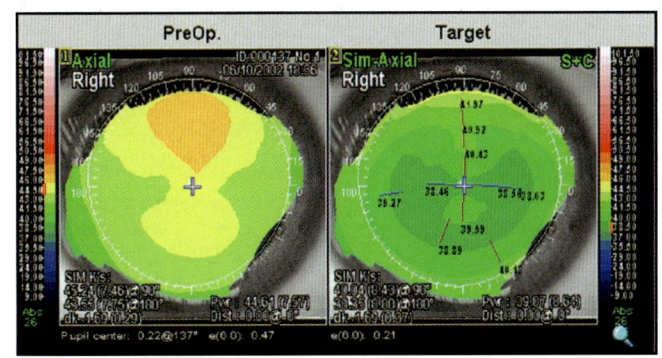

Figure 11-25. Same case of Figure 11-24. NIDEK Final Fit target axial map, right, shows pseudo-decentration after standard treatment.

We have tried to overcome this unpredictability with a particularly refined use of NIDEK Final Fit. The CATZ ablation pattern of NIDEK Final Fit imparts a refractive change in which all total OPD-detected ocular aberrations, and particularly spherical aberration, are optimized in the central 4.5 mm.[22] The curvature of the remaining cornea is then gradually modified in order to achieve a constant curvature gradient up to the external 10 mm margin of the ablation, maintaining at the same time the best possible reduction of ocular aberrations (Figures 11-23 and 11-24).

The central 4.5-mm area of ablation must not be confused with an OZ. An advanced use of NIDEK Final Fit was adopted for custom ablation in these cases. The segmental ablation for treatment of high-order components was applied first. This part of the treatment may change the axis and power of the cylinder; therefore, at this point, the new axis and power of astigmatism were estimated. Finally, the resulting spherical component to be treated was calculated (Figures 11-25 to 11-27). The amount of tissue removed by the excimer ablation was limited, even with a wide final TZ diameter, and it was distributed over most of the corneal surface, reducing

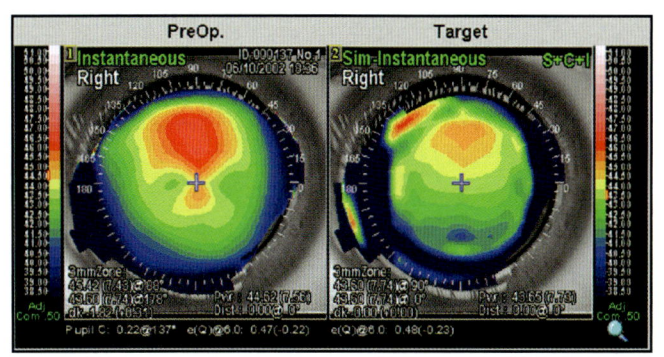

Figure 11-24. Right: an unacceptable custom ablation target map, instantaneous algorithm.

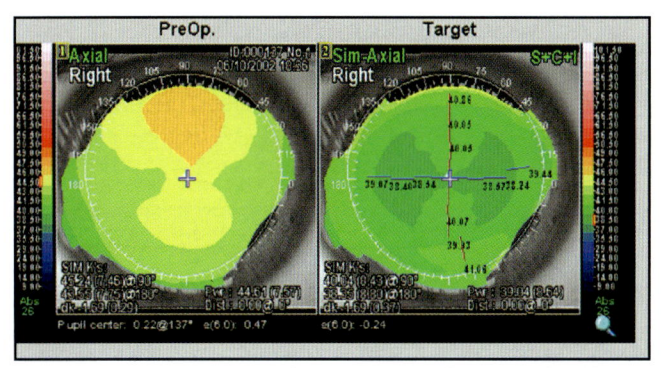

Figure 11-26. NIDEK Final Fit target axial map, right, shows residual astigmatism and refractive error.

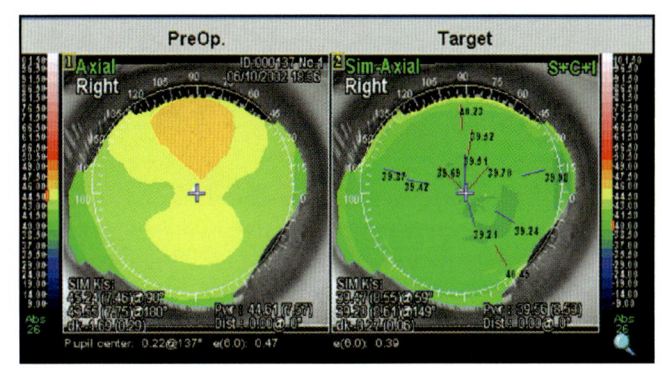

Figure 11-27. NIDEK Final Fit target axial map, right, shows proper determination and correction of unmasked astigmatism. Note the resulting size of optical zone.

the actual biomechanical effect. Improper ablation may thus result in pseudodecentration, residual astigmatism, induction of new high-order aberrations, residual refractive error, and eventually, poor vision.

The most important factor in our opinion is axis error because high-order aberrations are more sensitive to this factor. A 3-degree difference in axis correction leads to 10% correction of astigmatism but to almost 17% of uncorrected trefoil and to 31% of uncorrected tetrafoil when present. Our study indicates that torsion error is frequent and relevant, and its detection is also essential for true custom ablation treatment. Some custom treatments automatically solve these problems, but they may require marked corneal tissue ablation, double correction of higher-order aberrations, or

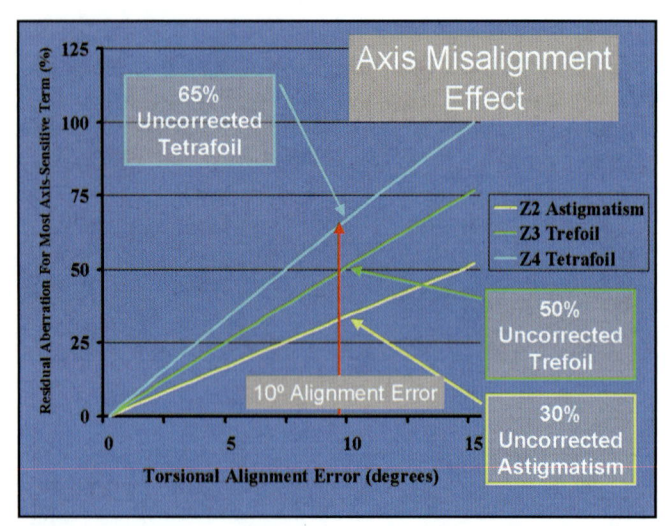

Figure 11-28. Axis misalignment effect on uncorrected astigmatism, trefoil, tetrafoil for a 10-degree alignment error.

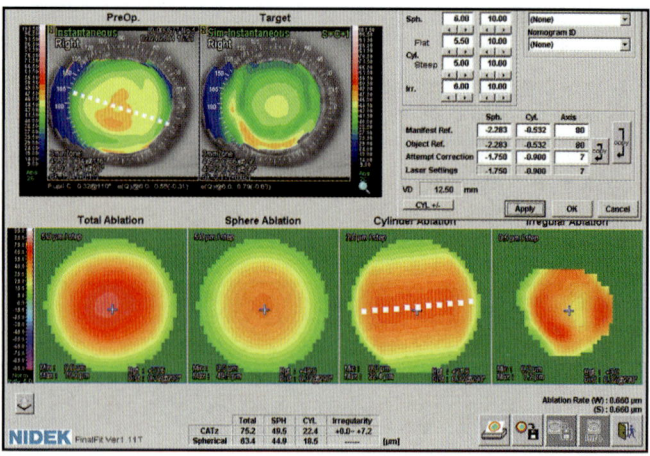

Figure 11-29. Treating high-order errors alters the axis of the unmasked astigmatism, with a change of 22 degrees.

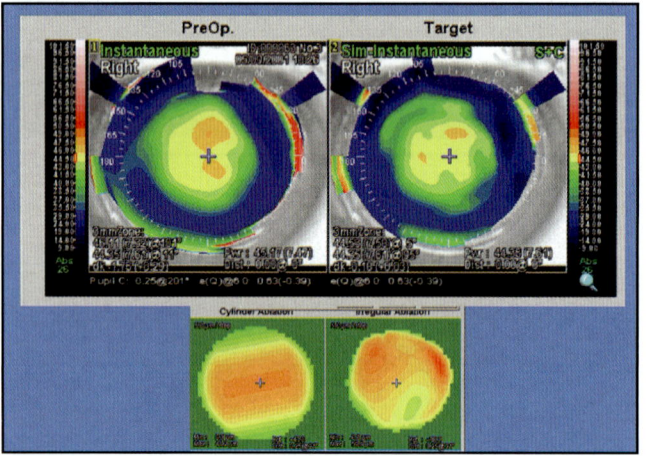

Figure 11-30. Difference in results due to a 3-degree error. Small axis errors could be considered insignificant, but they are usually coupled to power errors, and high-order aberrations are more sensitive to axis errors.

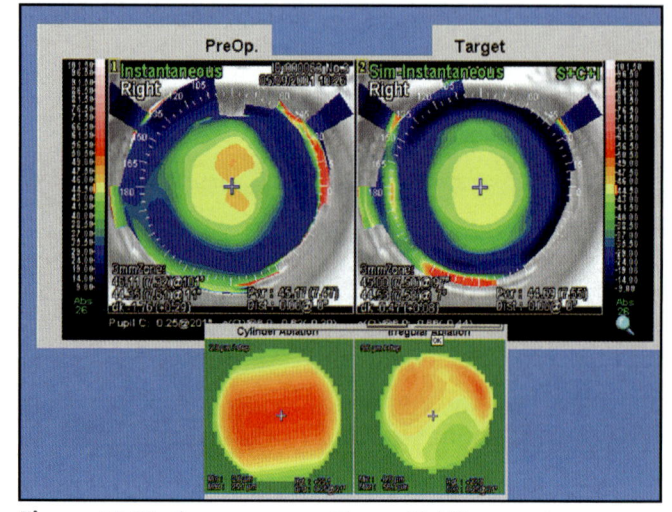

Figure 11-31. Same case as Figure 11-30, no axis error.

concentrating the correction in one area, weakening the biomechanics of the cornea.[18] Presently, for a high quality custom correction of refractive defects, we are convinced that the automatic approach may not always be the best and that an accurate check of the true astigmatism power and axis, after elimination of high-order aberrations, is mandatory.

Cyclotorsion

Since treatment of astigmatism can be frustrating, several factors must be carefully considered:
* Residual error may be present despite all efforts.
* The residual axis may be disturbingly different from the preoperative axis.
* Custom ablation has solved the problem only partially.

Extensive cyclotorsional movement is a clinical reality, and it can result in significant optical errors, as it is shown in Figure 28.

Underestimating the problem of cyclotorsion in the treatment of high astigmatism means compromising the Custom Ablation goal (Figures 11-28 through 11-31). Using the NIDEK Torsion Error Detector, we evaluated preoperative axis rotation in 68 eyes, finding a 24% negative axis rotation (ie, 10 to 5 degrees) and a 76% positive axis rotation (ie, 10 to 15 degrees) with a mean axis rotation of 3 degrees ± 2.64 degrees, a minimal rotation of 0 degrees, and a maximal rotation of 10 degrees.

Since custom ablation applies unaccounted eccentric focal ablations, cyclotorsion during ablation may cause inaccurate positioning of spots, hypocorrection, cylinder axis deviation, and induction of aberrations. The residual uncorrected cylinder, the axis error, and the new induced cylinder all cause new high-order aberrations (personal communication, Refr@ctive.online 2003 and 2004). Postoperative high-order aberrations may be less tolerated than residual refractive error and cannot be corrected with spectacles. Compensation

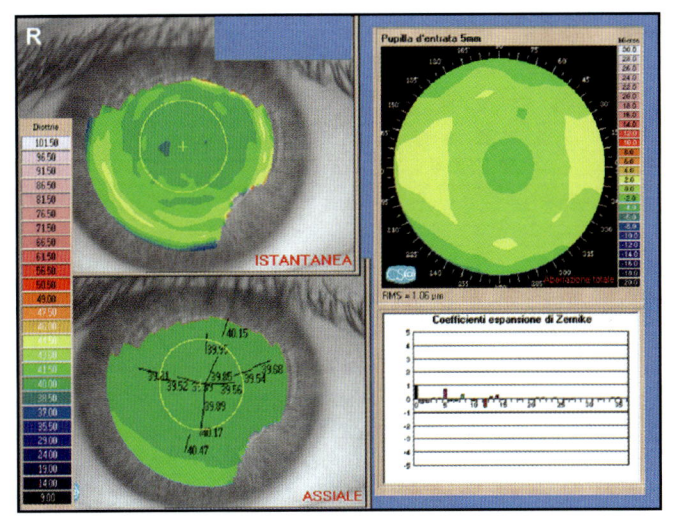

Figure 11-32. An almost monochromatic 1-year postoperative topographic map on the axial algorithm (below, left) with an effective optical zone much wider than the above-mentioned 4.5 mm as well as a general containment in induction of aberrations.

with automated cyclotorsional tracking is necessary to optimize the benefits of wavefront-driven ablations (McDonald MB, personal communication, AAO Refractive Surgery Subspecialty Day, 2003). Therefore, correct axis alignment is mandatory, and torsion error detectors enhance the possibilities of Custom Ablation.

Smoothing

Due to the ablation patterns of the different excimer lasers, as well as to the overlapping of the spots, any corneal ablation generates a surface with a certain degree of micro-irregularities (see Figure 7-7). Avoiding an increase in aberrations after refractive surgery is a difficult goal, and corneal irregularities induced by excimer ablation may cause aberrations, mostly relevant in scotopic conditions.[21] When high refractive defects are corrected, required ablations will be deep and induce more irregularities, and it is assumed that the predictability of the correction is inversely related to the amount of refractive defect corrected. These irregularities can be macroscopic (ie, related to centration and shape of ablation—rough or steep ablation margins—and induce mostly coma and spherical aberration) or microscopic (ie, related to microirregularities of the ablated cornea, inducing high-order aberrations).

In surface ablation, the epithelium attempts to solve these macro- and microirregularities through several layers of epithelial cells and/or collagen deposition.[14,16,17] Collagen deposition may lead to postoperative haze. Marked variation of curvature in the peripheral portion of the ablation also leads to collagen deposition, a phenomenon that reduces this curvature variation but induces regression. These phenomena reduce the predictability of the imparted correction.

In LASIK, the corneal flap covers and thus solves the stromal microirregularities present after ablation. However, it may not be able to follow all the ablation-generated macro-irregularities of the stromal bed, since this "blanket effect" can be reduced by markedly elevated stromal bed irregularity "peaks." Epithelial hyperplasia will then occur with reduction of refractive predictability and regression. Large epithelial profile changes after LASIK have been demonstrated using three-dimensional, very high-frequency digital ultrasound scanning systems.[22]

We have tried to overcome unpredictability linked to microirregularity and corneal biomechanics in several ways. Information on surface and total aberrometry provided in photopic, scotopic, and mesopic conditions by the NIDEK OPD integrated aberrometer, refractometer, topographer, and pupillometer is integrated through Final Fit software to provide a complete aberrometric optimization of the ablated corneal profile. The CATz ablation pattern of the Final Fit imparts a refractive change in which all total OPD-detected ocular aberrations, and particularly spherical aberration, are optimized in the central 4.5 mm. The curvature of the remaining cornea is then gradually modified in order to achieve a constant curvature gradient up to the external 10-mm margin of the ablation, maintaining at the same time the best possible reduction of ocular aberrations. The central 4.5-mm area of ablation must thus not be confused with an OZ. An advanced use of Final Fit is adopted for custom ablation. The segmental ablation for treatment of high-order components is applied first. This is a fundamental step, because this part of the treatment may change axis and power of the cylinder. In fact, it eliminates the coma- and trefoil-related portion of astigmatism. At this point the new axis and power of astigmatism need to be estimated and properly corrected. Once this is done, the resulting spherical component to be treated is calculated.

This surgical method offers several advantages. Removal of epithelium, LASEK, or Epi-LASIK generate no biomechanical effect, as can be seen from the negligible curvature changes detected by comparing corneal topography pre- and postflap creation (see Figure 7-10). The amount of tissue removed by the excimer ablation is limited, even with a wide final TZ diameter, and it is distributed all over most of the corneal surface, reducing the actual biomechanical effect.

With this technique, the final corneal curvature gradient is constant, as can be observed from an almost monochromatic postoperative topographic map on the axial algorithm, with an effective OZ much wider than the above-mentioned 4.5 mm, as well as a general containment of aberration increase (Figure 11-32). With Final Fit, the corneal curvature gradient from center to periphery is reduced and made more gradual. The gradient is positioned in the extreme periphery, beyond 9 mm, where the cornea is thicker and flatter. The above-mentioned topographical red ring will appear of limited width and intensity in diopters, thus not actually red but a paler color as well as being located very peripherally. Furthermore, spherical aberration will be reduced, providing excellent vision quality even with dilated pupils. This strategy

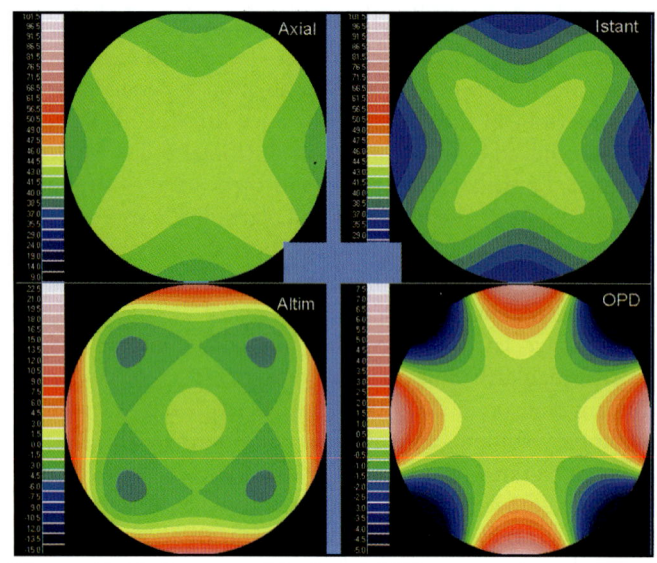

Figure 11-33. Topographical and OPD maps when tetrafoil is present.

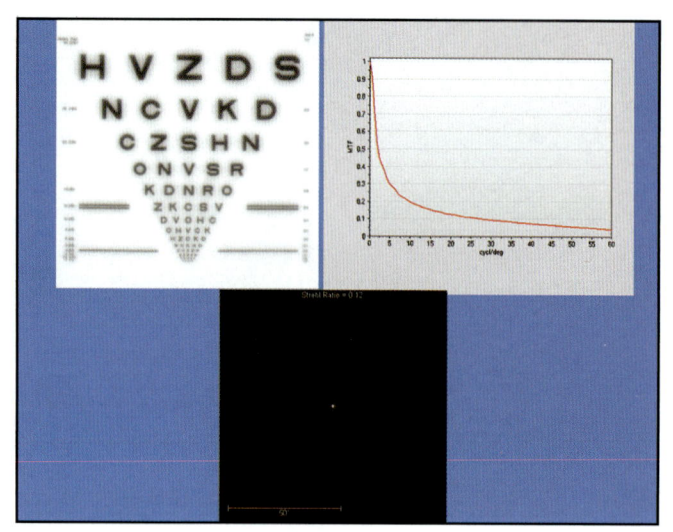

Figure 11-34. Visual function summary and Modulation Transfer Factor of tetrafoil.

will make the determination of pupil diameter less critical: at the corneal diameter corresponding to mesopic pupil—4 to 7 mm—the corneal curvature change will be constant with reduced aberrations for the incoming light.

With the OPD aberrometer, surface aberrations can be calculated up to the sixth order, when usually aberrations are considered only up to the fourth order. In our studies, surface aberrations at one year showed no substantial increase up to a 5-mm pupil, but spherical aberrations remained stable for a 3-mm pupil and increased by 52.6% in value for a 5-mm pupil.[22,24]

In a previous study, we showed a direct relationship between the immediate amount of postsurgical stromal surface irregularity and the 1-year haze and loss of one or more lines of visual acuity.[16] This led to the adoption of PTK-style smoothing as the final step of refractive laser surgery. We have addressed the advantages of this technique in Chapter 8

Treating Astigmatism

Low Compound Myopic Astigmatism (-0.50 to -2.0 D)

Low compound myopic astigmatism can still be corrected in a satisfactory manner with the crossed-cylinder technique if the astigmatism is regular (ie, the two segments of the bow-tie are symmetrical). Irregular astigmatism must be corrected with custom ablation.

High Compound Myopic Astigmatism (Greater Than -2.0 D)

High compound astigmatism requires a deeper ablation and, thus, a greater curvature gradient between center and periphery. Presently, the best way to treat this defect is custom ablation. Treatment of aberrations, with detection of true residual astigmatism power and axis, as mentioned above, will often show that aberrations cause a relevant portion of total astigmatism.

Mixed Astigmatism

Mixed astigmatism remains one of the most challenging defects for refractive surgery. Recent advancements in the correction of mixed astigmatism include pursuit of a postoperative corneal surface that is as symmetrical as possible, centrally as well as in the periphery.[3] Mixed astigmatism can be classified as regular, showing the typical bow-tie shape with lobes symmetrical in shape and dioptrical power, lying on the same axis. Irregular astigmatism, not showing these features and presently regarded as resulting from high-order optical aberrations, will ideally need custom ablation for proper correction.

In the past, several ablation patterns have been proposed for the treatment of mixed astigmatism: correction on the steep meridian (myopic cylinder ablation + hyperopic sphere ablation), correction on the flat meridian (hyperopic cylinder ablation + myopic sphere ablation), cross-cylinder ablation, and bitoric ablation (asymmetrically split on two meridians).[3,10,24,25] Azar, in a thorough analysis of various available methods, recommended correction on the hyperopic meridian only with the advantage of removing less cornea than with any other technique.[8] Astigmatic ablation on one meridian only induces tetrafoil. Figures 11-33 and 11-34 show the topographical pattern, visual function summary, and Modulation Transfer Factor of tetrafoil.

For a long time, cross-cylinder ablation with a multizone pattern and smoothing has been a mainstay of our treatment for mixed astigmatism. Before the introduction of Custom Ablation and torsion error detectors, in a personal series of 29 eyes in 20 patients with preoperative 0.84 ± 0.15 visual acuity (VA), with 1.73 ± 1.25 D sphere and -3.20 ± 0.90 D cylinder, treated with the multizone cross-cylinder technique, after a follow-up period of 327 ± 196 days, postoperative VA was 0.88 ± 0.11 with 1.11 ± 1.52 D sphere and -1.55 ± 1.42 D cylinder.

BSCVA was preserved, though with only a 56% reduction of spherical error and a 49% reduction of cylindrical error. Total wavefront error was understandably decreased, since astigmatism was the main component, and spherical aberration and coma remain unchanged.

However, when the problem of axis alignment was evaluated, mean resulting axis error in treatment was 9.6 ± 14.6 degrees. This meant a mean refractive error induced by axis misalignment of 0.92 ± 1.38 D sphere and -1.22 ± 1.06 D cylinder (personal communication, Refr@ctive.online 2003 and 2004). Presently, custom ablation with torsion error detection is our preferred treatment for mixed astigmatism.

Compound Hyperopic Astigmatism

Hyperopic astigmatism ablation aims to increase steepness on the flatter meridian while minimizing treatment of the steepest one. Following the same reasoning used for myopic astigmatism, in this case too, the end result is an irregular "four-leaf" astigmatism with undercorrection along the oblique meridians and a myopic shift. If regression occurs, we will have a cornea featuring mixed astigmatism. The aberrations induced by the myopic and the hyperopic astigmatism ablation are diametrically opposed and almost perfectly symmetric.

Since many of the considerations listed for mixed astigmatism apply to compound hyperopic astigmatism, custom ablation with torsion error detection is presently our preferred treatment for this defect, too.

Conclusions

After the introduction of LASIK, surface refractive surgery has received less interest due to observed regression, haze and postoperative pain. Surface refractive surgery remains an interesting option because it offers advantages such as a wider range of refractive correction and easier retreatments due to the limited amount of stromal tissue ablation. Creating a regular postoperative surface with smoothing can contain haze formation, and in our studies a progressive custom ablation approach with identification of true corneal astigmatism after elimination of the high-order aberration component, as well as accurate compensation for possible cyclotorsion, has proved to be a satisfactory method for the correction of astigmatism.

References

1. Vinciguerra P, Sborgia M, Epstein D, Azzolini M, McRae S. Photorefractive keratectomy to correct myopic or hyperopic astigmatism with a cross-cylinder ablation. *J Refract Surg.* 1999;15:S183-S185.
2. Danasoury MA, Waring GO, el-Maghraby A, Mehrez K. Excimer laser in situ keratomileusis to correct compound myopic astigmatism. *J Refract Surg.* 1999;13:511-520
3. Chayet AS, Montes M, Gomez L, Rodriguez X, Robledo N, McRae S. Bitoric laser in situ keratomileusis for the correction of simple myopic and mixed astigmatism. *Ophthalmology.* 2001;108:303-308.
4. Dierick HG, Missotten L. Is the corneal contour influenced by a tension in the superficial epithelial cells. *J Refract Corneal Surg.* 1992;8: 54-59.
5. Vinciguerra P, Epstein D, Azzolini M. Ablation of both meridians in LASIK and PRK—a new tissue-saving strategy for correcting astigmatism. *Invest Ophthalmol Vis Sci.* 1999;40:S782.
6. Vinciguerra P, Azzolini M, Radice P. A new corneal analysis after excimer laser ablation: digitized retroillumination. In: Pallikaris IG, Siganos DS. *LASIK.* Thorofare, NJ: SLACK Incorporated; 1997.
7. Vinciguerra P, Azzolini M, Airaghi P, Radice P, De Molfetta V. Effect of decreasing surface and interface irregularities after photorefractive keratectomy and laser in situ keratomileusis on optical and functional results. *J Refract Surg.* 1998;14:S199-S203
8. Azar DT, Primack JD. Theoretical analysis of ablation depths and profiles in laser in situ keratomileusis for compound hyperopic and mixed astigmatism. *J Cataract Refract Surg.* 2000;26:1123-1136.
9. Vinciguerra P. Cross-cylinder ablation for the correction of myopic or hyperopic astigmatism. In: Gimbel HV, Anderson Penno EE. *Refractive Surgery. A Manual of Principles and Practice.* Thorofare, NJ: SLACK Incorporated; 2000:105-113.
10. Epstein D, Vinciguerra P, Prussiani A, Camesasca FI. Cross-cylinder ablation in LASIK and PRK—A new tissue-sparing, accuracy-enhancing strategy for correcting astigmatism. *Invest Ophthalmol Vis Sci.* 2000;41:S690.
11. Vinciguerra P, Epstein D, Camesasca FI, Prussiani A. A new splitting technique to improve optical zone curvature in astigmatism correction in LASIK and PRK. *Invest Ophthalmol Vis Sci.* 2000;41:S688.
12. Piovella M, Camesasca FI, Fattori C. Excimer laser photorefractive keratectomy for high myopia. Four-year experience with a multiple zone technique. *Ophthalmology.* 1997;104:1554-1565.
13. Vinciguerra P. The correction of astigmatism with a cross-cylinder ablation. In: Buratto L, Brint S. *LASIK: Advanced Principles and Techniques.* 2nd ed. Thorofare, NJ: SLACK Incorporated; 2001.
14. Huang D, Tang M, Shekhar R. Mathematical model of corneal surface smoothing after refractive surgery. *Am J Ophthalmol.* 2003;135:267-278.
15. Balestrazzi E, De Molfetta V, Spadea L, et al. Histological, immunoistochemical, and ultrastructural findings in human corneas after photorefractive keratectomy. *J Refract Surg.* 1995;11:181-187.
16. Vinciguerra P, Azzolini M, Radice P, et al. A method for examining surface and interface irregularities after photorefractive keratectomy and laser in situ keratomileusis: predictor of optical and functional outcomes. *J Refract Surg.* 1998;14:S204-206.
17. Vinciguerra P, Azzolini M, Airaghi P, et al. Effect of decreasing surface and interface irregularities after photorefractive keratectomy and laser in situ keratomileusis on optical and functional outcomes. *J Refract Surg.* 1998;14:S199-S203.
18. Roberts C. Biomechanics of the cornea and wavefront-guided laser refractive surgery. *J Refract Surg.* 2002;18:S589-592.
19. Vinciguerra P, Camesasca FI. Butterfly laser epithelial keratomileusis for myopia. *J Refract Surg.* 2002;18:S371-373.
20. Vinciguerra P, Camesasca FI, Randazzo A. One-year results of butterfly laser epithelial keratomileusis. *J Refract Surg.* 2003;19:S223-226.
21. Oshika T, Klyce SD, Applegate AR, et al. Comparison of corneal wavefront aberrations after photorefractive keratectomy and laser in situ keratomileusis. *Am J Ophthalmol.* 1999;127:1-7.
22. Vinciguerra P, Camesasca FI, Torres IM. Transition zone design and smoothing in custom laser-assisted subepithelial keratectomy. *J Cataract Refract Surg.* 2005;31:39-47.
23. Reinstein DZ, Silverman RH, Raevsky T, et al. Arc-scanning very high-frequency digital ultrasound for 3D pachimetric mapping of the corneal epithelium and stroma in laser in situ keratomileusis. *J Refract Surg.* 2000;16:414-430.
24. Vinciguerra P, Camesasca FI, Urso R. Reduction of spherical aberration with the Nidek NAVEX customized ablation system. *J Refract Surg.* 2003;19:S195-S201.
25. Dausch D, Klein R, Landesz M, Schroder E. Photorefractive keratectomy to correct astigmatism with myopia or hyperopia. *J Cataract Refract Surg.* 1994 Mar;20 Suppl:252-257
26. Argento CJ, Cosentino MJ, Biondini A. Treatment of hyperopic astigmatism. *J Cataract Refract Surg.* 1997 Dec;23(10):1480-1490.

CHAPTER 12

Treatment of Hyperopia

Paolo Vinciguerra, MD; Fabrizio I. Camesasca, MD

Treatment of Hyperopia: Simply Frustrating?

More or less consciously, newly qualified refractive surgeons may consider treatment of hyperopia as a situation opposite to but similar and almost specular to myopia. Disappointingly, laser refractive surgery has often resulted in more unsatisfactory results and complications for hyperopia than for myopia.[1-4]

Apparently, hyperopia treatment simply increases the physiological curvature characteristics of the cornea, with a steep center and a flat periphery. Moreover, ablation is applied peripherally where the cornea is thicker and, theoretically, more tissue can be ablated. All this might make one think that surgical results of excimer laser refractive treatment of hyperopia would be more than satisfactory. In reality, while all agree that myopia can be treated up to -8.0 to 10.0 D, no one plans treatment for a +8.0 D hyperopia.

If we carefully examine a corneal surface after hyperopic ablation, we may notice some important peculiarities. We can begin by considering the transition zone (TZ); when treating myopia, we create just one TZ, but in the treatment of hyperopia, the central corneal curvature is increased and two TZs are needed, featuring a double change in curvature and a median flexus point. This double TZ is the most critical point of hyperopia treatment.[5] The most central of these two TZs cannot be considered as part of the optical zone (OZ) (Figure 12-1). This portion of the newly induced curvature generates a refractive effect but features a flexus with variation in curvature and is connected to the peripheral corneal curvature through the second curvature zone. Therefore, when comparing myopic and hyperopic treatments with the same ablation diameter, the functionally effective hyperopic OZ will be smaller than the myopic one because the ablated area encompasses two TZs. This makes hyperopic treatment more sensitive to decentration, with decreasing vision quality if the treatment is not perfectly centered.

The ablation diameter must be planned to fit the zone of curvature inversion precisely where the normal peripheral cornea flattens. Using the elevation map, the surgeon must calculate the maximal corneal diameter and place the flexus on the flat peripheral cornea, thus preserving normal corneal physiology (Figure 12-2). If the flexus area is positioned centrally, far from this peripheral area of physiological corneal flattening, multifocality and high-order optical aberrations will be induced. Also, hyperopic ablation generates a negative longitudinal spherical aberration (LSA) with worse with worse vision quality due to the fact that para-axial light rays will pass through the first curvature flexus that imparts a hyperopic shift.

However, it is important to remember that these problems are sometimes reduced by the anatomical characteristics of hyperopic eyes. This is because the hyperopic eye features smaller axial length, anterior chamber, corneal diameter, and pupil size.

* Corneal diameter. It is often small. When an OZ of normal diameter is applied on a small cornea, the effective functional OZ is wider.
* Pupil size. Since their infancy, hyperops are accustomed to accommodate constantly, by neural reflex, and simultaneous myosis.. Quite often, their pupil diameter is smaller than for a myopic same age peer. This means that these patients are less sensitive to a smaller OZ. Moreover, the two above-mentioned TZs will lie in the peripheral zone, positioned in a corneal area where the curvature is less marked and has a lower influence on refraction. In a hyperopic eye with low anterior chamber, the treatment results will be less influenced by pupil

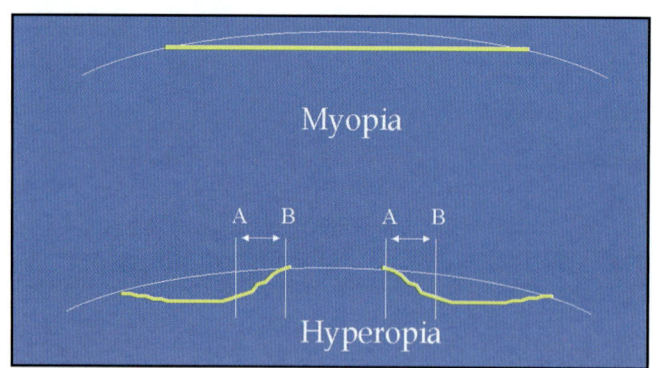

Figure 12-1. Hyperopic ablation. The central part of transition zone (A-B) cannot be considered part of the optical zone.

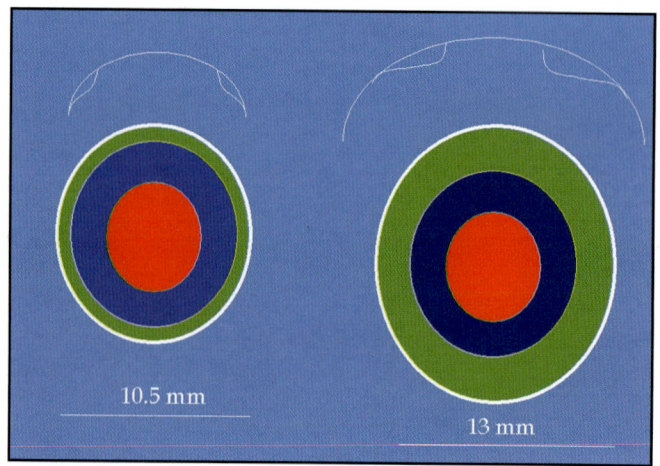

Figure 12-2. Importance of corneal diameter in hyperopic refractive surgery.

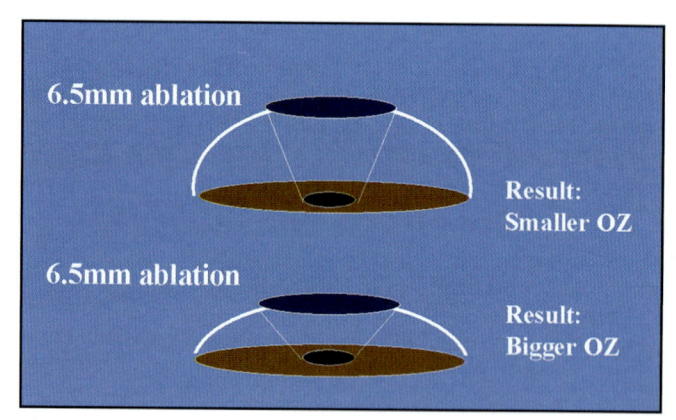

Figure 12-3. Importance of anterior chamber depth in hyperopic refractive surgery. Given a 6.5-mm optical zone ablation, an eye with a low chamber will enjoy a larger optical zone than one with a deep chamber, and even a small size optical zone may sufficiently cover the pupillary area.

diameter: even an OZ of small size may sufficiently cover the pupillary area, since the treated corneal arc will be closer to the pupillary area, and will thus be able to cover the pupillary margin during midriasis (Figure 12-3).

* Anterior chamber depth. Given the same ablation diameter, an eye with a low chamber will enjoy a larger OZ than one with a deep chamber (see Figure 12-3), and a larger portion of corneal surface will be involved in the treatment. This can be better understood by making a comparison with peeking through a keyhole. If the eye is very close to the keyhole, the visual field is wider, and it becomes smaller as the observer moves back from the keyhole.

Generally speaking, the size of the OZ is less important for a hyperopic patient than for a myopic one. These and the following observations can be assumed to be valid for PRK, LASEK, and LASIK treatments. Therefore, hereafter we will refer to refractive treatment as including PRK, LASEK, and LASIK, with some important exceptions that will be detailed.

Analyzing Hyperopic Treatment: Optical Zone, Corneal Eccentricity, and Spherical Aberration

Optical Zone and Ablation Zone

In refractive surgery, it is mandatory to understand the difference between the ablation zone (AZ) and OZ, as the two areas are often mistakenly attributed the same meaning. The AZ is the diameter of the area where the corneal tissue has been removed to achieve the desired refractive correction (ablation diameter). The OZ, on the contrary, defines the corneal area where the desired refractive effect has been obtained, and which features an almost constant refractive power. It is the functionally useful central area of the cornea (see Chapters 1, 7).

The peripheral limit of the AZ is often marked by the presence of a "blue ring" that indicates a sharp variation in corneal curvature. Topographically, the instantaneous algorithm highlights the AZ while the axial algorithm shows the useful OZ, although the latter is represented more accurately by a wavefront map. In theory, the OZ useful to vision should coincide with the laser setting, while the TZ should join the OZ to the nontreated cornea. In actual fact, not all lasers' ablation profiles provide the same refractive effectiveness. In some of them, the OZ resulting from ablation is larger than the setting; in others, due to the significant difference in curvature radius between the treated and the nontreated area, the final OZ is smaller than treatment settings.

Corneal Eccentricity (Q value)

Corneal eccentricity is the measure of corneal asphericity; it expresses the degree of change in corneal curvature (corneal curvature gradient) from a flatter periphery to a more curved central portion (see Chapter 1). Eccentricity values are positive when the cornea is prolate (ie, flatter around the periphery and more curved centrally) and negative when it is oblate (ie, more curved around the periphery and flatter centrally). Normal eccentricity values (e values) range between +0.4 and +0.6 (normally prolate cornea—curved in the center, flat in the periphery).[6] A different and commonly-used parameter to express the same concept is the Q value. For the sake of simplicity, we will use the e value. A hyperopic treatment increases the e value, thus approaching a keratoconus-like situation. Central keratoconus, featuring a high eccentricity with e values of +1.5 or more, amplifies the physiological situation of transition from a curved central cornea to a flat periphery. On the contrary, a myopic treatment induces negative eccentricity, inverting the normal morphology.

SPHERICAL ABERRATION

Spherical aberration (SA) is a property of spherical optic media, causing peripheral rays to be focused before axial rays (rays are only focused in the same point in aplanatic surfaces, where the dioptric power is identical in every point). From the point of view of subjective perception, the effect is that a point-like image appears surrounded by a halo of variable width, depending on the magnitude of the SA. The difference in diopters between central and marginal power of the pupil is called longitudinal spherical aberration (LSA). The SA of a normal eye is approximately 0.50 D (0.156 μm). LSA expresses the aberration induced by corneal multifocality. It is a measure of SA; its increase indicates a decrease in contrast sensitivity. If SA is measured according to the OSA system, as a component of the wavefront error, the cornea has a positive value and the crystalline lens a negative one, which in the young eye, increases its negativity during accommodation.

SPHERICAL ABERRATION AFTER REFRACTIVE SURGERY

SA is commonly observed after refractive surgery due to a marked change in the corneal profile, and is in the portion that demarcates the transition area between the ablated area and the untreated area (the red ring in the topographic map of myopic treatment as well as the blue ring in the hyperopic treatment, both highlighted by the instantaneous algorithm). Like other eye aberrations, SAs are influenced by many variables; for example, they increase as the pupil diameter expands and also vary according to age, accommodation, vitreous body properties, retina morphology, and other unknown factors.[7,8] The aberrometer is presently the ideal tool for the study of eye errors and aberrations through the analysis of the emerging wavefront. However, a SA can be detected using other investigation methods as in corneal topography—in the instantaneous map, if the red ring is visible, in the elevation map, and if corneal eccentricity values are negative.

SAs impair vision to variable extents, depending on their degree of seriousness. Minor SAs reduce vision quality only to a limited extent, as they cause a slight loss of sensitivity to contrast and contribute to providing greater depth of field and focus. Conversely, more substantial SAs interfere with the optical quality of the retinal image and manifest themselves with an excessive reduction of perceived contrast and with night halos. SAs have an influence on the size of the OZ and the quality of vision, and this influence can be clearly observed by subtracting only SAs from wavefront maps. The greatest relevance is attributable to SAs.

OPTICAL ZONE AND SPHERICAL ABERRATION IN HYPEROPIC ABLATION

If the OZ is planned merely as a function of the diameter of the AZ without taking SA into account, the results may be frustrating. In reality, if there is a high SA value, even a treatment with a very wide AZ may in fact feature a small OZ on the axial map. High SA in myopic treatment is indicated by red ring that is intense (high gradient), wide (larger cornea involved), and closer to the corneal apex (small TZ). The same red ring pattern will show both on the topographic (instantaneous algorithm) and aberrometric map. Hyperopic and myopic ablations change SA values, with myopic ablation increasing positive SA, and hyperopic ablation inducing negative SA. This difference has been noted in LASIK, too.[9]

In a hyperopic ablated eye, SA is induced by two rings showing corneal curvature variation (blue in hyperopic). The external ring may be harder to identify on topographical maps since it is positioned on the flatter, more peripheral cornea. A high corneal curvature gradient, with a blue ring closer to the corneal apex and, thus, a high SA, means a small OZ with an optical situation comparable to the notoriously poor central keratoconus optics. This may easily explain the lack of popularity of this treatment among hyperopic patients. Often, a 3.0-D correction on a hyperopic patient will be poor in quality with reduced night vision and noticeable halo perception. Furthermore, a corrected myopic patient will experience an enlargement of the retinal image, while a hyperopic patient will see it reduced.

In the past, it was generally thought that excessively high corneal curvature values would lead to a keratoconus-like situation. From our studies, it appears that an important factor for this complication is the eccentricity. Interestingly, we may meet patients with corneal curvature values of 46.0 D who show good visual acuity, while others with 45.0 D, for example, do not enjoy such good vision. In a patient with 46.0 D and normal eccentricity, there is no marked peripheral flattening, and visual acuity will be good. On the contrary, a keratoconus patient with a corneal curvature within normal values, such as 45.0 D, will inevitably show a high eccentricity and, therefore, marked SA, a very small homogeneous OZ, and reduced vision quality.

High eccentricity after hyperopic treatment performed with insufficient care may lead to an optical situation resembling that of central keratoconus; there will be a central dioptrically homogeneous area, but of small diameter. The patient enjoys a tolerable optical quality situation only in myosis, while when the pupil dilates multifocality and becomes unbearable. The corneal periphery features high dioptrical

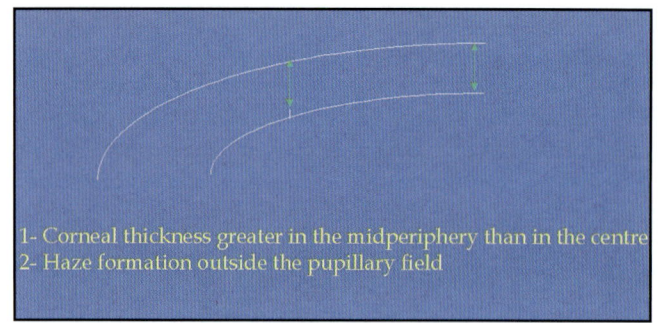

Figure 12-4. Lesser importance of ablation depth in hyperopic ablation. The corneal periphery offers the advantage of a greater thickness allowing deeper ablations. HAZ in the periphery will not hamper visual acuity.

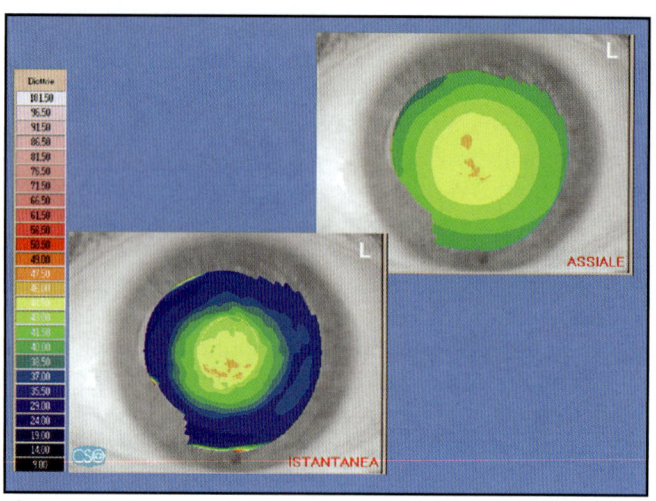

1- Corneal thickness greater in the midperiphery than in the centre
2- Haze formation outside the pupillary field

Figure 12-5. Hyperopic custom LASEK (+2.5 D). Note wide optical zone.

gradient from center to periphery (high eccentricity). This situation is typical of old-style treatments for hyperopia.

Correction of Hyperopia With LASIK, LASEK, and PRK

Correction of hyperopia with LASIK is more successful, even in the presence of high e values. In fact, the flap does not perfectly follow the new shape of the stromal bed, thus reducing the eccentricity created by the ablation. In LASEK and PRK, corneal epithelium faithfully follows the new imparted morphology. However, above certain values of eccentricity, even LASIK fails.

Treated hyperopic eyes may show a small, white, discrete nodular opacity on the corneal apex, whose etiology is described in the section "Hyperopic White Scar." This lesion appears irregular on topography, inducing marked corneal deformity and leading to poor vision. Eccentricity is usually markedly positive.

If corneal eccentricity remains positive ($e = 1.0$ to 1.5), PTK retreatment of these hyperopic nodular areas provides limited or no result at all with scar recurrence on the point of greatest corneal curvature. On the contrary, when eccentricity is decreased (eg, with corneal excimer laser smoothing), recurrence is prevented. A key point of hyperopic ablation is thus to maintain a corneal eccentricity as close as possible to physiological values.

Corneal topography offers the advantage of an accurate evaluation of the quality of hyperopic ablation. A wide, homogeneous central area is necessary for a better vision quality, and the surgeon must strive to achieve it while topographically monitoring the result. The aberrometric map permits evaluation of central corneal dioptrical homogeneity as well as detection of irregularities that may generate aberrations. The more peripheral the treatment, the less important the second peripheral part of the TZ (see Figure 12-1). Our experience with the OPD aberrometer shows that with good topographical indexes, we have a satisfactory aberrometric map; more than 80% of optical aberrations are caused by the first corneal surface.

Several recent reports of hyperopic PRK, LASIK, and LASEK follow-up, even on a long-term basis, are available but are sometimes conflicting with regard to results and stability.[10-17] There is general agreement, however, that low (<3.0 D) to moderate (3.0 to 5.0 D) hyperopia treatment is effective, both with LASIK and PRK. When greater amounts are corrected, the results are less convincing.[14]

The future is represented by a wider OZ (in relation to corneal diameter) of 7 mm or greater, with a first, smoother, and homogeneous TZ up to 10 mm and a second, limbal TZ of more than 10 mm. Let us remember that the corneal periphery also offers the advantage of a greater thickness (Figure 12-4).

Currently, no NIDEK software for custom ablation of hyperopia is available. Our approach is to correct high-order aberrations with the Final Fit custom software and subsequently apply the spherical ablation. Figure 12-5 shows the result of an hyperopic custom LASEK for +2.5 D with a typically-wide OZ. Figure 12-6 shows the wavefront of an hyperopic LASIK.

Complications of Hyperopia Treatment

Several possible causes may be considered as causes of complications in the treatment of hyperopia.

Decentration

Due to the accommodative effort required to focus on a near target, the hyperopic patient usually has greater problems in staring at the target light with the possibility of eye movement. Since the real OZ is smaller in the hyperopic treatment than in myopic, decentration leads to more severe consequences. The effect of the same amount of decentration in millimeters from the visual axis is quite different according to corneal curvature; steeper corneas are affected to a greater extent. The greater the corneal curvature, the more decentration is increased due to the greater corneal curvature gradient achieved in the hyperopic eye. The magnitude of this gradient

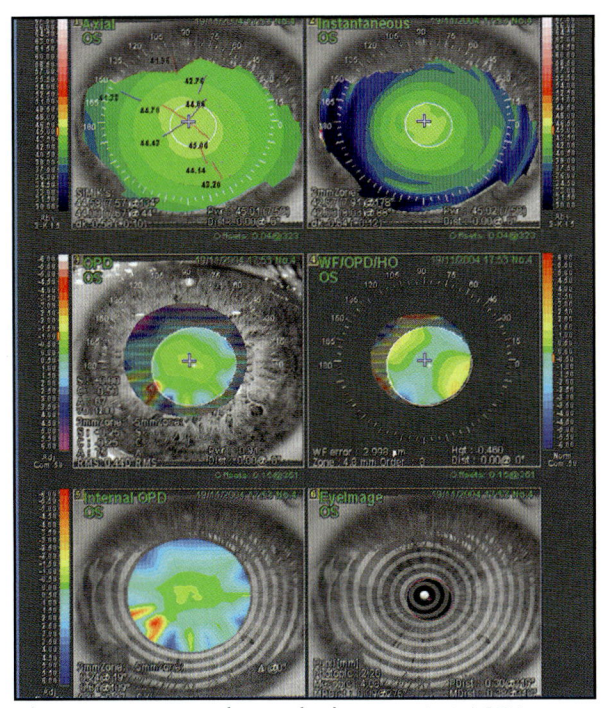

Figure 12-6. Wavefront of a hyperopic LASEK.

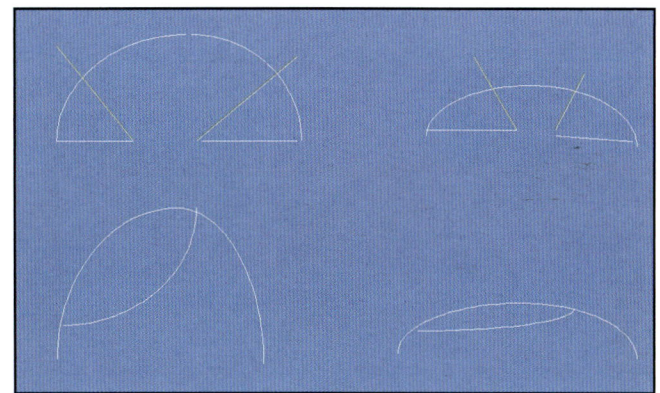

Figure 12-7. Influence of corneal curvature on decentration. The greater the corneal curvature, the more decentration is increased due to prismatic effect.

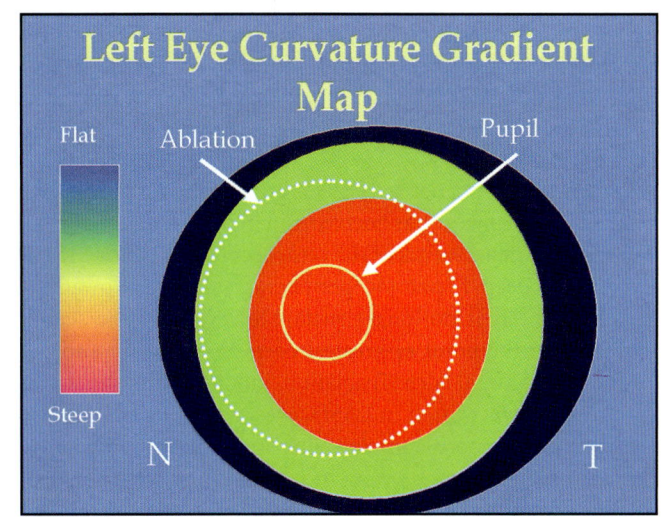

Figure 12-8. Influence of the transition zone in the temporal corneal region. In an eye with a nasal pupil, the transition zone will involve a paracentral, steeper corneal portion in the temporal region with consequent high postoperative dioptrical gradient. In the nasal region, the transition zone will involve a flatter peripheral cornea.

is far different from the same gradient obtained when treating a myopic eye for the same net amount of diopters. This induces more aberrations and poorer vision quality (Figure 12-7). Correction of decentration is possible but difficult and, nevertheless, induces relevant optical aberrations (eg, coma). Let us examine the keratoscopic appearance of a treatment for hyperopia that has been improperly administered. The rings will show extremely inhomogeneous intermediate spaces: some rings will show sudden intermediate space increase, expression of a sudden change in the ray of curvature. These curvature changes, especially if asymmetrical, induce aberrations of first, second, third and fourth order. Maintaining a constant ray of curvature is mandatory to achieve good visual quality. Conversely, an elevated SA reduces the contrast perceived by the patient. Furthermore, if this condition is asymmetrically distributed on the cornea, coma and other aberrations will be present, reducing the quality of vision, and causing a fastidious monocular double vision.

LACK OF ADEQUATE TRANSITION ZONE

This may be caused by inadequate analysis of the preoperative corneal topography, error in surgical strategy, and the limits of possible TZ size with a particular type of laser. The resulting complications include dimensionally insufficient OZ with fluctuations in visual acuity as well as rapid postoperative dioptrical variations induced by focal fourth-order optical aberrations and regression. The width of the TZ must be defined by considering the amount of correction to impart and the topographical features of the eye. The TZ has more influence in high corrections and in more "spherical" corneas as well as in the temporal corneal region. In an eye with a nasal pupil, the TZ will involve a paracentral, steeper corneal portion in the temporal region with consequent high postoperative dioptrical gradient. In the nasal region, the TZ will involve a flatter peripheral cornea (Figure 12-8). In LASIK patients, an inadequate TZ causes loss of vision quality with occurrence of halos and glare, easier regression, and loss of vision.

HYPEROPIC WHITE SCAR

Highly positive eccentricity values (above 1.0 to 1.2) are typical of keratoconus cases and of some cases of hyperopic ablations that share the presence of a subepithelial (PRK) or subflap (LASIK) whitish scar.[18,19] This scar, as mentioned previously, corresponds topographically to the point of maximal corneal curvature (Figures 12-9 and 12-10). In these cases, there is always a high eccentricity value and, thus, high SA. Presently, the etiology of this scar remains uncertain and includes an inhomogeneous lachrymal film as well as lid

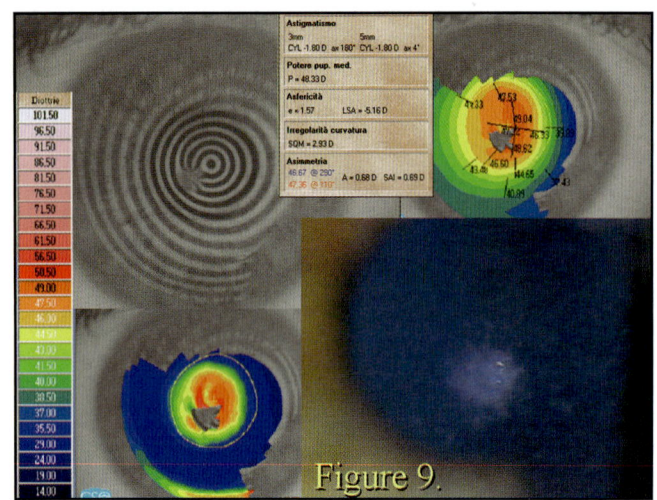

Figure 12-9. Biomicroscopy, keratoscopy, and topography of eyes with a subepithelial (PRK) whitish scar, corresponding topographically to the point of maximal corneal curvature.

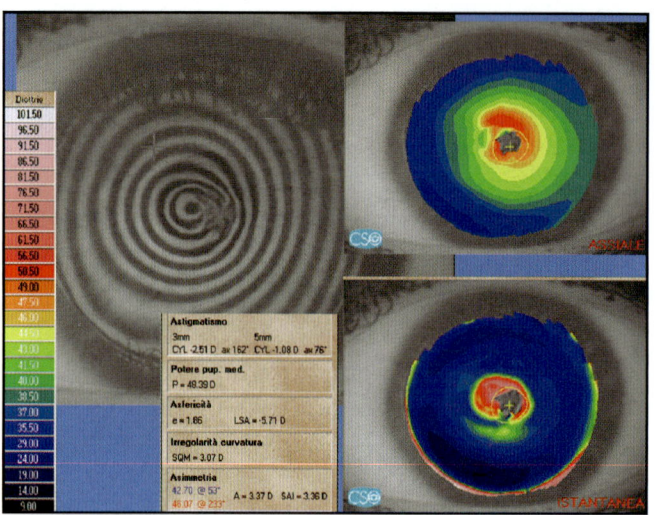

Figure 12-10. Biomicroscopy, keratoscopy, and topography of eyes with a subepithelial (PRK) whitish scar, corresponding topographically to the point of maximal corneal curvature.

trauma on that particularly steep portion of cornea. In the past, this type of scar has been considered the consequence of the selective denervation of the central corneal area due to the excessively deep hyperopic peripheral ablation. Nowadays, this hypothesis is no longer sustainable because the scar is observed in the point of greatest corneal curvature and not in that of maximal corneal ablation. Furthermore, the scar is not observed very often in LASIK eyes, where central corneal denervation is more complete due to the flap. However, a similar scar may be observed in post-traumatic corneal leukomas always in the point of greatest corneal curvature. Very often in these cases of corneal leukoma, topographic analysis may be misleading due to problems with the elaboration of the map. Keratoscopy must always be obtained and examined. In our opinion, the key factor is the corneal curvature gradient. The higher this gradient, the higher the curvature variation per millimeter will be—expressed by eccentricity and Q value—and the higher the probability that this problem will occur.

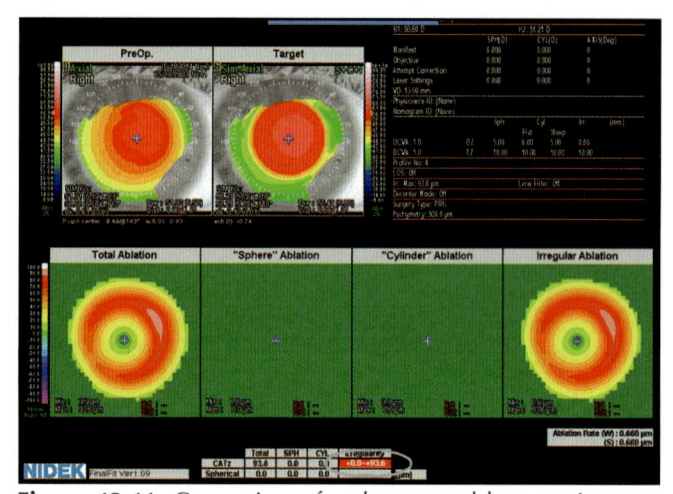

Figure 12-11. Correction of a decentered hyperopic treatment with custom ablation, using the NIDEK Final Fit software. Above right is the initial situation, above left is the final target, below is the irregular ablation pattern.

Retreatments

It is necessary to ablate the corneal apex selectively after precise identification with a pachimetric map. The diameter must be carefully measured before performing the ablation. Then, it is important to reduce the eccentricity. Ablation must be myopic in order to substantially widen the optical and TZs with use of a masking fluid and custom ablation, as detailed in Chapter 30 (Figure 12-11).

Successful treatment of white scars features a reduction of corneal eccentricity. Recently, we have introduced a transepithelial approach to these white hyperopic scars. The scar is the portion of cornea where the epithelium is thinnest. Ablation is calculated with a custom program and then directly applied on the dry epithelium. If the ablation is performed without illumination, the appearance of the stroma where the epithelium has been ablated will be readily visible as markedly darker areas. After a 50-μm ablation, the epithelium will be almost completely removed, and a smoothing phase with masking fluid can follow. If necessary, intraoperative topography can be performed and a new customized ablation planned and performed, again followed by smoothing.

Hyperopic Astigmatism

The goal of custom ablation is to achieve a corneal surface that is as symmetrical and similar as possible to a physiological corneal surface. Symmetry is an essential factor in order to prevent high-order optical aberrations (eg, coma).

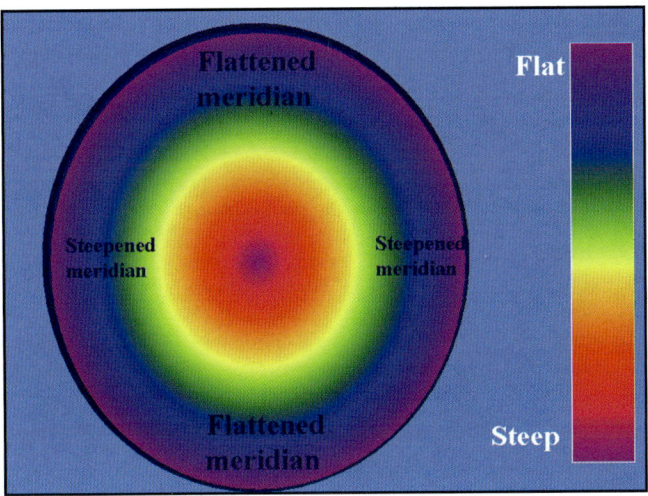

Figure 12-12. Scheme of physiologically prolate cornea after cross cylinder ablation for hyperopic astigmatism.

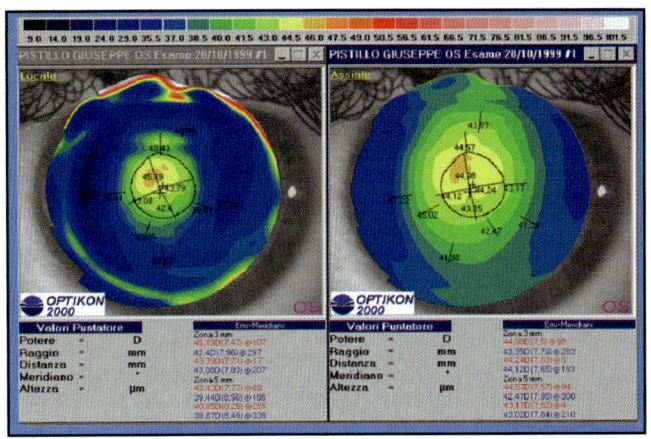

Figure 12-13. Postoperative topography after treatment for hyperopic astigmatism of -4.0 D. Cornea shows a prolate shape.

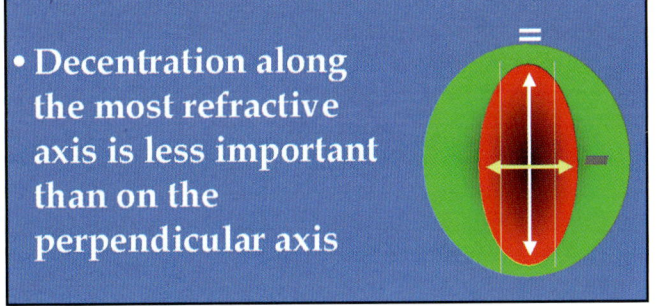

Figure 12-14. Decentration along the most refractive axis is less troublesome than decentration along the less refractive axis. The latter case may lead to hypocorrection, induction of fourth-order optical aberrations with loss in visual acuity, monocular diplopia, and halos.

Correction of hyperopic astigmatism with traditional techniques may lead to the onset of a central keratoconus with leukoma, especially if the spherical equivalent is positive.

CROSS-CYLINDER TECHNIQUE

A valid alternative is represented by the cross-cylinder technique.[20-25] If the spherical equivalent is negative, eccentricity does not increase but decreases, becoming negative, and no leukoma will appear. If the mean ray of curvature is preserved, mean eccentricity remains constant. Therefore, cross-cylinder technique does not increase eccentricity, and a corneal situation closer to normal physiology can be obtained (Figures 12-12 and 12-13).

If the spherical equivalent is positive and the postoperative increase in curvature is sudden, we will have a corneal area featuring an extreme curvature, just like a keratoconus. This area is more easily exposed to lid trauma as well as to an inhomogeneous distribution of lachrymal film, with risk of leukoma occurrence.

Complications of Hyperopic Astigmatism Treatment

Complications in the treatment of hyperopic astigmatism include the following:

DECENTRATION ALONG ONE OF THE TWO MAIN MERIDIANS

This situation differs depending on the axis of decentration: decentration along the most refractive axis is less troublesome than decentration along the less refractive axis. This last may lead to hypocorrection, and induction of fourth order optical aberrations, leading to loss in visual acuity, monocular diplopia, and halos (Figure 12-14).

AXIS VARIATION

This can be induced by incorrect patient positioning, error in laser setting of the astigmatism axis (TABO vs international), difference in objective vs. subjective axis, or a tracking problem. Axis variation may result in postoperative hyper-hypocorrection of sphere, hypocorrection of astigmatism, mixed astigmatism, irregular astigmatism, and pseudo-decentration.

References

1. Tabbara KF, El-Sheik HF, Monowarul-Islam SM. Laser in situ keratomileusis for the correction of hyperopia from +0.50 to +11.50 diopters with the keracor 117C laser. *J Refractive Surg*. 2001;17:123-128.
2. Ditzen K, Huschka H, Pieger S. Laser in situ keratomileusis for hyperopia. *J Cataract Refract Surg*. 1998;24:42-47.
3. Zadok D, Maskaleris G, Montes M, et al. Hyperopic laser in situ keratomileusis with the Nidek EC-5000 excimer laser. *Ophthalmology*. 2000;107:1132-1137.

4. Sher NA. Hyperopic refractive surgery. *Curr Opin Ophthalmol.* 2001; 12(4):304-308.
5. Williams DK. One-year results of laser vision correction for low to moderate hyperopia. *Ophthalmology.* 2000;107:72-75.
6. Vinciguerra P, Camesasca FI. Treatment of hyperopia: a new ablation profile to reduce corneal eccentricity. *J Refractive Surgery.* 2002; 18:S315-317.
7. Martinez CE, Applegate RA, Klyce SD, et al. Effect of papillary dilatation on optical aberration after Keratectomy. *Arch Ophthalmol.* 1998;116:1053-1062.
8. McLellan JS, Marcos S, Burns SA. Age related changes in monochromatic wave aberration of human eye. *Invest Ophthalmol Vis Sci.* 2001; 42:1390.
9. Kohnen T, Mahmoud K, Buhren J. Comparison of corneal higher-order aberrations induced by myopic and hyperopic LASIK. *Ophthalmology.* 2005;112:1692.
10. O'Brart DP, Patsoura E, Jaycock P, Rajan M, Marshall J. Excimer laser photorefractive keratectomy for hyperopia: 7.5-year follow-up. *J Cataract Refract Surg.* 2005; 31:1104-1113.
11. Jin GJ, Lyle WA, Merkley KH. Laser in situ keratomileusis for primary hyperopia. *J Cataract Refract Surg.* 2005;31:776-784.
12. Kermani O, Schmeidt K, Oberheide U, Gerten G. Hyperopic laser in situ keratomileusis with 5.5-, 6.5-, and 7.0-mm optical zones. *J Refract Surg.* 2005;21:52-58.
13. Jaycock PD, O'Brart DP, Rajan MS, Marshall J. 5-year follow-up of LASIK for hyperopia. *Ophthalmology.* 2005;112:191-199.
14. Varley GA, Huang D, Rapuano CJ, et al. LASIK for hyperopia, hyperopic astigmatism, and mixed astigmatism: a report by the American Academy of Ophthalmology. *Ophthalmology.* 2004;111:1604-1617.
15. Zadok D, Raifkup F, Landau D, Frucht-Pery J. Long-term evaluation of hyperopic laser in situ keratomileusis. *J Cataract Refract Surg.* 2003; 29:2181-2188.
16. Autrata R, Rehurek J. Laser-assisted subepithelial keratectomy and photorefractive keratectomy for the correction of hyperopia. Results of a 2-year follow-up. *J Cataract Refract Surg.* 2003;29:2105-2114.
17. Carones F, Vigo L, Scandola E. Laser in situ keratomileusis for hyperopia and hyperopic and mixed astigmatism with LADARVision using 7 to 10-mm ablation diameters. *J Refract Surg.* 2003;19:548-554.
18. Nagy Z, Krueger RR, Suveges I. Central bump-like opacity as a complication of high hyperopic photorefractive keratectomy. *Am J Ophthalmol.* 1999;128:636-638.
19. Sener B, Özdamar A, Aras C. Apical nodular subepithelial corneal scar after retreatment in hyperopic photorefractive keratectomy. *J Cataract Refract Surg.* 2000;26:352-357.
20. Vinciguerra P, Epstein D, Radice P, Azzolini M. Long-term results of photorefractive keratectomy for hyperopia and hyperopic astigmatism. *J Refract Surg.* 1998;14:S183-S185.
21. Vinciguerra P, Sborgia M, Epstein D, Azzolini M, MacRae S. Photorefractive keratectomy to correct myopic or hyperopic astigmatism with a cross-cylinder ablation. *J Refract Surg.* 1999;15:S183-S185.
22. Azar DT, Primack JD. Theoretical analysis of ablation depths and profiles in laser in situ keratomileusis for compound hyperopic and mixed astigmatism. *J Cataract Refract Surg.* 2000;26:1123-1136.
23. Vinciguerra P. Cross-cylinder ablation for the correction of myopic or hyperopic astigmatism. In: Gimbel HV, Anderson Penno EE. *Refractive Surgery. A Manual of Principles and Practice.* Thorofare, NJ: SLACK Incorporated; 2000.
24. Epstein D, Vinciguerra P, Camesasca FI, et al. Cross cylinder ablation in LASIK and PRK—A new tissue-sparing, accuracy-enhancing strategy for correcting astigmatism. *Invest Ophthalmol Vis Sci.* 2000;41: S690.
25. Vinciguerra P, Camesasca FI. Cross cylinder ablation. In: MacRae SM, Krueger RR, Applegate RA. *Custom Corneal Ablation.* Thorofare, NJ: SLACK Incorporated; 2001.

CHAPTER 13

TREATMENT OF PRESBYOPIA

*Fabrizio I. Camesasca, MD; Paolo Vinciguerra, MD;
Maria Ingrid Torres Munoz, MD*

Introduction

Presbyopia is age-related reduction in amplitude of accommodation with the loss of the ability to change the eye's focus from far to near. The mechanism by which the eye can change focus on near and distant objects or accommodation has been on the subject of speculation for centuries.

The Helmholtz theory indicates the impossibility of obtaining a variation in curvature of the lens in a crystalline lens sclerosis following atrophy of the ciliary muscle.[1]

The Schachar theory of accommodation[1-5] states that there is increased equatorial zonular tension during accommodation, and presbyopia is due to a decrease in the effective working distance of the ciliary muscle as a result of normal crystalline lens growth (increase in equatorial volume). On the basis of this mechanism, the amplitude of accommodation may be increased only by softening the lens stroma or capsule, reducing its mass, rejuvenating the ciliary muscle by somehow reversing ciliary muscle atrophy, or reversing ciliary body fibrosis. Since none of these methods are clinically possible, surgical therapy has emerged to increase the amplitude of accommodation and reverse the symptoms of presbyopia.

Correction of presbyopia with excimer lasers has always played second fiddle to the treatment of myopia, hyperopia, and astigmatism. The reasons for this subordinate role are fairly straightforward: substantial technical difficulties in determining the size and location of the area to be treated, the ensuing risk of severely debilitating visual complications, and the problem of defining when presbyopia first begins to trouble the patients.

Surgical Techniques

Since 1991, several different excimer laser surgical techniques have been introduced, including monovision with near correction for the nondominant eye, inferior off-center ablation to correct hyperopia and presbyopia, and the use of multiple masks to cover corneal portions during ablation to generate a profile fit for distance and near vision.[6-8] This last technique adopts a mask with a mobile diaphragm fitted with two blunt metal blades placed on the cornea for the creation of the semilunar ablation zone. The mask permits ablation with a variable number of laser scans creating two consecutive curvatures. The semilunar zone thus increases depth toward the untreated cornea. The upper part of the semilunar zone corrects hyperopia (ie, the presbyopia), and the lower area served as the transition to the untreated cornea. However, all these techniques lead to controversial results. Presently, two different principles are adopted, one acting on spherical aberration (SA) (Bartoli) and the other aimed to generate an increase in central corneal curvature (Telandro).[9,10]

CONTROL OF SPHERICAL ABERRATION

Wavefront analysis in normal eyes shows an increase in SA during accommodation. The almost neutral or slightly positive total ocular SA (0.156 ± 0.088 μm, OSA system) becomes more negative during accommodation.[11,12] Based on this observation, so-called "aberrometric" correction of presbyopia aims at reducing the amount of central SA and moving it towards negative values (eg, from +0.3 to -0.4, or from +0.7 to +0.2) after the correction of the initial underlying refractive defect. This is achieved with a hyperopic-like correction ring ablation in the corneal midperiphery. This method provides

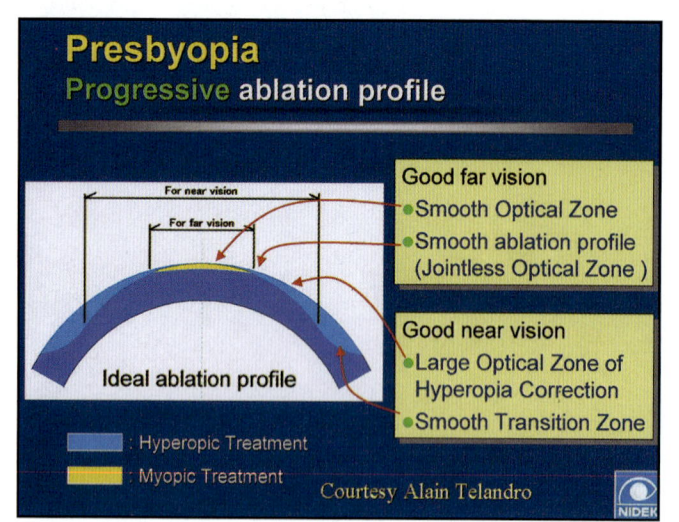

Figure 13-1. Progressive ablation profile for presbyopia, according to Dr. Alain Telandro's method.

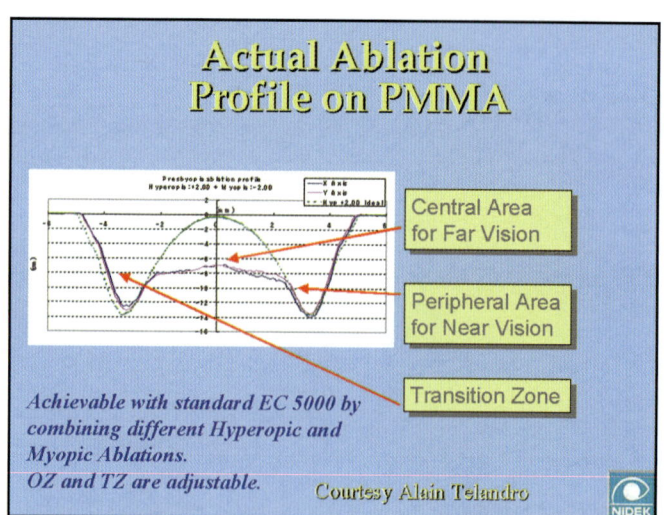

Figure 13-2. Actual ablation profile on PMMA, increased central corneal curvature.

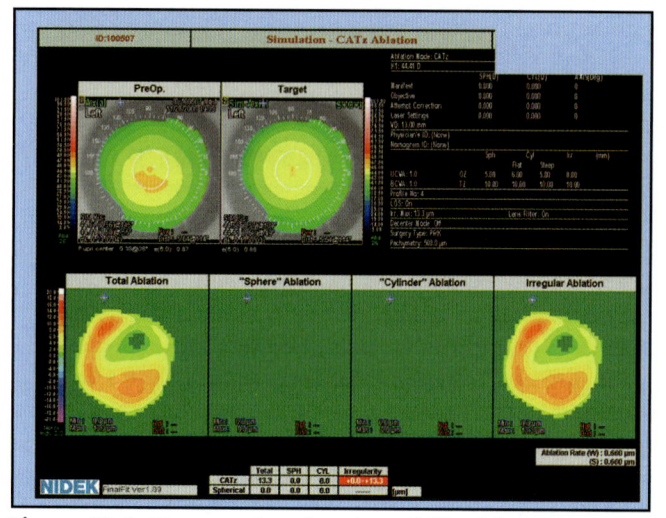

Figure 13-3. Preoperative situation, CATz ablation pattern, and target map, axial algorithm.

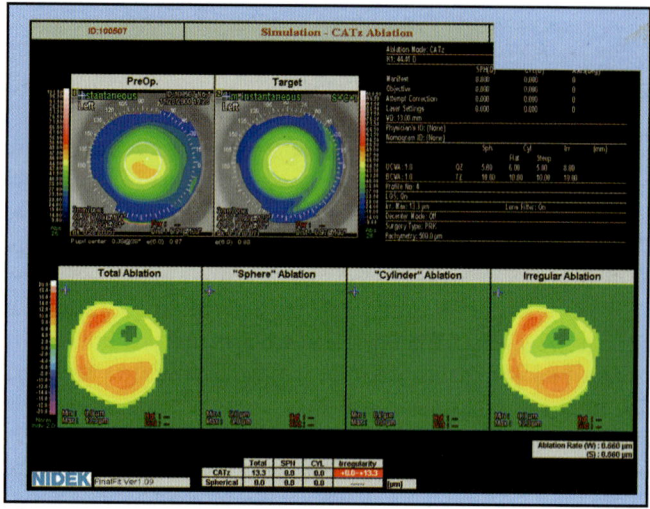

Figure 13-4. Same eye and situation as Figure 13-3, instantaneous algorithm.

interesting results in hyperopic or emmetropic eyes with a small plus refraction component. In myopic eyes, this standard photoablative pattern does not induce a negative but a positive SA. In these cases, determination of preoperative SA is mandatory. If positive, correction strategy will include an aberrometric hypercorrection.[10] Unfortunately, in myopic eyes, this treatment induces corneal multifocality, reducing distance vision quality whenever pupils dilate. The increase in negative SA and the asphericity / eccentricity index seems to increase the ocular depth of field, improving near vision and compensating the age-related presbyopic lens changes.[10]

INCREASED CENTRAL CORNEAL CURVATURE

The technique of progressive ablation profile for treatment of hyperopia developed by Dr. Alain Telandro consists in generating a multifocal ablation with several zones featuring different refractive powers. Central cornea provides distance vision and a concentric midperipheral zone for near vision. Pseudo-accommodative cornea (PAC) NIDEK software version 6T is used to calculate the multistep ablation profile.[9] This optical solution is similar to that of multifocal IOLs. The software generates a multiple zone ablation pattern, featuring hyperopic ablations with smaller diameters hypercorrecting the sphere and then a very small diameter central myopic correction (Figures 13-1 and 13-2).

Presently, our approach includes treatment of high-order aberrations with the NIDEK Final Fit. Figure 13-3 presents preoperative situation, CATz ablation pattern, and target map—axial algorithm. Figure 13-4 presents the same situation—instantaneous algorithm. The PAC software includes a questionnaire with fields on refractive and clinical data, as well as lifestyle (Figures 13-5 and 13-6) providing the ablation plan (Figure 13-7) with power as well as optical and transition zone size.

It is interesting to observe that this solution also gives varying results according to the preoperative refractive

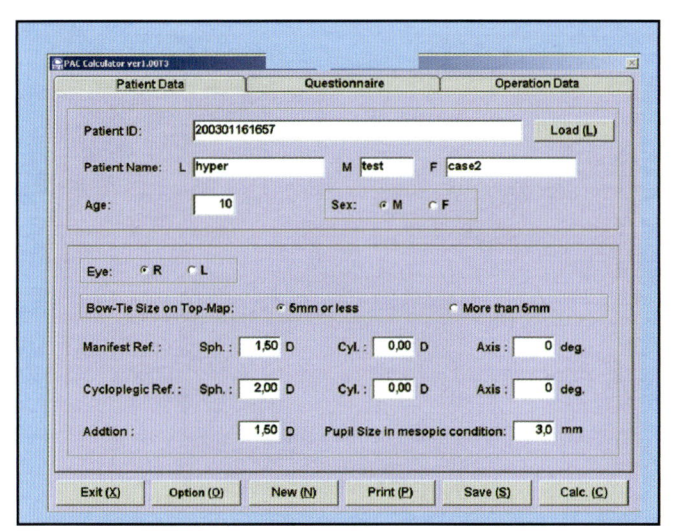

Figure 13-5. PAC software, patient data folder.

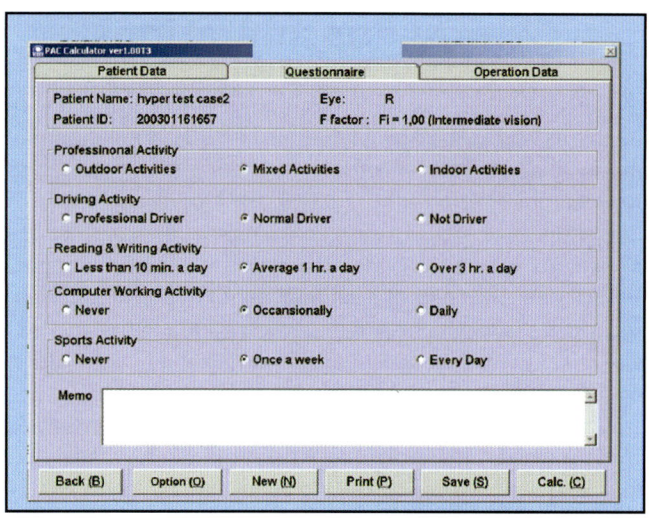

Figure 13-6. PAC software, questionnaire folder.

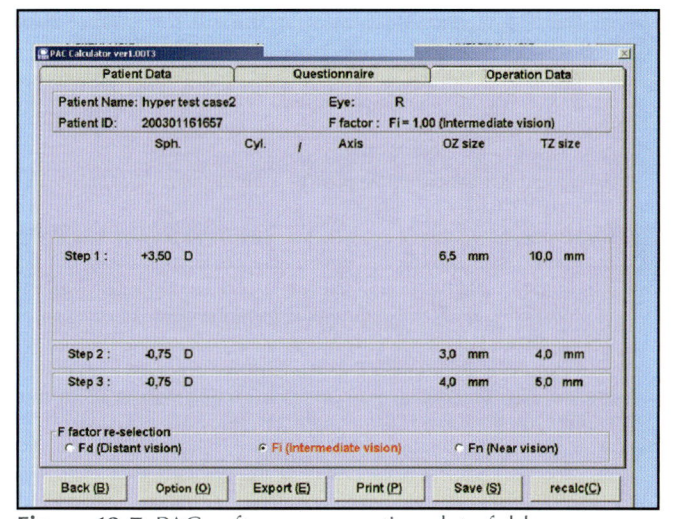

Figure 13-7. PAC software, operation data folder.

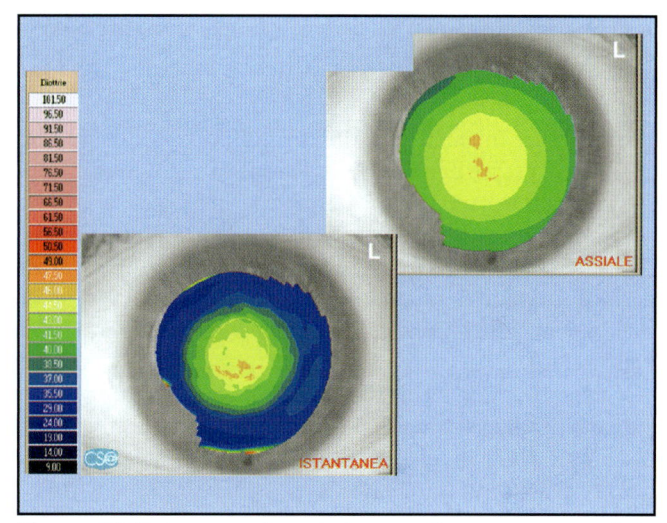

Figure 13-8. Increased central corneal curvature, result in a hyperopic eye, note wide optical zone.

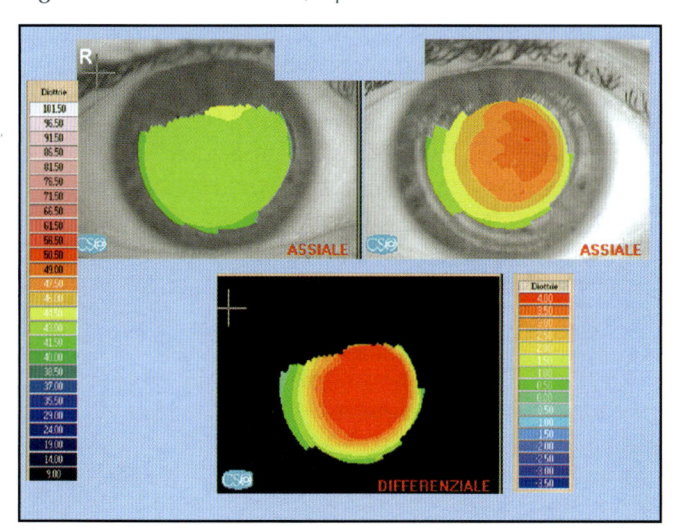

Figure 13-9. Increased central corneal curvature, result in a hyperopic eye, note very wide optical zone.

defect. Hyperopic eyes will have a wider optical zone since the central small myopic ablation will reduce the center-to-periphery optical gradient, and in the periphery, the red-ring generated by the myopic ablation will also increase the functional optical diameter of the previously applied hyperopic ablation. These two factors will improve the final result, a multifocal cornea with a very wide optical zone (Figures 13-8 and 13-9).[13,14] On the contrary, in myopic eyes, this approach will lead to a situation that can be properly analyzed with an instantaneous topographic algorithm, showing a marked mid-peripheral red-ring, clearly indicating a refractive situation with increased SA (Figure 13-10). Increase in SA generates an increase in depth of field, but unfortunately, whenever the pupil dilates and corneal portions with greater curvature are involved, the optical quality of the system decreases markedly. Thus, myopia correction with this approach worsens vision quality when the pupil is dilated.

Clinical Considerations

Both the above-mentioned techniques can be utilized with LASIK as well as surface ablation. Excimer laser treatment of presbyopia can still be considered in its initial phases, and we recommend carefully selecting the surgical patients. In our opinion, this treatment can presently be recommended to patients wishing to widen their spectacle-free vision possibilities but who do not need high quality vision for certain specific tasks (eg, night-driving, reading for a long-time, etc) and who are ready to accept partial worsening of their vision in certain conditions (eg, at sunset).

This requires an appropriate and well-considered informed consent to carefully explain to the patient that his visual performance may worsen in certain conditions. In plain words, promising too much may be harmful. Furthermore, this treatment is not recommended for eyes with very wide pupils in scotopic conditions (eg, 5 mm).

If the correction is applied on hyperopic eyes, it is important to remember what is stated in the Chapter 12 in connection with the influence of globe size on refractive surgery, and precisely that in small eyes the corneal portion involved by ablation is proportionally wider. Given that presbyopic correction leads to overcorrection in the periphery and a myopic correction in the central cornea, it is important, as usual in surface ablation, to avoid sudden and marked increases in corneal curvature, to prevent the typical complication of excessive hyperopic correction (eg, hyperopic white scar) (see Figure 10-9).

Currently, the ideal candidate for presbyopic treatment is a patient with hyperopia 3.0 D with normal corneal thickness, a scotopic pupil smaller than 5 mm, and no need for high quality vision in specific tasks.

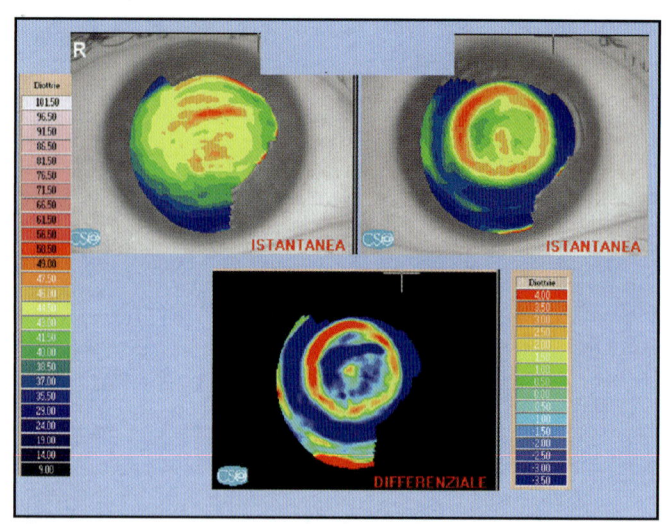

Figure 13-10. Increased central corneal curvature, result in a myopic eye, note increase in SA.

References

1. Bartoli F. Aberrometric correction of presbyopia: theory and results. In: Garg A, ed. *Mastering the Techniques of Presbyopia Surgery.* New Delhi, India: Jaypee Brothers; 2006.
2. Schachar RA, Cudmore DP, Black TD. Experimental support for Schachar's hypothesis of accommodation. *Ann Ophthalmol.* 1993; 25:404-409.
3. Schachar RA, Anderson DA. The mechanism of ciliary muscle function. *Ann Ophthalmol.*1995;27:126-132.
4. Schachar RA. Pathophysiology of accommodation and presbyopia: understanding the clinical implications. *J Fla Med Assoc.* 1994;81:268-271.
5. Schachar RA, Black TD, Kash RL, et al. The mechanism of accommodation and presbyopia in the primate. *Ann Ophthalmol.* 1995;27:58-67.
6. Bauerberg JM. Centered vs. inferior off-center ablation to correct hyperopia and presbyopia. *J Refract Surg.* 1999;15:66-69.
7. Vinciguerra P, Nizzola GM, Nizzola F, Ascari A, Azzolini M, Epstein D. Zonal photorefractive keratectomy for presbyopia. *J Refract Surg.* 1998;14:S218-221.
8. Vinciguerra P, Nizzola GM, Bailo G, Nizzola F, Ascari A, Epstein D. Excimer laser photorefractive keratectomy for presbyopia: 24-month follow up in three eyes. *J Refract Surg.* 1998;14:31-37.
9. Telandro A. Pseudo-accommodative cornea: a new concept for correction of presbyopia. *J Refract Surg.* 2004; 20: S714-717.
10. Bartoli F. Ipotesi di correzione aberrometrica della presbiopia. PRK. Trattamento refrattivo e aberrometrico. Minerva Medica; 2003.
11. Hofer H, Artal P, Singer B, Aragon JL, Williams DR. Dynamics of the eye's wave aberration. *J Opt Soc Am A Opt Image Sci Vis.* 2001; 18:497-506.
12. Cheng H, Barnett JK, Vilupuru AS, et al. A population study on changes in wave aberrations with accommodation. *J Vis.* 2004;4:272-280.
13. Cantu R, Rosales MA, Tepichin E, Curioca A, Montes V, Bonilla J. Advanced surface ablation for presbyopia using the Nidek EC-5000 laser. *J Refract Surg.* 2004;20: S711-13.
14. Rudakova TE, Kurenkov VV, Polunin GS. Characteristics of correction of myopia by photorefractive keratectomy in patients with presbyopia. *Vest Oftalmol.* 2000;116:31-33.

CHAPTER 14

Topographically Guided Transepithelial PRK for Refractive and Therapeutic Purposes

Leopoldo Spadea, MD; Angela Di Gregorio, MD

Every cornea has its own characteristics that make it different from all the others: thickness, shape, radius of curvature, profile, asphericity, and toricity. These are the main elements that new ablative strategies take into consideration with the help of informatics. Good software, therefore, should be able to adapt its surgical program to every kind of presurgically analyzed cornea.

In reality, standard software sets up the ablative strategy by taking into consideration the refractive modification that is worth pursuing, and this is calculated by referring to an ideal cornea model taken as a standard, virtually absolute value. From a physical viewpoint, this set-up may be correct, but often it does not correspond to the final outcome in which, even though refraction has achieved the desired theoretical target, the patient may complain of a less than optimal functional quality. The reason (decentralization, central island) for this is often revealed only by evaluation systems, such as computerized corneal topography.[1] These considerations lead to the conviction that it is necessary to devise a system that will permit the creation of a specific ablative pattern for each cornea that will lead, on the one hand, to the correction of the residual ametropia, and on the other, to the creation of a corneal surface that strays as little as possible from the natural physiological profile. Naturally, in theory, this would also be postulate for correction of irregular forms of astigmatism, which cannot be corrected by common surgical techniques. This is how the idea of the customized ablation, which permits the creation of a customized ablation program, originated.[2]

This program for customized ablation can be created by a corneal topographer that provides an altimetric algorithm. The choice of this kind of topographer is based on the fact that lasers carve the cornea working in microns, not diopters; it is, therefore, essential to think in heights so that the laser and the topographer can work in symbiosis. This idea stems from the assumption that the software conducting the photo ablation keeps to the refractive correction that it has been set to produce and calculates it based on an ideal cornea model.[3]

The excimer laser employed in this research, performed at our clinic, is MEL 70 G (Carl Zeiss Meditec, Dublin, California), a flying spot third-generation laser producing a kind of ablation that may be based on a circular scan or on a randomized scanning spot. The characteristics of the laser are a 193-nm wavelength, a 35-Hz frequency, a 180-mJ/cm^2 fluence, and a 0.25-µm ablation rate. The laser uses a 1.8-mm diameter flying spot with a Gaussian profile. A cone for controlled atmosphere (CCA) is employed on the laser output to remove smoke or particles in the way of the laser beam.[4]

This laser is an interfaceable workstation devised to analyze noticeable corneal map surgical data and, using the Topography Supported Customized Ablation (TOSCA) system (Figure 14-1), it produces a simulation of the effects that laser treatment will have in making a new corneal curvature outline. This system permits surgeons to perform photorefractive treatment supported by topographical data. In fact, a simple topographical image of the patient's eye is turned into a "customized" treatment profile. TOSCA software permits the rectifying of refractive mistakes even in asymmetric, irregular, and refractive defect corneas. After entering the patient's refractive data and calculating the difference between the patient's map and a reference sphere (best-fit sphere), a specific ablation pattern suited to that particular cornea and calculated by the special MEL 70 excimer laser program is obtained. In this case, ablation is performed by a pseudo-randomized scanning. The TOSCA system permits presurgical simulation of the laser ablation showing, step by step, the depth of the ablation in microns. Tissue Save Ablation (TSA) software, which permits up to 70% of ablative tissue to be saved, is associated with the TOSCA software. This customized technique with corneal

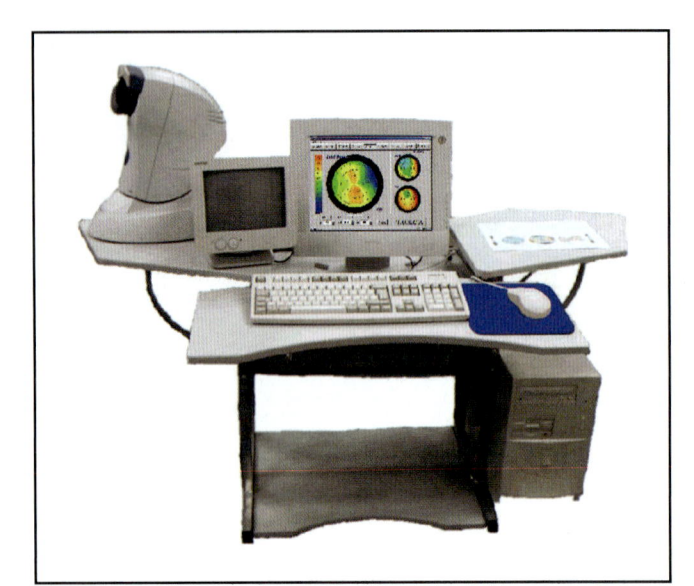

Figure 14-1. Representation of TOSCA software.

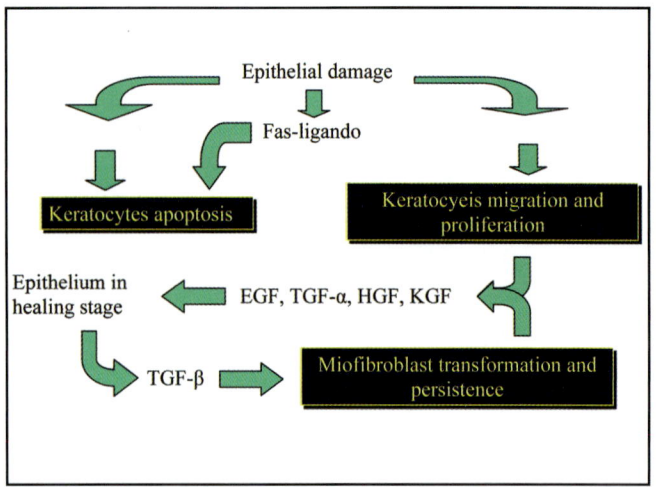

Figure 14-2. Molecular regulation of epithelial cells and keratocytes in corneal recovery process.

topography link has been employed by us to perform excimer laser photorefractive keratectomy (PRK) transepithelially (TE). Use of the TE-PRK technique gives the advantage of preventing chemical or mechanical removal from allowing stromal irregularity[5] to remerge. In fact, when topographically-linked PRK surgery is practiced, the datum used is a topographical map also including the epithelium that when the ablation is performed, behaves as a kind of a masking fluid. Another advantage of surface transepithelial ablation is that it promotes a lower incidence of events that may result in epithelial damage. In fact, during the corneal healing process, a molecular rearrangement of epithelial cells and keratocytes occurs. Epithelial damage determines the release both of interleukin 1, which provokes keratocytical apoptosis, and the platelet-derived growth factor (PDGF), which determines a proliferation and migration of keratocytes. The latter activates the release of other growth factors (EGF, TGS-α, HGF, KGF) that permit the epithelium to heal. Re-epithelization, by itself, determines the release of the growth factor TGF-β that provokes the transformation and the persistence of fibroblasts (Figure 14-2).[6-8]

The efficiency and safety of transepithelial topographically guided ablation in the treatment of an irregular corneal profile has been assessed on several corneal pathologies and postsurgery conditions such as irregular astigmatism after keratoplastic, enhancements, corneal opacity therapeutic treatment, and LASIK complications.

After a refractive corneal surgery, laser retreatment is always a rather difficult topic. A whole series of issues, such as patient expectations, the presurgery situation, the outcome obtained, etc, must be considered. The surgeon has to know the patient's history and understand which of the multiple variables have determined the unsuccessful result. Refraction, biomicroscopy, computerized videokeratography, and pachymetry are indispensable to identify every change in the corneal curvature that may have occurred during the follow-up as a result of the pharmacological therapy.[9,10]

If the initial refractive procedure has been correctly performed, the reason for failure must be related to a biologically anomalous response.[11] The choice of retreatment must be decided with the patient, explaining all possible risks and benefits.[12]

Nowadays, requests for excimer laser resurgery are due principally to the desire to achieve emmetropization or to improve the loss of vision in qualitative terms with respect to the presurgery condition, regardless of the refractive profit.

The reasons for performing excimer laser retreatment may be hypo/hypercorrections, regressions, decentralization, or small optical areas. When performing retreatment after a PRK surgery, the causes leading to visual damage must be carefully evaluated. Possible causes of regressions after PRK and LASIK surgery are classifiable as depending on the patient (eg, age, systemic pathologies), the kinds of instrument employed (eg, large beam, scanning and flying spot laser), the treatment parameters (kind of laser beam produced and possible ablation geometries), and differing postoperative therapy. Local postsurgery therapy can influence the refraction process during adaptation and minimize the appearance of corneal haze.[13]

In fact, at varying times after surface stromal ablation in areas subjected to photo ablation, it is possible to observe the formation of disorganized neocollagen that is co-responsible for haze. When this occurs at a high rate (>2 Heitzmann scale), it may determine an alteration both in the quality and the quantity of the vision, especially when assessed at a low contrast. Some studies have shown that epithelial hyperplasia after PRK modifies the normal thickness of the epithelium, sometimes doubling it. Disorganized subepithelial neocollagen is constituted *ex novo* by synthesized mucus polysaccharides and glycosamminoglicans.[14,15] Spadea et al, in research conducted on 50 eyes employing a high frequency ultrasound technique (50 MHz), noted a slightly above (or below) average increase of the corneal thickness equal to 6.5 µm after LASIK surgery to correct myopia between 5.0 and 12.0 D.[16] Finally, Chayet et al pointed out that regression causes corneal ectasia, corneal hydration, stromal synthesis, and epithelial hyperplasia.[17] This work may consequently cause hyper- or hypocorrection, astigmatism, and myopic regression leading to consideration of retreatment. Therefore, in consideration of our necessity for safety and effectiveness, it would be appropriate to apply a technique that reduces tissue leak and does not lead to the insurgence of haze.[18]

Photo therapeutic keratectomy (PTK) is a laser technique useful for treating superficial corneal pathologies such as cicatrix, dystrophy, epithelial erosion, and regular band keratopath; fibrosis after radial keratectomy (RK) or penetrating keratoplasty (PKP); and opacity after PRK, delaying or eliminating the need for a corneal transplant.[19-22]

The success of PTK is related to the corneal transparency, the regularity of the corneal profile, and the refraction obtained, but the predictability of PTK is poor due to the lack of standardization. Therefore, the possibility of achieving good refractive outcomes in pathological corneas is firstly dependent upon the surgeon's ability and, sometimes, unpredictable factors.[23,24] In fact, PTK is an efficient method for obtaining corneal transparency by removing the opacity situated in the anterior third of the stromal thickness; however, it is a difficult technique with a low predictability due to lack of standardization.[25-27] On the contrary, the procedure becomes easier and faster when topographically guided PTK is applied. In recent research conducted on 29 eyes with post-surgery corneal irregularities the introduction of excimer laser customized ablation proved to be a technique suitable for treating such irregularities, with an improvement of the visual acuity (VA).[28,29] Transepithelial customized PTK seems to be a powerful technique for treating corneal irregularities, ensuring good corneal transparency, and preventing haze formation.[30-32]

The appearance of high and irregular astigmatism after PKP is often difficult to correct with glasses, and it is not always possible to apply contact lenses because they may determine peripheral corneal vascularization with a consequent increased risk of a rejection.[33,34] In some research, it has been reported that about 20% of the patients successfully subjected to PKP later had to undergo refractive surgery. In spite of the improvement of suture techniques and their modulation, postsurgery astigmatism is still a problem connected to keratoplasty. Several surgical techniques have been devised to treat post-PKP astigmatism.

Over recent years, LASIK has been tested as a treatment for ametropia in post-PKP: this procedure has one remarkable advantage because, by maintaining the anatomical integrity of the Bowmann membrane, it does not excessively modify physiology of the cornea; however, this surgical procedure has been associated with complications causing significant alterations to vision.[35,36] Several studies have highlighted that complications may occur, especially during creation of the flap: the percentage ranges from 0.3% to 10%. These risks may depend either on the mechanical action or on the surgeon's lack of experience.[37-40] The risks include the creation of buttonholes, free-caps, and incomplete or irregular flaps.[41,42]

Several authors have proposed alternative surgical techniques to treat flap-shaping complications. One is to replace the flap and retreat after at least 3 months; another is transepithelial ablation.[43]

The advantage of using the transepithelial PRK technique is that it avoids the possibility that mechanical or chemical removal of the epithelium will give rise to stromal irregularity resulting from an unsuccessful cut. In fact, during topographically linked PRK surgery, a topographical map is applied that also includes the epithelium, which behaves as a kind of masking fluid during the ablation procedure, subsequently producing a homogeneous surface.[44-46]

Technical Characteristics of TOSCA

TOSCA is an advanced system for acquiring data on the morphology of a corneal surface required to plan the subsequent MEL 70 excimer laser surgery. Using a CCD video camera, the TMS-3 (Tomey, Nagota, Japan) topographer evaluates the corneal surface of the patient's eye and measures the correct corneal profile curvature. The memorized images are visualized in real time on the monitor. The connected computer works out the data and permits the software to interpret the results obtained afterwards as well as analyzing the collected images. These TMS-3 recorded images are chosen and sent to the TOSCA software; finally, the data are further elaborated and transferred to the MEL 70 excimer laser to perform a customized treatment. The software processes the data inside the MEL 70 excimer laser to "pilot" the ablation pattern.

Before the treatment, the depth of ablation required to remove corneal opacity is measured; subsequently, the corneal epithelial thickness measured by ultrasound pachymetry is added by the TSA software to the ablation planned with the TOSCA system. This is necessary to perform a correct transepithelial procedure.

To avoid the hyperopic effect of central PTK ablation, we employ a rectification factor to prevent an excessive hyperopization. In effect, by calculating the ablation thickness, assessed at 5 mm in the central cornea area according to Munnerlyn's (diopters = ablation x 3/ optical area^2) formula, a hyperopic rectification factor is added.[47]

Surgical Technique

A patch is placed over the eye that will not be operated, while a sterile eyelid speculum is inserted into the eye to be treated after topical anesthesia by instillation with 0.4% oxyprobocaine drops. The patient is instructed to stare at a coaxial light (yellow diode), and the surgeon performs the ablation transepithelially, using the center of the pupil as the focus point. An active eye-tracking system, oriented on a metal ring, monitors centration. After photoablation, a therapeutic soft contact lens is used until complete re-epithelization

Table 14-1. Preoperative Data Before Topographically Guided Transepithelial PRK Retreatments (33 eyes)

	Age Mean ± SD (range)	UCVA Mean ± SD (range)	BSCVA Mean ± SD (range)	MRSE Mean ± SD (range)	Corneal Thickness Mean ± SD (Range)	Time Mean ± SD (Range)
Myopic Re-PRK (21)	38.27 ± 8.04 (28 to 55)	20/28 ± 20/28 (20/60 to 20/25)	20/100 ± 20/28 (20/60 to 20/20)	-2.54 ± 2.60 (-0.50 to -6)	457.39 ± 50.05 (387 to 570)	26.14 ± 28.77 (6 to 108)
Hyperopic Re-PRK (12)	41 ± 9.65 (28 to 55)	20/67 ± 20/28 (20/100 to 20/25)	20/20 (20/30 to 20/20)	+2.23 ± 0.65 (+1.25 to 3.25)	487.18 ± 64.61 (400 to 565)	14.25 ± 12.38 (6 to 48)

Table 14-2. Postoperative Uncorrected and Best Spectacle-Corrected Visual Acuity and Corneal Thickness After Topographically Guided Transepithelial PRK Retreatments (33 eyes)

	UCVA Mean ± SD (range)	BSCVA Mean ± SD (range)	MRSE Mean ± SD (range)	Corneal Thickness Mean ± SD (range)
Myopic Re-PRK (21)	20/20 ± 20/28 (20/50 to 20/20)	20/20 ± 20/30 (20/50 to 20/20)	-0.07 ± 0.38 (-0.50 to +0.75)	423.47 ± 24.84 (333 to 432)
Hyperopic Re-PRK (12)	20/20 ± 20/25 (20/25 to 20/20)	20/20 (20/20)	+0.09 ± 0.26 (-0.25 to +0.50)	423.36 ± 53.10 (356 to 525)

(from 4 to 8 days), antibiotic drops, and artificial teardrops are administered. Subsequently, corticosteroid-based drops are prescribed three times a day for at least a month, and later they are scaled down depending on the corneal haze and the refractive outcome. In the group of transepithelial topo-customized PRK retreatments, 25 eyes of 22 patients (12 male and 10 female), aged between 21 and 55 years (mean, 39.2 ± 8.6 SD), 14 patients had a myopic refractive defect (-2.50 ± 0.7 SD), and 11 patients had a hyperopic defect (+2.2 ± 0.6 SD) (Table 14-1).

Mean uncorrected visual acuity (UCVA) changed from 20/50 ± 20/67 SD to 20/28 ± 20/67 SD. Mean best spectacle-corrected visual acuity (BSCVA) that presurgically was 20/22 ± 20/100 SD changed to 20/20 ± 20/100 SD postsurgically (Table 14-2).

The mean of the presurgery refractive data expressed in spherical equivalent was -0.8 ± 0.9 SD, whereas the postsurgery mean was 0.4 ± 0.9 SD (Figure 14-3 and 14-4).

The presurgery mean of the average central corneal power was 40.01 ± 2.38 D and after repeat PRK treatment was 38.97 ± 1.9 D. Keratometric astigmatism mean in presurgery was 1.6 ± 1.51 D, while in postsurgery it was 0.87 ± 0.3 D.

Haze was assessed on the Heitzmann scale (0 to 5). None of the patient's eyes were retreated for significant opacities due to primary treatment (haze >2). In our patients, corneal haze showed a sudden rise between 3 and 6 months after retreatment and, in the aftermath, gradually diminished. No patient has a haze score higher than 2 (Figure 14-5).

Phototherapeutic Keratectomy

Twenty-six eyes of 24 patients were selected, all 24 patients (22 male and 2 female) with a mean age of about 50.8 ± 17 SD (range, 20 to 74 years old). The preoperative corneal pathologies treated during our research were caused by postinfectious scarring in 6 eyes, post-traumatic scarring in 18 eyes, and post-PRK scarring in 2 eyes (Figure 14-6). In all the eyes, the trauma or infection had occurred more than 2 years previously, whereas for those damaged by PRK, the treatment had been performed at least 1 year before. Each patient was treated once, and complications such as re-epithelialization delays, recurrent infections, and increased intraocular pressure induced by topical corticosteroid use were not noted (Table 14-3).

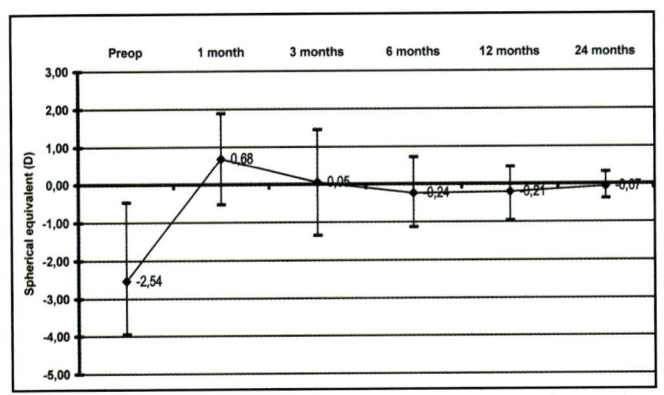

Figure 14-3. Change in spherical equivalent of manifest refraction over time after topographically guided trans-epithelial PRK myopic retreatment (21 eyes).

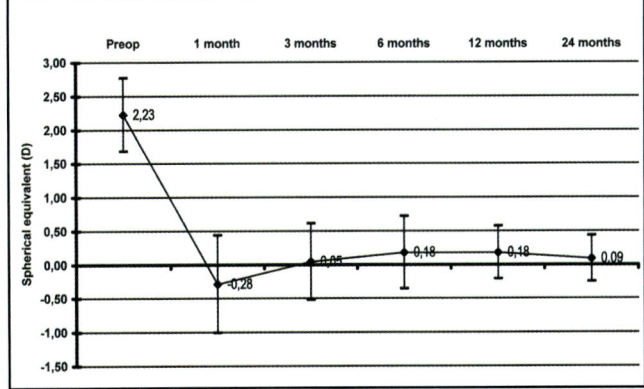

Figure 14-4. Change in spherical equivalent of manifest refraction over time after topographically guided transepithelial PRK hyperopic retreatment (12 eyes).

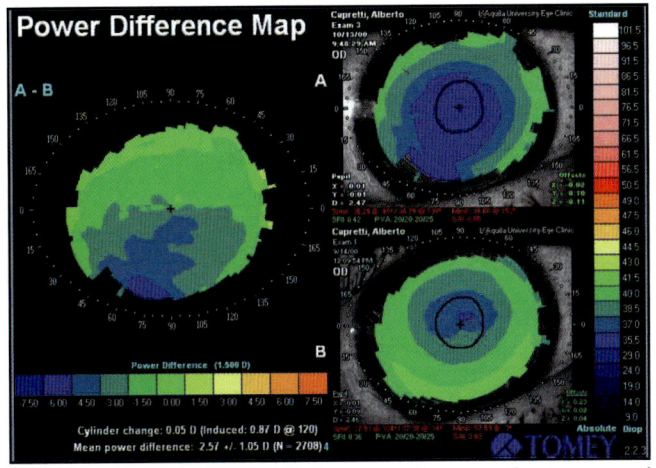

Figure 14-5. The differential map (left) shows the improved corneal profile obtained from before (bottom right) and after (top right) (plano; VA 20/20) topographically guided transepithelial treatment.

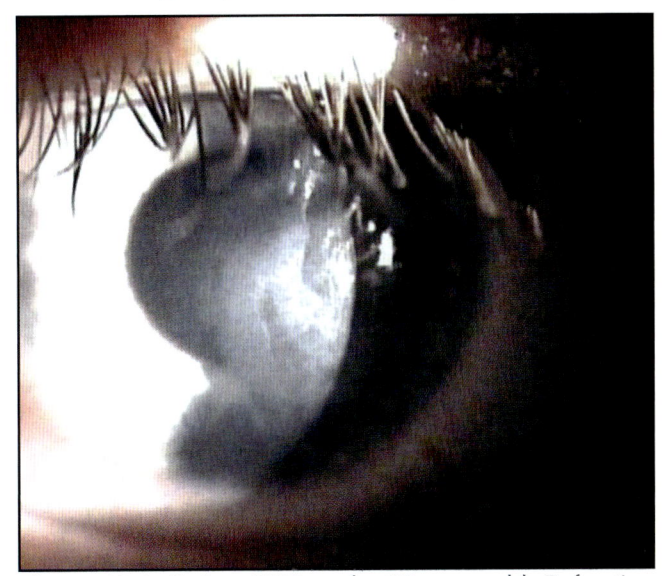

Figure 14-6. Patient DBS, male, 20 years old. Refraction LE +1 sph. November 1999: postinfectious (herpes virus) superficial corneal opacities.

Haze always proved to be inferior to 1, on the Heitzmann scale (from 0 to 5). Corneal transparency was shown to have improved in every eye by comparing presurgery biomicroscope images with the postsurgery ones (Figures 14-7 and 14-8). Both the UCVA and the BSCVA increased and the differences were statistically significant (respectively $p=0.008$ and $p<0.001$).

Spherical equivalent refractive data can be seen in Figure 3. By comparing the presurgery spherical equivalent data to the final refractive outcome, statistically significant differences have not been shown by the Student t test ($p > 0.05$). The UCVA showed a statistically significant improvement ($p = 0.008$), from a presurgical mean value of 20/200 ± 20/200 SD (range, 20/1200 to 20/30) to a postsurgical mean value of 20/50 ± 20/100 SD (range, 20/600 to 20/20), whereas the BSCVA went from 20/50 ± 20/100 SD (range, 20/1200 to 20/25) to 20/25 ± 20/100 SD (range, 20/63 to 20/20) ($p <0.001$). BSCVA increased in every eye by 2 or more lines in 76.9% of the eyes and by 1 line in the remaining 23.1% (Figure 14-9).

Spherical equivalent refraction went from a presurgical mean value of -0.125 ± 2.77 SD (range, -4.5 to +5.5 D) to a postsurgical mean value of +1.33 ± 1.28 SD (range, 1.0 to +3.5 D) with a mean refraction value significantly modified ($p = 0.019$) of +1.45 ± 2.61 SD (range, -4.5 to +6.0 D); 34.6% of the eyes (9/26) showed a hyperopic shift ≥1.0 D (Table 14-4). Spherical equivalent refractive data is shown in Figure 14-10. Twenty-three percent of the eyes (6/26) had a final refraction within ±0.5 D from emmetropia, 50% (13/26) within ±2.0 D, and 100% (26/26) within ±4.0 D.

PRK After LASIK Complication

Two patients were evaluated. Each one had previously undergone PKP surgical: one for a keratoconus and one for an unsatisfactory outcome of the previous PRK. The two male patients had an average age of 30 ± 4 SD (range, 28 to 32 years old).

Eighteen months after PRK surgery in each eye, we removed the sutures and, after a further 6 months, due to

Preoperative Data Before Topographically Guided Transepithelial PTK Treatments

Table 14-3

Patient	Corneal Pathology	S.E.	UCVA	BCVA	Corneal Thickness	Maximum Ablation
# 1	Post-traumatic	-3.5	20/200	20/63	464	137
# 2	Post-traumatic	+3.75	20/600	20/25	572	150
# 3	Postinfectious	+1	20/100	20/32	415	132
# 4	Post-traumatic	0	20/1200	20/1200	580	120
# 5	Post-traumatic	-4	20/600	20/32	455	150
# 6	Postinfectious	-4.5	20/100	20/50	547	160
# 7	Post-traumatic	+2.5	20/600	20/25	563	128
# 8	Post-traumatic	+1.75	20/50	20/25	582	141
# 9	Post-traumatic	+5.5	20/600	20/100	587	101
# 10	Postinfectious	-1	20/50	20/32	539	147
# 11	Post-traumatic	0	20/32	20/32	424	154
# 12	Post-traumatic	-1.5	20/200	20/63	481	132
# 13	Post-PRK	-2	20/200	20/25	406	149
# 14	Post-PRK	-3	20/600	20/25	426	88
# 15	Post-traumatic	-2.5	20/200	20/63	474	127
# 16	Postinfectious	-1	20/50	20/32	536	137
# 17	Post-traumatic	+3.25	20/600	20/25	583	150
# 18	Postinfectious	-1	20/100	20/32	417	132
# 19	Post-traumatic	0	20/1200	20/1200	545	122
# 20	Post-traumatic	-3.75	20/600	20/32	465	150
# 21	Postinfectious	-1.5	20/100	20/50	555	120
# 22	Post-traumatic	+3.5	20/600	20/25	568	128
# 23	Post-traumatic	+1.75	20/50	20/25	574	131
# 24	Post-traumatic	+4.5	20/200	20/100	578	101
# 25	Post-traumatic	0	20/32	20/32	442	154
# 26	Post-traumatic	-1.5	20/200	20/63	418	112

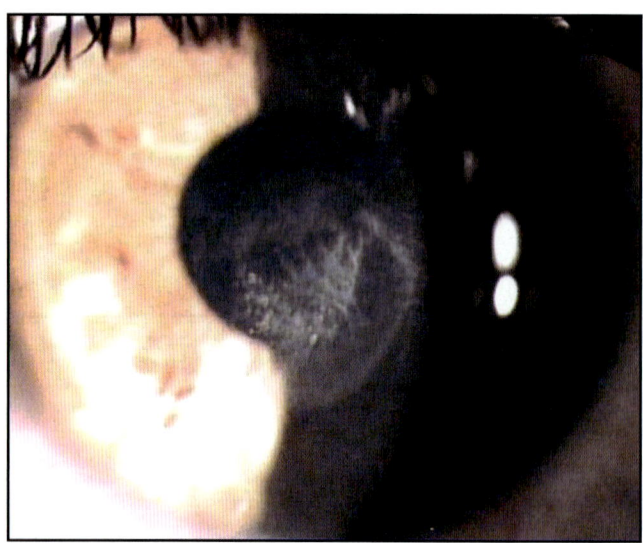

Figure 14-7. Patient DBS, male, 20 years old. Refraction LE +2 sph = +2.50 cyl (70°). December 2000: remarkable reduction of superficial corneal opacities.

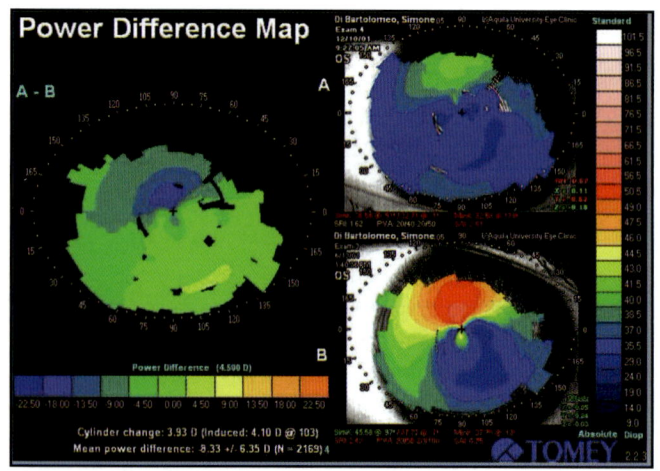

Figure 14-8. Comparison between imagines before (bottom right) and after (top right), the better corneal clarity permit a gain of 4 Snellen lines, obtaining 20/20 of BCVA; differential map (left).

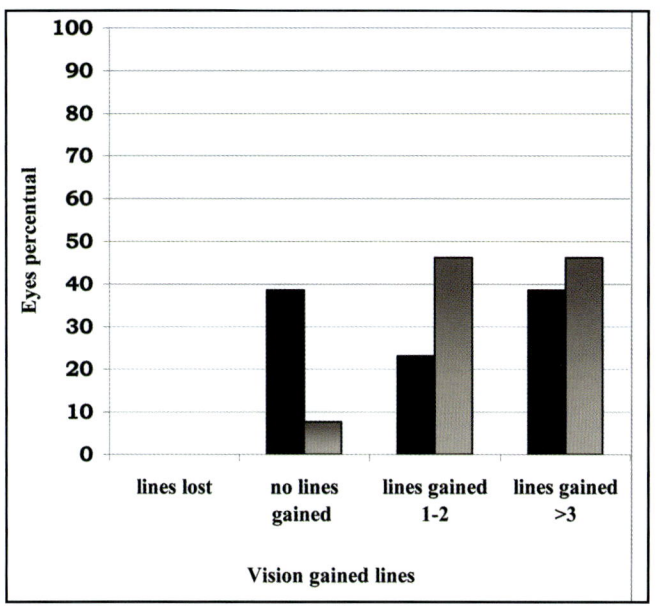

Figure 14-9. Gained line after topographically guided transepithelial PTK.

POSTOPERATIVE DATA AFTER TOPOGRAPHICALLY GUIDED TRANSEPITHELIAL PTK TREATMENTS

Patient	SE	UCVA	BCVA	Corneal Thickness
# 1	+2.5	20/200	20/25	374
# 2	+3.5	20/600	20/20	522
# 3	+3.25	20/100	20/20	395
# 4	+2	20/200	20/63	530
# 5	0	20/20	20/20	305
# 6	+1	20/25	20/20	457
# 7	+0.25	20/40	20/20	543
# 8	+2	20/40	20/20	532
# 9	+1	20/63	20/32	547
# 10	+1	20/50	20/25	462
# 11	0	20/25	20/25	394
# 12	0	20/50	20/50	429
# 13	-1	20/25	20/20	347
# 14	-1	20/25	20/20	387
# 15	+2	20/200	20/25	404
# 16	+1.5	20/50	20/25	456
# 17	+3	20/600	20/20	525
# 18	+3.25	20/100	20/20	359
# 19	+2.5	20/200	20/63	502
# 20	+0.25	20/20	20/20	308
# 21	+0.75	20/25	20/20	433
# 22	+2	20/40	20/20	534
# 23	+2	20/40	20/20	526
# 24	+1	20/63	20/32	542
# 25	0	20/25	20/25	349
# 26	+1.75	20/50	20/50	368

Table 14-4

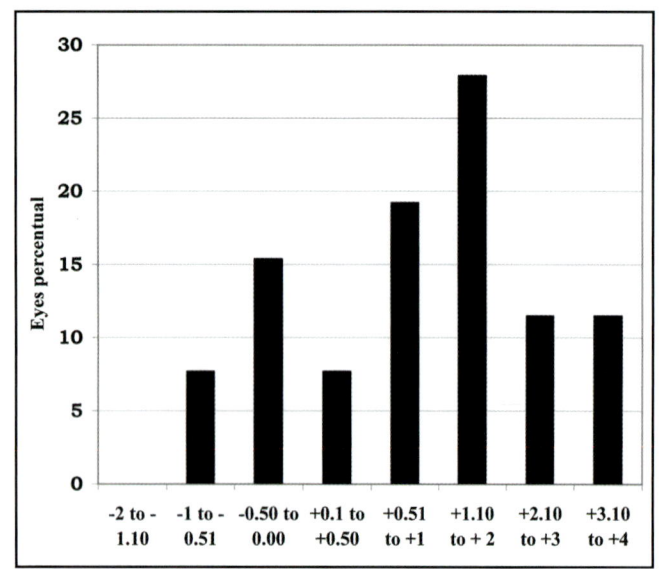

Figure 14-10. Change in spherical equivalent of manifest refraction over time after topographically guided transepithelial PTK.

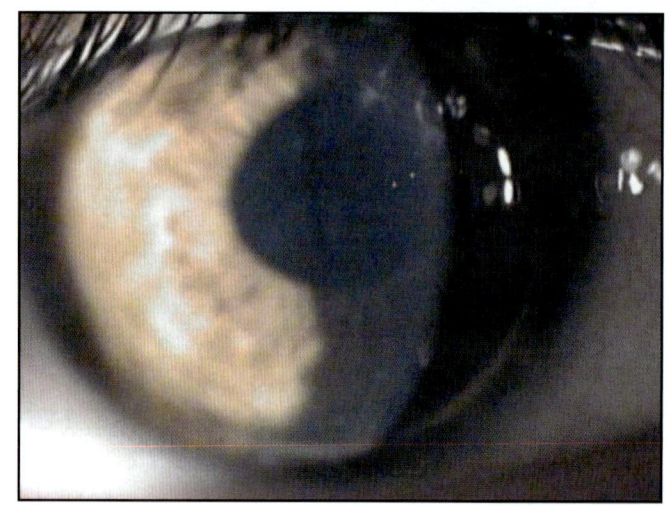

Figure 14-11. Patient RZ, male, 31 years old. Preoperative Refraction RE -1.50 sph = +6 cyl (110 degrees). October 2003: outcome after buttonhole complication.

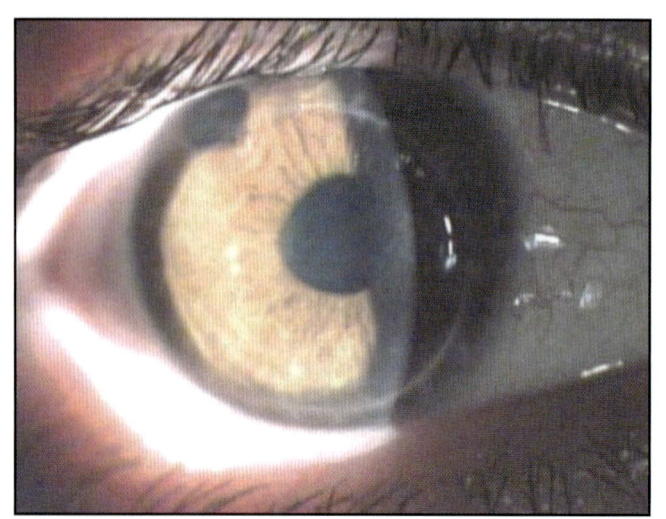

Figure 14-12. Patient R.Z., male, 31 years old. Refraction RE +0.75 sph = -2 cyl (10 degrees). May 2004: improvement of clinic features.

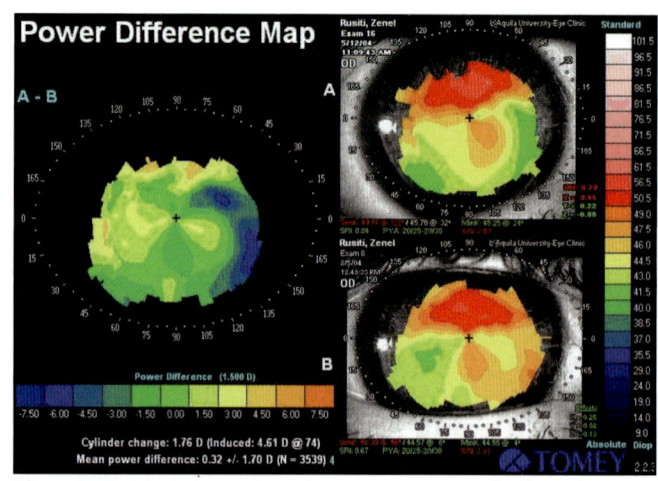

Figure 14-13. Comparison between images before (bottom right) and after (top right), the best corneal transparence permits a gain of 1 Snellen line, obtaining 20/20 of BCVA; differential map (left).

the presence of a high-order astigmatism, we decided to perform LASIK surgery. In both cases, the LASIK procedure was aborted because of the formation of a buttonhole (Figure 14-11). The flap has been carefully replaced, and a soft therapeutic lens has been applied. After transepithelial topo-customized PRK, both patients presented an improvement in both corrected and uncorrected VA.

CASE 1

After LASIK treatment, during which a buttonhole complication occurred, the refraction shown went from -2 sph = -3.5 cyl (180 degrees) to -3.5 sph = -4 cyl (180 degrees). The UCVA changed from 20/67 to 20/100 and the corrected one from 20/20 to 20/30. After the transepithelial customized PRK surgery (Figure 14-12) was performed, the refraction shown was -1 sph = -0.50 cyl (25 degrees), the UCVA was 20/30 and the corrected one was 20/20, and there was an improvement of 4 lines in both the UCVA and BSCVA. The mean of the average central corneal power presurgically was 42.69 D, while after transepithelial customized PRK treatment, it was 41.0 D (Figure 14-13). The presurgical keratometric astigmatism mean was 8.3 D, becoming 2.01 D after surgery.

CASE 2

For some days after LASIK, when a buttonhole occurred, subjective refraction remained unaltered, equal to -1.5 sph = +6 cyl (110 degrees). Neither UCVA nor BSCVA underwent any change, remaining respectively at 20/600 and 20/50. After transepithelial customized PRK surgery, the refraction shown was +0.75 sph = -2 cyl (10 degrees), UCVA was 20/67, and corrected VA was 20/50 with an improvement in UCVA of 3 lines. The mean of the average central corneal power presurgically, was 45.1 D and after transepithelial customized PRK treatment was 46.6 D. Presurgically, the keratometric astigmatism average was 8.4 D, and postsurgically, it was 6.1 D. The customized technique excimer laser PRK with a transepithelial computerized corneal topographer link is a new procedure, not yet completely standardized but that has been employed in our experience to correct refraction defects in the corneal morphological component too.[48,49]

The decision to perform transepithelial ablation is secondary to the consideration that the epithelial bed modifies and covers corneal surface irregularities. However, the risk of performing an ablation that may produce some minor irregularities has to be accepted, since in some points, laser spots characterized by a different ablation rate, work on epithelium, whereas in other points, they work on the stroma.[50,51]

In our experience, the efficiency and safety of customized PTK proves high when seeking to improve an irregular corneal profile caused by several corneal pathologies and postsurgical conditions with irregular astigmatism.

Moreover, with standard PTK, the well-known hyperopic shift is a high price to pay to achieve corneal transparency. Therefore, the main application for this technique is the treatment of myopic eyes, but refractive changes are very unpredictable. Starr has reported an average hyperopic shift of 2.81 D, with 63% of the eyes showing hyperopia of ≥1.0 D and a maximum of 15.75 D.[52]

In our experience, after trans-epithelial customized PRK, the average hyperopic shift was only 1.45 D, with 34.6% of the eyes showing hyperopia of ≥1.0 D and a maximum of 6.0 D.

In conclusion, the topo-customized PRK technique performed transepithelially has produced a range of positive data, but it has some limits too: a lack of direct and sure connection between the topographical map and the ablation center. Moreover, ablation percentage for opaque and pathological corneal tissue differs from that of the normal stromal components, and this may cause irregular and asymmetric ablation.[53,54]

References

1. Spadea L, Bianco G, Balestrazzi E. Four techniques for retreatment after excimer laser photorefractive keratectomy. *J Refract Surg.* 1996; 12:693-696.
2. Alessio G, Boscia F, La Tegola MG. Topography-driver excimer laser for the retreatment of decentralized myopic Photorefractive Keratectomy. *Ophthalmology.* 2001;108(9):1695-1703.
3. Alessio G, Boscia F, La Tegola MG, Sborgia C. Topography-driven photorefractive keratectomy: results of corneal interactive programmed topographic ablation software. *Ophthalmology.* 2000;107 (8):1578-1587.
4. Wygledowska-Promienska D, Zawojska I, Gierek-Ciaciura S. Correction of irregular astigmatism using excimer laser MEL 70 G-SCAN with the TOSCA program introductory report. *Klin Oczna.* 2000;102(6):443-447.
5. Dausch D, Schroder E, Dausch S. Topography-controlled Excimer Laser Photorefractive Keratectomy. *J Refract Surg.* 2000;16(1):13-22.
6. Spadea L, Sabetti L, Balestrazzi E. Effect of centering excimer laser PRK on refractive results: a corneal topography study. *J Refract Corneal Surg.* 1993;9(2):S22-25.
7. Spadea L, Colucci S, Bianco G, Balestrazzi E. Long term results of excimer laser photorefractive keratectomy in high myopia: a preliminary report. *Ophtamic Surgery and Lasers.* 1998;29:490-496.
8. Heitzmann J, Binder PS, Kassar BS, Nordan LT. The correction of high myopia using the excimer laser. *Arch Ophthalmol.* 1993;111:1627-1634.
9. Spadea L, Cantera I, Cantera E, et al. Progressive iatrogenic keratectasia following laser in situ keratomileusis. *IOVS.* 2000;44(4):S464.
10. Chayet AS, Assil KK, Montes M, et al. Regression and its mechanism after laser in situ keratomileusis in moderate and high myopia. *Ophtalmology.* 1998;105:1194-1199.
11. Gimbel HV, Stoll SB. Photorefractive Keratectomy with customized segmental ablation to correct irregular astigmatism after Laser in Situ Keratomileusis. *J Refract Surg.* 2001;17(2):S229-232.
12. Spadea L, Bianco G, Masini MC, Balestrazzi E. Videokeratographic changes after excimer laser in situ keratomileusis for correction of high myopia. *J Cataract Refract Surg.* 1999;25(12):111-120.
13. Spadea L, Bianco G. The corneal endothelium after excimer laser in situ keratomileusis for correction of high myopia. *Ocular Surgery News.* 2001;17:12-27.
14. Balestrazzi E, De Molfetta V, Spadea L, et al. Excimer Laser Photorefractive Keratectomy: histological, immunoistchimical and ultrastructural study on human corneas. *Ital J Ophth.* 1992;VI/2:95-100.
15. Gartry DS, Larkin FP, Hill AR, et al. Retreatment for significant regression after excimer laser photorefractive keratectomy. *Ophthalmology.* 1998;105:131-141.
16. Spadea L, Fasciani R, Necozione S, Balestrazzi E. Role of the corneal epithelium in refractive change following laser in situ keratomileusis for high myopia. *J Refract Surg.* 2000;16:133-139.
17. Chatterej A, Shah S, Bessaut DA, Doyle SJ. Results of excimer laser retreatment of residual myopia after previous photorefractive keratectomy. *Ophthalmology.* 1997;104:1321-1326.
18. Young L, Chen G, Li W, et al. laser in situ keratomileusis enhancement after radial keratotomy. *J Refract Surg.* 2000;16:187-90.
19. Carones F, Vigo L, Carones AV, Brancato R. Evaluation of photorefractive keratectomy retreatments after regressed myopic laser in situ keratomileusis. *Ophthalmology.* 2001;108(10):1732-7.
20. Hahn TW, Sah WJ, Kim JH. Phototherapeutic keratectomy in nine eyes with superficial corneal diseases. *Refract Corneal Surg.* 1993;9 (suppl): S115-S118.
21. Dausch D, Landesz M, Klein R, Schroder E. Phototherapeutic keratectomy in recurrent corneal epithelial erosion. *Refract Corneal Surg.* 1993;9:419-424.
22. O'Brart DPS, Gatry DS, Lohmann CP, et al. Treatment of band keratopathy by excimer laser phototherapeutic keratectomy: surgical techniques and long term follow up. *Br J Ophthalmol.* 1993;77:702-708.
23. Fong YC, Chuck RS, Stark WJ. McDonnel PJ. Phototherapeutic keratectomy for superficial corneal fibrosis after radial keratectomy. *J Cataract Refract Surg.* 2000;26:616-619.
24. Vrabec MP, Anderson JA, Rock ME, et al. Electron microscopic findings in a cornea with recurrence of herpes simplex keratites after excimer laser phototherapeutic keratectomy. *CLAO J.* 1994;20:41.
25. Faschinger CW. Phototherapeutic keratectomy of a corneal scar due to presumed infection after photorefractive keratectomy. *J Cataract Refract Surg.* 2000;26:296-300.
26. Dogru M, Katakami C, Yamanaka A. Refractive changes after excimer laser phototherapeutic keratectomy. *J Cataract Refract Surg.* 2002; 28(2):207-8.
27. Orndahl M, Fagerholm P, Fitzsimmons T, Tengroth B. Treatment of corneal dystrophies with excimer laser. *Acta Ophthalmol.* 1994;72: 235-240.
28. Spadea L, Bianco G, Balestrazzi E. Topographically guided excimer laser photorefractive keratectomy to treat superficial corneal opacities. *Ophthalmology.* 2004;111(3):458-62.
29. Knorz MC, Jendritza B. Topographically guided laser in situ keratomileusis to treat corneal irregularities. *Ophthalmology.* 2000;107: 1138-1143.

30. Alessio G, Boscia F, La Tegola MG, Sborgia C. Corneal interactive programmed topographic ablation customized photorefractive keratectomy for correction of postkeratoplasty astigmatism. *Ophthalmology.* 2001;108(11):2029-2037.
31. Tamayo Fernandez GE, Serrano MG. Early clinical experience using custom Excimer Laser ablations to treat irregular astigmatism. *J Cataract Refract Surg.* 2000;26(10):1442-1450.
32. Daush D, Schroder E, Dausch S. Topography-controlled excimer laser keratectomy. *J Refract Surg.* 2000;16:13-22.
33. Seiler T, Kriegerowski M, Schnoy N, Bende T. Ablation rate of human corneal epithelium and Bowman's layer with the excimer laser (193 nm). *Refract Corneal Surg.* 1990;6:99-102.
34. Dada T, Vajpayee RB. Laser in situ keratomileusis after penetrating keratoplasty. *J Cataract Refract Surg.* 2002;28:7.
35. Lin RT, Maloney RK. Flap complications associated with lamellar refractive surgery. *Am J Ophthalmology.* 1999;127:129-136.
36. Jabbur NS, Myrowitz E, Wexler JL, O'Brien TP. Outcome of second surgery in LASIK cases aborted due to flap complications. *J Cataract Refract Surg.* 2004; 30:993-999.
37. Carones F, Vigo L, Carones AV, Brancato R. Evaluation of photorefractive keratectomy retreatments after regressed myopic laser in situ keratomileusis. *Ophthalmology.* 2001;1732-1737.
38. Gimble H., Penno E, Van Westenbrugge J, et al. Incidence and management of intraoperative and early post operative complication in 1000 consecutive laser in situ keratomileusis cases. *Ophthalmology.* 1998;104:1839-1848.
39. Tham VM, Maloney RK. Microkeratome complications of laser in situ keratomileusis. *Ophtalmology.* 2000;107;920-924.
40. Pallikaris IG, Katsanevaki VJ, Panagopoulou SI. Laser in situ keratomileusis intraoperative complications using one type of microkeratome. *Ophthalmology.* 2002;109:57-63.
41. Koay PYP, McGhee CNJ, Weed KH, Craig JP. Laser in situ keratomileusis for ametropia after penetrating keratoplasty. *J Refract Surg.* 2000;16:140-146.
42. Jason M, Jacobs MD, Michael J, Taravello MD. Incidence of intraoperative flap complications in laser in situ keratomileusis. *J Cataract Refract Surg.* 2002;28:23-28.
43. Leung ATS, Rao SK, Cheng ACK, Yu EWY, Fan DSP, Lam DSC. Pathogenesis and management of laser in situ keratomileusis flap buttonholes. *J Cataract Refract Surg.* 2000;26:358-362.
44. Zadok D, Mascaleris G, Garcia V, et al. Outcomes of retreatment after Laser in Situ Keratomileusis. *Ophthalmology.* 1999;106(12):2391-2394.
45. Güell JL, Lohmann CP, Malecaze FA, et al. Intraepithelial photorefractive keratectomy for regression after laser in situ keratomileusis. *J Cataract Refract Surg.* 1999;25:670-674.
46. Chalita MR, Roth AS, Krueger R. Wavefront-guided surface ablation with prophylactic use of mitomycin C after a buttonhole laser in situ keratomileusis flap. *J Refract Surg.* 2004;20:176-181.
47. Munnerlyn R, Kooms SJ, Marshall J. Photorefractive keratectomy: a technique for laser refractive surgery. *J Cataract Refract Surg.* 1988;14: 46-52.
48. Jain VK, Abell TG, Bond WI, Stevens Jr G. Immediate transepithelial photorefractive keratectomy for treatment of laser in situ keratomileusis flap complications. *J Refracti Surg.* 2002;18:109-112.
49. Hjortdal O, Ehlers N. Treatment of post keratoplasty astigmatism by topography supported customized laser ablation. *Acta Ophthalmology Scand.* 2001; 79:376-380.
50. Knorz MC, Jendritza B. Topographically guided laser in situ keratomileusis to treat corneal irregularities. *Ophthalmology.* 2000;107: 1138-1143.
51. Wilson SE, Mohan RR, Hong JW, Lee JS, Choi R, Mohan RR. The wound healing response after laser in situ keratomileusis and photorefractive keratectomy: elusive control of biological variability and effect on custom laser vision correction. *Arch Ophthamol.* 2001; 119(6):889-896.
52. Starr M, Donnenfeld E, Newton M, Tostanoski J, Muller J, Odrich M. Excimer laser phototherapeutic keratectomy. *Cornea.* 1996;15(6): 557-565.
53. Spadea L, DiGregorio A. Enhancements of retreatment after photorefractive keratectomy and LASIK using topographically guided excimer laser photoablation. *J Cataract Refract Surg* (in press).
54. Spadea L, Di Gregorio A, Balestrazzi E: PRK topo-customizzata transepiteliale negli esiti di button-hole: tecnica e risultati a lungo termine. 84° Congresso Nazionale della Società Oftalmologia Italiana; Roma, 24-27 Novembre 2004..

CHAPTER 15

THE ROLE OF AMINO ACIDS IN CORNEAL HEALING

A NEW METHOD FOR EVALUATING CELLULAR DENSITY AND EXTRACELLULAR MATRIX DISTRIBUTION

Maria Ingrid Torres Munoz, MD; Paolo Vinciguerra, MD;
Fabrizio I. Camesasca, MD; Fabio Grizzi, PhD;
Francesco Saverio Dioguardi, MD; Nicola Dioguardi, MD

Introduction

The corneal wound healing response is of particular relevance for refractive surgical procedures since it is an important determinant of efficacy and safety. A number of common complications are directly related to the healing process. These complications (overcorrection, undercorrection, regression, delayed re-epithelialization, corneal stroma opacification, and many others) have their roots in the biologic response to surgery.[1] The corneal epithelium, stroma, nerves, inflammatory cells, and lacrimal glands (and tear film) are the main tissues and organs involved in the wound healing response to corneal surgical procedures.[2-4] Complex cellular interactions mediated by cytokines, growth factors, chemokines, and their receptors occur among the cells of the cornea, resulting in a highly variable biologic response.[5,6] The process occurs immediately after the initial epithelial injury, caused by microkeratome blade, alcohol exposure, or mechanical scrape. The initial insult results in the release of many cytokines responsible for triggering a variety of responses in keratocytes. Among these processes are keratocyte apoptosis, keratocyte necrosis, keratocyte proliferation, migration of inflammatory cells, and myofibroblast generation.[1,7,8,9-11] These cellular interactions are involved in extracellular matrix reorganization, stromal remodeling, wound contraction, and several other responses to surgical injury.

The tear film appears to coregulate the metabolism of the corneal epithelium through the delivery and removal of epithelial metabolic substance, and the tear film appears to act like a master modulator of many of the events involved in corneal wound healing. Mediators and growth factors produced by the lacrimal glands are important in regulating epithelial healing and epithelial cell differentiation.[3,4,9,12,13] The acqueous layer of the tear film contains the water-soluble contents of the tear film. Seventeen amino acids have been isolated from human tears, either in mg/mL or traces[14] (Table 15-1). The tear film has an amino acid concentration of 7.5 mg/100 ml, three to four times higher than the serum concentration. Despite this quantitative difference, serum and tear film are qualitatively identical in terms of types of detectable amino acids. Serum and tear concentrations of amino acids are directly related. A decrease of serum amino acids leads to a similar decrease in tears, and vice versa.

Re-epithelialization is an energy-consuming, substrate-demanding process. Cellular division and extracellular matrix synthesis require intense protein synthesis. Corneal epithelium synthesizes protein and glycoprotein at a faster rate during corneal epithelial wound healing.[15] Re-epithelialization is possible and qualitatively optimal only if amino acids are available in the substrate in the adequate amounts and correct composition.

Effects of Amino Acids in Corneal Healing

EFFECTS ON THE CORNEAL EPITHELIUM

Studies conducted *in vitro* on eye bank eyes as well as *in vivo* suggest that re-epithelialization improves when an increase of serum and tear film amino acids is obtained.[16,17]

Eye Bank Cornea Study

A study was conduced on human eye bank corneas where epithelium had been removed. The corneas were kept for 7 days in standard storage medium, either simple or enriched with amino acids. After 3 days of incubation, all de-epithelialized human eye bank corneas showed complete re-epithelialization,

Table 15-1. Amino Acids in Human Reflex Tears

Glycine
Alanine
Glutamine
Asparagine
Serine
Threonine
Argirine
Leucne and isoleucine
Lysine
Valine
Taurine
a-Aminobutiric acid
Histadine
Phenylalanine
Proline
Tyrosine

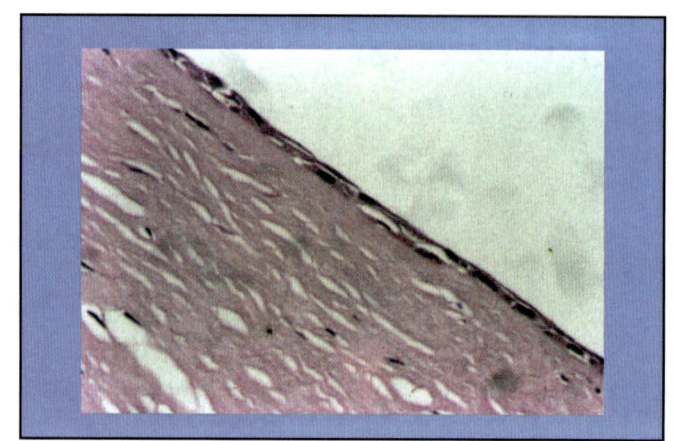

Figure 15-1. Human eye bank cornea with epithelium removed, after 2 days in standard storage medium.

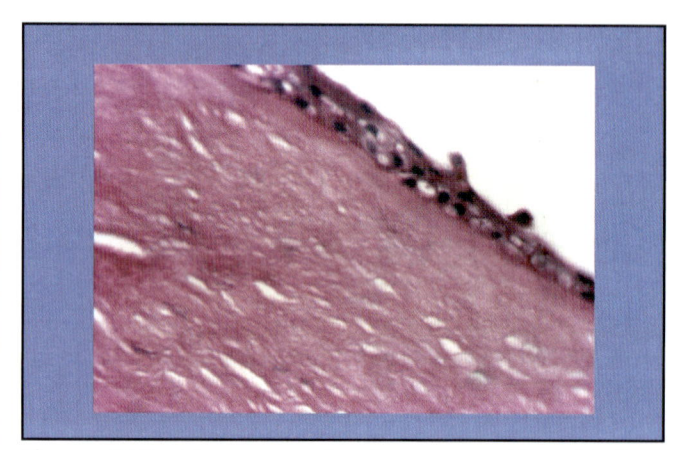

Figure 15-3. Human eye bank cornea with epithelium removed, after 7 days in standard storage medium.

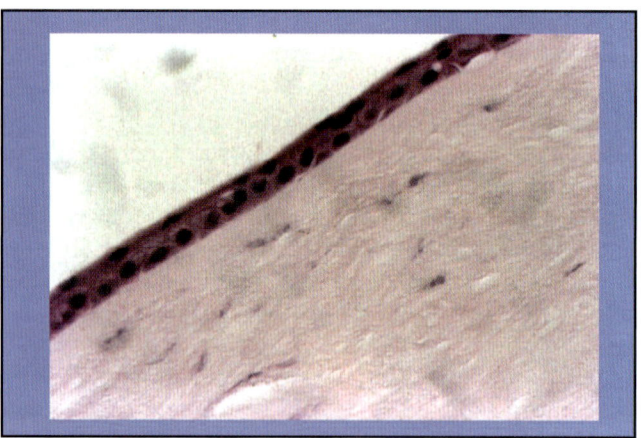

Figure 15-2. Human eye bank cornea with epithelium removed, after 2 days in standard storage medium plus amino acids.

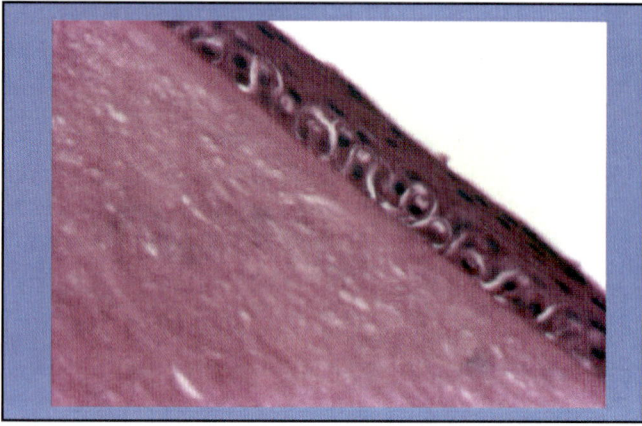

Figure 15-4. Human eye bank cornea with epithelium removed, after 7 days in standard storage medium plus amino acids.

but those incubated with amino acids had thicker and better organized epithelium. After 7 days of exposure to supplements with amino acids, the corneas still had much thicker and better organized epithelium when compared to corneas incubated in the simple standard storage media[16] (Figures 15-1 through 15-4).

In Vivo Studies

Clinical studies conducted in patients with chronic corneal ulcers resistant to usual treatment and patients subjected to refractive surgery (PRK) who had delayed re-epithelialization after PRK in the first eye have shown that an increased amino acid concentration in serum and the tear film, obtained through oral supplementing (Table 15-2), improves re-epithelialization.[16]

An extensive medical history was taken after delayed re-epithelialization was noted in the first eye, and the patients were taking drugs to suppress appetite or reduce intestinal adsorption for dieting purpose. This dysfunctional food intake situation may have reduced serum and tear film amino acids concentrations, thus delaying the corneal re-epithelialization process. Obtaining information about dietary habits as part of the preoperative evaluation for refractive surgery appears to be highly indicated.

The results of these studies show that supplementing epithelial cells and keratocytes with amino acids, either *in vitro* or *in vivo*, increases their duplication rate and the speed with

Table 15-2. COMPOSITION OF AMINO ACIDS ADMINISTERED

Dosage: 4.8 g 3 times daily

Amino Acid	Amount
L-Glycine	1000 mg
L-Cystine	79.7 mg
L-Histidine	79.9 mg
L-Phenylalanine	53.1 mg
L-Methionine	26.6 mg
L-Tyrosine	15.9 mg
L-Tryptophan	10.6 mg
L-Threonine	185 mg
L-Proline	875 mg
L-Leucine	664 mg
L-Lysin	345 mg
L-Isoleucine	332 mg
L-Valine	332 mg

which the normal corneal surface is restored. The *in vitro* study showed a plateau effect with progressive addition of amino acids: the effect on their growth reaches a maximum and then stabilizes. An excess of the amino acids substrate does not lead to hypertrophy, hyperplasia, or metaplasia of the newly deposed tissue.[16]

EFFECTS ON THE CORNEAL STROMA

The extracellular matrix serves as a structural support for the corneal stroma and mediates signaling events that regulate the intracellular environment of stromal keratocytes. Keratocytes remodel disordered collagen that is produced by activated keratocytes during the wound healing process.[18] Thus, they play a key role in the repair response after refractive surgery, determining the refractive results in term of hypo- or hypercorrections, regression, residual optical aberrations, or new treatment-related aberrations. During the healing process, keratocyte proliferation and collagen synthesis took place, and the keratocytes showed a higher amino acid incorporation.[19] A corneal injury mediates signal transduction events causing the phosphorylation of tyrosine residues of specific adhesion proteins and that phosphorilation is required for cellular adhesion and migration.[20] An amino acid and protein substrate is necessary for the healing process of corneal stroma.

Studies conducted in vitro on eye bank eyes showed that progressively increasing amino acid supplements led to an increase in the percentage of fibroblasts.[16] Amino acid supplementing may modify the behavior of both stroma keratocytes and of other stroma components and induce an increase in keratocyte density as well as changes in intercellular matrix structure and cell distribution pattern.[21]

To measure the changes in stroma keratocytes and intercellular matrix in patients on an oral amino acid treatment, an innovative method has been used for evaluating the complexity of the stromal structure. A brief description of this method is provided below (for a more detailed description, see Chapter 37).

A New Method for Measuring the Stroma Structure

To evaluate the differences and changes in stroma structure, patients were examined with the confocal microscopy technique, which records images of cornea scans providing *in vivo* views of cornea cross sections with resolution levels comparable to histological sections. So far, studies to measure stroma keratocyte density through confocal microscopy have been based on the manual count of keratocytes on some of the scans performed.[22,23] This gives a keratocyte density value expressed as number of cells per cubic millimeter, obtained using an extremely subjective method. In fact, the process of calculating stroma keratocyte density is far from easy, as it is not done on a clear-cut monomolecular film, like the cornea endothelium.

The corneal stroma is a highly complex biological system. Stroma keratocytes, as observed through the confocal microscope, appear as cells with dimly defined contours, arranged on a number of cell layers according to a precise pattern and surrounded by an intercellular matrix having its own characteristics. In order to formulate a correct evaluation of the corneal structure, we must consider all of these factors. Indeed, the main problem we had to address during this study was how to measure the corneal structure objectively.

On the basis of these criteria, we used a calculation strategy based on the application of mathematics to the study of complex biological systems through the calculation of fractal dimensions. Fractal geometry makes it possible to measure highly complex structures such as corneal stroma, taking into account not only cellular density but also all the other factors composing the stroma. The high level of complexity of tissues studied, and the accuracy with which they are measured suggested the idea of applying this methodology to the study of the cornea. Moreover, we used this measurement method on histological specimens of human corneas in order to compare calculated values against those obtained using Confoscan corneal scans.

The application of this method involves a series of steps described as follows:

* The first stage is the acquisition of stroma images through confocal microscopy. The scan was performed using Confoscan 3.0 (NIDEK, Irvine, Calif). Three hundred fify images were taken for each patient, with scans every 12 µm (Figure 15-5).

* Computer-assisted image analysis system: the second stage is the digitizing and processing of stroma images. Using the computer, each image was transformed into a two-dimensional image composed of a set of pixels; this process highlights image diversity and enables us to quantify the light intensity of each pixel according to a grey scale (Figure 15-6).

146　Chapter 15

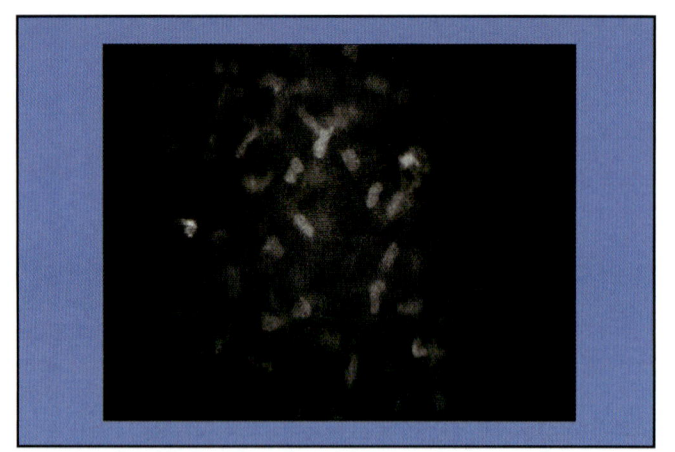

Figure 15-5. Acquisition of stroma images through confocal microscopy; 350 images were taken from each point. The interval between two images was 12 µm.

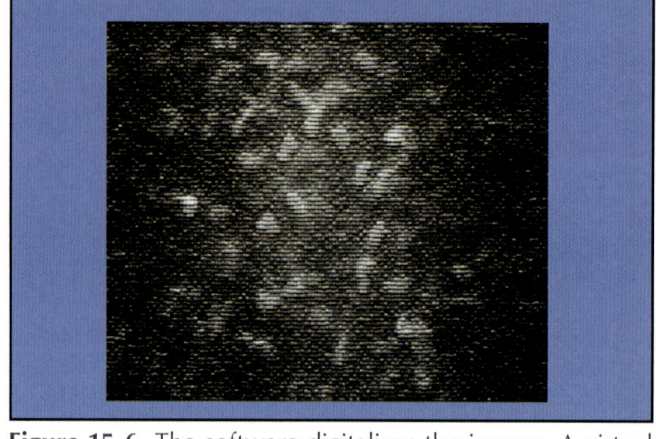

Figure 15-6. The software digitalizes the images. A virtual image is obtained where light intensity can be quantified for each pixel.

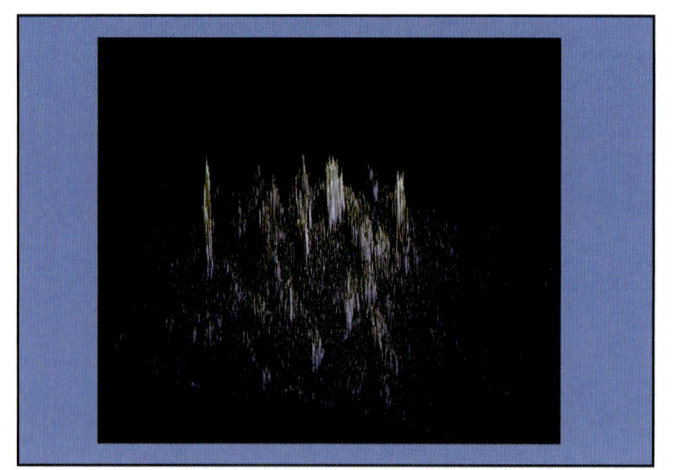

Figure 15-7. Light intensity values transformed into peaks to obtain a pseudo three-dimensional image; each peak represents a pixel.

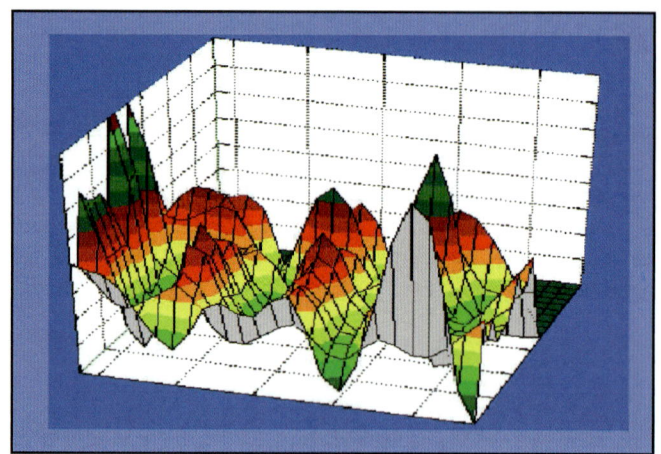

Figure 15-8. Fractal surface dimension, processing of the fractal surface from a stroma scan.

* In the third stage, a peak value is attributed to each pixel, according to its light intensity value on the grey scale. Thus, we obtain a pseudo three-dimensional image resulting from the processing of the stroma confocal scan. This image has been called stroma subunit (Figure 15-7).
* In the final stage, the stroma subunit is measured through the fractal dimension calculation. The fractal calculation system measures the size of the stroma subunit (ie, the space occupied by this structure) through a mathematical formula whose result is the index representing the stromal fractal dimension (fractal surface dimension).

$$D = \lim_{\varepsilon \to 0} \frac{Log N(\varepsilon)}{Log(1/\varepsilon)}$$

This measurement system is able to calculate an index for each stroma scan (stroma subunit) obtained with confocal microscopy. The significant advantage offered by this measurement system is the possibility to quantify corneal stroma complexity with a single numeric value obtained in an objective manner through the computer.

The index obtained is a numeric value indicated with the letter D, fractal surface dimension. This value is a fractional number comprised between 2 and 3, and depends directly on three factors: keratocyte density, intercellular matrix structure, and cell distribution pattern (Figure 15-8). Each stroma image of each patient was computer processed as described above, and a fractal dimension index D was calculated (Figure 15-9). Currently, we are not able to determine to what extent each of these factors contributes to the D index value. The formulation of a three-dimensional model based on each patient's cornea scans will enable us to calculate the number of cells forming the stroma and provide us with a quite accurate knowledge of their distribution and intercellular matrix structure.

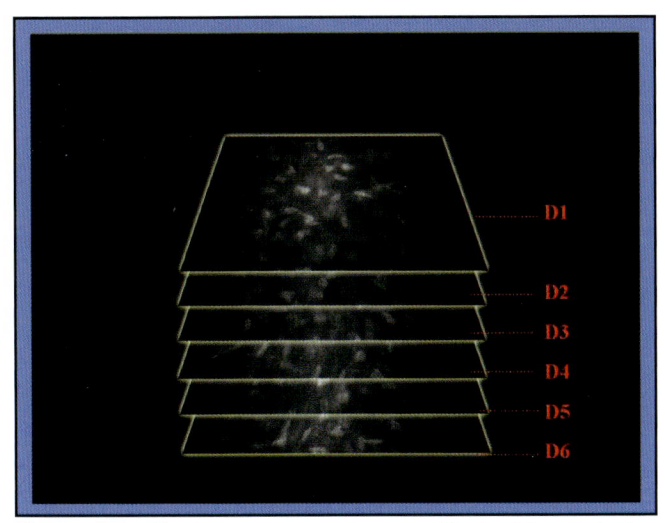

Figure 15-9. Each stroma scan is quantified with a D index (fractal surface dimension).

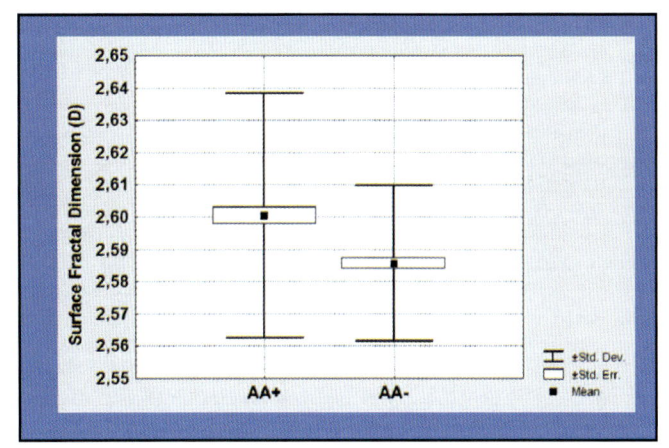

Figure 15-10. Group 1 (AA+) has a mean surface fractal dimension (D) value significantly higher than Group 2 (AA-). The D values of Group 1 (AA+) have a higher SD than Group 2 (AA-), indicating a variable response to AA treatment.

A further advantage is the introduction of a simulation program; thanks to this program, it is possible to modify several parameters (eg, stroma hydration conditions or the percentage of collagen tissue existing in the intercellular matrix) and to view D index (fractal surface dimension) variations as a result of changes in these parameters. This calculation system has already been validated for the study of pulmonary fibrosis and liver cirrhosis, for bone tissue structure evaluation, and for the morpho-structural study of precancerous and cancerous breast lesions.[24-28]

Significance of the D Index, Fractal Surface Dimension, Applied to Corneal Stroma Measurement

Clinical results of this study indicate that an oral supplement with amino acids may change the corneal stroma structure increasing keratocytes density and modifying the intercellular matrix. Using this new method for the measurement of these changes, providing quantification of the stromal structure complexity with a single numerical value, showed that the group of patients treated with amino acids had higher keratocyte density values than the group untreated with amino acids (control patients) and observed differences in cell distribution patterns and intercellular matrix structures of the two study groups.

The difference between groups proved to be statistically significant. In terms of percentage, it translates in a difference of 10% between the two groups, which means that the patients treated with amino acids have a corneal stroma with a D index value 10% higher than patients not treated with amino acids[21] (Figure 15-10).

Conclusions

Most advances in refractive surgery are currently aimed at improving the quality of refractive treatments by reducing optical aberrations or at least by avoiding the creation of new aberrations. This is undoubtedly the right direction to pursue in order to achieve visual excellence as a result of our procedures. Any medication capable of modulating the repair response to restore corneal physiology may help greatly in this direction, and clinical research should pay special attention to these adjuvant drugs.

References

1. Netto MV, Mohan RR, Ambrosio R Jr, Hutcheon AE, Zieske JD, Wilson SE. Wound healing in the cornea: a review of refractive surgery complications and new prospects for therapy. *Cornea.* 2005;24(5):509-522.
2. Wilson SE, Netto M, Ambrosio Jr R. Corneal cells: chatty in development, homeostasis, wound healing, and disease. *Am J Ophthalmol.* 2003:136;136:530-536.
3. Tervo T, Vesakuoma M, Bennett GL, et al. Tear hepatocyte growth factor (HGF) availability increases markedly after excimer laser surface ablation. *Exp Eye Res.* 1997;64:501-504
4. Wilson SE, Liang Q, Kim W-J. Lacrimal gland HDF, KGF, and EGF mRNA levels increase after corneal epithelial wounding. *Invest Ophthalmol Vis Sci.* 1999;40:2185-2190.
5. Wilson SE, Liu JJ. Stromal epithelial interactions in the cornea. *Prog Retin Eye Res.* 1999;18:293-309.
6. Carrington LM, Boulton M. Hepatocyte growth factor and keratincyte growth factor regulation of epithelial and stromal wound healing. *J Cataract Refract Surg.* 2005;31(2):412-423.
7. Kuo TC. Corneal wound healing. *Curr Opin Ophthalmol.* 2004;15(4): 311-315.
8. Netto M, Wilson SE. Corneal wound healing relevance to wavefront guided laser treatments. *Ophthalmol Clin North Am.* 2004;17(2): 225-31,vii.

9. Mohan RR, Ambrosio R Jr, Zieske JD, Wilson SE. Apoptosis, necrosis, proliferation, and myofibroblast generation in the stroma following LASIK and PRK. *Exp Eye Res.* 2003;76(1):71-87.
10. Wilson SE. Analysis of the keratocyte apoptosis, keratocyte proliferation, and myofibroblast transformation responses after photorefractive and laser in situ keratomileusis. *Trans Am Ophthalmol Soc.* 2002; 100:411-433
11. Szentmary N, Nagy ZZ, Resch M, Szende B, Suveges I. Proliferation and apoptosis in the corneal stroma in longterm follow-up after photorefractive keratectomy. *Pathol Res Pract.* 2005;201(5):399-404.
12. O'Brien T, Li Q, Ashraf MF, Matteson DM, Stark WJ, Chang CC. Inflammatory response in the early stages of wound healing after excimer laser keratectomy. *Arch Ophthalmol.* 1998;116:1470-1474.
13. Ambròsio R Jr, Kalia R, Mohan RR, et al. *Early Wound Healing Response to Epithelial Scrape Injury in the Human Cornea.* Abstract #4206. ARVO 2002.
14. Flachmeyer R, Wiechert P. Die Freien Amino-sauren in demenschen Tranenflussigkeit. *Graefes Arch Clin Ex Ophthalmol.* 1963;165:516.
15. Zieske JD, Gipson IK. Protein synthesis during corneal epithelial wound healing. *Invest Ophthalmol Vis Sci.* 1986; 27(1): 1-7.
16. Vinciguerra P, Camesasca FI, Ponzin D. Use of amino acids in refractive surgery. *J Refract Surg.* 2002; (suppl)18.
17. Rivaud C, Negrel AD. Monobloc Lamellar autokeratoplasty (MLAK) and Corneal Cicatrization. A propos of a comparative trial in a control group and a group treated with a L-cystine and pyridoxine hydrochloride combination. *J Fr Ophthalmol.* 1987;10 (1):35-40.
18. Kim W-J, Helena MC, Mohan RR, Wilson SE. Changes in Corneal Morphology Associated with Chronic Epithelial Injury. *Invest Ophtalmol Vis Sci.* 1999;40:35-42.
19. Katakami C, Sahori A, Kazusa R, Yamamoto M. Keratocyte Activity in Wound Healing after Epikeratophakia in rabbits. *Invest Ophtkalmol Vis Sci.* 1991;32(6):1837-1845.
20. Haq F, Trinkaus-Randall V. Injury of stromal fibroblasts induces phosphorylation of focal adhesion proteins. *Curr Eye Res.* 1998;17(5):512-523.
21. Torres Munoz I, Grizzi F, Russo C, Camesasca FI, Dioguardi N, Vinciguerra. the role of amino acids in corneal stromal healing. a new method for evaluating cellular density and extracellular matrix distribution. *J Refract Surg.* 2003;19(2 Suppl):S227-30. Erratum in : *J Refract Surg.* 2003;19(3):288.
22. Mitooka K, Ramirez M, Maguire LJ, et al. Keratocyte density of central human cornea after in situ keratomileusis. *Am J Ophthalmol.* 2002; 307-314,133.
23. Mc LarenJW, Nau CB, Kitzmann AS, Bourne WM. Keratocyte density: comparison of two confocal microscopes. *Eye Contact Lens.* 2005; 31(1):28-33.
24. Dioguardi N, Grizzi F, Bossi P, Roncalli M. Spectral dimension to quantify liver fibrosis in needle biopsy specimens. *Analytical and Quantitative Cytology and Histology.* 1999;21:262-266.
25. Grizzi F, Dioguardi N. A fractal scoring system for quantifying active collagen synthesis during chronic liver disease. *International Journal of Chaos Theory and Applications.* 1999;4:2-3,39-44.
26. Dioguardi N, Grizzi F. Fractal dimension exponent for quantitative evaluation of liver collagen in bioptic specimens. In: *Mathematics and Biosciences in Interaction.* Boston, Mass: Birkhauser Press; 2001.
27. Grizzi F, Colombo P, Barbieri B, et al. Correspondence. E. Sabo et al., Microscopic analysis and significance of vascular architectural complexity in renal cell carcinoma. *Clin Canc Res.* 2001;7(10): 3305-3307.
28. Grizzi F, Muzzio PC, Di Maggio A, Dioguardi N. Geometrical analysis of benign and malignant breast lesions. *Radiol Med (Torino).* 2001; 101(6):432-435.

SECTION IV

The Evolution of Surface Ablation: LASEK, Epi-LASIK, and Custom Ablation

CHAPTER 16

LASEK

Thomas V. Claringbold II, DO; Lee Shahinian Jr, MD

Introduction

In laser assisted sub-epithelial keratectomy (LASEK), excimer laser stromal ablation is performed under a hinged flap of corneal epithelium. No microkeratome is used, and no stromal lamellar cut is made. In this chapter, we first summarize the history of LASEK and the rationale for LASEK. We then discuss preoperative evaluation and preparation, the standard surgical technique, postoperative management, pain management, potential complications, postoperative haze, and clinical results. In the Appendices you will find a sample LASEK consent form, information on LASEK instrumentation and a recipe for the preparation of autologous serum eye drops.

History

LASEK was first described in print by Dr. Massimo Camellin of Rovigo, Italy. Dr. Camellin's LASEK acronym (for "laser epithelial keratomileusis") has become widely adopted. However, many surgeons, including the authors, now use "laser assisted sub-epithelial keratectomy" to more accurately describe the LASEK procedure.

In March 1999, Dr. Sunil Shah of Birmingham, England presented his technique and 6-month data for PRK with an epithelial flap at a meeting of the British Society of Refractive Surgery. His technique was essentially the same as that described by Dr. Camellin. In this study, subsequently published in the *British Journal of Ophthalmology*,[2] 36 patients had traditional PRK on one eye and PRK with epithelial flap on the other eye, with 1-year follow-up. Less corneal haze was seen in the epithelial flap eyes.

Since the pioneering work of Camellin and Shah, many refractive surgeons have adopted LASEK. However, few surgeons perform this procedure exclusively, and LASEK still accounts for a relatively small percentage of all laser vision correction surgery. Two main factors account for this lack of wider acceptance. First, LASEK cannot match LASIK for postoperative comfort and rapid vision recovery. Second, some surgeons are not convinced that clinical results are any better with LASEK than with PRK.

Rationale for LASEK

Any examination of the rationale for LASEK must compare this procedure with LASIK and PRK.

As noted by the authors,[3,4] LASEK is a safer procedure than LASIK because all stromal flap complications are eliminated. LASIK complications related to the stromal flap include buttonhole,[5,6] thick flap making full laser treatment impossible,[7] decentered flap, incomplete flap,[8] free cap, corneal perforation,[9] optic atrophy,[10] glaucomatous field loss,[11,12] poor flap adherence,[13] poor epithelial adherence,[14,15] striae,[16] epithelial ingrowth,[17,18] flap melt,[19] diffuse lamellar keratitis (DLK),[20] secondary DLK,[21,22] interface infections,[23,24] interface blood or debris, and late traumatic flap dislocation.[25-31] By eliminating these problems and greatly reducing the incidence of corneal ectasia,[32-36] LASEK significantly improves the risk/benefit ratio of refractive surgery.

Furthermore, LASEK can be performed in some cases where LASIK may be contraindicated, as in patients with thin, steep, or flat corneas; anterior basement membrane dystrophy; large pupils; high myopia; deep-set eyes or tight orbits; glaucoma; filtering bleb; scleral buckle; previous vitrectomy; and optic nerve drusen. LASEK may also be a safer procedure than LASIK with activities (eg, public safety, contact sports, machining) that increase the likelihood of eye trauma postoperatively.

Thus, while both LASIK and LASEK give excellent vision results in most patients, LASEK is emerging as a safer procedure with broader indications than LASIK. While LASIK remains the more popular procedure, the authors suspect that many patients do not adequately understand the risks of LASIK. Today there is an irrational exuberance for LASIK. It is worth remembering that stromal flap complications occur in approximately 4% of eyes.[37] Whenever safety issues are down-played or ignored, there is a risk that when a change in attitude finally occurs, it may be sudden and wrenching, with significant financial and professional liability implications.

Comparing LASEK and PRK, considerable laboratory and clinical evidence suggests that less postoperative haze is seen with LASEK than with PRK. It has been known for almost 40 years that stromal keratocytes disappear after corneal abrasion.[38] Wilson and coworkers[39] suggested that these stromal changes are caused by cytokines released by the injured epithelium. An alternative mechanism was proposed by Zhao, Nagasaki, and Maurice.[40] They demonstrated that merely exposing the bare stroma to normal tears caused a loss of stromal keratocytes. Either hypothesis suggests a protective role for a layer of epithelium/basal lamina overlying the ablated stroma postoperatively as a tissue bandage.

The need to apply less laser treatment for LASEK than for PRK to achieve the same correction indicates a decreased stromal healing response in LASEK compared with PRK.

Choi et al[41] found that the application of amniotic membrane after PRK reduces keratocyte proliferation and corneal haze in a rabbit model, possibly by reducing the infiltration of inflammatory cells and loss of keratocytes in the ablation area during the early postoperative period.

Confocal microscopy has been used to study and compare the healing responses of PRK[42] and LASIK[43] and might be a method to study the tissue-bandage effect of the epithelial flap in LASEK.

As for clinical studies, Lee et al[44] found less corneal haze in LASEK eyes than PRK eyes ($p = 0.02$), although the follow-up was only 3 months.

Shah et al[2] found significantly less haze in LASEK eyes compared with PRK eyes in 36 patients who were followed for a year after PRK on one eye and LASEK on the fellow eye.

In a prospective study, Autrata and Rehurek[45] compared PRK in one eye with LASEK in the fellow eye of 92 myopic patients. They found significantly less haze in the LASEK eyes at 1, 3, 6, 12, and 24 months postoperative. In a subsequent study,[46] the same authors compared PRK and LASEK in a hyperopic population. Again they found significantly less postoperative corneal haze in the LASEK eyes over 2 years.

Astle, Huang, and coauthors[47] found less postoperative haze in a pediatric LASEK population than they had previously experienced with PRK.

While visually significant postoperative haze has been reported with both PRK and LASEK, the authors have the clinical impression[3,4] that less haze is seen with LASEK, and the routine use of MMC can be avoided.

Preoperative Evaluation and Preparation

The patient's motives for LASEK should be carefully noted. It is important that patients have realistic expectations and a mature understanding of the potential risks and benefits of this elective procedure. Laser vision correction should be presented as a method to reduce rather than to eliminate the patient's dependence on glasses and contact lenses.

Preoperative evaluation should include general medical and eye history, contact lens history, corrected and uncorrected visual acuity, keratometry, corneal topography, photopic and scotopic pupil measurements, manifest and cycloplegic refractions, external eye and slit lamp examination, intraocular pressures, Schirmer tear test, corneal pachymetry, and dilated fundus examination.

LASEK should not be performed on persons:
* With herpes eye infection
* With severely dry eyes
* With excessive corneal scarring or keloid formation
* With ectatic corneal dystrophies
* With autoimmune disease, rheumatoid arthritis, or systemic lupus erythematosis
* With uncontrolled diabetes
* Taking Accutane (Roche Laboratories, Nutley, NJ) or amiodarone (Cordarone [Collegeville, Pa])
* Who are pregnant or are nursing, or who expect to become pregnant within 6 months following the LASEK procedure
* Who are not available for postoperative care or who have unrealistic expectations or a poor understanding of the procedure and its risks

There may be additional contraindications.

Soft contact lenses should be discontinued 1 week before the examination. Toric soft lenses and hard contact lenses should be discontinued 3 weeks before the examination. For the latter group, serial refractions should be performed every 2 weeks until stable.

Although the patient should be given a detailed written consent (see Appendix A), that information accompanies but does not replace the surgeon's discussions with the patient before and after LASEK. Also, American surgeons should explain to their patients that LASEK is an off-label use of the excimer laser.

Makeup and perfume should be avoided on the day of surgery. Patients with rosacea facial changes should be started on doxycycline 100 mg BID 1 week preoperatively, continuing until there is good remodeling of the epithelial surface postoperatively. Surgeons can follow their usual regimen for preoperative sedation.

Standard Surgical Technique

PREPARATION OF THE 20% ALCOHOL SOLUTION

1. Glass ampoule of dehydrated 98% ethyl alcohol injection, USP 1.0 cc. Available from: Priority Healthcare.
2. Sterile water for injection, preservative-free (or balanced salt solution [BSS]) 4.0 cc.
3. Mix the alcohol and water in a syringe. Pass the resulting 19.6% alcohol solution through a 0.2-µm filter into a 10-cc sterile multidose vial. Store refrigerated.
4. Draw up 0.4 cc of the dilute alcohol solution in a tuberculin syringe, remove needle, push 0.1 cc through cannula to clear any autoclave moisture and avoid further dilution.

LASEK NOMOGRAMS

Camellin/Shahinian: VISX (Plus Cylinder Format) and NIDEK (Minus Cylinder Format)

≤8 D: 10% to 15% off sphere (spectacle plane)
8 to 10 D: 15% off sphere
≥10 D: 20% off sphere
Cylinder: VISX: treat full cylinder
NIDEK: Increase by 25% and further decrease absolute value of sphere by 40% of cylinder
Hyperopia: VISX: Decrease sphere by 20% to 30%

Claringbold: VISX (Plus Cylinder Format)

Step One:
Determine refraction at corneal plane (ie, similar to fitting contacts):
* For refractions less than -4.75 D, use manifest refraction
* For refractions greater than -4.75 D: With the patient still in the phoropter, the vertex distance to the corneal surface is measured using the phoropter side mirrors. Using a distometer wheel (House of Vision Inc., Chicago, Illinois), the patient's refraction at the corneal plane is determined.

Step Two:
For patients <40 years of age, an additional 0.25 D is subtracted from the value determined in Step 1. For patients >40, an additional 0.5 D is subtracted from the value determined in Step 1. This value is used for the spherical correction.

Step Three:
Cylindrical correction is treated for 100% of the value. (*All treatments performed in PLUS cylinder). **Leave VISX default vertex at 12.5 mm **

These nomograms are general guidelines, and must be customized based on the individual surgeon's equipment, location, environment (especially operating suite temperature and humidity), and experience.

LASEK INSTRUMENTS

See Appendix B.

LASEK PROCEDURE STEPS, INCLUDING SPECIFIC PEARLS BASED ON OUR EXPERIENCE

1. Proparacaine 0.5% every 5 min x 5. The multiple doses are important to loosen the epithelium. Topical antibiotic. Oral sedation prn.
2. Betadine prep, 3M Tegaderm drape (1624W), lid speculum.
3. Drip ice-cold BSS onto the cornea, 50 drops.
4. Trephine the epithelium, centered on the pupil. Use 8.0 or 9.0 mm, 270-degree dull trephine. Moderate downward pressure is applied to score the corneal epithelium. The trephine can also be slightly rotated. Because the blade extends only 270 degrees, a hinge is created at 12:00.
5. Center the alcohol cone (9.0 or 10.0 mm) on the trephine mark, pressing down gently with uniform pressure to create a good seal.
6. Fill cone with 20% alcohol solution (approx. 0.1 cc) for 30 to 40 seconds. Timing may be altered, depending on the patient (slightly longer for younger patients and contact lens wearers) and experience with the fellow eye. During the period of alcohol application, continuously observe the light reflex on the alcohol surface. Any movement of the light reflex indicates that a leak is occurring.
7. Remove alcohol from cone with Merocel sponge, allowing the alcohol solution to come up to the sponge rather than touching the delicate epithelium. Rinse cornea and conjunctiva with BSS.
8. Dry the peripheral cornea with a Merocel sponge to reveal the trephine mark.
9. Starting at 6:00, create the edges of the epithelial flap with the microhoe, pressing down; Bowman's membrane will not be damaged. Use short chopping strokes inferiorly, like a garden hoe. Use a sliding action temporally and laterally, like a capsulorrhexis. Reapply well and alcohol for 10 seconds if flap edge is adherent.
10. Elevate the epithelial flap with the epithelial detaching spatula ("hockey stick" spatula) or bow dissector. It is important to press DOWN as you advance the spatula or dissector, to avoid separating the epithelium from its basement membrane. The flap will lift more easily if there is a narrower front to work with, that is, if the flap is brought in from the sides as you advance it from 6:00

toward 12:00. When using the bow dissector, STOP if the epithelium begins to move, as this indicates the epithelium is separating from its basement membrane. Do not continue with the bow dissector unless the basement membrane detaches easily from the underlying Bowman's. Care should be taken not to advance the dissection beyond the hinge. The epithelial flap is gathered on its hinge at 12 o'clock, exposing a glassy-smooth Bowman's membrane.

11. Sweep Bowman's with the same spatula to remove any epithelial debris or excess moisture.

12. Apply laser according to your nomogram. Note: the bed (eg, Bowman's) is smoother than the usual bed seen after a LASIK microkeratome incision. Care should be taken to assure the focal plane is indeed at the stromal surface.

13. Immediately drip chilled BSS onto the cornea, about 10 drops for every diopter of treatment. Do not dry the cornea.

14. Replace the epithelial flap with the smooth epithelial replacement spatula. Unlike traditional LASIK, flap alignment is **not** critical. The flap usually overlaps the edges of its bed, but that is OK.

15. Apply a bandage soft contact lens (the authors' preference is the Bausch & Lomb Soflens 66, F/M).

16. Instill antibiotic and NSAID drops. Apply eye shield.

Postoperative Management

Patients use antibiotic eye drops QID until the epithelium is healed. Fluorometholone is also started QID immediately postoperatively, continued for 1 month, and then selectively tapered. In one practice (TC), the fluorometholone is tapered beginning at postoperative day 14 in mild to moderate myopes (< -5.0 D). A shield should be worn at night until the epithelium is healed and the bandage soft lens is removed, typically on postoperative day 4. Eye cosmetics, strenuous exercise, gardening, and dusty environments should be avoided for 1 week after the procedure, and swimming should be avoided for 2 weeks.

The eye is examined the first day after LASEK. The central epithelial defect usually closes by day 4, although occasionally epithelial healing is delayed. Best visual acuity follows remodeling of the healed epithelial surface. Vision is often worse on days 2 to 3 than on day 1 but returns to approximately 20/20 to 20/30 by 7 to 10 days. Vision usually stabilizes within 1 month.

Initial overcorrections are common with LASEK. Refract all patients at 1 month. For low to moderate myopia, stop the steroid drops if there is overcorrection >0.5 D. For high myopia, stop the steroids if there is overcorrection >1.0 D and recheck in 1 to 2 weeks. If overcorrection persists, consider inserting an 8.4/14.0 soft contact lens to induce regression. If refraction is near plano, restart the steroids, tapering 1 drop per day per month over 3 months. This regimen should be taken as a general guideline to postoperative steroid use, to be adjusted according to the individual surgeon's experience.

Pain Management

It is important that patients understand that some pain occurs in the first 24 to 72 hours after LASEK. Specific preoperative, intraoperative, and postoperative steps can be taken to minimize or eliminate the pain associated with LASEK.

Preoperative counseling of patients is a very important, if not *the most* important, step. One must be proactive in discussing the likelihood of postoperative pain with the patient. LASIK and LASEK patients will compare notes, and LASEK patients must have a clear understanding of what to expect postoperatively. Here is an example of what one might say to the patient preoperatively:

"You will likely have some discomfort for a day or 2 after your laser procedure. That's one of the downsides of LASEK. Let me tell you about some specific steps we are going to take to manage any discomfort you might have, because there are some distinct advantages to LASEK and that's why we are choosing this procedure."

Preoperative medications include diazepam 5 to 10 mg sublingually 30 to 60 minutes before the procedure. While a single dose of topical anesthetic (proparacaine or tetracaine 0.5%) is usually adequate for anesthesia, multiple doses help loosen the corneal epithelium, making it easier to elevate during surgery. This is in distinct contrast to LASIK, where minimal preoperative medication is used to protect the epithelium. Therefore, for LASEK, we typically apply a drop of topical anesthetic every 5 minutes times 5 with an additional drop when starting the procedure.

Proper contact lens selection can minimize postoperative discomfort. Tight-fitting lenses should be avoided. Dr. Durrie[47] has demonstrated better results with low-water, nonionic soft lenses. Our lens of choice is the Bausch and Lomb Soflens 66 (Rochester, NY), F/M (flat medium base curve). This lens does not come in plano power, so we usually select a -0.5 D lens. It is thin, fits flattened corneas well, and is easy to handle during insertion; in addition, it is flexible (so it does not pop out during healing). Alternative lenses include the CIBA Night and Day silicone hydrogel lens (Duluth, Ga) and the Biomedics 55 ocufilcon D lens (BC 8.9) (CooperVision, Fairport, NY).

After surgery, let patients know the surgeon is on their team 100%. We give each patient our pager, cell, and home phone numbers and encourage them to reach us directly at any time with questions or concerns. We do not want a patient in pain to have to go through an answering service or the on-call doctor. Just as they are warned to expect some pain after LASEK, patients also know the surgeon is available if they need help.

Second, patients should limit their activities in the first 3 to 4 postoperative days. Excessive activity seems to be associated with more eye pain. Specifically, patients should avoid gardening, going out for dinner and evening entertainment, travel, and exposure to wind and dust (eg, cleaning out the attic). This admonition should be repeated on the second and third postoperative days, even if a patient is feeling better, as increased activity in the first 3 to 4 days seems to correlate with relapses of pain.

Third, check the bandage contact lens. A tight lens can cause pain. There should be 1 to 3 mm of vertical lens movement with blinking. If no other reason can be identified when examining a patient with increased postoperative pain, simply exchanging the contact lens in the office can sometimes alleviate the discomfort. The contact lens should be left in place until the central epithelial defect is healed, usually 3 to 4 days. If only blotchy or punctate fluorescein staining remains, the eye is usually more comfortable with the contact lens removed. If the contact lens falls out at home, instruct patients not to try to reinsert the old contact lens but to return to the office for a new lens.

Fourth, there are specific therapeutic measures patients should use to reduce postoperative pain. Ice packs applied to the temples are sometimes helpful, and ibuprofen 400 to 600 mg should be taken TID. Additionally, the patient is given 3 Vicodin (Abbott, Abbott Park, Ill) tablets, to be used 1 PO Q 4 to 6 hours for severe pain and/or to help with sleep the first night or two. While topical nonsteroidal anti-inflammatory drops (NSAIDs) have been advocated to mitigate postoperative pain, some surgeons avoid these medications because of reported corneal complications. We have found dilute topical anesthetics to be a useful adjunct in controlling postoperative pain in LASEK patients. Studies have shown that topical anesthetics at one-tenth their normal concentration have an analgesic effect without inducing anesthesia or toxicity.[48] These drops can be used as often as every 30 minutes for several days without apparent toxicity. Tetracaine preparations have proven to be more stable than proparacaine in dilute concentrations. A stabilized preparation of dilute (0.05%) tetracaine is available on the market.

In summary, despite the advantages of LASEK, patients should be counseled to expect pain postoperatively. Intraoperatively, chilled BSS should be applied before and after laser ablation and a proper bandage soft contact lens selected. Bonding with the patient, limiting activity, temple ice packs, contact lens management, oral pain medication, and dilute topical anesthetics are all important in ameliorating the postoperative pain and improving patient acceptance of this procedure.

Potential Complications

Intraoperatively, it is important to avoid alcohol leaks onto the conjunctiva, as that will cause postoperative pain. The risk of leaks is increased in patients with higher amounts of astigmatism, and care should be taken to apply even, downward pressure on the holding well. After the dilute alcohol solution has been instilled into the well, the surface meniscus should be carefully observed through the operating microscope for any movement or change in light reflex. If a substantial alcohol leak occurs, immediately remove the remaining alcohol from the well with a cellulose sponge, remove the well, and then thoroughly rinse the eye surface with chilled BSS. Reapply the well and alcohol solution if additional alcohol exposure is necessary to loosen the epithelium.

Small to moderate size tears in the epithelial flap do not impact the clinical result and can be ignored. If the epithelial flap is inadvertently detached from its hinge, care should be taken to reposit the flap in its original location, basement membrane down, following laser ablation. If the flap is badly damaged or lost, the operation is merely converted to PRK.

Potential postoperative complications include problems related to topical steroid use (glaucoma, cataract, ptosis), infection, mild recurrent erosion symptoms, delayed epithelial healing, and stromal haze.

Increased intraocular pressure can occur with fluorometholone, and periodic pressure checks are mandatory as long as steroids are continued. A single case of fluorometholone-induced cataract has been reported,[50] and that was after prolonged heavy dosage. This risk is greater in young patients. Infections have been reported after LASEK, but the incidence is unknown. The authors have not noted any infections during the immediate postoperative period in their respective practices. A low incidence of mild recurrent erosion symptoms without frank epithelial defect was reported in one series.[4]

Treatment options for delayed epithelial healing include bandage contact lens, patching, artificial tears, punctal plugs, oral doxycycline 100 mg BID, elimination of toxic eye drops (antibiotics, preservatives), and autologous serum eye drops.[51,52]

Postoperative Haze

Any discussion of surface ablation techniques such as LASEK needs to include the current concepts regarding post-surgical haze. One of the main concerns regarding PRK is that some patients develop visually significant corneal haze. Of particular concern is the sometimes-severe haze that can develop 4 to 12 months after the procedure, which has been termed late-onset corneal haze (LOCH). New insight into the mechanism of haze formation has led to new prophylactic regimens and decreased risk of vision loss following laser vision correction.

After any surface ablation procedure, the *wound healing response* prior to epithelial healing is thought to play a significant role in the formation of haze.[53] Stromal healing immediately after keratorefractive surgery occurs in three main phases.[39,53] Various biochemical factors are released during these phases and can play a role in the development of LOCH. In the initial phase, keratocyte apoptosis is thought to initiate the healing response.[54] This response appears to be regulated by transforming growth factor-ß1 (TGF-ß1).[55] The second phase of healing is characterized by proliferation of the keratocytes adjacent to the wound area. These keratocytes transform into fibroblasts and migrate into the area of cell apoptosis.[56] During the third phase of stromal wound healing, fibroblasts may become myofibroblasts. The extent to which this occurs is thought to be related to the type of corneal wound as well as the amount of stromal tissue removed.[57,58] These cells deposit extracellular matrix (ECM) material below the surface of the epithelium. The reflective properties of the ECM deposits are thought to be responsible for the development of LOCH.

Studies comparing LASEK to PRK indicate that the presence of the *epithelial flap* in LASEK may help protect the stroma during this early period of wound healing. Less TGF-ß1 is released in the early postoperative period following LASEK than following PRK.[59] LASEK, which leaves the epithelial basement membrane relatively intact within the flap, creates less of a wound response and, therefore, may decrease the transformation of fibroblast into myofibroblasts. The authors speculate that the epithelial flap acts as a "tissue bandage" in the early postoperative period and plays a key role in the absence of LOCH in their personal LASEK results.[3,4]

The association between *UV exposure* and the development of LOCH has recently gained increased acceptance. Alexander Stojanovic, MD of Tromso, Norway was first to report this connection.[60] Tromso is located above the Artic Circle and, therefore, has periods when it is dark for 24 hours per day during the winter and light for 24 hours per day during the summer. Dr. Stojanovic reviewed 314 cases of PRK and found a 3.7% LOCH rate. When these cases were analyzed, they were found to all occur during the summer months and were correlated with increased levels of environmental UV radiation.

In an effort to prevent postoperative haze caused be UV exposure, Dr. Stojanovic studied the use of *vitamin C prophylaxis*. The rationale for using vitamin C was based on animal studies showing that diurnal animals had higher levels of ascorbic acid in their corneas compared to nocturnal animals. In particular, reindeer (an animal whose habitat is primarily above the Artic Circle) had some of the highest levels found in nature. This observation has been interpreted as an environmental adaptation that protects the eye from UV radiation. Vitamin C has been ascribed a protective role as a UV filter as well as a scavenger of free radicals (ie, antioxidant).

In a prospective study,[61] Dr. Stojanovic prescribed vitamin C to all of his patients undergoing PRK or LASEK. Each patient received vitamin C 500 mg BID orally for 1-week preoperatively and 2-weeks postoperatively. After 1 year, no patients (>250 PRK/>100 LASEK) developed LOCH.

Bilgihan and coworkers[62] have demonstrated a significant decrease in the normal levels of ascorbic acid in human tears during the first 5 postoperative days following all laser refractive procedures. These findings led us to utilize vitamin C prophylaxis for high myopes (LS) or all patients (TC) undergoing LASEK. No studies have quantified the dose or time period to obtain maximum benefit from taking vitamin C. Currently, our LASEK patients are asked to begin taking 1000 mg vitamin C orally QD as soon as the decision to proceed with surgery is made. They are then asked to continue this regimen for at least 3 months after the procedure.

Mitomycin C (MMC) has been shown to be very efficacious when used to treat patients who have developed visually significant LOCH.[63] Recently, MMC has also been proposed to prophylactically prevent the formation of postoperative haze.[64,65] MMC's antineoplastic properties inhibit fibroblast function and proliferation. Early studies show that this use of MMC is safe and effective. However, anecdotal cases of complications due to incorrect dilution of the MMC as well as over- and undercorrections from intended refraction have been reported. To date, no studies have demonstrated the long-term safety of MMC used in this setting. Currently, given the extremely low incidence of haze reported when LASEK is performed correctly (ie, good epithelial flap creation and replacement) and when such prophylactic measures as oral vitamin C and topical steroids are used appropriately, the authors do not advocate the prophylactic use of MMC in LASEK for the prevention of LOCH.

Clinical Results

Claringbold, in a retrospective, single-surgeon interventional case series,[3] reported outcomes of 222 consecutive eyes with myopia ranging from -1.25 to -11.25 D and astigmatism up to +2.25 D treated with LASEK. Results were analyzed at 4 days, 2 weeks, 3 months, 6 months, and 12 months after surgery. Postoperatively, uncorrected visual acuity (UCVA) was 20/40 or better in 84% of eyes at Day 4 and in 98% of eyes at 2 weeks. In 84 eyes followed for 12 months, UCVA was 20/15 in 16 eyes (19.0%), 20/20 in 53 eyes (63.1%), and 20/25 in 15 eyes (17.9%). There was no loss of best spectacle-corrected visual acuity (BSCVA), and no eyes required retreatment.

In a prospective study,[4] Shahinian reported LASEK results in 146 eyes with myopia (range -1.25 to -14.38 D) or myopic astigmatism. No mitomycin C was used. After 6 and 12 months, no eye lost 2 or more lines of BSCVA. After 6 months, UCVA was 20/20 in 57% and 20/40 or better in 96% of eyes. After 12 months, UCVA was 20/20 in 56% and 20/40 or better in 96% of eyes. No eye developed corneal haze affecting visual acuity. There were no serious or vision-threatening complications.

Taneri et al[66] reviewed literature reporting 21 LASEK series, 1421 eyes in total. LASEK provided long-term stable results without serious complications such as infection or late haze formation. Postoperative discomfort and prolonged visual recovery until the epithelium closes remain the biggest disadvantages of LASEK compared to LASIK.

Summary

LASEK, first described in 1999, has proven to be a useful form of surface ablation. Visual results are comparable to those of LASIK. Most importantly, all stromal flap complications are eliminated. However, LASEK still represents a relatively small percentage of laser vision correction procedures, principally because it cannot match LASIK for postoperative comfort and rapid vision recovery.

Although corneal haze affecting vision has been reported after LASEK, the authors have seen no visually significant haze, treating up to -14.0 D of myopia. Published comparative studies indicate that LASEK produces less postoperative haze than PRK.

While patient preparation, instrumentation, surgical technique, and postoperative management vary somewhat from surgeon to surgeon, the authors have detailed a specific approach designed to shorten the learning curve and aid the transition from PRK and LASIK to LASEK.

References

1. Cimberle M. LASEK may offer the advantages of both LASIK and PRK. *Ocular Surgery News*. 1999; March:28.
2. Shah S, Sebai Sarhan AR, Doyle SJ, et al. The epithelial flap for photorefractive keratectomy. *Br J Ophthalmol*. 2001;85:393-396.
3. Claringbold T. Laser-assisted subepithelial keratectomy for the correction of myopia. *J Cataract Refract Surg*. 2002;28:18-22.
4. Shahinian L. Laser-assisted sub-epithelial keratectomy (LASEK) for low to high myopia and astigmatism. *J Cataract Refract Surg*. 2002; 28:1334-1342.
5. Leung AT, Rao SK, Cheng AC, et al. Pathogenesis and management of laser in situ keratomileusis flap buttonhole. *J Cataract Refract Surg*. 2000;26:358-362.
6. Pulaski JP. Etiology of buttonhole flaps. *J Cataract Refract Surg*. 2000;26:1270-1271.
7. Hori Y, Watanabe H, Maeda N, et al. Medical treatment of operative corneal perforation caused by laser in situ keratomileusis. *Arch Ophthalmol*. 1999;117:1422-1423.
8. Holland SP, Srivannaboon S, Reinstein DZ. Avoiding serious corneal complications of laser assisted in situ keratomileusis and photorefractive keratectomy. *Ophthalmology*. 2000;107:640-652.
9. Wong VW, Zhu CC, Rao SR, Lam DS. Corneal perforation during laser in situ keratomileusis. *J Cataract Refract Surg*. 2000;26:1103-1104.
10. Lee AG, Kohnen T, Ebner R, et al. Optic neuropathy associated with laser in situ keratomileusis. *J Cataract Refract Surg*. 2000;26:1581-1584.
11. Bushley DM, Parmley VC, Paglen P. Visual field defect associated with laser in situ keratomileusis. *Am J Ophthalmol*. 2000;129:668-671.
12. Weiss HS, Rubinfeld RS, Anderschat JF. LASIK-associated visual field loss in a glaucoma suspect. *Arch Ophthalmol*. 2001;119:774-775.
13. Gimbel HV, Penno EE, van Westenbrugge JA, et al. Incidence and management of intraoperative and early postoperative complications in 1000 consecutive laser in situ keratomileusis cases. *Ophthalmology*. 1998;105:1839-1847.
14. Dastgheib KA, Clinch TE, Manche EE, et al. Sloughing of corneal epithelium and wound healing complications associated with laser in situ keratomileusis in patients with epithelial basement membrane dystrophy. *Am J Ophthalmol*. 2000;130:297-303.
15. Ti SE, Tan DT. Recurrent corneal erosion after laser in situ keratomileusis. *Cornea*. 2001;20:156-158.
16. von Kulajta P, Stark WJ, O'Brien TP. Management of flap striae. *Int Ophthalmol Clin*. 2000;40:87-92.
17. Walker MB, Wilson SE. Incidence and prevention of epithelial growth within the interface after laser in situ keratomileusis. *Cornea*. 2000;19:170-173.
18. Waring GO, Epithelial ingrowth after laser in situ keratomileusis. *Am J Ophthalmol*. 2001;131:402-403.
19. Castillo A, Diaz-Valle D, Gutierrez AR, et al. Peripheral melt of flap after laser in situ keratomileusis. *J Refract Surg*. 1998;14:61-63.
20. Smith RJ, Maloney RK. Diffuse lamellar keratitis. A new syndrome in lamellar refractive surgery. *Ophthalmology*. 1998;105:1721-1726.
21. Haw WW, Manche EE. Late onset diffuse lamellar keratitis associated with an epithelial defect in six eyes. *J Refract Surg*. 2000;16:744-748.
22. Weisenthal RW. Diffuse lamellar keratitis induced by trauma 6 months after laser in situ keratomileusis. *J Refract Surg*. 2000;16:749-751.
23. Quiros PA, Chuck RS, Smith RE, et al. Infectious ulcerative keratitis after laser in situ keratomileusis. *Arch Ophthalmol*. 1999;117:1423-1427.
24. Garg P, Bansal AK, Sharma S, Vemuganti GK. Bilateral infectious keratitis after laser in situ keratomileusis. *Ophthalmology*. 2001;108:121-125.
25. Melki SA, Talamo JH, Demetriades AM. Late traumatic dislocation of laser in situ keratomileusis corneal flaps. *Ophthalmology*. 2000;107:2136-2139.
26. Booth MA, Koch DD. Late laser in situ keratomileusis flap dislocation caused by a thrown football. *J Cataract Refract Surg*. 2003;29:2032-2033.
27. Aldave AJ, Hollander DA, Abbott RL. Late-onset traumatic flap dislocation and diffuse lammellar inflammation after laser in situ keratomileusis. *Cornea*. 2002;21:604-607.
28. Franklin QJ, Tanzer DJ. Late traumatic flap displacement after laser in situ keratomileuisis. *Mil Med*. 2004;169:334-346.
29. Tumbocon JA, Paul R, Slomovic A, Rootman DS. Late traumatic displacement of laser in situ keratomileusis flaps. *Cornea*. 2003;22:66-69.
30. Patel CK, Hanson R, McDonald B, Cox N. Case reports and small case series: late dislocation of a LASIK flap caused by a fingernail. *Arch Ophthalmol*. 2001;119:447-449.
31. Sridhar MS, Rapuano CJ, Cohen EJ. Accidental self-removal of a flap—a rare complication of laser in situ keratomileusis surgery. *Am J Ophthalmol*. 2001;132:780-782.
32. Seiler T. Iatrogenic keratectasia after laser in situ keratomileusis. *J Refract Surg*. 1998;14:312-317.
33. Koch DD. The riddle of iatrogenic keratectasia. *J Cataract Refract Surg*. 1999;25:453-454.
34. Geggel HS, Talley AR. Delayed onset keratectasia following laser in situ keratomileusis. *J Cataract Refract Surg*. 1999;25:582-586.
35. Joo CK, Kim TG. Corneal ectasia detected after laser in situ keratomileusis for correction of less than -12 diopters of myopia. *J Cataract Refract Surg*. 2000;26:292-295.
36. Amoils SP, Deist MB, Gous P, Amoils PM. Iatrogenic keratectasia after laser in situ keratomileusis for less than -4.0 to -7.0 diopters of myopia. *J Cataract Refract Surg*. 2000;26:967-977.
37. Sugar A, Rapuano C, Culbertson W, et al. Laser in situ keratomileusis for myopia and astigmatism: safety and efficacy. *Ophthalmology*. 2002;109:175-187.
38. Dohlman CH, Gasset AR, Rose J. The effect of the absence of corneal epithelium or endothelium on stromal keratocytes. *Invest Ophthalmol Vis Sci*. 1968;7:520-534.
39. Wilson SE, Mohan RR, Hong JW, et al. The wound healing response after laser in situ keratomileusis and photorefractive keratectomy. *Arch Ophthalmol*. 2001;119:889-896.
40. Zhao J, Nagasaki T, Maurice D. Role of tears in keratocyte loss after epithelial removal in mouse cornea. *Invest Ophthalmol Vis Sci*. 2001;42:1743-1749.
41. Choi YS, Kim JY, Wee WR, Lee JH. Effect of the application of human amniotic membrane on rabbit corneal wound healing after excimer laser photorefractive keratectomy. *Cornea*. 1998;17(4):389-95.
42. Moller-Pedersen T, Cavanagh HD, Petroll WM, Jester JV. Stromal wound healing explains refractive instability and haze development after photorefractive keratectomy. *Ophthalmology*. 2000;107:1235-1245.
43. Vesaluoma M, Perez-Santonja J, Petroll WM, et al. Corneal stromal changes induced by myopic LASIK. *Invest Ophthalmol Vis Sci*. 2000;41:369-376.
44. Lee JB, Seong GJ, Lee JH, et al. Comparison of laser epithelial keratomileusis and photorefractive keratectomy for low to moderate myopia. *J Cataract Refract Surg*. 2000;27:565-570.
45. Autrata R, Rehurek J. Laser-assisted subepithelial keratectomy for myopia: two-year follow-up. *J Cataract Refract Surg*. 2003;29:661-668.

46. Autrata R, Rehurek J. Laser-assisted subepithelial keratectomy and photorefractive keratectomy for the correction of hyperopia: results of a 2-year follow-up. *J Cataract Refract Surg.* 2003;29:2105-2114.
47. Astle WF, Huang PT, Ingram AD, Farran RP. Laser-assisted subepithelial keratectomy in children. *J Cataract Refract Surg.* 2004;30(12):2529-2535.
48. Durrie DS, personal communication, 2005.
49. Shahinian L, Jain S, Jager R, et al. Dilute topical proparacaine for pain relief after photorefractive keratectomy. *Ophthalmology.* 1997;104:1327-1332.
50. Bilgihan K, Gurelik G, Akata F, et al. Fluorometholone-induced cataract after photorefractive keratectomy. *Ophthalmologica.* 1997;211(6):394-396.
51. Young AL, Cheng AC, Ng HK, et al. The use of autologous serum tears in persistent corneal epithelial defects. *Eye.* 2004;18:609-614.
52. Geerling G, MacLennan S, Hartwig D. Autologous serum eye drops for ocular surface disorders. *Br J Ophthalmol.* 2004;88:1467-1474.
53. Li DQ, Tseng SC. Three patterns of cytokine expression potentially involved in the epithelial-fibroblasts interactions of human ocular surface. *J Cell Physiol.* 1995;163:61-79.
54. Baldwin HC, Marshall J. Growth factors in corneal wound healing following refractive surgery: a review. *Acta Ophthalmol Scand.* 2002; 80:238-247.
55. Jester JV, Petroll WM, Cavanaugh HD. Corneal stromal wound healing in refractive surgery: the role of myofibroblasts. *Prog Retin Eye Res.* 1999;18:311-356.
56. Wilson SE, He YG, Weng J, et al. Epithelial injury induces keratocyte apoptosis: hypothesized role for the interleukin-1 system in the modulation of corneal tissue organization and wound healing. *Exp Eye Res.* 1996;62:325-327.
57. Mohan RR, Hutcheon AEK, Choi R, et al. Apoptosis, necrosis, proliferation, and myofibroblasts generation in the stroma following LASIK and PRK. *Exp Eye Res.* 2003;76:71-87.
58. Lin N, Yee SB, Mitra S, et al. Prediction of corneal haze using an ablation depth/corneal thickness ratio after laser epithelial keratomileusis. *J Refract Surg.* 2004;20:797-802.
59. Lee JB, Seong GJ, Lee JH, et al. Comparison of TGF-beta1 in tears following laser in situ keratomileusis and photorefractive keratectomy. *J Refract Surg.* 2002;18:130-134.
60. Stojanovic A, Nitter T. Correlation between ultraviolet radiation level and the incidence of late-onset corneal haze after photorefractive keratectomy. *J Cataract Refract Surg.* 2001;27:404-410.
6!. Stojanovic A, Ringvold A, Nitter, T. Ascorbate prophylaxis for corneal haze after photorefractive keratectomy. *J Refract Surg.* 2003;19:338-343.
62. Biligihan A, Biligihan K, Toklu Y, et al. Ascorbic acid levels in human tears after photorefractive keratectomy, transepithelial photorefractive keratectomy, and laser in situ keratomileusis. *J Cataract Refract Surg.* 2001;27:585-588.
63. Majmudar PA, Forstot SL, Dennis RF, et al. Topical mitomycin-C for subepithelial fibrosis after refractive corneal surgery. *Ophthalmology.* 2000;107:89-94.
64. Carones F, Vigo L, Scandola E, Vacchini L. Evaluation of the prophylactic use of mitomycin-C to inhibit haze formation after photorefractive keratectomy. *J Cataract Refract Surg.* 2002;28:2088-2095.
65. Porges Y, Ben-Haim O, Hirsh A, Levinger S. Photorefractive keratectomy with mitomycin-C for corneal haze following photorefracive keratectomy for myopia. *J Refract Surg.* 2003;19:40-43.
66. Taneri S, Zieske JD, Azar DT. Evolution, techniques, clinical outcomes, and pathophysiology of LASEK: review of the literature. *Surv Ophthalmol.* 2004;49:576-602.

CHAPTER 17

BUTTERFLY LASEK

Paolo Vinciguerra, MD; Fabrizio I. Camesasca, MD

LASEK

The first presentation of LASEK dates to 1999.[1,2] Due to favorable comparison with the other two excimer refractive techniques available—LASIK and PRK—LASEK popularity has been slowly but steadily increasing.[3,4]

With the increase in medico-legal problems related to refractive surgery all over the Western World, ophthalmologists pay great attention to surgical techniques that may reduce complications and provide reliable results. Even LASEK, however, may have complications that hamper rapid postoperative recovery such as postoperative low epithelial viability. The clinical appearance of this reduced viability is a greyish appearance of the epithelial flap, featuring reduced transparency. In the immediate postoperative period, epithelial cell adhesion to the corneal stroma is reduced, and corneal debris can be observed under the protective contact lens. This nonviable, grey flap can be lost in the immediate postoperative period; therefore, reducing the advantages offered by LASEK. Stromal protection is decreased with consequent ocular discomfort. Visual acuity is reduced, and this situation improves only when the epithelial flap reattaches to the limbus.

We developed a modification of LASEK technique, the "butterfly" LASEK, aimed to preserve the connection between corneal flap and limbus, essential for re-establishing corneal epithelial adhesion and stratification.[5]

SURGICAL TECHNIQUE

Preoperative anesthesia consists of two applications of oxybuprocaine chlorhydrate eyedrops. The patient is prepped and draped, and a lid speculum is applied. Lidocaine 4% eyedrops are instilled. Using a specifically designed spatula (Vinciguerra Spatula [ASICO, Westmont, Ill]), a thin abrasion of 0.75 mm is imparted to the paracentral corneal epithelium, from 8:00 to 11:00, sparing the optical zone. After positioning the LASEK fluid-holding ring, a 20% solution of alcohol and BSS is applied to the cornea for a time ranging from 5 to 10 seconds, adjusted according to the firmness of epithelial adhesion noted during removal of the thin paracentral line.

With the above-mentioned spatula, the epithelium, with its basal membrane, is gently dissected from Bowman's membrane up to the limbus (Figure 17-1). After application of the alcohol solution, it is mandatory to keep the epithelium well hydrated in order to preserve the obtained loosening effect. If hydration is not properly maintained, in the time required to dissect the first flap, the second one will become dehydrated, thus hampering easy dissection. Furthermore, care must be taken not to inadvertently perforate the flap during flaps creation. The spatula must, thus, be tangential to the corneal surface, not vertical.

Before ablation, the stromal surface is carefully dried. The flap must be kept moist. To keep the flap safely folded peripherally and prevent its ablation, a specially designed retractor/protector is positioned (Vinciguerra Retractor Forceps [ASICO]) until excimer ablation is completed (Figure 17-2).

We used a NIDEK EC 5000 excimer laser (Gamagori, Japan). All treatments were performed with multizone ablations with the widest possible diameters, and the cylinder component of the defect was treated with the cross cylinder technique. After the refractive laser ablation, a smoothing phase was performed to achieve a regular stromal bed as similar as possible to the physiological Bowman membrane. Smoothing was performed by continuously applying a hyaluronic acid masking fluid (Laservis, Chemedica, Munich, Germany) on the surface with a special spatula (Buratto Spatula [ASICO]). In order to prevent a possible hyperopic shift, the smoothing diameter should be at least 9.5 mm, involving the entire corneal surface. Smoothing requires

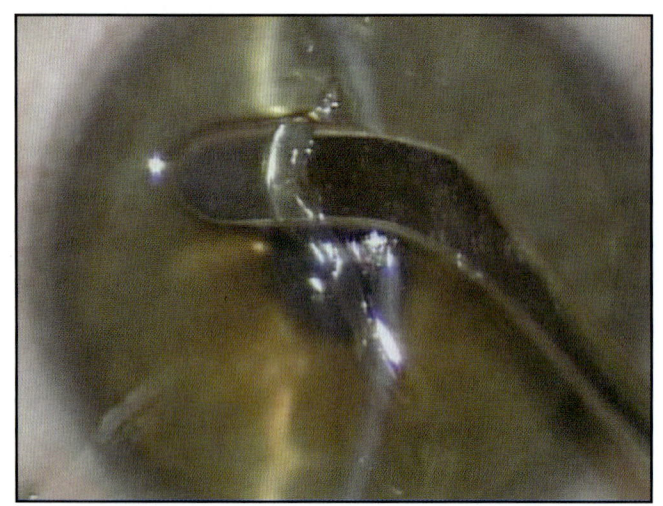

Figure 17-1. Using a specifically designed spatula (Vinciguerra's spatula [ASICO, Calif]), a thin abrasion of 0.75 mm is performed on the paracentral corneal epithelium, from 8:00 to 11:00, sparing the optical zone. After applying a 20% solution of alcohol and BSS, with the same spatula the epithelium is gently dissected from Bowman's membrane up to the limbus.

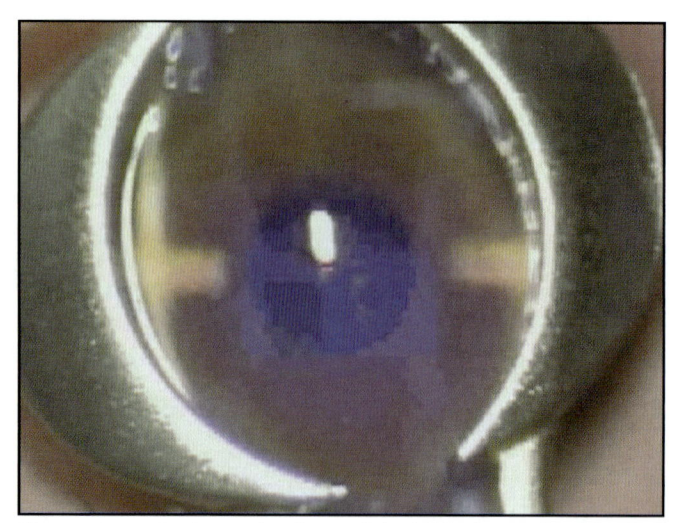

Figure 17-2. To keep the flap safely folded peripherally and prevent its ablation, a specially designed retractor/protector is positioned, (FCPS retractor of Vinciguerra [ASICO, Calif]) until excimer ablation is completed.

continuous application with even distribution of the masking fluid to avoid formation of dry areas. Ablation on a dry area would not create the desired smoothing but just a localized ablation. To avoid overheating the tissue, the ablation is set at 30 µm, with a frequency of 10 Hz. The actual ablation is only 8 µm, due to the presence of the masking fluid.

Once the smoothing phase is completed, the retractor/protector is removed, and the epithelial flaps are gently repositioned over the Bowman membrane using the Vinciguerra/Carones spatula (ASICO) with their margins overlapped. Finally, a protective contact lens is applied, and cyclopentholate 1%, tobramycin, and betamethasone eye drops instilled. The patients were then treated with netilmicyn eye drops 4 times a day for 5 days; after removal of the contact lens, the treatment consisted of fluorometholone eye drops 3 times daily for 15 days and hyaluronic acid 0.15% 5 to 6 times daily for 6 months.

In two studies on butterfly LASEK, we observed that this new technique led to improved postsurgery cell vitality and refractive recovery compared with the traditional technique.[5,6]

We evaluated butterfly LASEK technique in 773 eyes of 452 patients with mean age of 34.3 ± 16.5 years, mean SE preoperative refraction of -5.3 ± 3.7 D (mean sphere -4.8 ± 3.6 D; mean cylinder -1.0 ± 1.4 D), ranging from -22.5 to +5.5 D. The follow-up examination was performed at day 1, 2, 3, and 4 (or until removal of the contact lens) and thereafter, at months 1, 3, 6 and 12. Tests performed during late follow-up examinations included corneal topography (CSO, Florence, Italy), autorefractometry, anterior segment biomicroscopy, and a complete ophthalmologic examination.

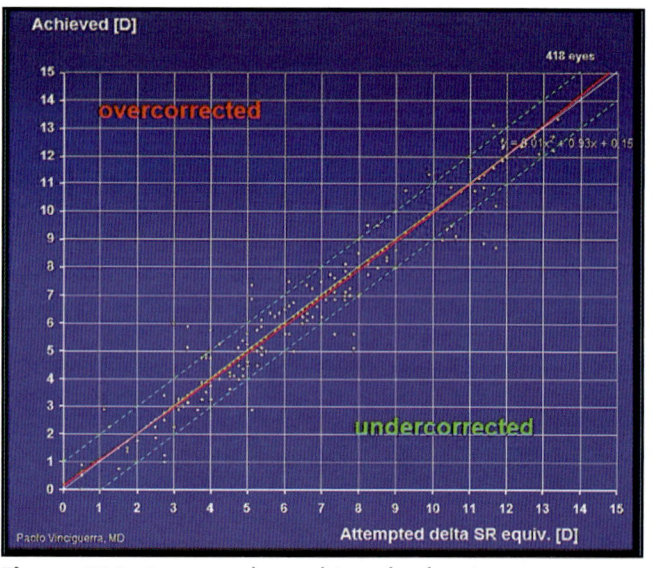

Figure 17-3. Attempted vs achieved refraction.

After 12 months, we could examine 542 (70.1%) of the treated eyes. Mean spherical equivalent was -0.2 ± 1.4 D (sphere -0.1 ± 1.3 D; cylinder -0.1 ± 0.6 D) ranging from -2.5 to 0.75 D. In 83% of the eyes treated, refraction within ±0.5 D of the desired correction was achieved (Figures 17-3 and 17-4). In 19% of the eyes treated, uncorrected visual acuity was greater than or equal to 1.2, in 56% greater than or equal to 1.0 and in 19% equal to 0.8 (Figure 17-5). In 83.0% of treated eyes, the achieved refraction ranged between ±0.5 D of the desired correction. Concerning visual acuity, we found a loss of 1 line in 0.3% of treated eyes; in 49.8% of cases, there was no postsurgery variation, while we recorded a gain of 1 line of visual acuity in 41.8%, of 2 lines in 9.8%, and of more than 2 lines in 1.6%.

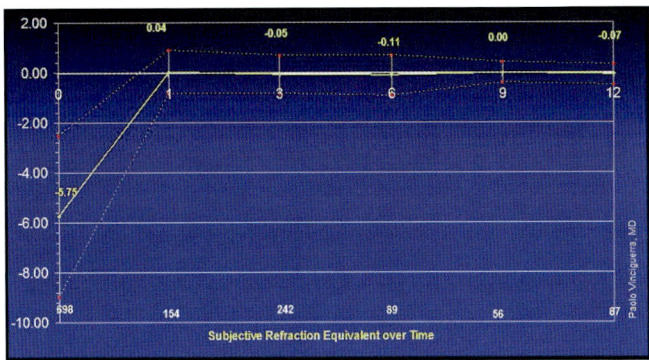

Figure 17-4. Pre- and postoperative refraction, spherical equivalent.

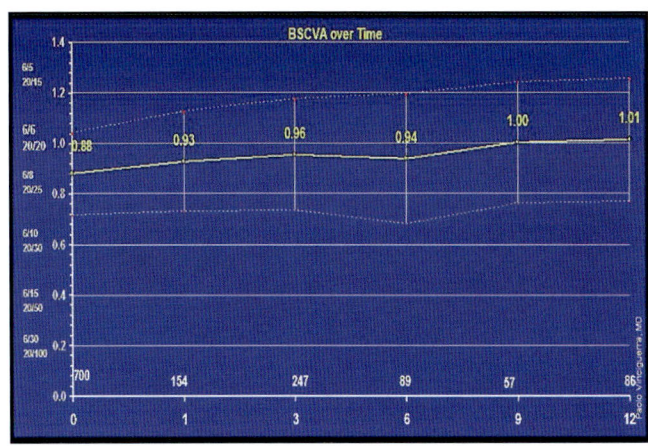

Figure 17-5. Best spectacle-corrected visual acuity over the entire follow-up period.

Discussion

The results of our clinical study confirmed that butterfly LASEK is a safe surgical procedure with an excellent refractive outcome that remains stable over time. These results were comparable to or even better than those obtained with PRK and LASIK.

In a randomized comparative clinical study on LASEK vs PRK for the treatment of low and medium myopia (between -3.0 and -6.5 D), Lee concluded that in LASEK there is a reduction of postsurgery pain (p = 0.047), a lower degree of mean haze after 1 month (p = 0.02), and 63% of patients report that they prefer the eye treated with LASEK to the one treated with PRK.[7] In a prospective LASEK vs LASIK comparative study after 6 months, Scerrati concluded that patients treated with the former surgical technique show better results in terms of corneal topography, noncorrected visual acuity, sensitivity to contrast, and refractive results as compared to patients treated with LASIK.[8] In several studies, Azar pointed out the excellent refractive results achieved through LASEK with a noncorrected visual acuity of 5/10 after 1 week in all patients with absence of postsurgery pain in 43% of cases.[3,9] In a noncomparative retrospective study on 84 eyes operated on consecutively by the same surgeon, Claringbold concluded that 1 year after the LASEK surgery, 16 eyes (19.0%) had achieved noncorrected visual acuity of 12/10, 53 eyes (63.1%) of 10/10, and 15 eyes (17.9%) of 8/10.[10] There were no losses of visual acuity lines, and no repeated surgery was necessary. Lee attributed the lower amount of haze compared with PRK to a reduced production of TGF-1 in post LASEK tear film.[11]

In our opinion, the main limitation of traditional LASEK is that preliminary trephination of epithelial flap severs it from the limbus, the source of new epithelial cells. Butterfly LASEK maintains this connection on a wide portion of the limbus minimizing the epithelial damage created, thus increasing the probabilities of maintaining epithelial vitality in the postsurgery period. Mechanical stability of the flap is also increased. We recommend having a dry stromal surface after ablation to improve flap adhesion and reduce postoperative epithelial edema. Adjustable alcoholization time also reduces epithelial damage.

In our experience, the more rapid return to epithelial transparency with butterfly LASEK indicated improved flap vitality, with consequent faster visual recovery. Less postoperative flap loss in butterfly LASEK is related to the more extensive connection of flap to the limbus. This reduces visual recovery time as well as postsurgery pain.

The different procedure to create the epithelial flap makes butterfly LASEK even easier to perform and to standardize, reducing training time for surgeons who intend to approach LASEK. The present study showed that the variation in the epithelial flap creation technique did not alter refractive results after 12 months, with an achieved refraction comprised between ±0.5 D of the desired correction in 83% of treated eyes in moderate myopia; such data are in line with the results reported in recent literature. Also to be noted is the lower degree of mean haze compared with PRK.

LASEK advantages over LASIK are well-known.[12] Flap complications are less dreadful than those observed with LASIK, more stroma is available for retreatment when necessary, and less biomechanical changes are induced, as pointed out by Cynthia Roberts in a previous chapter.

Higher amounts of myopia can be treated with LASEK rather than with LASIK, with a smaller risk of long-term ectasia because of the greater amount of corneal tissue that can be used for ablation.[5,13]

In conclusion, the experience acquired in recent years with the butterfly LASEK technique makes us confident in the development of photorefractive surgery and in the progressive elimination of the problems that have been found so far in this type of surgery.

References

1. Camellin M, Vinciguerra P, Nizzola GM. LASEK: laser epithelial keratomileusis. A new technique for improving healing and decreasing postoperative pain. (Communication, 1999 ASCRS, Best Paper of the Section).
2. Camellin M. Laser epithelial keratomileusis for myopia. *J Refract Surg.* 2003;19:666-670.

3. Taneri S, Feit R, Azar DT. Safety, efficacy, and stability indices of LASEK correction in moderate myopia and astigmatism. *J Cataract Refract Surg.* 2004;30:2130-2137.
4. Duffey RJ, Leaming D. US trends in refractive surgery:2003 ISRS/AAO survey. *J Refract Surg.* 2005;1:87-91.
5. Vinciguerra P, Camesasca FI. Butterfly laser epithelial keratomileusis for myopia. *J Refract Surg.* 2002;18(S):S371-3.
6. Vinciguerra P, Camesasca F, Randazzo A. One-year results of butterfly laser epithelial keratomileusis. *J Refract Surg.* 2003;19(S):S223-226.
7. Lee JB, Seong GJ, Lee JH, et al. Comparison of laser epithelial keratomileusis and photorefractive keratectomy for low to moderate myopia. *J Cataract Refract Surg.* 2001;27(4):565-570.
8. Scerrati E. Laser in situ keratomileusis vs. laser epithelial keratomileusis (LASIK vs LASEK). *J Refract Surg.* 2001;17(2 Suppl):S219-221.
9. Azar DT, Ang RT, Lee JB, et al. Laser subepithelial keratomileusis: electron microscopy and visual outcomes of flap photorefractive keratectomy. *Curr Opin Ophthalmol.* 2001;12(4):323-328.
10. Claringbold TV 2nd. Laser-assisted subepithelial keratectomy for the correction of myopia. *J Cataract Refract Surg.* 2002;28(1):18-22.
11. Lee JB, Choe CM, Kim HS, Seo KY, Seong GJ, Kim EK. Comparison of TGF-beta1 in tears following laser subepithelial keratomileusis and photorefractive keratectomy. *J Refract Surg.* 2002;18(2):130-134.
12. Shahinian L Jr. Laser-assisted subepithelial keratectomy for low to high myopia and astigmatism. *J Cataract Refract Surg.* 2002;28:1334-1342.
13. Esquenazi S, He J, Bazan NG, Bazan HE. Comparison of corneal wound-healing response in photorefractive keratectomy and laser-assisted subepithelial keratectomy. *J Cataract Refrac Surg.* 2005;31:1632-1639.

CHAPTER 18

LASEK WITH CUSTOM ABLATION AND SMOOTHING

Paolo Vinciguerra, MD; Fabrizio I. Camesasca, MD

Introduction

After being hailed as the new frontier of excimer laser surgery, aberrometry-based custom ablation is now entering in its mature phase with a constantly increasing number of positive reports.[1-5] However, several factors may still play an important role in impeding full achievement of planned refractive results. Irregularities of the ablated corneal surface may enhance collagen deposition and, therefore, produce variations in the final refractive results.[6-8] On the contrary, a smooth ablated surface induces less reparatory response, leading to less haze formation and better refractive predictability.[6,9] We introduced corneal smoothing in the final phase of refractive treatment following the results of studies performed in 1998.[8,9] The results of a recent study by Wilson demonstrate a relationship between the level of corneal haze formation after PRK and the level of stromal surface irregularity.[10]

The transition zone is a particularly delicate point in the creation of a new optical surface with excimer laser ablation. In this portion of the ablation, the new central curvature must be connected with the unchanged peripheral corneal curvature. In excimer laser refractive surgery, marked variation of curvature in this peripheral portion may induce a reparatory response that reduces curvature variation physiologically but may induce regression and restriction of the effective optical zone.

We considered the above-mentioned concepts and the results of our previous studies and designed a surface corneal ablation strategy for custom LASEK to increase predictability by reducing the biomechanical and reparative responses of the cornea.

Surgical Technique

In a recent study, we prospectively evaluated myopic and hyperopic eyes undergoing LASEK refractive surgery.[11] Selection criteria included age greater than 18 years, no known systemic, metabolic, or collagen diseases, no tear film defect, and a cornea with no asymmetry features that could indicate the presence of a form-fruste keratoconus.

All patients underwent complete preoperative ophthalmologic examination, with determination of refractive defect by cycloplegia, pupillometry, endothelial cell counts, corneal topography with CSO topographer (Florence, Italy), and evaluation with the NIDEK OPD aberrometer (Gamagori, Japan). The NIDEK OPD is a time-based aberrometer, detecting the time and intensity difference between the light ray projected inside the eye (scanning slit) and the reflected ray (reflection light). This instrument provides refraction, a topographic map, an aberrometric map, as well as an OPD map that conveys information on the shape of the wavefront expressed in diopters, thus with an eagle's view of all involved refractive defects (see Chapter 6).

All patients signed an informed consent. Starting with the first preoperative week, and continuing through the postoperative re-epithelialization period, all the patients received oral supplements containing amino acids.[12] The butterfly LASEK technique has been described in the previous chapter.[13,14]

Surgery was always performed with the NIDEK EC 5000 excimer laser by the same surgeon (PV), who elaborated the ablation plan with the Final Fit ablation software featuring the Custom Ablation Transition Zone (CATz) software (NIDEK), on the basis of the topographical and aberrometric data. Ablation included an aspherical component, for treatment of the spherical defect (radially symmetric aberrations),

Figure 18-1. Final Fit ablation software with Custom Ablation Transition Zone software. Ablation includes a component for treatment of spherical defects (radially symmetric aberrations), a toric component for treatment of astigmatism (linearly symmetric aberrations), and a flying spot component for treatment of high-order aberrations (irregular components).

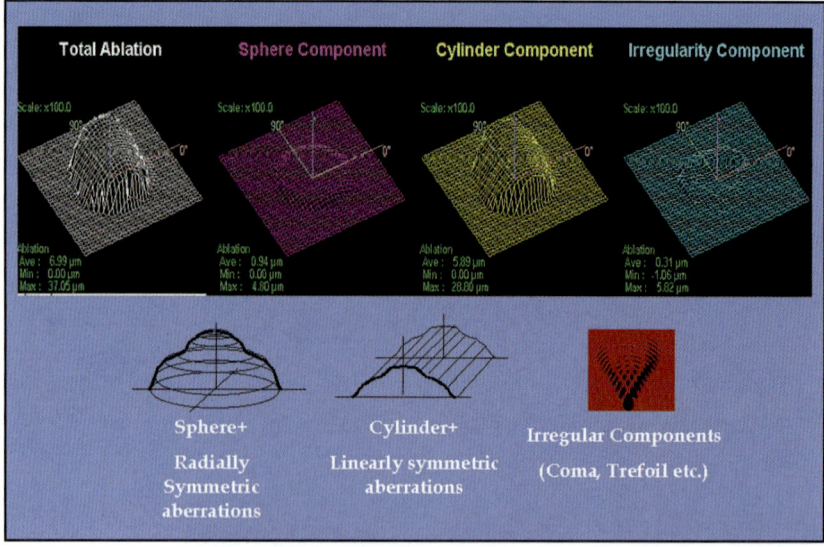

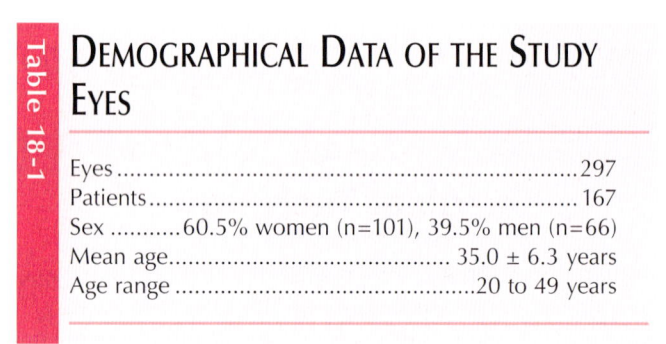

Table 18-1	DEMOGRAPHICAL DATA OF THE STUDY EYES
	Eyes 297
	Patients 167
	Sex .... 60.5% women (n=101), 39.5% men (n=66)
	Mean age .... 35.0 ± 6.3 years
	Age range .... 20 to 49 years

a toric component for treatment of the astigmatism (linearly symmetric aberrations), and a flying spot component for treatment of high order aberrations (irregular components) (Figure 18-1). The transition zone featured a diameter of 10 mm.

After the ablation, smoothing was performed to remove corneal microirregularities of a size inferior to the spot size (0.89 mm) and to the height of ablation (0.25 μm), and achieve a regular stromal bed as similar as possible to the physiological Bowman's layer. Smoothing was performed by applying a hyaluronic acid masking fluid (LASERVIS, Chemedica, Munich, Germany) and continuously distributing it over the corneal surface with a special spatula (Buratto Spatula [ASICO, Westmont, Ill]). The smoothing diameter was 10 mm, thus involving the entire corneal diameter. To avoid overheating the tissue, frequency was set at 10 Hz, and the ablation at 30 μm. After completing the smoothing, the epithelial flaps were gently repositioned over the corneal surface, the retractor/protector was removed, a protective contact lens was placed in position, and cyclopentholate chlorhydrate 1%, netilmycin sulphate 0.3%, and tobramycin-dexamethasone association eyedrops were administered before removal of the lid speculum. All patients underwent complete ophthalmologic examination with corneal topography at 30, 90, 180, and 360 days. Refractive data was managed with the Datagr@ph Med (Wendelstein, Germany) software. Statistical evaluation was performed with Student's t-test.

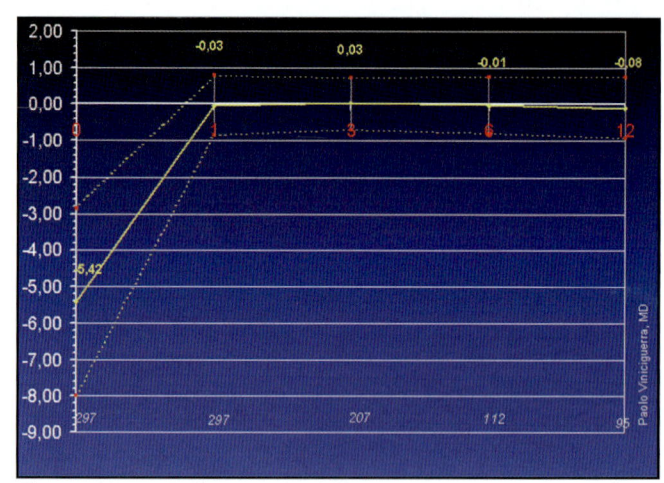

Figure 18-2. Refractive stability: postoperative SE refraction at follow-up examinations.

We treated 297 eyes in 167 patients. Table 18-1 reports demographic and refractive data. Pre- and postoperative refraction at all follow-up intervals is presented in Figure 18-2 and Table 18-2. Mean preoperative SE refraction was -5.46 ± 2.57 D ranging from -14.13 D to +3.5 D. At a final 1-year examination, the mean SE refraction was -0.15 ± 0.5 D, ranging from -4.0 D to +1.0 D. No eye required retreatment. Two eyes with initial refraction greater than -10.5 D SE reached final-moderately myopic (-3.0 and -4.0 D SE) refraction, as planned preoperatively due to limited corneal thickness and myopia in the fellow eye. The safety of the procedure, showing lines of visual acuity gained, unchanged, or lost, is presented in Figure 18-3. Efficacy, with percentage of UCVA calculated in Log Mar units, is presented in Figure 18-4. A scattergram of attempted vs achieved correction is presented in Figure 18-5. Corneal haze—graded according to Epstein—was absent at the 1-year control.[15]

Table 18-2. Pre- and Postoperative Refraction at the Different Follow-Up Intervals

Time	Eyes	Mean Sphere ± S.D. (D)	Range, Sphere (D)	Mean Cylinder ± SD (D)	Range, Cylinder (D)	Mean SE ± SD (D)	Range, SE (D)
Preop.	297	-5.03 ± 2.57	-13.50 to +4.00	-0.88 ± 0.76	-4.50 to +1.00	-5.46 ± 2.57	-14.13 to +3.50
1 month	297	+0.12 ± 0.65	-3.00 to +2.00	-0.39 ± 0.82	-1.00 to +1.50	-0.08 ± 0.72	-4.00 to +3.00
3 months	207	+0.06 ± 0.54	-2.50 to +2.00	-0.17 ± 0.55	-1.00 to +1.00	-0.03 ± 0.56	-2.75 to +2.00
6 months	112	0.00 ± 0.46	-3.00 to +1.00	-0.15 ± 0.35	-1.50 to +1.00	-0.08 ± 0.48	-3.50 to +1.75
12 months	95	-0.05 ± 0.50	-3.00 to +1.00	-0.21 ± 0.41	-1.50 to +0.00	-0.15 ± 0.50	-4.00 to +1.00

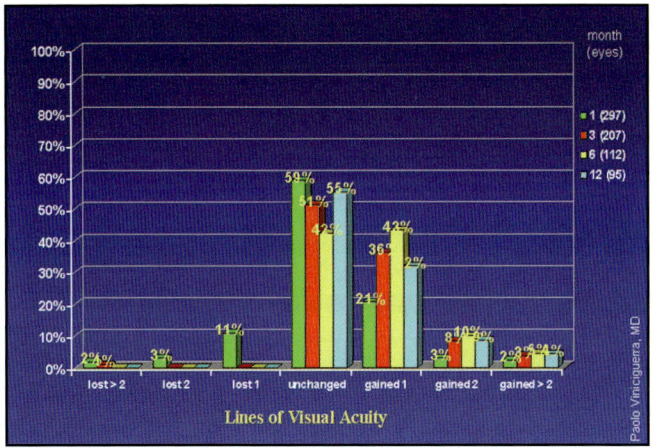

Figure 18-3. Safety of the procedure. Percentage change of BSCVA at the different follow-up intervals.

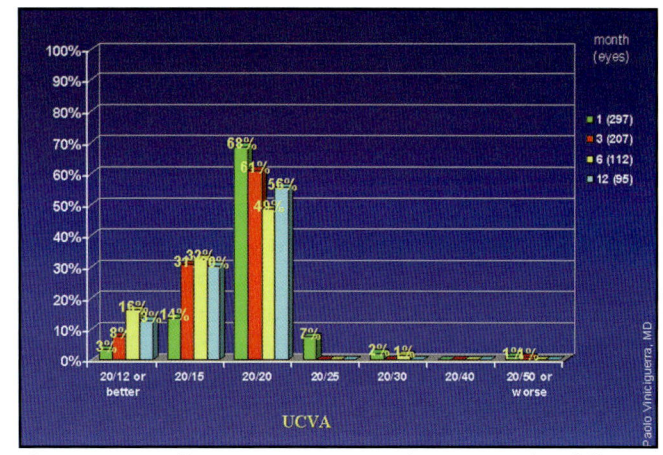

Figure 18-4. Efficacy: Percentage of UCVA at the different follow-up intervals.

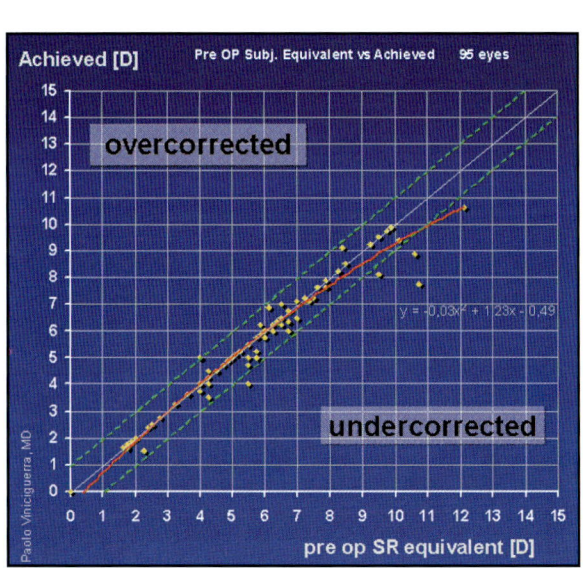

Figure 18-5. Attempted vs achieved refractive correction, at 1 year.

Custom LASEK

Customized ablation, either based on surface or on total aberrometry, is arousing increasing interest among refractive surgeons. Nevertheless, the target of a perfectly predictable treatment often remains elusive. Several factors may be taken into account when examining the limits of custom ablation.

The ablation patterns of the different excimer lasers, as well as the overlapping of their spots, always generate a corneal surface with microirregularities. Avoiding increase in aberrations after refractive surgery is a difficult goal, and corneal irregularities induced by excimer ablation may cause aberrations.[16] After surface ablation, the corneal epithelium attempts to solve macro- and microirregularities through several layers of epithelial cells and/or collagen deposition.[6,8,9] Variation of curvature in the peripheral portion of the ablation may also lead to collagen deposition, a phenomenon that is aimed at reducing this unnatural variation in the curvature but induces regression. All these phenomena reduce the prevedibility of the imparted correction.

Cynthia Roberts has presented an interesting theory on the influence of corneal biomechanical properties on refractive result after surface or stromal surgery, proposing that the central severing of elastic corneal lamellae following surface or stromal surgery induces relaxation of the peripheral residual lamellae, with decompression of the extracellular matrix and increase in curvature and thickness of peripheral stroma. This apparently results in tangential traction forces on the underlying lamellae, which in the central cornea, constitute the postoperative corneal surface, resulting in a central flattening not related to the ablation profile. This would lead to a hyperopic shift. Results of myopic treatments will thus be increased, while in hyperopic ones they will be decreased. This phenomenon will be more marked in LASIK, where the number of severed lamellae is tenfold that of PRK, and contribute to the unpredictability of refractive surgery (see Chapter 6).[17]

We have tried to overcome unpredictability due to microirregularity and corneal biomechanics in custom ablation in several ways. Information on surface and total aberrometry generated in photopic, scotopic, and mesopic conditions by NIDEK OPD integrated aberrometer, refractometer, topographer, and pupillometer was integrated through Final Fit software to provide a complete aberrometric optimization of the ablated corneal profile. The NIDEK Final Fit software presents the surgeon with the preoperative situation, and with the ablation divided in the sphere, cylinder, and irregular component. The software simulates the resulting corneal and examines its topographical features, thus providing information on the actual resulting optical zone. These important features guide the surgeon in defining the proper steps towards the best attainable postoperative cornea. High corneal curvature gradients can be modulated. The surgeon can choose among a family of curves expressing different ablation profiles and leading to different spherical aberrations that can be used in situations such as retreatments.

This new way to perform customized ablation works distributing the curvature change with a more gradual and peripheral pattern. The CATZ ablation pattern of the Final Fit optimizes all OPD-detected ocular aberrations in the central 4.5-mm, particularly spherical aberrations. The curvature of the remaining cornea is then gradually modified in order to achieve a constant curvature gradient up to the external 10-mm margin of the ablation, maintaining at the same time the best possible reduction of ocular aberrations. An advanced use of Final Fit was adopted for custom ablation in our study. The segmental ablation for treatment of high-order components was applied first. This part of the treatment may change axis and power of the cylinder, thus at this point the new axis and power of astigmatism were estimated (see Chapter 11). Finally, the resulting spherical component to be treated was calculated.

This surgical method offers several advantages. The amount of tissue removed was limited, even with a wide final transition zone diameter, and it was distributed all over most of the corneal surface, reducing the biomechanical effect. The final corneal curvature gradient was constant.[18] In conventional myopic ablations, the sudden and marked variation

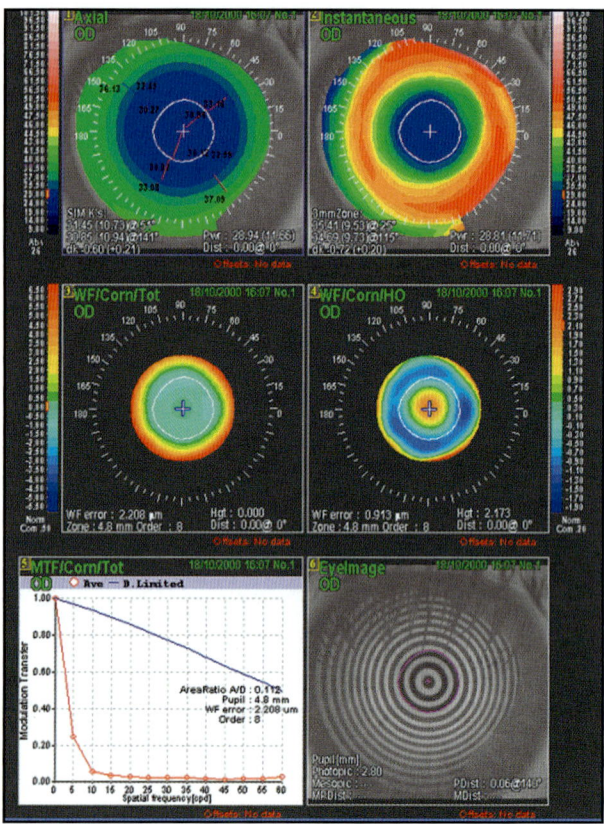

Figure 18-6. Results of custom ablation, conventional. Note how the optical zone is wide (axial, upper left), but the ablation zone is smaller (red ring on instantaneous map, upper right). Aberrometry on corneal wavefront (center right) shows induction of spherical aberration.

in corneal curvature gradient between central treated and peripheral untreated cornea is expressed topographically by a red ring visible on an instantaneous algorhythm as well as by the aberrometric red ring of spherical aberration (Figure 18-6). With Final Fit, the corneal curvature gradient from center to periphery is reduced, made more gradual, and positioned in the extreme periphery, beyond 9 mm, where the cornea is thicker and flatter. Thus, the topographical red ring will appear of limited width and intensity in diopters— not actually red but paler colors—as well as being located very peripherally. Furthermore, spherical aberration will be reduced, providing excellent vision quality even with dilated pupils (Figures 18-7 and 18-8).

Apparently, smoothing at the end of surgery provides a regular stromal bed for the corneal epithelium, reducing collagen deposition as well as haze formation with consequent possible reduction of imparted correction.[9] This has been confirmed by PRK and LASEK studies.[14,19-21] The positive results of LASEK surgery reported in this study are comparable to those of other LASEK studies evaluating a large number of eyes as well as to LASEK with postoperative aberrometric analyses.[1,22-25]

After the introduction of LASIK, surface refractive surgery has received less interest due to observed regression, haze,

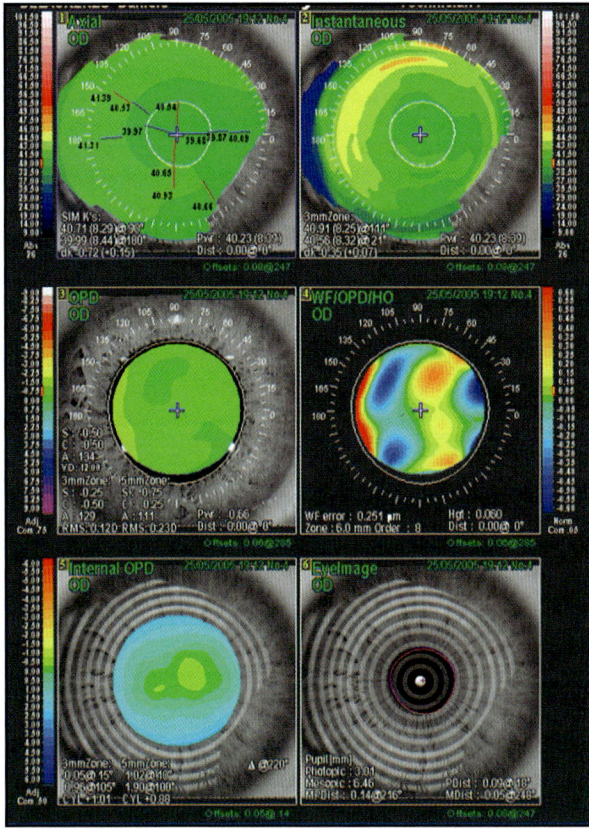

Figure 18-7. Results of custom ablation, NIDEK Final Fit with reduction of corneal curvature gradient from center to periphery, inconspicuous red ring on instantaneous (upper right) and no spherical aberration on wavefront maps (center).

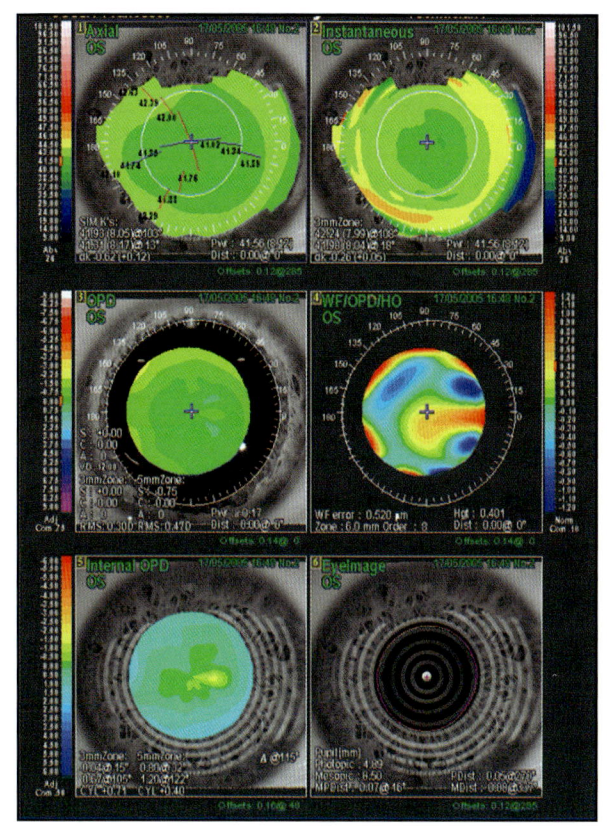

Figure 18-8. Another case of custom ablation, NIDEK Final Fit with reduction of corneal curvature gradient from center to periphery.

and postoperative pain. However, due to possible variations in flap size and thickness, the biomechanical factor at play in LASIK may render custom ablation less predictable, as well as making containment of induction of aberrations less effective. The risk of late-onset postoperative corneal ectasia remains a rare but troublesome possibility.[26]

With the advent of LASIK, surface excimer laser refractive surgery was abandoned mostly due to problems related to postoperative pain, haze formation, regression, and poor vision. Nevertheless, it retained part of its interest because it offered advantages such as a wider range of refractive correction and easier retreatments due to contained stromal tissue that the ablation maintained. It would appear that by creating a regular postoperative surface with smoothing haze formation can be contained, the regression problem can now be solved by treating the transition zone differently and a better understanding of biomechanical forces at play in the cornea. If confirmed by further studies, it is our opinion that the refractive surgery strategy presented in this paper may increase the recently renewed interest in surface refractive surgery.

References

1. Yul SK, Bum LJ, Jaeyoung KJ, et al. Comparison of higher-order aberrations after LASEK with a 6.0 mm ablation zone and a 6.5 mm ablation zone with blend zone. *J Cataract Refract Surg.* 2004;30:653-657.
2. Gimbel HV, Sofinski SJ, Mahler OS, et al. Primary multipoint (segmental) custom ablation. *J Refract Surg.* 2003;19:S202-208.
3. Sarkisian KA, Petrov AA. Clinical experience with the customized low spherical aberration ablation profile for myopia. *J Refract Surg.* 2002;18:S352-356.
4. Marcos S, Barbero S, Llorente L, Merayo-Lloves J. Optical response to LASIK surgery for myopia from total and corneal aberration measurements. *Invest Ophthalmol Vis Sci.* 2001;42:3349-3356.
5. Marcos S. Aberrations and visual performance following standard laser vision correction. *J Refract Surg.* 2001;17:S596-601.
6. Huang D, Tang M, Shekhar R. Mathematical model of corneal surface smoothing after refractive surgery. *Am J Ophthalmol.* 2003;135:267-278.
7. Balestrazzi E, De Molfetta V, Spadea L, et al. Histological, immunohistochemical, and ultrastructural findings in humans corneas after photorefractive keratectomy. *J Refract Surg.* 1995;11:181-187.
8. Vinciguerra P, Azzolini M, Radice P, et al. A method for examining surface and interface irregularities after photorefractive keratectomy and laser in situ keratomileusis: predictor of optical and functional outcomes. *J Refract Surg.* 1998;14:S204-206.
9. Vinciguerra P, Azzolini M, Airaghi P, et al. Effect of decreasing surface and interface irregularities after photorefractive keratectomy and laser in situ keratomileusis on optical and functional outcomes. *J Refract Surg.* 1998;14:S199-S203.

10. Netto MV, Mohan RR, Sinha S, Sharma A, Wilson SE. Stromal haze, myofibroblasts, and surface irregularity after PRK. *Exp Eye Res.* 2005;19 (in press).
11. Vinciguerra P, Camesasca FI, Torres I. One-year results of custom laser epithelial keratomileusis with the NIDEK system. *J Refract Surg.* 2004;20:S699-7040.
12. Vinciguerra P, Camesasca FI, Ponzin D. Use of amino acids in refractive surgery. *J Refract Surg.* 2002;18:S374-377.
13. Vinciguerra P, Camesasca FI. Butterfly laser epithelial keratomileusis for myopia. *J Refract Surg.* 2002;18:S371-373.
14. Vinciguerra P, Camesasca FI, Randazzo A. One-year results of butterfly laser epithelial keratomileusis. *J Refract Surg.* 2003;19:S223-226.
15. Epstein D, Fagerholm P, Hamberg-Nyström H, Tengroth B. Twenty-four-month follow-up of excimer laser photorefractive keratectomy for myopia. Refractive and visual acuity results. *Ophthalmology.* 1994;101:1558-1564.
16. Oshika T, Klyce SD, Applegate AR, et al. Comparison of corneal wavefront aberrations after photorefractive keratectomy and laser in situ keratomileusis. *Am J Ophthalmol.* 1999;127:1-7.
17. Roberts C. Biomechanics of the cornea and wavefront-guided laser refractive surgery. *J Refract Surg.* 2002;18:S589-592.
18. Vinciguerra P, Camesasca FI, Torres I. Transition zone design and smoothing in custom laser-assisted subepithelial keratectomy. *J Cataract Refract Surg.* 2005;31:39-47.
19. Vinciguerra P, Torres I, Camesasca FI. Applications of confocal microscopy in refractive surgery. *J Refract Surg.* 2002;18:S378-381.
20. Vinciguerra P, Camesasca FI. Treatment of hyperopia: a new ablation profile to reduce corneal eccentricity. *J Refract Surg.* 2002;18:S315-317.
21. Vinciguerra P, Camesasca FI, Urso R. Reduction of spherical aberration with the Nidek NAVEX customized ablation system. *J Refract Surg.* 2003;19:S195-S201.
22. Autrata R, Rehurek J. Laser-assisted subepithelial keratectomy for myopia: two-year follow up. *J Cataract Refract Surg.* 2003;29:661-668.
23. Shahinian L Jr. Laser-assisted subepithelial keratectomy for low to high myopia and astigmatism. *J Cataract Refract Surg.* 2002;28:1334-1342.
24. Anderson NJ, Beran RF, Schneider TL. Epi-LASEK for the correction of myopia and myopic astigmatism. *J Cataract Refract Surg.* 2002;28:1343-1347.
25. Claringbold TV. Laser-assisted subepithelial keratectomy for the correction of myopia. *J Cataract Refract Surg.* 2002;28:18-22.
26. Wang Z, Chen J, Yang B. Posterior corneal surface topographic changes after Laser In Situ Keratomileusis are related to residual corneal bed thickness. *Ophthalmology.* 1999;106:406-410.

CHAPTER 19

REFRACTIVE, ABERROMETRIC, AND PACHYMETRIC STABILITY AND PATIENT'S SATISFACTION IN REFRACTIVE STATUS AND VISION PROFILE AFTER CUSTOMIZED TREATMENT

Mario R. Romano, MD

Introduction

In the last few years, there has been an increasing interest in the personalization of photoablative corneal treatment to correct refractive errors. Aberrometry has thus become a new diagnostic instrument in refractive surgery.[1] The concept of personalized correction on the wavefront has become of topical interest with the result that attempts are made to correct optical defects, too, such as coma, oblique astigmatism, and other Seidel aberrations beyond the low radial orders;[2] just some years ago, these concepts were confined to theory and not to clinical practice. Customized ablation aims at optimizing the optical system through the use of spherical, cylindrical, and asymmetric treatments with aspheric profile. The parameters coming into play in the planning of an appropriate customized aspherical profile are manifold, and include anatomic factors (corneal thicknesses, pupillometry, AC depth), optical factors (corneal topography, wavefront measurement), and the individual patient's preferences and requirements (presbyopia, occupation, psychological tolerance).

The introduction of a photoablative refractive surgery of this kind has produced a radical change in the approach to the eye optical system. In this complex process, which includes several variables and whose final aim is the optimization of the patient's aberrometric and visual results, the only variable we can control is the ablation algorithm. The goal is to get an ablation algorithm purposing the most appropriate tissue removal based on topographical and/or aberrometric links in order to get homogeneous and stable ablation profiles. If we assume that the planning of our treatment is suitable to the aberrometric/refractive error we want to correct, it is natural to ask ourselves what follows: how much of the planning of an appropriate customized treatment will turn into a real advantage for the patient in terms of vision quality? Can the results in terms of aberrations and satisfaction got by the patient in the first months be considered stable? The excimer laser induces biomechanical structural changes to the cornea, correlated in a nonlinear way to the ablation depth and the number of the ablated lamellas.[3] Therefore the corneal biomechanical structure involves some predictability limits on the real form of the cornea after the photoablative procedure. Could a more homogeneous profile, such as the customized one, make the corneal response after the photoablative treatment more predictable? Can an aspherical profile with a smaller peripheric thickening influence the changes on the corneal central curvature in the long run?

This chapter deals with aims at analyzing the results obtained after customized treatment by NIDEK EC5000 (Gamagori, Japan) compared to the results from a standard multizone isodioptric treatment. The efficacy, the reliability, and the stability of the refractive, aberrometric, and pachymetric results compared in the long run shall be evaluated. We shall further evaluate the patient's satisfaction index and, above all, the subjective troubles that mostly affect the daily activities of the patients who underwent a customized treatment.

Efficacy and Safety of Customized Treatment

At present, photorefractive surgery (PRK) is considered an effective method to correct refractive errors, assuring the possibility to be successfully repeated and avoid postoperative regressions[4] and haze.[5] Last generation customized treatments, in particular, myopic treatments, further reduce the incidence of these unfavorable events. Thus, we carried out a

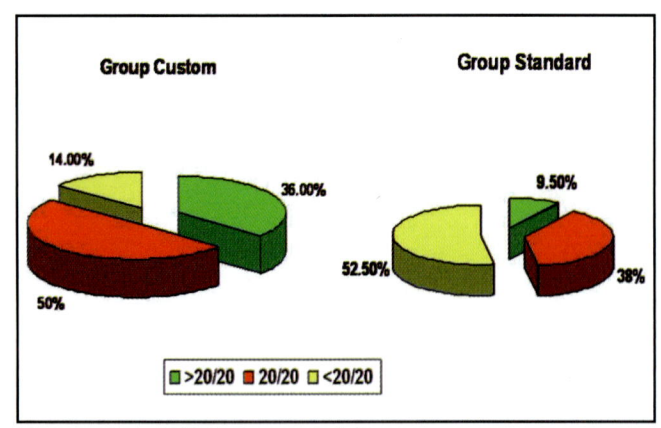

Figure 19-1. UCVA 1-month follow-up.

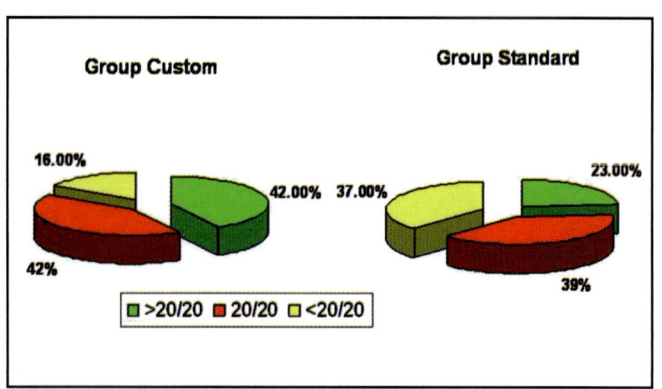

Figure 19-2. UCVA 18-months follow-up.

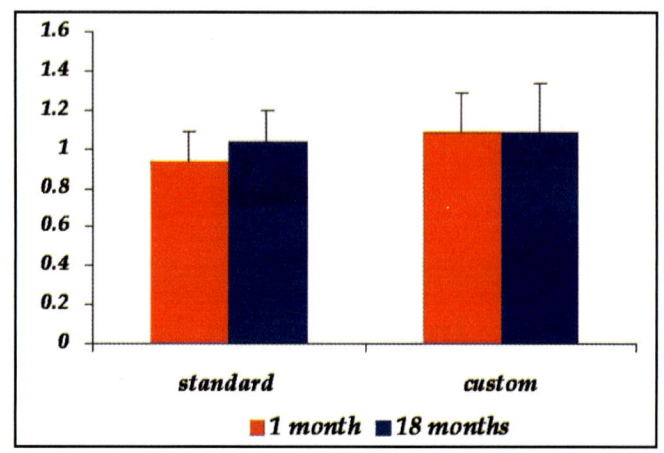

Figure 19-3. The efficacy index of the treatment at 1-month follow-up is less than 1 in the standard group, but at 18-month follow-up it was over 1 and reached the custom group.

perspective randomized clinical study in order to determine the efficacy, reliability, and stability of the customized treatment vs the standard one—both were performed with the NIDEK EC5000. The study was carried out on 54 eyes of 27 patients, who were randomized in two groups:

1. The custom group included 27 eyes (mean spherical equivalent refraction -3.26 ± 1.35 D; range -1.75 to -6.5 D) treated with the custom guided corneal ablation system by NIDEK, which included OPD-Scan, Final Fit program, and Nidek Multipoint EC5000 excimer laser. A custom ablation transition zone (CATZ) was used in all eyes (profile 4) with large transition zone (10 mm).

2. The standard group included 27 eyes (mean spherical equivalent refraction -4.78 ± 2.95 D; range -2.0 to -12.0 D) that underwent conventional PRK using the same laser, with multizone isodioptric photoablative strategy with step of 0.3 mm and transition zone of 2.5 mm.

In both groups, we performed visual acuity, manifest refraction, wavefront analysis, and pachimetry preoperatively and postoperatively at 1 and 18 months. The Refractive Status and Vision Profile (RSVP) was self-administered by participants at each control.[6-7] The RSVP is a questionnaire that measures self-reported vision-related health status (symptoms, functioning, expectations, and concern) in persons with refractive error. We measured scores on overall RSVP scale and on eight RSVP subscales (functioning, driving, concern, expectations, symptoms, glare, optical problems, and problems with corrective lens). There were no statistically significant differences between the customized ablation groups in terms of preoperative uncorrected visual acuity (UCVA) and best spectacle corrected visual acuity (BSCVA). At 1-month follow-up in the standard group, the mean spherical equivalent refraction was -0.006 ± 0.3739 D with UCVA of 0.92 ± 0.13 D and BSCVA of 1.005 ± 0.12 D, and in the custom group, the mean spherical equivalent refraction was -0.0284 ± 0.267 D with UCVA of 1.07 ± 0.26 D and BSCVA of 1.182 ± 0.211 D. In the standard group, the UCVA of the eyes was >20/20 in 9.5%, = 20/20 in 38%, and <20/20 in 52.5%; in the custom group, the UCVA of the eyes was >20/20 in 36%, =20/20 in 50%, and <20/20 in 14% (Figure 19-1). At 18-months follow-up in the standard group,

the mean spherical equivalent refraction was -0.044 ± 0.223 D with UCVA of 1.01 ± 0.19 D and BSCVA of 1.05 ± 0.14 D; in the custom group, the mean spherical equivalent refraction was -0.021 ± 0.26 D with UCVA of 1.01 ± 0.25 D and BSCVA of 1.143 ± 0.206 D. In the standard group, the UCVA of the eyes was >20/20 in 23%, =20/20 in 38.5%, and <20/20 in 38.5%; in the custom group, the UCVA of the eyes was >20/20 in 42%, =20/20 in 42%, and <20/20 in 16% (Figure 19-2). The efficacy index (UCVA postop/BSCVA preop) of the treatment was at 1-month follow-up 0.93 in the standard group and 1.08 in the custom group. At 18-months follow-up, it was 1.08 in the standard group and 1.08 in the custom group (Figure 19-3). The safety index (BSCVA postop/BSCVA preop) of the treatment at 1-month follow-up was 1.07 in the standard group and 1.22 in the custom group. At 18-months follow-up, it was 1.02 in the standard group and 1.26 in the custom group (Figure 19-4). The differences in spherical equivalent refractive error observed in the two groups at 1 month (P>0.05) and 18 months (P>0.05) following surgery were not statistically significant. Therefore, the amount of eyes having a visual acuity ≥20/20 at 1-month follow-up was 47.5% in the standard group vs 86% of the custom group; the numbers reached at 18-month follow-up was 62% in the standard group vs 84% of the custom group. In the same way, the

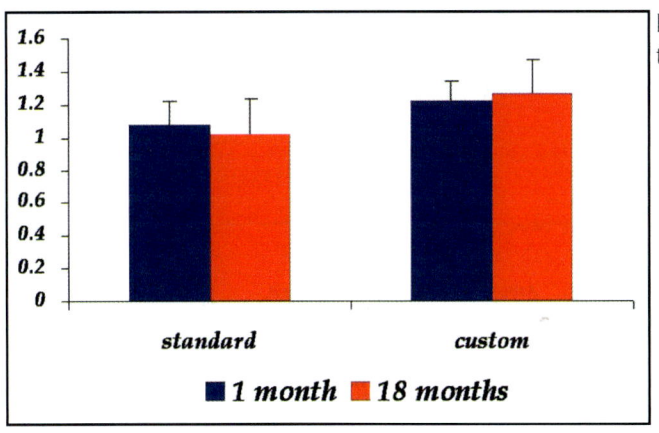

Figure 19-4. The safety index was over 1 in both groups from the first control.

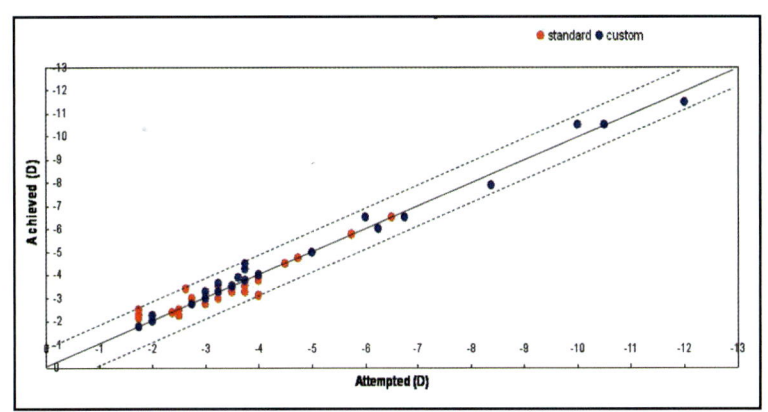

Figure 19-5. The scattergram of the attempted versus achieved correction after 18 months shows a high predictability of the refractive results which were within ±1.0 D.

efficacy index of the treatment at 1-month follow-up was less than 1, and at 18-months follow-up it was over 1 and reached the custom group. The safety index was over 1 in both groups from the first control. The scattergram of the attempted versus achieved correction after 18 months for both groups is shown in Figure 19-5. It shows a slight overcorrection of the refractive target in the custom group as opposed to a slight undercorrection in the standard group; both groups show a high predictability of the refractive results that were within ±1.0 D. The difference between regression coefficient values was not statistically significant (P>0.05). We can therefore assert that photoablative strategies are both efficacious and reliable, with a long-term predictability. Moreover, we found that the custom group reached a refractive stability and an efficacy over 1 already in the first month after surgery.

Wavefront Error After Customized Treatment

After PRK, high-order aberrations increase significantly.[8-9] We performed the custom guided corneal ablation (by CATZ) with expectation of a reduction of increase in ocular aberrations in the custom group as compared to the standard one. In particular, we compared the single low order and high-order aberrations in both groups. Furthermore, we measured how the root mean square (RMS) error changes from 1 to 18 months after surgery in both groups. In a comparison of Zernike polynomials, the increase of postoperative defocus, astigmatism of second radial order, coma of third radial order, spherical aberration of fourth radial order, and high-order aberration in customized ablation group was smaller than those in the conventional ablation group at 1 month (Figure 19-6) and 18 months (Figure 19-7) follow-up, but they did not reach statistical significance (P>0.05). An interesting datum noticed by us is the RMS error change from the first to the 18th month after surgery above all in the standard group. As a matter of fact, each of the aberrations considered by us showed a stable progress up to 18-month follow-up in the custom group, while in the standard group it had a more unpredictable profile which tended to an RMS error smaller than the one of the first month after surgery (Figure 19-8). Therefore, the custom group reached a stability of the aberrometric error earlier than the standard group, which resulted in an efficacy and refractive stability of the custom group from the first month after surgery.

Depth of the Laser Photoablation

In researching the ideal corneal ablation, the main parameter to be considered is given by the corneal thickness available to photoablation. The present ablation algorithms have the dual purpose of keeping an ablation profile with a coefficient of aspherical aberration as physiological as possible

Figure 19-6. The RMS error in the customized ablation group is smaller than that in the conventional ablation group at 1-month follow-up.

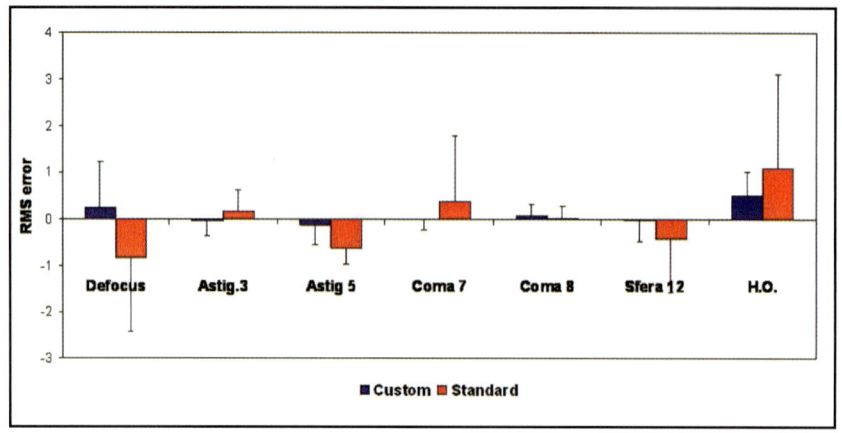

Figure 19-7. RMS error at 18-month follow-up.

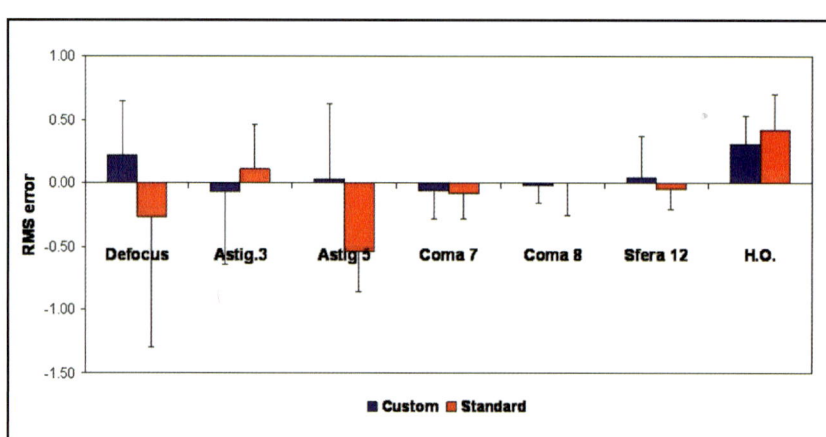

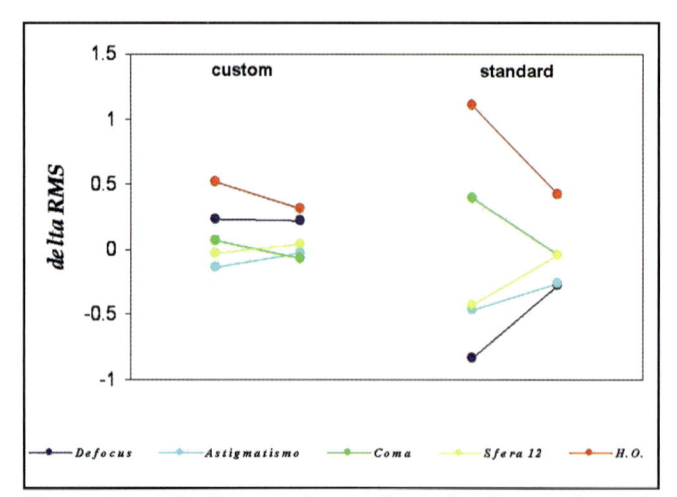

Figure 19-8. RMS error change from the first to the 18th month after surgery above all in the standard group.

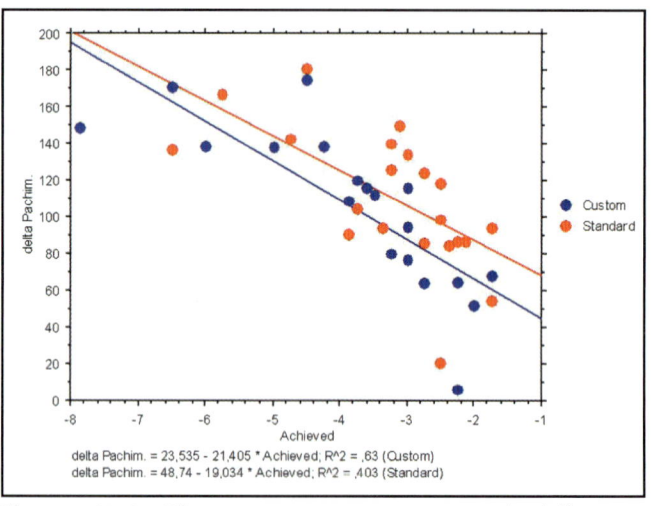

Figure 19-9. The scattergram at 18-month follow-up showed that the intercept had a lower mean value in the custom group, but the difference of regression coefficient in both groups is not statistically significant ($P>0.05$).

while limiting the depth of the photoablated corneal tissue. The present ablation algorithms are not based on the simple geometric approach of tissue removal and secondary variation of curvature (Munnerlyn model). They aim at a customized profile of aspherical type in order to limit the increase in aberrations after surgery and to respect the potential biomechanical changes, which can have a significant impact on the curvature variations within the ablation zone.[3] In order to evaluate the ablation depth both in the custom and in the standard group, we determined the correlation between the photoablated pachymetric thicknesses and the corrected refractive error (Figure 19-9). The scattergram at 18-month follow-up showed that the intercept had a lower mean value in the custom group (custom a = 23.53 vs standard a = 48.74), which means that the initial photoablated corneal thicknesses are lower in the custom group. Therefore, we can start from

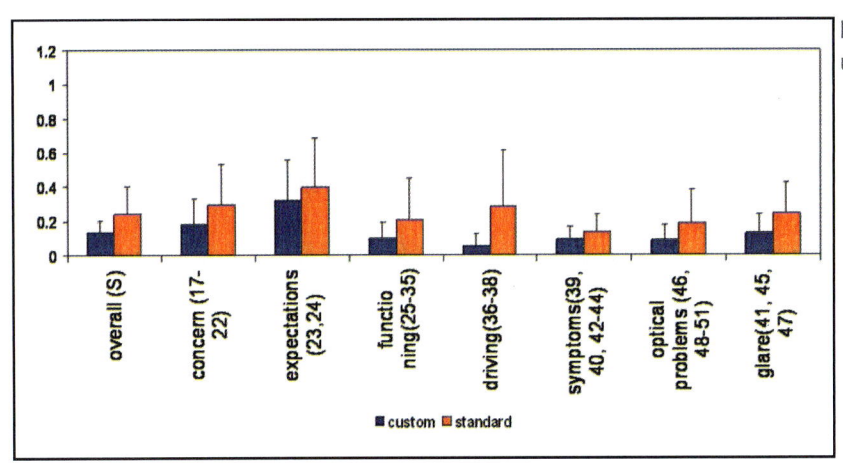

Figure 19-10. RSVP data at 1-month follow-up.

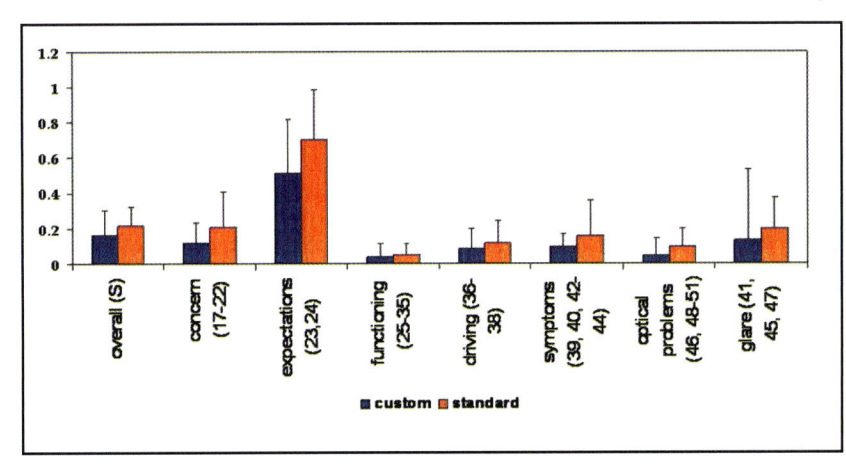

Figure 19-11. The RSVP at 18-month follow-up, the subjective symptomatology stays lower in the custom group.

ablation optical zones with smaller diameters. Furthermore, we can see that the regression coefficient was 21.405 in the custom group and 19.034 in the standard group, but the difference between said values was not statistically significant (P>0.05). This means that the photoablated corneal thicknesses tend to be the same in both groups, with the advantage that in the custom group we start from small optical zones and keep wide transition zones (10 mm) allowing us an aspherical profile and a higher respect of the biomechanical structural changes of the cornea.

Refractive Status and Vision Profile

Research has shown that patient-reported assessments of functioning, satisfaction, and symptoms capture aspects not detected by traditional clinical measures of the need for outcomes of surgery.[10] At present, we realize the necessity of a subjective systematic evaluation of refractive surgery candidates in order to compare the results received in connection with different therapeutic options. Reduced visual performance after refractive corneal surgery, halos, and loss of contrast visual acuity are attributed to an increase in optical aberrations from refractive surgery. The main goal of our study was to evaluate how the refractive results and the variations of induced aberrations can affect the patients' symptomatology. Patients had to answer a questionnaire named RSVP,[6-7] which is a questionnaire that measures self-reported, vision-related health status in persons with refractive error. Items are grouped into domains based on judgments regarding the particular aspect of health-related quality of life.[11] These areas include functioning (ability to carry out activities in daily life), symptoms (sensations experienced by an individual), health perceptions (satisfaction with health), and expectations (beliefs about future health states). Figure 19-10 shows the RSVP data at 1-month follow-up. The custom group shows a subjective symptomatology lower than in the standard group in each domain, above all, in the ones concerning the functioning (P>0.05), driving (P<0.05), and glare (P>0.05). At 18-months follow-up, the subjective symptomatology stays lower in the custom group, but the differences between the two groups are fewer (Figure 19-11). As a matter of fact, at 18-months follow-up, the score on overall RSVP scale and on each RSVP subscale decreases, whereas the score of each subscale in the custom group is stable. Hence, these data show a greater subjective satisfaction of the patient in the custom group compared to the one in the standard group. In the latter, however, there is a long-term subjective improvement, which is almost the same as in the custom group. Such data can be considered in line with what was previously seen in the change of the aberrations and the efficacy of the standard treatment at 18-months follow-up. In other words, the custom treatment reaches refraction and a stable aberrometric error from the first month after surgery, whereas the standard group requires a longer time to make the aberrometric and refractive result stable. Afterwards, there is a parallel improvement of the patient's subjective symptomatology and satisfaction.

groups was not statistically significant in terms of treatment efficacy, aberrations, and symptomatology. However, in the custom group we saw a tendency to a greater satisfaction in line with a lower RMS error and with a stable efficacy from the first month.

Conclusions

It is known that the cornea responds biomechanically to the structural changes induced by refractive surgery by excimer laser in correlation with the number of ablated lamellas.[3] The fact that there are two forces (besides the one exerted by the simple tissue removal) that come into play in the determination of the final cornea form is well known. In addition to the biomechanical response of the cornea, the epithelial hyperplasia and the ablation profile affect the final form of the cornea.

The present study has shown that the postoperative refraction and RMS error continue to be unstable for up 18 months after conventional ablation (standard group). Such observations have been confirmed by other studies of PRK, which have shown that refractive stability was achieved between 6 months and 1 year.[12] The instability observed in our series treated in a conventional way might be due to topographic steepening, which is followed by a slight epithelial hyperplasia. A literature review of corneal wound healing demonstrated that the improved outcome and stability of refraction were the slope of the wound surface over the entire area of the ablation.[13] Small ablation zones with a greater rate of change in power at the edge of the ablation zone were associated with an increase in epithelial hyperplasia.[14]

Our treatments for the custom group were customized at the corneal surface in order to make the profile as homogeneous as possible. We elected not to correct the internal aberrations, when their correction might have caused a imperfect regular corneal profile. Therefore, we applied a custom ablation transition zone (CATZ), getting aspherical surfaces with a homogeneous ablation profile and wide optical zones. As a result, the custom treatment proved to be efficacious and, most of all, stable in refractive and aberrometric terms from the first month after surgery. The difference between both

References

1. Mierdel P, Wiegard W, Krinke HE, Kaemner M, Seirler T. Measuring device for determining monochromatic aberrations of the human eye. *Ophthalmology.* 1997;6:441-445.
2. McDonald MB. Summit Autonomus custom cornea LASIK outcomes. *J Refract Surg.* 2000;16:S617-618.
3. Roberts C, Mahmoud A, Herderick EE, Chan G. Characterization of cornea curvature changes inside and outside the ablation zone in LASIK. Abstract. *Invest Ophathalmol Vis Sci.* 2000;4:S679.
4. Pietila J, Makinen P, Uusitolo H. Repeated photorefractive keratectomy for undercorrection and regression. *J Refract Surg.* 2002;18:155-161.
5. Sigonos DS, Katsanevaki VJ, Pallicaris IG. Correlation of subepithelial haze and refractive regression 1 month after photorefractive keratectomy for myopia. *J Refract Surg.* 1999;15: 338-342.
6. Vitale S, Shein OD, Meinert CL, Steinberg EP. A questionnaire to measure vision-related quality of life in persons with refractive error. *Ophthalmology.* 2000;107:1529-1539.
7. Schein OD, Vitale S, Cassard SD, Steinberg EB. Patient outcomes of refractive surgery. The refractive status band vision profile. *J Cataract Refract Surgery.* 2001;27:665-673.
8. Thibos LN, Hong X. Clinical applications of Shack-Hartmann aberrometer. *Optom Vis Sci.* 1999;76:817-825.
9. Seiler T, Kaemmerer M, Mierdel P, Krinke H-E. Ocular optical aberration after photorefractive keratectomy for myopia and myopic astigmatism. *Arch Ophthalmol.* 2000;118:17-21.
10. Steinberg EP, Tielsch JM, Schein OD, et al. The UF-14. An index of functional impairment in patients with cataract. *Arch Ophthalmol.* 1994;112:630-638.
11. Patrick DL, Erickson P. *Health Status and Health Policy: Quality of Life in Health Care Evaluation and Resource Allocation.* New York, NY: Oxford University Press; 1993:76-106.
12. Nakamishi M, Suzuki M, Shimizu K. Long-term clinical course of excimer laser photorefractive keratectomy. *Nippon Gauka Gakkai Zasshi.* 2003;107:94-98.
13. Corbett MC, Verma S, O'Brart DP, et al. Effect of ablation profile on wound healing and visual performance 1 year after excimer laser photorefractive keratectomy. *Br J Ophthalmol.* 1996;80(3):224-234.
14. Hamberg-Nystrom H, Gauthier CA, Holden BA, et al. A comparative study of epithelial hyperplasia after PRK: Summit versus VISX in the same patient. *Acta Ophthalmol Scand.* 1996;74(3):228-231.

CHAPTER 20

ADVANCED SURFACE ABLATIONS FOR MYOPIA: EPI-LASIK

Vikentia J. Katsanevaki, MD, PhD; Maria I. Kalyvianaki, MD;
Irini I. Naoumidi, PhD; Ioannis G. Pallikaris, MD, PhD

Laser in situ keratomileusis (LASIK) has been widely accepted and is currently the most popular surgical approach for the photorefractive correction of ametropias, providing fast visual recovery and minimal postoperative discomfort.[1,2] However, complications that have been related[3-8] to the method, such as flap-related complications, dry eye, reported postoperative mechanical instability of the cornea, and vision-threatening inflammations have turned many surgeons back to surface ablation.

Advanced surface ablations refer to photorefractive surface surgical modalities that were developed to manage the drawbacks of traditional photorefractive keratectomy (PRK)[9,10] (ie, the postoperative pain and the formation of subepithelial haze).

Laser assisted subepithelial keratectomy (LASEK)[11] was the first procedure that involved preservation of the epithelium in order to control corneal wound healing. The procedure involves the use of an alcohol solution for the successful *en toto* separation of the epithelium as a sheet. The ablation takes place on the exposed stroma and the epithelial flap is then repositioned on the top of the cornea. Although the beneficial effect of the replaced epithelial sheet (as compared to the conventional PRK method) is still is still under question,[26] many studies[12-22] have shown LASEK to be a safe and effective approach for the correction of myopia and myopic astigmatism, proposing LASEK to be superior to PRK. Drawbacks of LASEK that have been reported are the dose- and time-dependent[25] toxic effect of alcohol on the corneal epithelium,[23,24] the interpatient variability of the ease of making epithelial flaps[26] necessitating variable application times of the alcohol solution,[27] and the long learning curve[28] of the technique.

Epi-LASIK[29-31] as an amalgam of LASIK and surface treatment much like LASEK also involves preservation of an intact epithelial sheet in order to control corneal wound healing. In Epi-LASIK however, the epithelial separation is achieved by means of a customized device that can achieve the successful epithelial separation mechanically without requiring the use of alcohol. As compared to LASEK, Epi-LASIK provides a completely automated way to perform advanced surface ablation and avoids the toxic effect of alcohol on the separated epithelium.

Histological Findings of Mechanically Separated Epithelial Sheets

During the evolution of Epi-LASIK, one of the initial goals was to determine whether mechanical separation provided any advantages as compared to alcohol-assisted separated epithelial sheets.

In a study that was conducted in the University of Crete, we cross-examined epithelial sheets that were obtained either with corneal preparation with alcohol or after mechanical separation using a prototype device. We found that due to a shallower cleavage plane, the basement membrane of alcohol-assisted epithelial sheets was destroyed upon separation—a finding that was also confirmed by other investigators.14,[32] However, transmission electron microscopy of mechanically separated sheets showed that mechanical separation of the corneal epithelium preserved the epithelial basement membrane, providing a slightly deeper cleavage plane as compared to that of alcohol[29] (Figure 20-1). As has been shown by in vitro studies,[33] the presence of an intact basement membrane is important for the control of corneal wound healing, thereby minimizing the fibrotic activation of keratocytes. Under this consideration, we assume that mechanically separated epithelial sheets are expected to be more effective in the

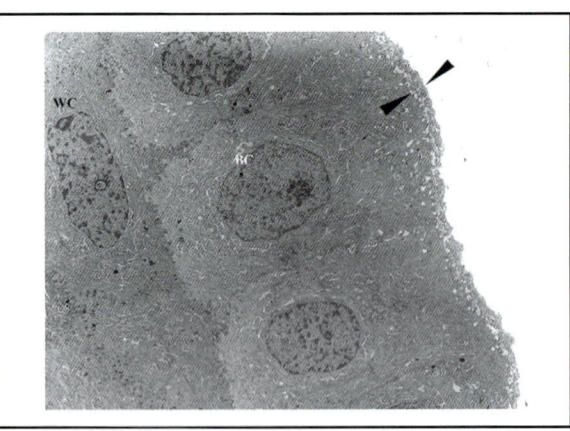

Figure 20-1. Electron microscopy of the basal part of the epithelial sheet. A small portion of Bowman's is included within the sheet (between arrows). BC = Basal cells. WC = Wing cells.

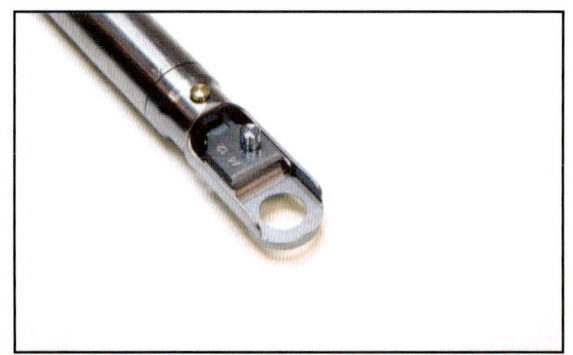

Figure 20-2. Centurion SES Epikeratome for epithelial separations (Norwood Abbey, Australia).

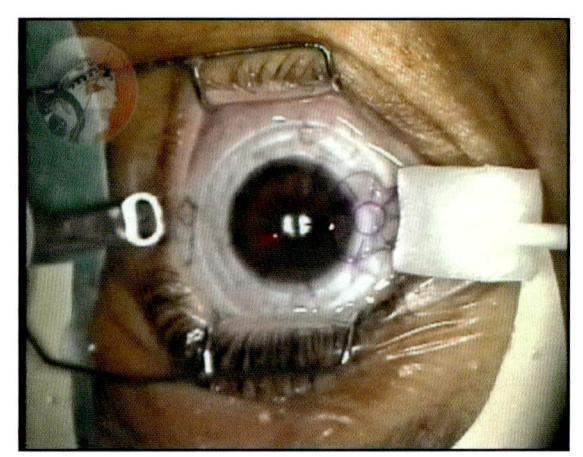

Figure 20-3. Manipulation on the epithelial flap with a moistened Merocel sponge.

control of postoperative inflammation and corneal wound response after photorefractive keratectomy as compared to those separated with alcohol.

Furthermore, the basement membrane is important for the viability of the epithelial sheet that is expected to act as a mechanical barrier between the corneal stroma and the tear film after the surgery. A histopathology study of a small number of sheets that were harvested and examined 24 hours after the surgery[34] showed that the epithelium was morphologically viable at that interval. Although it is clinically evident that the replacement of the epithelial sheet does not cancel the migratory phase of epithelial healing and that it is replaced within the first days after the surgery, histopathology data provide supporting evidence that at least for the first postoperative hours, the mechanically separated sheets remain viable, providing a "living contact lens" to cover the ablated cornea.

Epi-LASIK: The Surgical Technique

The operative eye is prepared with povidone-iodine and 3 drops of topical tetracaine hydrochloride 0.5% (applied every 5 minutes before the procedure) and is covered with a sterile drape.

The epithelial separations are currently performed in our center with the use of a commercially available epithelial separator (Centurion EpiEdge Epikeratome, Norwood Abbey, Australia), which is an electrically powered device (Figure 20-2) that operates under low suction in a manner similar to a conventional microkeratome. Instead of a blade, it features a disposable, oscillating polymethylmethacrylate (PMMA) separator with an advance speed of 3.5 mm/sec. The resulting separated epithelial sheet has a nasal hinge and a diameter of 9.5 to 10 mm.

Although the replacement of the epithelial sheet is not mandatory as with the classic LASIK flap, preoperative corneal marking enables the surgeon to replace of epithelium without any stress. Before the epithelial separation, the cornea is marked with a customized marker (Epi-LASIK marker, Duckworth & Kent, Baldock, UK) that features two concentric circles crossed by eight radial arms. Upon the replacement of the epithelial sheet, any deformity of the concentric circles dictates the sheet's proper repositioning.

The manipulations on the epithelial flap can be conducted either by a moistened Merocel sponge (Medtronic, Jacksonville, Fla) (Figure 20-3) or a customized spatula (Epi-LASIK spatula, Duckworth & Kent, Baldock, UK). The lift and the replacement of the separated epithelial sheet are often achieved with a single movement. Any inward or outward folds of its edges can be restored with the use of the spatula after irrigation with balanced salt solution. Once the epithelial sheet is stuck to the underlying stroma in accordance with the preoperative marks, a therapeutic contact lens is applied onto the operative eye (Figure 20-4).

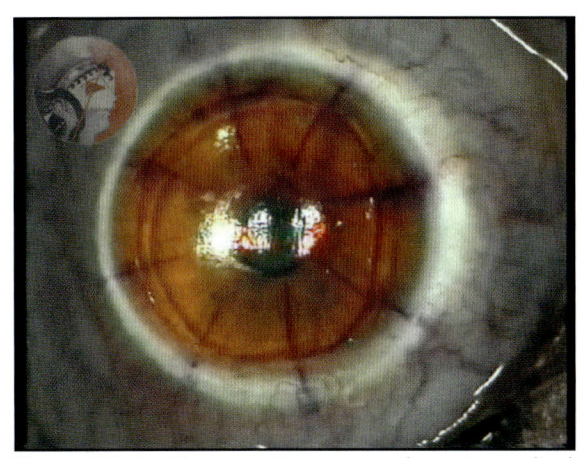

Figure 20-4. Therapeutic contact lens is applied onto the operative eye.

Clinical Results After Myopic Epi-LASIK

Early Postoperative Course

At the end of the surgery, the replaced epithelial sheet often overlays its initial gutter, probably due to the intraoperative mechanical stretch on the epithelial sheet upon separation. Immediately after the operation the epithelial sheet is transparent. During the healing process of the corneal surface, the borders between the newly synthesized epithelium and the remnants of the separated sheet are easily observed at slit lamp biomicroscopy. The migrating cells gradually replace the separated epithelial sheet, which is subsequently constricted in the central area. Starting from its peripheral part around the edges, on the first postoperative day, the sheet becomes hazy in its total area until about the third day after the treatment. At that time, the hazy area measures about the central 1 to 2 mm, whereas a front of newly synthesized, transparent epithelium migrates from the corneal periphery toward the center of the corneal surface. After that stage, the transparency of the corneal epithelium is restored within 24 to 48 hours and the therapeutic contact lens is removed. A central healing line is often apparent after the removal of the therapeutic contact lens. The time of epithelial healing ranges from 3 to 5 days between the treated eyes.

As with LASEK,[18,19] Epi-LASIK is not a totally pain-free procedure. Postoperative pain of the treated eyes is currently assessed in our center with the use of a subjective questionnaire that patients grade pain in a scale from 0 to 4 in 2-hour intervals on the operative day and once daily in the following days.

The postoperative regimens after the procedure include eye drops of Diclofenac sodium 0.1% QID for 2 days and combined eye drops of tobramycin-dexamethasone QID until the removal of the therapeutic lens. After the removal of the lens, all treated eyes receive fluorometholone eye drops QID for 5 weeks in a tapered dose. Artificial tears are prescribed for use at the patients' discretion.

In a preliminary study of 44 eyes,[29] we found that 16% of the treated eyes had burning feeling or worse within the first 2 postoperative hours. The pain subsided within the following hours and on the first postoperative day 26% of the eyes had only minor discomfort. In order to deal with this finding, we included intraoperative corneal cooling with the instillation of prefrozen balanced salt solution (BSS) before the epithelial separation and after the ablation. After this alteration of the technique in the more than 200 eyes that we followed, only 12% had a burning feeling that subsided after the first 2 hours after the treatment (data under publication). Even with lower pain grading, however, the vast majority of the patients report mild discomfort and photophobia, especially during the first couple of days after the treatment.

In regard to the visual performance, the mean uncorrected visual acuity (UCVA) of the treated eyes corresponded well with the progress of the epithelial healing and the transparency of the replaced epithelial sheet. More particularly, UCVA is better on the first postoperative day when the epithelial sheet is still transparent. This decreases around the third postoperative day, as the epithelial sheet becomes hazy, and, finally rises again when the epithelial healing is complete. In a series of 243 eyes treated with the wavelight Allegretto for up to -8.0 D, the mean log MAR UCVA on the day of re-epithelization was of 0.25 ± 0.14, ranging from 0.7 to 0.0 according to the placement of the epithelial healing line in regard to the visual axis.

Late Refractive and Visual Results

Since May 2003 when we received the latest version of the separator, we have performed 243 surgeries. The preoperative spherical equivalent of the treated eyes was up to -8.0 D, with cylinder up to -2.25 D.

One year after the treatment, the spherical equivalent of the treated eyes ranged from -1.25 to +0.625D (-0.18 ± 0.6D) with 80.32% of the eyes within 0.5 D (96.72% within 1 D) of the attempted correction having either clear corneas (90%) or clinically insignificant trace haze (10%).

One year after the treatment, 60% of the eyes had line gain of one or more Snellen lines, whereas 2% had 1 line loss of best corrected vision. Contrast sensitivity of the higher examined spatial frequencies was found increased 1 year after the treatment.

Complications

In a series of 403 separations that were performed with the initial version of the epithelial separator up to May 2003, we recorded seven (1.3%) incursions of the separator within the anterior stroma. In all the cases, the incursion was very superficial and the operation was completed in accordance of the placement of the stromal crease in relation to the visual axis. In five eyes, the stromal penetration occurred outside the treatment zone and the operation was completed at the same session as planned, whereas in two eyes, the irregularity implicated the treatment zone and the cases were aborted. The epithelial sheets were carefully replaced and the eyes were treated on a later date with LASIK with no further complications. The eyes were followed for 10 to 14 months. At the last follow-up visit, all the eyes were within 0.5 D of the attempted correction with no loss of BCVA.

Comment

The expected beneficial effect of the replaced epithelial sheet is still controversial. Comparative clinical trials of PRK and LASEK have shown LASEK-treated eyes to have lower pain scores during the first postoperative days and lower haze scores at the first postoperative month[12] and 1 year postoperatively.[13] Litwak et al[27] questioned these results and noticed greater discomfort, longer epithelial healing period, and lower uncorrected visual acuity during the first 3 days in the LASEK-treated eyes. A probable reason could be the longer alcohol application the authors used for the epithelial separation in this study. Two recent prospective, randomized studies[26,35] comparing PRK and LASEK came to no favorable outcome for the latter. Both studies included patients that had one eye treated with LASEK and the contralateral eye treated with PRK. Pirouzian et al[26] studied 30 patients and compared the subjective pain level, the rate of epithelial defect recovery, and the visual acuity in both their eyes. They observed no differences between the LASEK- and the PRK-treated eyes. They noticed a different epithelial healing pattern in both groups, but the time needed for the epithelial healing was similar. They also applied the alcohol solution for 45 seconds and emphasized the unpredictability in the ease of making the epithelial flap during the LASEK procedure. Hashemi et al[35] included 42 patients in their comparative study with spherical equivalent in the range -1.0 to -6.5 D and a follow-up of 3 months. They demonstrated that LASEK was an effective, safe, and predictable technique, but found out that it had no advantages over PRK regarding pain, epithelial healing time, or the refractive or visual outcome. In another study, Lee et al[36] compared epithelial healing, postoperative pain scores, and refractive results following three different epithelial removal techniques: conventional PRK, excimer laser (transepithelial PRK), and alcohol (LASEK). They found no significant differences in clinical outcomes, subepithelial opacity at 6 months postoperatively, and pain scores on the first 2 postoperative days. They noticed the fastest epithelial healing rate in LASEK group. The LASEK group also demonstrated a slight undercorrection probably due to hydration of the cornea. We could assume that the different alcohol concentrations used and the variable duration of alcohol application needed for the epithelial separation result in various effects of alcohol on the epithelial sheet itself and, therefore, different results of the technique.

An issue that has arisen is whether the alcohol-assisted separated epithelial sheet is vital in order to protect the stroma during the epithelial healing process. Some authors supported that a longer period than 20 seconds is sometimes needed for the loosening of the epithelial layer during the LASEK procedure.[17,25,27] Gabler et al[34] showed that after a 45-second exposure to alcohol solution 20%, only half of the epithelial cells remained vital. Therefore, a longer exposure of the cornea to alcohol may be threatening for the viability of the epithelial flap. Hazarbassanov et al[37] used hypertonic saline solution 5% in a group of eyes and 20% alcohol solution in another group to create the epithelial flap and compared the healing time, the visual recovery, and the refractive outcome in both groups. Both techniques showed similar results, but the eyes treated with the hypertonic solution had a faster epithelial healing time than the alcohol treated eyes. The authors concluded that in order to avoid the toxic effect of alcohol on the epithelium and the surrounding tissues, a more epithelium-friendly method is needed. Numerous authors[16-18] agreed that epithelial separation with no use of alcohol would be more preferable.

Our initial clinical results after Epi-LASIK for myopia have shown the efficacy, safety, and predictability of this technique. These results are comparable to many studies of LASEK-treated eyes.[12-22] Epi-LASIK is an alternative method of separating an epithelial sheet with no use of alcohol. Except for avoiding the toxic effect of alcohol on the epithelial sheet and the corneal stroma, Epi-LASIK offers an automated way of epithelial separation with a device that resembles a microkeratome. Therefore, it may have a shorter learning curve than LASEK for an experienced LASIK surgeon.

Since the initial description of Epi-LASIK by Pallikaris and the University of Crete, almost every major microkeratome manufacturing company launched an epikeratome for Epi-LASIK treatments. This response from the industry highlights the necessity within the refractive community for a method that can safely and effectively complement LASIK in the armament of the refractive surgeon. Involvement of more surgeons and analysis of clinical results of a larger number of eyes is expected to clarify the place of Epi-LASIK in the future refractive practice.

References

1. Pallikaris IG, Papatzanaki ME, Siganos DS, Tsilimbaris MK. A corneal flap technique for laser in situ keratomileusis. Human studies. *Arch Ophthalmol*. 1991;109(12):1699-702
2. Hersh PS, Brint SF, Maloney RK, et al. Photorefractive keratectomy versus laser in situ keratomileusis for moderate to high myopia: a randomized prospective study. *Ophthalmology*. 1998;105:1512-1522.
3. Pallikaris IG, Katsanevaki VJ, Panagopoulou SI. Laser in situ keratomileusis intraoperative complications using one type of microkeratome. *Ophthalmology*. 2002;109(1):57-63.
4. Carpel EF, Carlon KH, Shannon S. Folds and striae in laser in situ keratomileusis flaps. *J Refract Surg*. 1999;15(6):687-690.
5. Melki SA, Azar DT. LASIK complications: etiology, management, and prevention. *Surv Ophthalmol*. 2001;(2);46:95-116.
6. Smith RJ, Maloney RK. Diffuse lamellar keratitis. A new syndrome in lamellar refractive surgery. *Ophthalmology*. 1998;105(9):1721-1726.
7. Wang MY, Maloney RK. Epithelial ingrowth after laser in situ keratomileusis. *Am J Ophthalmol*. 2000;129(6):746-751.
8. Pallikaris IG, Kymionis GD, Astyrakakis NI. Corneal ectasia induced by laser in situ keratomileusis. *J Cataract Refract Surg*. 2001;27(11):1796-1802.
9. Seiler T, Wollensak J. Myopic photorefractive keratectomy with excimer laser: one-year follow up. *Ophthalmology*. 1991; 98:1156-1163.

10. Epstein D, Fagerholm P, Hamberg-Nystroem H, Tengroth B. Twenty-four-month follow up of excimer laser photorefractive keratectomy for myopia, refractive, and visual outcome results. *Ophthalmology*. 1994;101:1558-1563.
11. Camellin M, Cimberle M. LASEK technique promising after 1 year of experience. *Ocular Surg News*. 2000;18(1):14-17.
12. Lee JB, Seong GJ, Lee JH, Seo KY, Lee YG, Kim EK. Comparison of laser epithelial keratomileusis and photorefractive keratectomy for low to moderate myopia. *J Cataract Refract Surg*. 2001;27(4):565-570.
13. Shah S, Sebai Sarhan AR, Doyle SJ, et al. The epithelial flap for photorefractive keratectomy. *Br J Opthalmol*. 2001;85:393-396.
14. Azar DT, Ang RT, Lee JB, Kato T, Chen CC, Jain S, Gabison E, Abad JC. Laser subepithelial keratomileusis: electron microscopy and visual outcomes of photorefractive keratectomy. *Curr Opin Ophthalmol*. 2001;12(4):323-328.
15. Camellin M. Laser epithelial keratomileusis for myopia. *J Refract Surg*. 2003;19:666-670.
16. Anderson NJ, Beran RF, Schneider TL. Epi-LASEK for the correction of myopia and myopic astigmatism. *J Cataract Refract Surg*. 2002;28:1343-1347.
17. Claringbold VT. Laser-assisted subepithelial keratectomy for the correction of myopia. *J Cataract Refract Surg*. 2002;28:18-22.
18. Shahinian L. Laser-assisted subepithelial keratectomy for low to high myopia and astigmatism. *J Cataract Refract Surg*. 2002;28:1334-1342.
19. Rouweyha RM, Chuang AZ, Mitra S, Phillips CB, Yee RW. Laser Epithelial Keratomileusis for myopia with the Autonomous Laser. *J Refract Surg*. 2002;18:217-224.
20. Taneri S, Zieske JD, Azar DT. Evolution, techniques, clinical outcomes, and pathophysiology of LASEK: review of the literature. *Surv Ophthalmol*. 2004;49:576-602.
21. Partal AE, Rojas MC, Manche EE. Analysis of the efficacy, predictability and safety of LASEK for myopia and myopic astigmatism using the Technolas 217 excimer laser. *J Cataract Refract Surg*. 2004;30:2138-2144.
22. Taneri S, Feit R, Azar DT. Safety, efficacy and stability indices of LASEK correction in moderate myopia and astigmatism. *J Cataract Refract Surg*. 2004;30:2130-2137.
23. Kamm O. The relation between structure and physiological action of the alcohols. *Journal of the American Pharmaceutical Association*. 1921;10:87-92.
24. Kim SY, Sah WJ, Lim YW, Hahn TW. Twenty percent alcohol toxicity on rabbit corneal epithelial cells: electron microscopic study. *Cornea*. 2002;21(4):388-392.
25. Chen CC, Chang JH, Lee JB, Javier J, Azar DT. Human corneal epithelial cell viability and morphology after dilute alcohol exposure. *Invest Ophthalmol Vis Sci*. 2002;43(8):2593-2602.
26. Pirouzian A, Thornton JA, Ngo S. A randomized prospective clinical trial comparing Laser Subepithelial Keratomileusis and Photorefractive Keratectomy. *Arch Ophthalmol*. 2004;122:11-16.
27. Litwak S, Zadok D, Garcia-de Quevedo V, Robledo N, Chayet AS. Laser-assisted subepithelial keratectomy versus photorefractive keratectomy for the correction of myopia. A prospective comparative study. *J Cataract Refract Surg*. 2002;28:1330-1333.
28. Chalita MR, Tekwani NH, Krueger RR. Laser epithelial keratomileusis: outcome of initial cases performed by an experienced surgeon. *J Refract Surg*. 2003;19:412-415.
29. Pallikaris IG, Naoumidi II, Kalyvianaki MI, Katsanevaki VJ. Epi-LASIK: Comparative histological evaluation of mechanical and alcohol-assisted epithelial separation. *J Cataract Refract Surg*. 2003;29(8):1496-1501.
30. Pallikaris IG, Katsanevaki VJ, Kalyvianaki MI, Naoumidi II. Advances in subepithelial excimer refractive surgery techniques: Epi-LASIK. *Curr Opin Ophthalmol*. 2003;14(4):207-212.
31. Pallikaris IG, Kalyvianaki MI, Katsanevaki VJ, Ginis HS. Preliminary clinical results of an alternative surface ablation procedure. *J Cataract Refract Surg*. 2005;31:879-885.
32. Espana EM, Gruetereich M, Mateo A, Romano AC, Yee SB, Yee RW, Tseng SCG. Cleavage plane of corneal basement membrane components by ethanol exposure in laser-assisted subepithelial keratectomy. *J Cataract Refract Surg*. 2003;29:1192-1197.
33. Stramer BM, Zieske JD, Jung JC, Austin JS, Fini ME. Molecular mechanisms controlling the fibrotic repair phenotype in cornea: implications for surgical outcomes. *Invest Ophthalmol Vis Sci*. 2003;44(10):4237-4246.
34. Katsanevaki VJ, Naoumidi II, Kalyvianaki MI, Pallikaris IG. Epi-LASIK: histological findings of epithelial sheets 24 hours after the treatment. *J Refract Surg*. 2006;22:151-154.
35. Hashemi H, Fotouni A, Foudazi H, Sadeghi N, Payvar S. Prospective, randomized, paired comparison of laser epithelial keratomileusis and photorefractive keratectomy for myopia less than -6.50 diopters. *J Refract Surg*. 2004;20:217-222.
36. Lee HK, Lee KS, Kim JK, et al. Epithelial healing and clinical outcomes in excimer laser photorefractive surgery following three epithelial removal techniques: mechanical, alcohol and excimer laser. *Am J Ophthalmol*. 2005;139:56-63.
37. Hazarbassanov R, Ben-Haim O, Varssano D, et al. Alcohol-vs. hypertonic saline-assisted laser-assisted subepithelial keratectomy. *Arch Ophthalmol*. 2005;123:171-176.
38. Kim JK, Kim SS, Lee HK, Lee IS, et al. Laser in situ keratomileusis versus Laser-assisted subepithelial Keratectomy for the correction of high myopia. *J Cataract Refract Surg*. 2004;30:1405-1411.

CHAPTER 21

LASEK AND Epi-LASIK Excimer Surface Ablation

Elena Albè, MD; Dimitri T. Azar, MD

Various methods of surface ablation have been developed since laser-assisted subepithelial keratomileusis (LASEK) was demonstrated to be a safe and effective procedure for the treatment of low to moderate refractive errors.[1] LASEK was first performed in 1996 by one of us (DTA); the procedure was independently conceived and popularized by Camellin, who coined the term LASEK.[2] Epi-LASIK (laser in situ keratomileusis) has emerged as a novel refractive procedure that eliminates the need for alcohol in creating the epithelial flap before surface ablation is performed. LASEK and Epi-LASIK are corneal surface ablative refractive procedures that combine several of the advantages of both LASIK and photorefractive keratectomy (PRK).[3] The advantages of LASEK and Epi-LASIK over PRK include the reduction of postoperative pain,[4] faster visual recovery, and decreased corneal wound healing.[5] The LASEK technique seems to avoid typical drawbacks of LASIK including iatrogenic ectasia[6] and flap-related complications,[7] such as irregular flaps, flap striae, and epithelial ingrowth.[8]

During LASEK, an alcohol solution is instilled on the cornea creating an epithelial flap that is repositioned over the laser-ablated corneal surface at the end of the procedure.[4] Despite the encouraging clinical results of LASEK, concerns about the toxic effect of alcohol on the epithelium and the underlying stroma[9] have led to the investigation of different approaches to try to preserve the epithelial sheet, chief among them being Epi-LASIK.

In Epi-LASIK, epithelial separation does not require the use of alcohol for epithelial loosening. The corneal epithelium is mechanically separated from the underlying stroma with the use of an epikeratome that features a blunt oscillating blade.[10] The epithelial sheet can be replaced on the operated cornea after photoablation. We have successfully employed another epikeratome in which the blade design consistently avoids epithelial tearing and Bowman's cutting.

Indications and Contraindications

LASEK and Epi-LASIK are mainly indicated in cases of low to moderate myopia and myopic astigmatism, corneal thinning, steep and flat corneas, and in cases where the patient's avocational activities predispose his or her eyes to ocular trauma.

Contraindications for LASEK and Epi-LASIK are severe dry eye (Sjögren syndrome), keratoconus, monocular patients, herpes zoster ophthalmicus, and exposure keratopathy.[11] Relative contraindications are a history of herpes simplex keratitis, previous ocular surgery, any active/residual/recurrent ocular disease, unstable/progressive myopia, irregular astigmatism, corneal scarring, and forme fruste keratoconus. It is important to rule out the presence of glaucoma or suspected glaucoma that may make the eye vulnerable to raised intraocular pressure (IOP) and any other previous ocular problem, such as significant lagophthalmos, uveitis, cataract, retinal vascular change, or lattice degeneration, that may interfere with the patient's visual acuity.

LASEK and Epi-LASIK Surgical Techniques

PREOPERATIVE EVALUATION

It is important to consider the patient's vocational and recreational refractive needs, discuss his or her surgical expectations, and review the risks and benefits of LASEK and Epi-LASIK. During the clinical examination, the patient undergoes a clinical evaluation consisting of uncorrected visual

Figure 21-1. Azar LASEK technique. (a) Corneal marking. (b) 18% alcohol is released in the dispenser. (c) The epithelium is cut using Vanna scissors. (d) Loosened epithelium is peeled as a single sheet. (e) A hinge of 2 to 3 clock hours of intact epithelium is left at the temporal margin. (f) Laser ablation is applied over the corneal stroma.

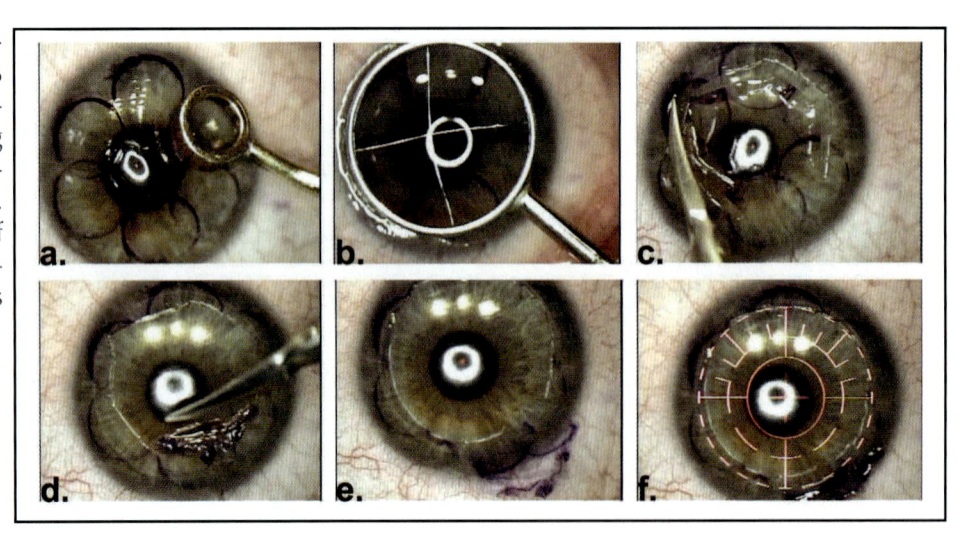

acuity (UCVA), best-corrected visual acuity (BCVA), manifest and cycloplegic refraction, ocular dominance, pachymetry, orthoptic examination, contact lens wear, tonometry, pupil size, slit lamp examination, corneal aesthesiometry, fundus examination, computerized videokeratography, and wavefront analysis.

LASEK Surgical Technique (Figure 21-1)

Topical nonsteroidal anti-inflammatory drugs (NSAIDs) could be used preoperatively for pain relief. A lid speculum is applied after topical 0.5% proparacaine anesthesia. The cornea is marked with overlapping 3-mm circles around the corneal periphery, simulating a floral pattern to allow the surgeon to have the precise reference points to realign the flap in the corneal beds.

An alcohol dispenser consisting of a customized 9-mm semi-sharp marker (ASICO, Westmont, Ill) attached to a glass syringe or a hollow metal handle serving as an alcohol reservoir is used. Firm pressure is exerted on the central cornea, and a button is pushed on the side of the handle, releasing the alcohol into the well of the marker. Alternatively, a 7-mm optical marker (Model E9011 3.0, Storz, St Louis, Mo) is used to delineate the area centered on the pupil. Gentle pressure is applied on the cornea while the barrel of the marker is filled with two drops of 18% ethanol (dehydrated alcohol, 1 mL ampules, American Reagent Laboratories, Shirley, NY). After 25 to 35 seconds, the ethanol is aspirated back into the syringe or absorbed with a dry cellulose sponge (Weck-Cel or Merocel, Xomed, Jacksonville, Fla) to prevent alcohol spillage onto the epithelium outside the marker barrel. If necessary, the ethanol application may be repeated for an additional 10 to 15 seconds.

One arm of a modified curved Vannas scissors or a jeweler's forceps is inserted under the epithelium and traced within or around the delineated margin of the epithelium, leaving 2 to 3 clock hours of intact margin. The loosened epithelium is peeled as a single sheet using the jeweler's forceps, a Merocel sponge, or a dedicated spatula, leaving a flap of epithelium with the hinge still attached. We use a superior hinge for patients having with-the-rule astigmatism; otherwise, we attempt a temporal hinge whenever possible.

The laser ablation is then initiated using either a scanning or excimer laser wide-area ablation.

After ablation, a 30-gauge anterior chamber cannula is used to hydrate the stroma and epithelial sheet with balanced salt solution (BSS). The epithelial sheet is replaced on the stroma using the straight part of the cannula under intermittent irrigation. Care is taken to realign the epithelial flap using the previous marks and to avoid epithelial defects. The flap is then allowed to dry for 2 to 5 minutes.

Epi-LASIK Surgical Technique (Figure 21-2)

Topical 0.5% tetracaine hydrochloride eye drops are used for the anesthesia. A sterile drape is applied, and a lid speculum is inserted. After irrigation with BSS using an anterior chamber cannula, the corneal epithelium is dried using a Merocel sponge, and the cornea is marked with a standard LASIK marker. The subepithelial separator is applied to the eye, and the suction is activated by a foot pedal. The oscillating blade separates the epithelium, leaving a 2- to 3-mm nasal hinge, the suction is released, and the device is removed from the eye. The epithelial sheet is reflected nasally using a moistened Merocel sponge to reveal the corneal stroma for ablation. After application of the excimer laser, the cornea is irrigated with BSS and the epithelial sheet is repositioned and left to dry for 2 to 3 minutes. After that time, the epithelial sheet has adhered to the corneal stroma. Anti-inflammatory and antibiotic eyedrops are instilled, and a therapeutic contact lens is applied to the eye.

Postoperative Management

After epithelial flap repositioning, the patient receives a combination of either diclofenac sodium 0.1% and tobramycin 0.3% dexamethasone 0.1% ointment or diclofenac sodi-

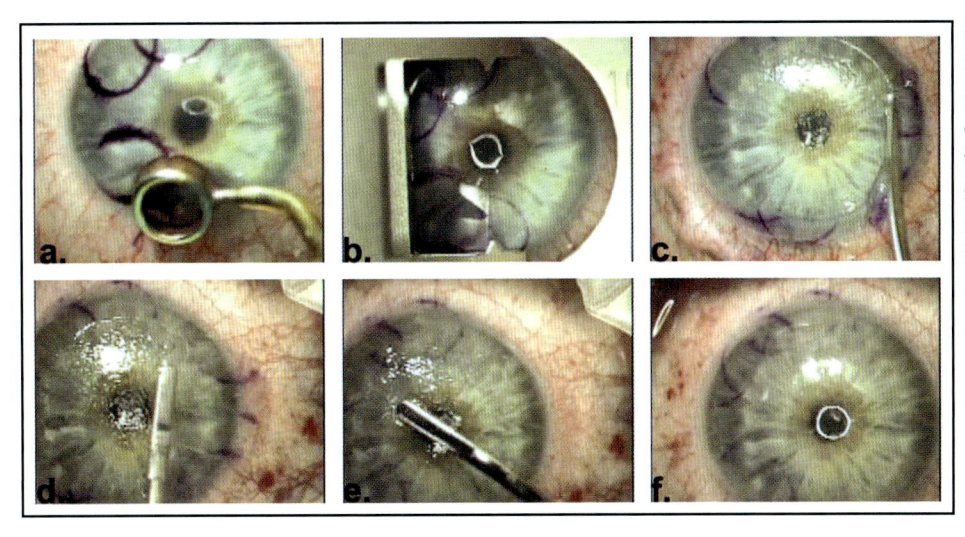

Figure 21-2. Epi-LASIK technique. (a) Corneal marking. (b) Epikeratome positioning over the corneal epithelium. (c) Epithelial flap lifting. (d) Epithelial flap repositioning after laser treatment. (e) Epithelial flap smoothing. (f) Bandage contact lens positioning.

um 0.1%, ciprofloxacin, and prednisolone acetate 1% drops immediately after surgery. A bandage contact lens (Softlens 66, Bausch & Lomb, Rochester, NY) is placed to reduce the friction between the eyelid and the corneal epithelium and to minimize postoperative pain. The bandage contact lens should remain in place until complete re-epithelialization of the corneal surface. Frequent lubrication with preservative-free artificial tears is advised. The usual postoperative regimen after lens removal includes topical fluoroquinolone (ciprofloxacin, ofloxacin, or levofloxacin) and steroid (prednisolone acetate 1%) drops four times per day for 1 week. The topical steroid is continued twice per day for another week and gradually reduced for 2 months.

Patients are seen on day 1 and day 3 or until complete epithelialization of the surface. They are seen again at 1 week, 1 month, 3 months, 6 months, and 1 year after the procedure.

Alcohol-Assisted Epithelial Removal

Manual epithelial debridement, which was used in the past to remove the corneal epithelium in PRK and phototherapeutic keratotomy (PTK), was shown to produce scratches and nicking in Bowman's layer and was found to be inaccurate as variable amounts of epithelium were left in place.[12,13]

Chemical agents such as 0.5% proparacaine, iodine, cocaine, alkali n-heptanol, and ethanol have been used to remove the corneal epithelium in experimental studies.[12,14] For centuries, alcohols have been appreciated for their antimicrobial properties;[15] they are fast-acting, barely toxic with topical application, nonstaining, nonallergic, and they readily evaporate. For infection control purposes, ethyl alcohol (ethanol) and isopropyl alcohol (isopropanol) are the alcoholic solutions most often used.

Concentrations of ethanol ranging from 10% to 30% were widely used to remove the corneal epithelium before PRK.[16-18] Today 18% to 20% ethanol is commonly utilized in LASEK.

The use of 100% ethanol for 2 minutes in rabbit corneas led to a significant decrease in stromal keratocytes after 24 hours.[19] Similarly, when using 70% isopropyl alcohol for 2 minutes for epithelium removal in rabbit eyes, Agrawal et al[20] found an increased inflammatory response and damaging effects on corneal keratocytes. Helena et al[21] observed increased keratocyte loss but decreased inflammation after using 50% ethanol for 1 minute compared to mechanical debridement.

Abad et al[16] showed that alcohol-assisted epithelial removal was a simple and safe alternative to mechanical epithelial removal before PRK. Applying 25% ethanol for 3 minutes, Stein et al[18] were able to grasp, lift, pull apart, and split the corneal epithelium using two McPherson forceps. These early reports revealed that epithelial removal using 18% to 25% alcohol for 20 to 25 seconds was faster, easier, and safer compared to mechanical debridement. They also showed that this concentration can produce sharp wound edges and a clean, smooth Bowman's layer and that central epithelium can be translocated in part or completely.[17] Carones et al[19] found significantly better results in terms of haze and corneal regularity in epithelial debridement using a 20% alcohol solution compared to mechanical debridement. The ethanol could be diluted in distilled water[3,4,15-17] and BSS.[18,19] Theoretically, the ethanol would be more effective in water solution. However, the epithelial protection may be greater in BSS. Camellin[2] strongly points out the importance of a hypotonic solution obtained by diluting alcohol in distilled water for facilitating epithelial detachment, whereas Vinciguerra uses BSS for dilution.[22] Hazarbassanov et al[23] showed that hypertonic saline (50% sodium chloride)-assisted LASEK provides good postoperative accuracy and safety and a similar rate of complication when compared with the results of 20% alcohol-assisted LASEK. The method of preparing 18% ethanol is drawing 2 mL of dehydrated alcohol (American Reagent Laboratories, Shirley, NY) from ampules into a 12-mL syringe. Add the sterile water for injection to 11 mL and mix well.[3] Cheng et al[24] demonstrated that ethanol 20% does not affect laser fluency, whereas a higher concentration does and should therefore be avoided.

Effect of Alcohol on Epithelial Cell Survival *In Vitro*

Alcohol has been known to have direct toxic effects on cells. It induces protein denaturation and lipid dissolution with the loss of specific cellular functions. Chen et al[15] detected a dose- and time-dependent effect of dilute alcohol on cultured corneal epithelial cells. The 25% concentration of dilute alcohol was the inflection point of epithelial survival. Significant increase in cellular death occurred after 35 seconds of 20% alcohol exposure; 40 seconds of exposure further increased apoptosis after 8 hours of incubation. These findings are consistent with the clinical observations of varied epithelial attachment to the stromal bed after LASEK surgery.

The *in vitro*, mono-layered results may apply to *in vivo*, multi-layered epithelia. The critical alcohol concentration and its exposure duration are thus frequently exceeded during surgery. Increased duration of alcohol application can be used intentionally to weaken the epithelial adhesions, which contributes to the variability in alcohol-induced toxicity that is observed *in vivo*.

Electron Microscopy

The aim of diluted alcohol application is to temporarily dissociate the corneal epithelial-stromal adhesion complex composed of intermediate filaments, hemidesmosomes, anchoring filaments, lamina densa, and anchoring fibrils.[25-27]

To study the effect of alcohol exposure and mechanical manipulation on the corneal epithelium, Azar et al[3] carried out electron microscopy studies on specimens obtained after conventional alcohol-assisted PRK. The images revealed that the epithelial cell layer is intact with a compact and regular arrangement, and the epithelial cells are still viable immediately after exposure to alcohol and surgical peeling. The presence of fragmented hemidesmosomes and basement membrane remnants still attached to the basal epithelial cell layer indicates that the point of separation was likely to be within the basement membrane. Neither the Bowman membrane nor the corneal stroma was found in the epithelial flap. Browning et al[28] determined that the corneal epithelial anatomic cleavage plane after alcohol-assisted epithelial removal was determined to be at the hemidesmosomal attachments, including the most superficial part of the lamina lucida of the basement membrane. Gabison et al[29] hypothesize that alcohol weakens the adhesions between epithelium and stroma, and assuming that the separation of the corneal epithelial layer from the stromal layer is within the basement membrane, they propose that the intact basement membrane may reduce the alteration of fibrotic phenotype.

Kim et al[9] evaluated the toxicity of 20% ethanol exposure for 30 seconds, 1 minute, and 3 minutes on rabbit corneal epithelia with scanning and transmission electron microscopy. They found widespread partial or total damage of microvilli, focal breaks of intercellular junction, and cellular edema. The damage increased with exposure time. After 1 minute of ethanol exposure, a slough of superficial epithelium was observed, which progressed with time.

In a study by Pallikaris et al,[30] transmission electron microscopy of six epithelial sheets obtained mechanically with a subepithelial separator (developed by Duckworth & Kent, Baldock, UK) showed that the separation was not within but underneath the basement membrane, which remained attached to the basal layer of the epithelium. Lamina densa and lamina lucida were preserved and the hemidesmosomes had normal morphology along almost the entire length of the basement membrane. The basal epithelial cells of the separated epithelial disks showed minimal trauma and edema.

The adherence of the basement membrane to the basal layer of the epithelium is significant because it is believed that the basement membrane provides the stability and support that keeps the epithelium intact even with manipulation, thereby preserving the integrity and viability of the entire epithelium. Specimens obtained using 15% and 20% alcohol concentrations showed formation of cytoplasmic fragments of the basal epithelial cells, enlargement of the intracellular spaces, and extensive discontinuities in the basement membrane, which was excised at the level of the lamina lucida, confirming that the alcohol-assisted cleavage plane was within the basement membrane.

Clinical Outcomes

LASEK vs PRK

In a comparative prospective study of 27 patients, Lee et al[4] provided the first clinical evidence that patients treated with LASEK for low and moderate myopia had lower postoperative pain and haze scores than PRK-treated eyes. Although Litwak et al[31] conducted a similar study that questioned these results, an increasing number of authors suggest that LASEK may provide advantages over PRK for the correction of myopia.[3,4,32-39] Taneri et al[1] evaluated 171 eyes with moderate myopia and astigmatism. One week postoperatively, 96% of eyes had UCVA of 20/40 or better but definitive visual recovery took more than 4 weeks in some eyes. Approximately 95% of eyes were within ±1.0 D of emmetropia after 4 to 52 weeks; the remaining 5% did not show major deviations. At 4 to 52 weeks, only one eye was uncorrected by more than 1.0 D of manifest refraction. On postoperative day 1, 57% patients complained of mild pain; severe pain was reported in 4% of eyes on day 1. Corneal haze appeared later than SPK and remained in two eyes at 2 years follow-up. The presence of trace to mild corneal haze peaked at 3 months, occurring in 18% of patients examined. No serious complications (including recurrent erosion syndrome) were encountered.

Owing to the large percentage of LASEK patients who have pain, a better understanding of epithelial adhesion with the stroma is important, although 50% of LASEK patients may have less pain than PRK patients in the immediate postoperative period.

LASEK vs Epi-LASIK

The fundamental difference between Epi-LASIK and LASEK is that the separation of the epithelial sheet is obtained mechanically without requiring the preparation of the cornea with alcohol or other chemical agent. Mechanical separation not only avoids the probable toxic effect of alcohol on the separated epithelial sheet,[9,15] but also provides an automated surgical procedure with a short learning curve for LASIK surgeons. Preliminary clinical results[40] suggest that Epi-LASIK is a safe and efficient method for the correction of low myopia. Pallikaris et al treated 44 eyes with Epi-LASIK for the correction of low myopia (range -1.75 to -7.0 D). The mean epithelial healing time was 4.86 ± 0.56 days (range 3 to 5 days),[40] 1 day later than after LASEK treatments.[33,35] Thirty-eight percent of the treated eyes had UCVA of 20/40 or better on day 1;[40] the percentage of eyes with UCVA of 20/40 or better on day 1 after LASEK ranges between 10%[33] and 45%.[34]

Similar to LASEK,[35] Epi-LASIK was not a totally pain-free procedure: during the first 2 hours after treatment 16% of patients reported burning pain that required medication; 65% reported no pain and 19% reported mild discomfort.[40] Twenty-six percent of the patients reported mild discomfort on the first postoperative day.[40]

At 1 month, the mean spherical equivalent of the treated eyes was -0.3 ± 0.6 D (range -1.0 to 0.87 D) and at 3 months it was -0.10 ± 0.4 D (range -0.75 to 0.75 D).[40] Ninety-seven percent of eyes had clear corneas or only a trace of haze 3 months after treatment.[40] In their study, Anderson et al[37] noted haze in 1.6% of patients in the first 3 months after treatment. Results at 6 months indicated that UCVA was 20/40 or better in 98% of patients.[37]

One of us showed that Epi-LASIK can be used for treating LASIK flap-related complications.[41] Despite the uneven stromal contour at the site of the original hinge and the irregular stromal surface after amputation of the LASIK flap, the Epi-LASIK procedure was successfully performed with a LASITOME microkeratome (Gebauer, Neuhausen, Germany) equipped with an EPI-head and an EPI-blade.

Case 1: LASEK

A 38-year-old man, who had no history of ocular diseases, underwent an uncomplicated bilateral surface procedure. His preoperative manifest refraction was -5.00 DS and -1.5 DC x 180 degrees in OD and -2.25 DS and -1.0 DC x 180 degrees in OS; best-spectacle corrected visual acuity (BSCVA) was 20/20 in both eyes. Pachymetry was 466 µm in OD and 468 µm in OS. IS values were 1.07 in OD and 1.18 in OS. Extraocular motilities and pneumotonometry were normal. His dominant eye was OD. Given the low pachymetric values in both eyes, LASIK was not recommended. The patient underwent uncomplicated LASEK in OD and uncomplicated Custom LASEK in OS.

At 1 day after surgery, the patient reported no pain in OS and severe pain in OD due to an epithelial abrasion. The flap was repositioned and a bandage contact lens was replaced. Both eyes presented a trace of haze for 5 months after surgery. At 13 months follow up, his UCVA was 20/25 in OD and 20/30 in OS and his refraction was -0.25 DS and -0.50 DC x 180 degrees in OD and plano -0.50 DC x 135 degrees in OS with BSCVA of 20/20 in both eyes. Pre-and postoperative topographies and wavefront analysis are shown in Figures 21-3a through 21-3d.

Case 2: Epi-LASIK

A 39-year-old woman, who had no history of ocular diseases, underwent an uncomplicated bilateral Epi-LASIK procedure aiming at mini-monovision in the non-dominant eye. Her preoperative manifest refraction was -4.5 DS and -0.25 DC x 145 degrees in OD and -3.75 DS and -0.25 DC x 53 degrees in OS; BSCVA was 20/20 in both eyes. K readings were 44.6/45.3 @ 78 degrees in OD and 44.7/45.3 @ 109 degrees in OS. Pachymetry was 561 µm in OD and 566 µm in OS. Shirmer test without proparacaine was 1 mm in 5 minutes in both eyes. Extraocular motilities and pneumotonometry were normal. Her dominant eye was OD. At 1 day after surgery, the patient reported severe pain, which required medication. Her epithelial healing time was 5 days in OS.

At 4 months follow-up, her UCVA was 20/25 in OD and 20/30 in OS, and her refraction was +0.75 DS and -1.0 DC x 15 degrees in OD and -0.5 DS and -0.5 DC x 35 degrees in OS with BSCVA of 20/20 in both eyes. The patient could read at J 1 with both eyes. Her right eye presented only a trace of haze. Pre- and postoperative Orbscan corneal topographies are shown in Figures 21-4a through 21-4d. No postoperative complications were observed.

Complications of LASEK and Epi-LASIK

Early postoperative complications of LASEK and Epi-LASIK include flap-related complications (such as free or incomplete epithelial flap, dissolution, fragmentation, fold, and slip) and pain, which decrease over time as the epithelium heals. Complications in the days following surgery include superficial punctuate keratitis and subepithelial foreign body.[36]

A common complication in patients with delayed healing of the corneal epithelium is corneal haze, which has been found in 31% of patients at 3 months.[36] It appears that there is a relation between TGF–β1 expression due to trauma and corneal haze. The integrity of the healing epithelium is also determined by the presence of the bandage contact lens in the first few days of recovery. Inadvertent displacement of the bandage contact lens can lead to slower healing of epithelial defects as well as increased risk of corneal haze in the future.

Less frequent complications include diplopia, which appears to be caused by decentralization or nonhomogeneous ablation, regression, significant haze, alcohol leakage, and steroid-induced glaucoma.

Figure 21-3. (a) Preoperative corneal topography in OD. (b) Preoperative corneal topography in OS. (c) Preoperative wavefront analysis in OD. (d) Preoperative wavefront analysis in OS. (e) Postoperative corneal topography in OD. (f) Postoperative corneal topography in OS.

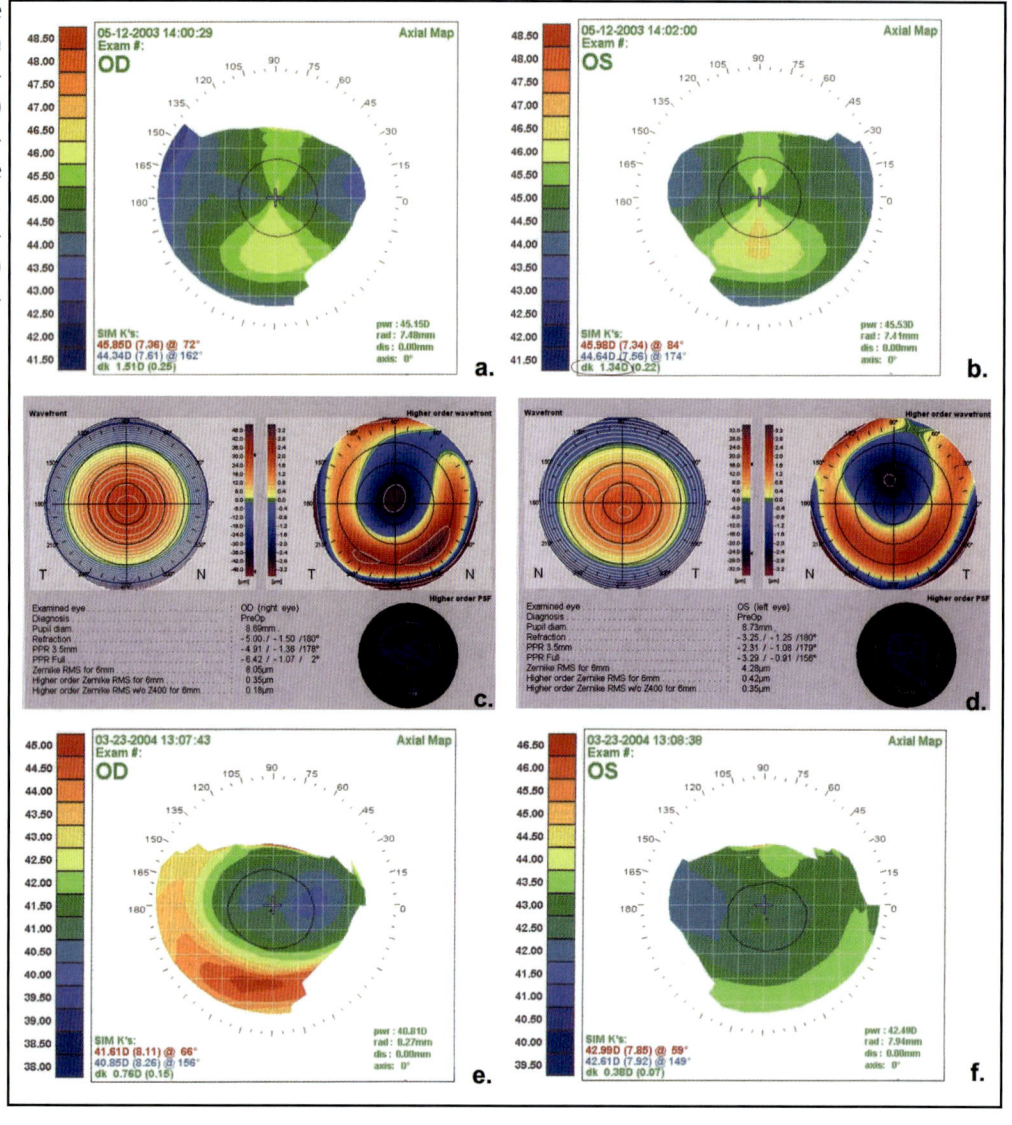

References

1. Taneri S, Feit R, Azar DT. Safety, efficacy, and stability indices of LASEK correction in moderate myopia and astigmatism. *J Cataract Refract Surg.* 2004;30(10):2130-2137.
2. Camellin M, Cimberle M. LASEK technique promising after 1 year of experience. *Ocular Surg News.* 2000(18):14-17.
3. Azar DT, et al. Laser subepithelial keratomileusis: electron microscopy and visual outcomes of flap photorefractive keratectomy. *Curr Opin Ophthalmol.* 2001;12(4):323-328.
4. Lee JB, et al. Comparison of laser epithelial keratomileusis and photorefractive keratectomy for low to moderate myopia. *J Cataract Refract Surg.* 2001;27(4):565-570.
5. Park CK, Kim JH. Comparison of wound healing after photorefractive keratectomy and laser in situ keratomileusis in rabbits. *J Cataract Refract Surg.* 1999;25(6):842-850.
6. Pallikaris IG, Kymionis GD, Astyrakakis NI. Corneal ectasia induced by laser in situ keratomileusis. *J Cataract Refract Surg.* 2001;27(11):1796-1802.
7. Pallikaris IG, Katsanevaki VJ, Panagopoulou SI. Laser in situ keratomileusis intraoperative complications using one type of microkeratome. *Ophthalmology.* 2002;109(1):57-63.
8. Melki SA, Azar DT. LASIK complications: etiology, management, and prevention. *Surv Ophthalmol.* 2001;46(2):95-116.
9. Kim SY, et al. Twenty percent alcohol toxicity on rabbit corneal epithelial cells: electron microscopic study. *Cornea.* 2002;21(4):388-392.
10. Pallikaris IG, et al. Advances in subepithelial excimer refractive surgery techniques: Epi-LASIK. *Curr Opin Ophthalmol.* 2003;14(4):207-212.
11. Taneri S, Zieske JD, Azar DT. Evolution, techniques, clinical outcomes, and pathophysiology of LASEK: review of the literature. *Surv Ophthalmol.* 2004;49(6):576-602.
12. Campos M, et al. Keratocyte loss after different methods of deepithelialization. *Ophthalmology.* 1994;101(5):890-894.
13. Griffith M, et al. Evaluation of current techniques of corneal epithelial removal in hyperopic photorefractive keratectomy. *J Cataract Refract Surg.* 1998;24(8):1070-1078.
14. Hirst LW, et al. Comparative studies of corneal surface injury in the monkey and rabbit. *Arch Ophthalmol.* 1981;99(6):1066-1073.
15. Chen CC, et al. Human corneal epithelial cell viability and morphology after dilute alcohol exposure. *Invest Ophthalmol Vis Sci.* 2002;43(8):2593-2602.
16. Abad JC, et al. A prospective evaluation of alcohol-assisted versus mechanical epithelial removal before photorefractive keratectomy. *Ophthalmology.* 1997;104(10):1566-1574; discussion 1574-1575.
17. Abad JC, et al. Dilute ethanol versus mechanical debridement before photorefractive keratectomy. *J Cataract Refract Surg.* 1996;22(10):1427-1433.

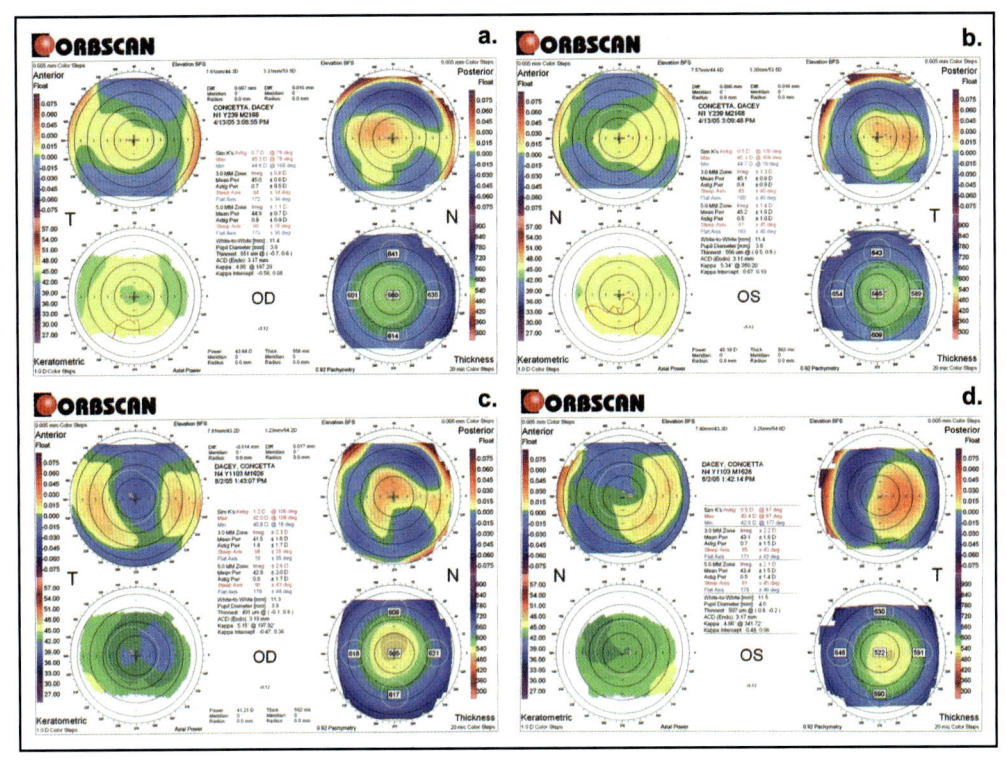

Figure 21-4. Orbscan corneal topography. (a) Preoperative in OD. (b) Preoperative in OS. (c) Postoperative in OD. (d) Postoperative in OS.

18. Stein HA, et al. Alcohol removal of the epithelium for excimer laser ablation: outcomes analysis. *J Cataract Refract* Surg. 1997;23(8):1160-1163.
19. Carones F, Fiore T, Brancato R. Mechanical vs. alcohol epithelial removal during photorefractive keratectomy. *J Refract Surg.* 1999;15(5):556-562.
20. Agrawal VB, et al. Alcohol versus mechanical epithelial debridement: effect on underlying cornea before excimer laser surgery. *J Cataract Refract Surg.* 1997;23(8):1153-1159.
21. Helena MC, et al. Effects of 50% ethanol and mechanical epithelial debridement on corneal structure before and after excimer photorefractive keratectomy. *Cornea.* 1997;16(5):571-579.
22. Vinciguerra P, Camesasca FI. Butterfly laser epithelial keratomileusis for myopia. *J Refract Surg.* 2002;18(3 Suppl):S371-373.
23. Hazarbassanov R, et al. Alcohol- vs hypertonic saline-assisted laser-assisted subepithelial keratectomy. *Arch Ophthalmol.* 2005;123(2):171-176.
24. Cheng AC, et al. Effect of alcohol on the efficacy of excimer laser power. *J Cataract Refract Surg.* 2004;30(7):1545-1548.
25. Gipson IK, Spurr-Michaud SJ, Tisdale AS. Anchoring fibrils form a complex network in human and rabbit cornea. *Invest Ophthalmol Vis Sci.* 1987;28(2):212-220.
26. Gipson IK, Spurr-Michaud SJ, Tisdale AS. Hemidesmosomes and anchoring fibril collagen appear synchronously during development and wound healing. *Dev Biol.* 1988;126(2):253-262.
27. Espana EM, et al. Cleavage of corneal basement membrane components by ethanol exposure in laser-assisted subepithelial keratectomy. *J Cataract Refract Surg.* 2003;29(6):1192-1197.
28. Browning AC, et al. Alcohol debridement of the corneal epithelium in PRK and LASEK: an electron microscopic study. *Invest Ophthalmol Vis Sci.* 2003;44(2):510-513.
29. Gabison EE, et al. Biochemical basis of epithelial dehiscence and reattachment after LASEK. In: Azar DA, Camellin M, Yee RW, eds. *LASEK, PRK, and Excimer Laser Stromal Surface Ablation.* New York, NY: Marcel Dekker: 2005;253-262.
30. Pallikaris IG, et al. Epi-LASIK: comparative histological evaluation of mechanical and alcohol-assisted epithelial separation. *J Cataract Refract Surg.* 2003;29(8):1496-1501.
31. Litwak S, et al. Laser-assisted subepithelial keratectomy versus photorefractive keratectomy for the correction of myopia. A prospective comparative study. *J Cataract Refract Surg.* 2002;28(8):1330-1333.
32. Shah S, et al. The epithelial flap for photorefractive keratectomy. *Br J Ophthalmol.* 2001;85(4):393-396.
33. Shahinian L Jr. Laser-assisted subepithelial keratectomy for low to high myopia and astigmatism. *J Cataract Refract Surg.* 2002;28(8):1334-1342.
34. Rouweyha RM, et al. Laser epithelial keratomileusis for myopia with the autonomous laser. *J Refract Surg.* 2002;18(3):217-224.
35. Camellin M. Laser epithelial keratomileusis for myopia. *J Refract Surg.* 2003;19(6):666-670.
36. Claringbold TV 2nd. Laser-assisted subepithelial keratectomy for the correction of myopia. *J Cataract Refract Surg.* 2002;28(1):18-22.
37. Anderson NJ, Beran RF, Schneider TL. Epi-LASEK for the correction of myopia and myopic astigmatism. *J Cataract Refract Surg.* 2002;28(8):1343-1347.
38. Autrata R, Rehurek J. Laser-assisted subepithelial keratectomy for myopia: two-year follow-up. *J Cataract Refract Surg.* 2003;29(4):661-668.
39. Chalita MR, Tekwani NH, Krueger RR. Laser epithelial keratomileusis: outcome of initial cases performed by an experienced surgeon. *J Refract Surg.* 2003;19(4):412-415.
40. Pallikaris IG, et al. Epi-LASIK: preliminary clinical results of an alternative surface ablation procedure. *J Cataract Refract Surg.* 2005;31(5):879-885.
41. Taneri S. EPI-LASIK after amputation of a LASIK flap, ESCRS, Editor. Lissabon; 2005.

CHAPTER 22

Wavefront Customized PRK: Zyoptix

Stefano Baiocchi, MD, PhD; Marco Lazzarotto, MD;
Claudia Sforzi, MD, PhD; Aldo Caporossi, MD

Introduction

The model of photorefractive ablation with an excimer laser was developed with the use of optical physics studies by Munnerlynn,[1] and the algorithms that guide the release of photonic energy[2-4] (delivery system) were studied on the basis of the equations proposed by this same author. In this ablative model, tissue removal centered on the geometrical center of the cornea is produced according to a spherical model, which can be associated with an integrated or sequential toric ablation.[5,6]

This valid and repeatable ablative model has a series of limitations, some not exactly intrinsic to the theoretical formulation of Munnerlynn and therefore able to be overcome with a different formulation or a modification of ablative and other algorithms, connected with asymmetry and the genesis of the defect to be removed, which require a different approach.

After the studies of the Rochester group[7,8] and the application of adaptive lenses in space optics[9-11] (the Hubble telescope), Bausch & Lomb began, during the second half of the 1990s, a project on refractive ablation with a laser guided by surveys of the deviations of the focalization of luminous rays of the eye in examination, with the objective of selectively removing from the cornea the cause of aberrations of the optical path from an individual eye and, therefore, to generate a new optical system without aberrations.[12] The first applications were exclusively for LASIK techniques[13,14] and it was possible, only after our insistent request (Videorefractive 1999, ASCRS 2000) to perfect a personalized procedure of frontal guided wavefront surface during the first treatments at the end of 2001.

The personalized Zyoptix system is an integrative system of surgical survey, elaboration, and planning that is carried out with a 217z spot flying laser with a variable diameter (2 and 1 mm) with a Gaussian truncated beam profile and an emission frequency of 50 and 100 Hz. The whole process of acquisition is critical and the correct positioning of the ablative program on the cornea requires accurate and effective ocular pursuit and centering (eye tracker) to avoid unsatisfactory results.

Acquisition of Data and Construction of Ablation File

The system of acquisition of data uses linear light scan tomography (Orbscan Iiz, Figure 22-1)[15-17] with a multiple acquisition system (acquisitions from 3 to 6), from which an elaboration of the mean values are deduced. The data obtained by Orbscan acquisition are then exported under the form of a file (.OTE) to the elaboration-integration system of the ablative file (treatment planner). The pachymetric data, together with the data of the central curvature and eccentricity (Figure 22-2) that appear on the screen, are used from the tomographic and pupillographic evaluation the end of the production of the ablation file carried out with this examination, while the pupillometric-pupillographic data (Figure 22-3) are acquired from the system which manages intraoperative eye-tracking. Elevation data, without any reference to the dioptrics map, and filtering keratoscopic data, are part of the file. OTE files are not included in the standard ablative process guided by the wavefront, while some of these make up part of the aspheric treatment and tissue savings file.

The second parameter is acquired first in the photopic pupil and then in the pharmacological scotopic pupil obtained with the Zywave aberrometer (Figure 22-4). The device chosen by Bausch & Lomb is based on the Hartmann-Shack principle,

Figure 22-1. (A) Orbscan IIz (left) and Zywave Aberrometer (right) workstation. (B) Orbscan focalization image (italic S) help the operator to obtain a well-centered, well-focused acquisition. (C) Orbscan Light slit during acquisition.

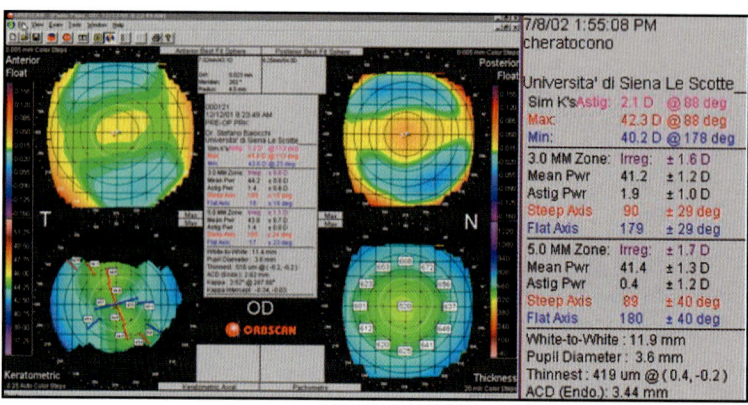

Figure 22-2. Left image shows the quad map Orbscan IIz image, and the right image represents the refractive and pachymetric summary.

Figure 22-3. Orbscan IIz pupillometric-pupillographic and centration data, image registration in .OTE file.

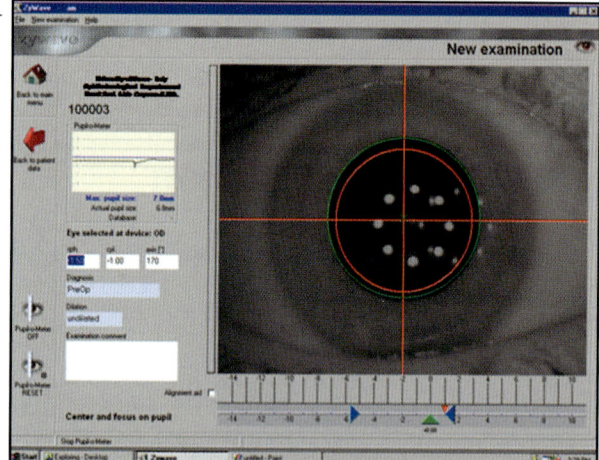

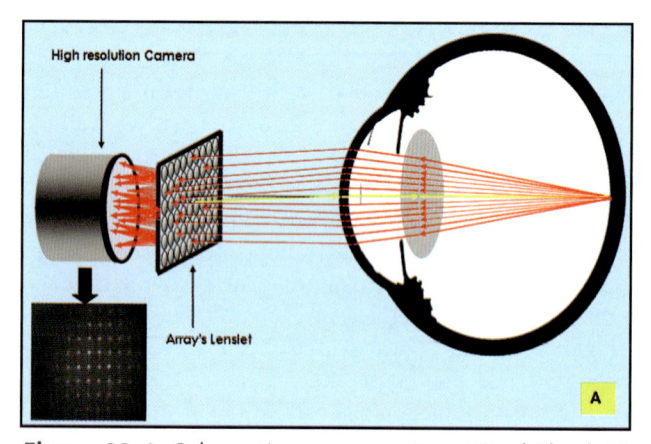

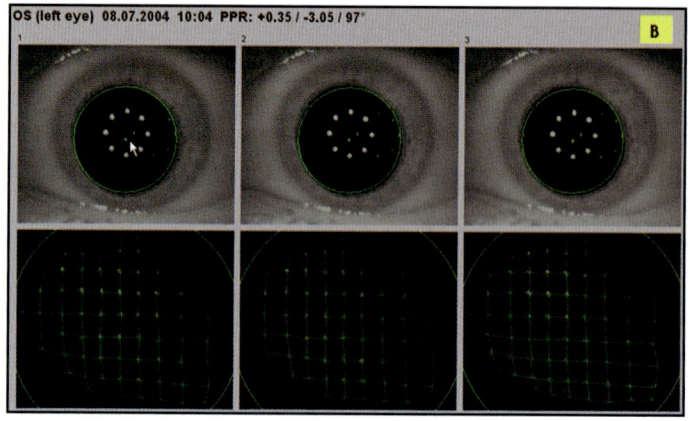

Figure 22-4. Schematic representation (A) of Shack-Hartmann aberrometer (Bausch & Lomb Zywave). Yellow arrow is the monochromatic light and the red arrow represents the retinal reflected rays (static in exit relevation). (B) Shows the Zywave photographic acquisition raw in astigmatic eye before the Zernike's coefficient expansion and its graphical transduction.

which is static exit aberrometry in which the puntiform monochromatic luminous[18-20] ray strikes the retina without undergoing modifications. From this, the ray is reflected toward the exterior as a beam of radiations that are modified in the course of the vitreous body, by the crystalline lens (vitreous lens interface, stroma, and aqueous lens interface), from the corneal-aqueous interface to that of the cornea-air, in that order. The exiting ray reformed by roughly parallel radiations travels through a lenslet array which divides the luminous bundle into a network, then is photographed by a

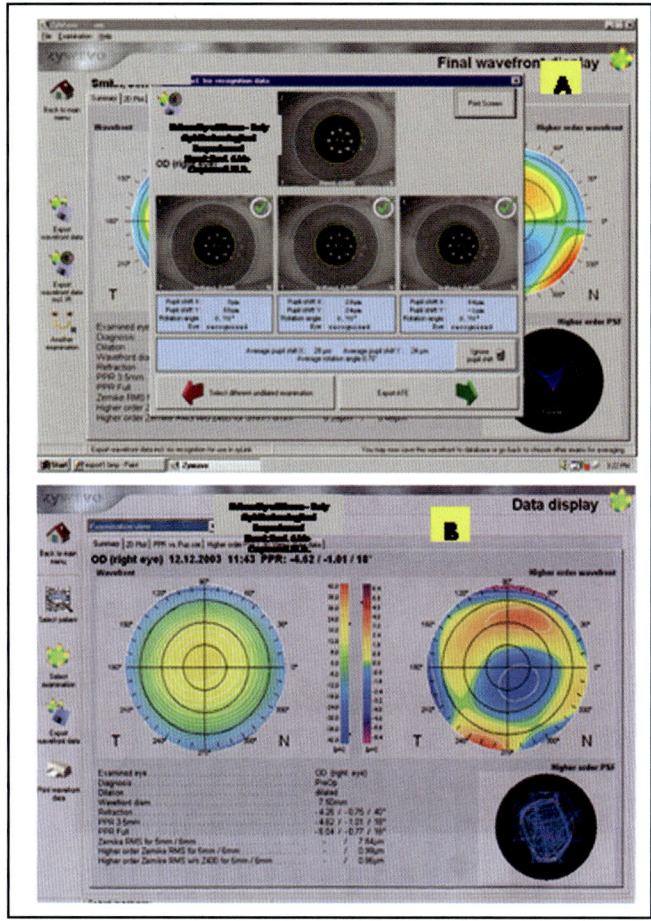

Figure 22-5. Centration acquired raw (A) and aberrometric maps in decentered regressed PRK (B). Total aberrometric is the left map, and high-order aberrometric map is the right map. The small inferior picture shows a simulated high-order point spread function.

high-resolution camera. The photographically gathered data are compared with the network produced by an ideal optical system, and the differences are calculated through the expansion of Zernike's coefficients.[21,22] The Zywave system sequentially carries out five measurements (acquired and sent with five successive impulses) for each examination, discarding the two least reliable acquisitions, farthest from the mean. From the three accepted measurements, it carries out a mean calculation of the single Zernike coefficients from which it reconstructs a total aberrometric map of the eye and a map of only the high-order (from the third on) aberrations (Figure 22-5). The execution of the aberrometric evaluation, in both myotic undilated pupil and in dilated with noncycloplegic mydriatics pupil (isonefrine 5% to 6%) has two aims: 1) the evaluation of the pupillary kinetic and the decentration that the pupil undergoes during the course of the midriasis, supplying data from the eye-tracking system and 2) the evaluation of the existence of second order aberrations (refractive defect) in photopic and scotopic conditions, and evaluation with the pupil at more than 6 mm of high-order aberrations.

Beyond these comparative evaluations, which are useful to the surgeon for evaluating the stability of the defect with variations of the pupil and the final analysis to confirm the choice of a guided ablation in connection with the wave of analysis with a pupillary diameter as wide as possible and without a considerable cycloplegic effect, it supplies information regarding a broader corneal area and allows for the treatment of a corneal surface (optical zone) that is broader and always superior to 6 mm and therefore broader than the scotopic pupil of the patient.

Once a valid acquisition is obtained with the pupil dilated pharmacologically, the exportable file (.ATE) is created for the elaboration system (Zylink treatment planner). Once this procedure begins, it provides a matching of the .OTE file with the .ATE file. Based on the subjective refractive, cycloplegic, and aberrometric data, together with the correction factor that we have elaborated for our system (each system has its own corrective factor, also depending upon climatic conditions of the laser equipment), it provides the quantification of the sphere to be corrected (from 85% to 100% of the aberrometric data depending upon the above mentioned parameters), leaving, however, still at 100% the values of the cylinder and its axis, because a significant part of these values influenced by the high-order aberrations that we must correct. Successively, based on the pupillometric data obtained (with the Orbscan or other pupillographics-pupillometers), one proceeds to the determination of the optical area of ablation (Figure 22-6A) and therefore carries out the simulation of the treatment (Figure 22-6B) carefully evaluating the elevative modifications that are simulated by the treatment planner. If there is any disagreement between the subjective or cycloplegic defect with the aberrometric data that exceeds 0.75/1 D in the Zywave survey, or a difference between the axis of the topographic/subjective cylinder and the value found by aberrometry of more than 10 degrees, the patient should be reevaluated and one should not proceed to treatment with these refractive discrepancies. However, in the case in which the parameters of difference between the measurements are below these values, one proceeds to the registration of the ablative file (.TLS) on the floppy disk in order to transfer it to the laser.

Results of Primary PRK Wavefront-Guided Zyoptix Treatments

As we have described, the procedure of the acquisition of data for the wavefront-guided treatments is fairly complex and requires a long period of time. It is also able to supply numerous data about the eye to be treated, which, if adequately carried forward onto the ocular surface, are able to modify the corneal surface asymmetrically and in a locally different manner in order to produce a significant improvement in optical quality of the system. The more asymmetrical and irregular the wavefront generated by the eye appears in examination, the greater the benefit that a treatment of this type can supply, compared to a preestablished symmetrical

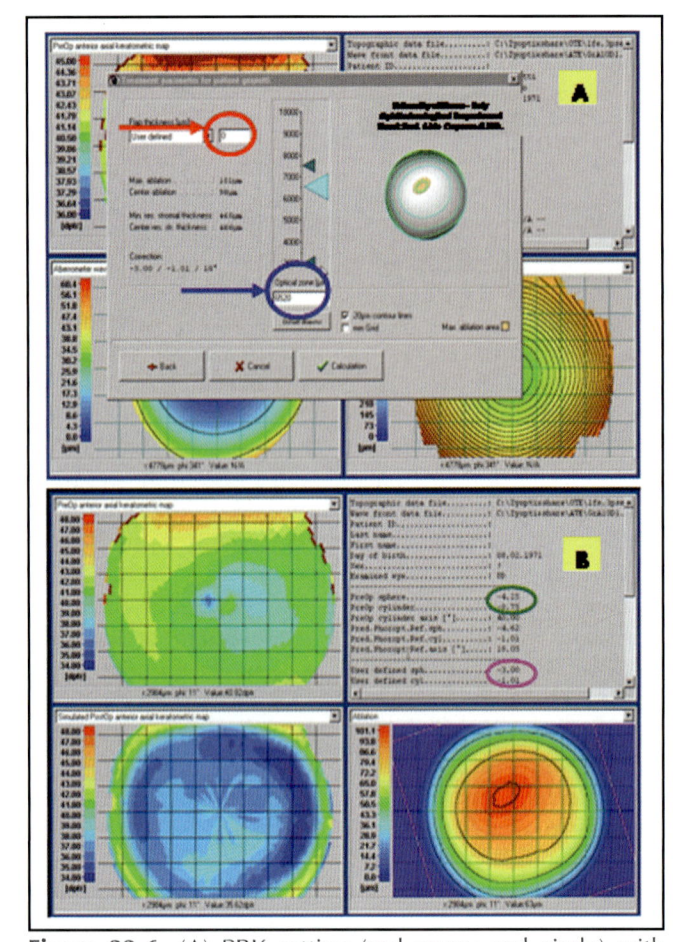

Figure 22-6. (A) PRK setting (red arrow and circle) with flap thickness=0 µm and optical zone diameter (blue arrow and circle) 6.520 mm in myopic spherocylindrical wavefront guided PRK. (B) Treatment simulation in PRK enhancement: the green circle shows wavefront measured data and the pink circle shows the treated data: 65% of the measured sphere was treated.

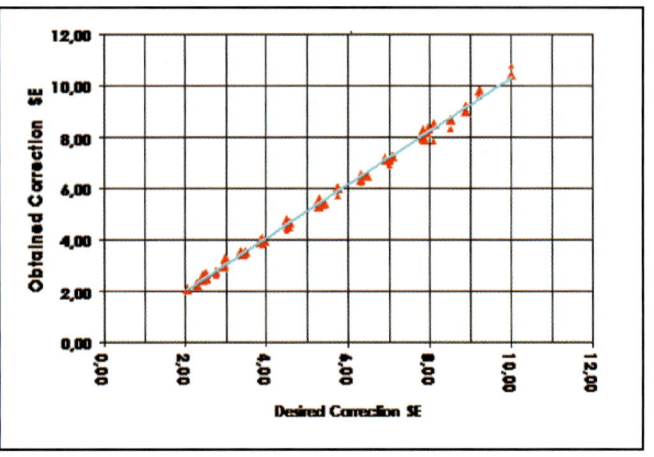

Figure 22-7. Scattergram of Zywave measured spherical equivalent in a series of consecutive 104 eyes with 12 months minimum follow-up. Undilated pupil in all cases, PPR (3.5-mm diameter) value.

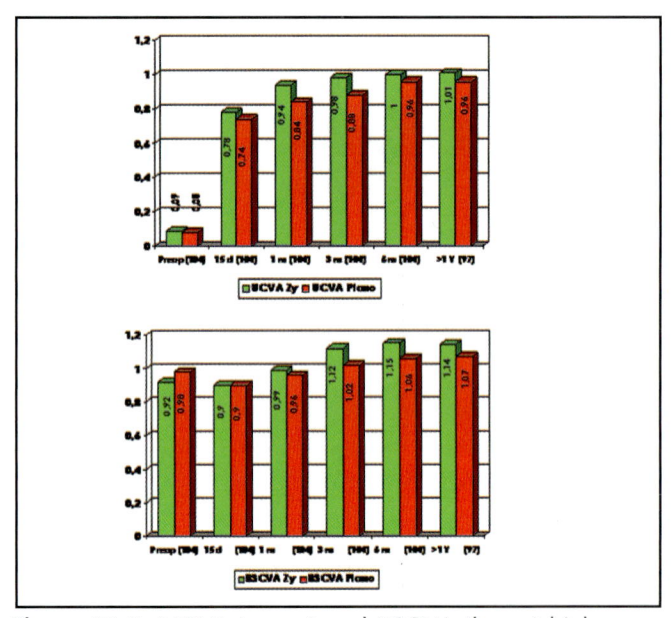

Figure 22-8. UCVA (upper) and BSCVA (lower) high contrast visual acuity in unselected consecutive serie of 104 Zyoptix PRK treated eyes (green bar) vs 104 uselected Planoscan PRK treated eyes. The difference between the two series was statistically significant at 1 and 3 months (p<0.05) in UCVA and at 3 and 6 months in BSCVA (p<0.05). Insignificant other follow-up time.

treatment. In fact, in our case study of 104 consecutive eyes in first surgery, we were able to observe better overall results compared to treatments based on preestablished symmetrical treatments (Planoscan) both from the point of view of instrumental aberrometric mapping and in functional performance. These data demonstrate how one has better accuracy in the correction of the refractive defect, both spherically and cylindrically, in both objective (aberrometrical) (Figure 22-7) and subjective evaluation with a significantly improved predictability both in the sphere and in the cylinder only for the aberrometrical data (p=0.086), while these data remain statistically significant for cylindrical correction (p=0.001). This difference also reflects on the functional performances that show an overall better result both in uncorrected visual acuity (UCVA) and in best corrected visual acuity (BSCVA) (Figure 22-8) which does not have a statistically significant importance during the entire follow-up, during the first 3 months for UCVA and in the follow-up at 3 and 6 months for BSCVA. Better statistical significance and higher constancy of results was obtained by analyzing the high-order aberrations as a total. In the whole population, one observes that both the HOA and the comatic aberrations are slightly, and in a statistically significant manner, inferior for the wavefront-guided treatments compared to conventional treatments for the components of the fourth order.[23] Above all, the Z_{400} primary spherical aberrations do not show statistically significant differences, as they showed inferior results in customized wavefront treatments compared to standard treatments[24] (Figure 22-9). The observed reduction of spherical aberration components does not show a significant statistical difference unless it is linked to the nonstratification of the cases. In fact,

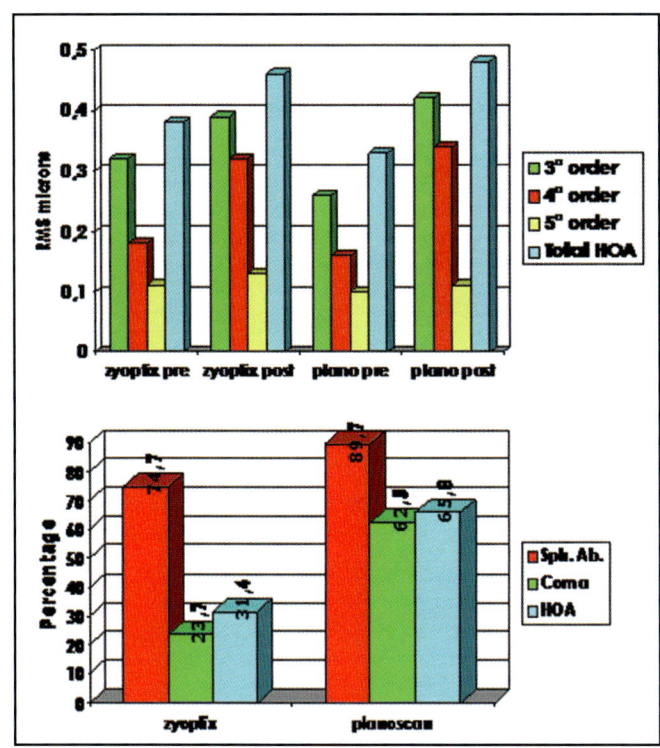

Figure 22-9. Unselected 104 Zyoptix PRK treated eyes vs unselected 104 Planoscan. The superior graph shows single order variations of RMS (microns) and the inferior shows the percentage variation before and 1 year after surgery of spherical aberration, coma, and total high-order aberrations.

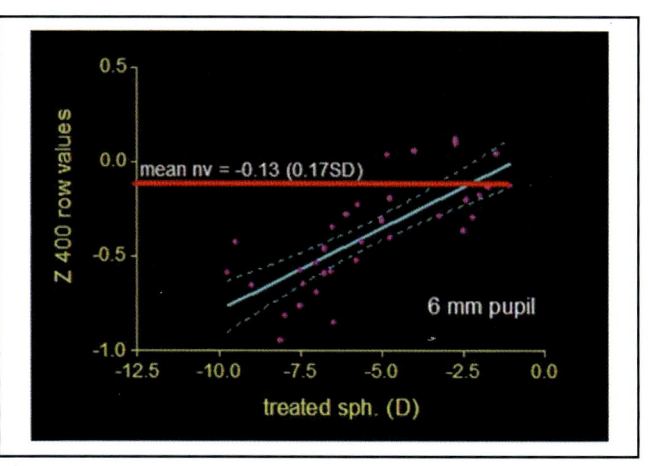

Figure 22-10. Six-mm pupil Zywave measured monochromatic longitudinal primary spherical aberration (A) in Zyoptix PRK-treated patients related with treated myopic spherical defect. Continuous and interrupted sky blue lines represent respectively linear regression and its 95% confidence limits. Red line indicates the preoperative mean value.

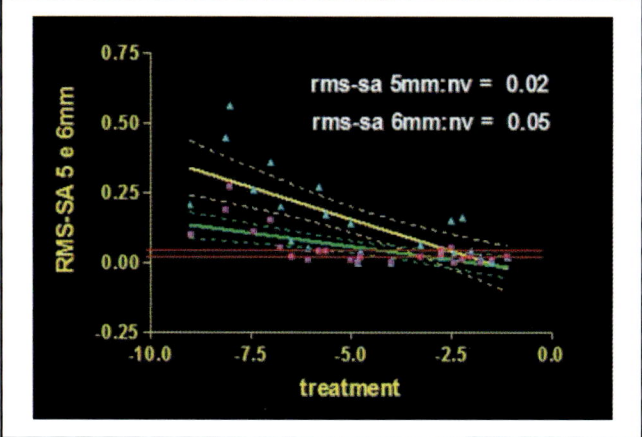

Figure 22-11. Five-(purple dot) and six-(sky blue triangle) mm pupil surgically induced spherical aberration Z400. The difference between before and after Zyoptix PRK in Zywave measured monochromatic longitudinal primary spherical aberration (μ RMS) shows that every sphere myopic treated diopters, in 6.2 optical zone treatment, induce meanly 0.02 μ RMS (at 5-mm pupil) and 0.05 μ RMS (at 6-mm pupil). Continuous and interrupted lines represent respectively linear regression and its 95% confidence limits, green for 5-mm pupil and yellow for 6-mm pupil.

if we analyze the distribution of the quantity of spherical aberrations present before surgery, we note that about 92% of the eyes that will undergo first surgery had primary spherical aberration values inferior to 0.3, and about 80% of cases had RMS values inferior to 0.15 (Figure 22-10). This means that we would still have a final increase in the same value also removing this component, keeping in mind that the treatment of 1 D of myopia with an optical zone of 6.2 mm involves an average induction of 0.05 of primary spherical aberration calculated on a 6-mm pupil diameter (Figure 22-11). Therefore, for treatments of less than 3 D of correction, there would not be a significant increase in this aberration, which tends to increase after surgery in all other cases. Obviously, the increase in spherical aberrations induced by conventional treatments involves the same amount of primary spherical aberrations without removing the preoperative value of spherical aberration. Therefore, these data explain the better instrumental results of wavefront-guided ablations that do not reach a statistical significance in unselected populations or with mean spherical corrections of an average of over 50% compared to the threshold of the cited 3 D (the examined population had an average spherical defect of 4.83 D ± 2.77).

Comatic aberrations behave differently: in fact, in populations undergoing first surgery, around 75% of cases have a value of third order aberrations of less than 0.5 RMS, but only 50% of the total is under 0.25 RMS. Therefore, only this population has results that are nearly equal between standard and personalized treatment, while all of the other cases positively feel the effect of a wavefront-guided treatment that is able to work asymmetrically on the corneal surface and therefore reduce the amount of asymmetry organically present and responsible for the comatic aberrations. This condition of reduction of the coma of the personalized ablation occurs only when the weight exceeds a value of 0.5 RMS, but starting from a value of 0.25, it does not increase to a postoperative value of third order aberrations, and this is the reason for the

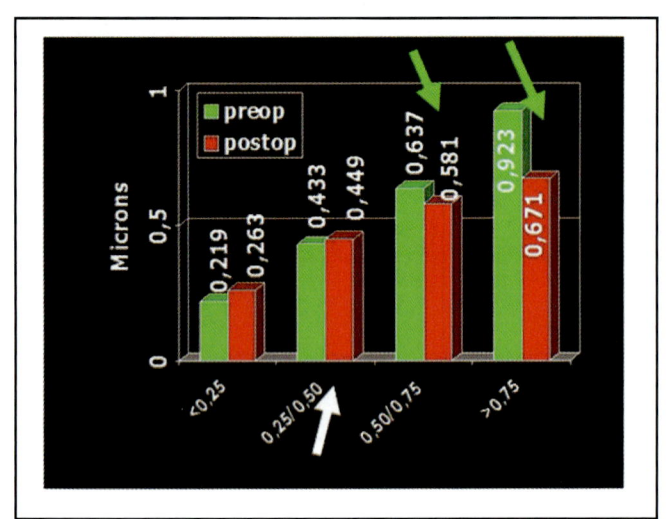

Figure 22-12. Comatic aberration RMS in 104 unselected Zyoptix PRK before and 12 months after treatment. The patients were stratified for preoperative third-order aberration RMS value. The bars shows a slight increasing in the lower two groups (<0.25 and 0.25/0.50 μ RMS) with a significant difference in the lower group (p=0.039 red arrow) and without significant difference in the second group (p=0.123 white arrow). In the high and very high aberrated eyes (0.5/0.75 and >0.75 μ RMS preoperative) we have a significant reduction in the first group (p=0.023 short green arrow) and a very significant reduction in the most aberrated group (p<0.001 long green arrow).

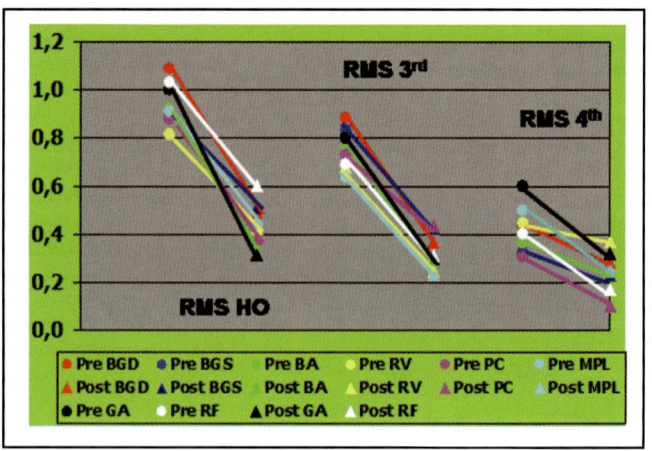

Figure 22-13. Aberrometric analysis in eight selected high preoperative aberrated eyes (HOA RMS >0.75 μm). The graph shows a significative reduction in all analyzed parameter. Comatic aberration shows a very repeatable reduction model.

statistically significant difference in unselected populations treated with wavefront-guided ablations compared to similar populations treated with standard ablations (Figure 22-12). The origin of comatic aberrations induced by treatment is not strictly tied to the entity of the treated spherical defect as much as correct centering, pupil location, and eyetracker efficacy in compensating ocular movements, particularly on level Z (tilting) and in compensating the shift that is present during the variations of diameter of the pupil. Analyzing the refractive and aberrometric results, it appears evident that a wavefront treatment is able to produce better results than Planoscan treatment, particularly regarding the correction of cylindrical defects due to the better aptitude in reducing asymmetries of the ocular optical system able to generate comatic aberrations. However, this does not produce on unselected populations significant differences in terms of predictability, and it does not determine significant differences in terms of high contrast visual acuity. However, in order to highlight the advantages of the treatment, we must evaluate contrast sensitivity in mesopic light conditions. Zyoptix PRK is able to supply results that are equal to preoperative values for medium to low frequencies (3 and 6 cycles/degree) and even to furnish better results compared to preoperative values in higher frequencies (12 and 18 cycles/degree) in contrast with what occurs with a similar population (with equal low and high-order aberration values) treated with Planoscan and evaluated at the same follow-up period of 6 months.

However, when analyzing a population with high preoperative aberrations (HOA >0.75 RMS), we note the overall advantages of the personalized treatment. In fact, in this case, beyond the instrumental data of the reduction of the aberrations based on both low and high-orders (limited to third and fourth orders) (Figure 22-13), one notes a considerable increase in functional ocular performance, including the values of high contrast visual acuity. In this case, we observed, on a selected case series of eight eyes, an increase in postoperative UCVA, up to and surpassing the preoperative BSCVA of an average of 1 Snellen line, and also an increase in BSCVA, which showed an average improvement of 1.8 Snellen lines (range 1 to 3) compared to preoperative examination.

Indications and Limits of PRK Zyoptix Treatment

Tissue removal based on the wavefront throughout the use of a flying spot laser with a 2- to 1-mm adjustable diameter undoubtedly allows for an ablative flexibility and an adaptability to different corneal morphologies that is much higher than preestablished ablation based on Munnerlynn's law.[25,26] These special characteristics obviously make the procedure highly recommended in situations in which the high-order aberrations are important enough to not allow complete vision, even with the best correction of the spherical and cylindrical[27,28] components, and even with the good ability demonstrated in the correction of preexisting spherical and comatic aberrations of a significant value. It should be noted that conditions of an elevated presence of HOA (superior to 0.75 RMS) in the populations of candidates for first surgery is a relatively slight number of cases, not exceeding 5% to 8% of the total (see Figure 22-13). Another important indication for Zyoptix treatment is average elevated astigmatism and topographically irregular astigmatism or symmetrical astigmatism, both simple and associated with myopic or

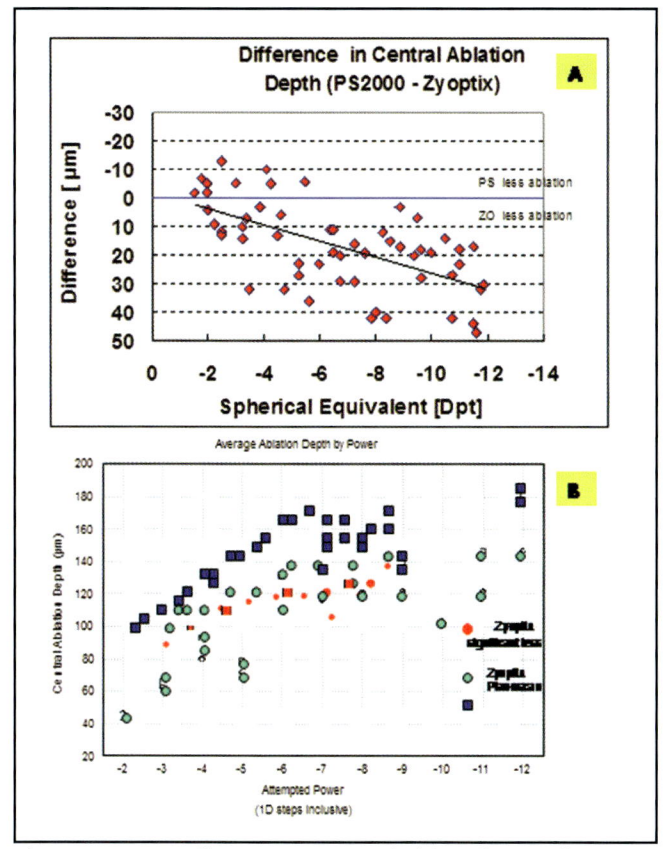

Figure 22-14. Difference in central ablated tissue between (A) Planoscan and Zyoptix PRK for same correction, same optical zone: correction increasing shows tissue saving increasing in Zyoptix procedure. Scatterplot of ablated tissue in Planoscan (blue square) and Zyoptix myopic PRK. Evident a nonlinear distribution of Zyoptix ablated tissue and a lesser ablated tissue for every correction (B).

mixed defects and with less electiveness, in mixed hyperopic astigmatism. This indication, beyond the flexibility and the adaptability of the Zyoptix procedure for corrections, is significantly justifiable in the ability shown by PRK-guided wavefront to save tissue and also for the possibility of carrying out tissue removal correcting the positive cylinder or a double-crossed cylinder which allows for a tissue savings that varies between 6% to 8%, which is associated with a capacity of tissue savings through the reduction of the transition area of 10% to 12%, leading to an approximate savings of 20%.[29,30] This savings allows, in the case of thin corneas, for treatments that would otherwise not be possible, and in the case of abundant tissue, one can enlarge the optic area, obtaining a reduction of induced spherical aberration. These last data are consequent at positive spherical aberration induced by the treatment of the positive cylinder, for which, in the case of myopic treatments superior to 4 to 5 D, one notes a considerable reduction of the amount of the negative spherical aberrations induced compared to simple spherical treatments for compensation (also only partial) of the positive spherical aberration induced by positive cylindrical treatment and negative spherical aberration due to myopic spherical treatment. Another condition that is highly indicated is the presence of not particularly thick corneas or with the presence of large (broad) pupils and average-elevated spherical-cylindrical defects, or rather all conditions in which there is an imbalance between tissue required for treatment and available corneal thickness. In these conditions one can take advantage of the ability of wavefront-guided ablation to save between 16% and 22% of tissue, depending upon the type of defect to be treated and the amount of preexisting aberrations (see Figure 22-12). In our unselected case series, we observed an average value of 18.4%.

Another condition in which surface wavefront ablation shows important advantages is enhancement procedures of previous ablations of the surface with transparent cornea, both in the presence and the absence of residual refractive defect. Wavefront-guided enhancement allows for recentering of decentered treatments and for enlarging reduced optical zones, above all considering the ability that the procedure has in correcting high preexisting aberrations of the third or fourth order.

It is less accurate and predictable in the correction of residual refractive defects with a tendency to overcorrection, which, in the existing small case record, provides for a correction of low order aberrations, on the order of 65% to 75% of the aberrometrically measured defocus data.

From international experience based on LASIK and our experience (more than 3 years), we believe that wavefront-guided treatment is undoubtedly a safe (in no case have we had the loss of 2 or more Snellen lines of BSCVA and we have observed a total safety index of 1.29) and effective solution (in over 90% of cases we have obtained a postoperative UCVA of equal to or less than the preoperative BSCVA with a total effectiveness index of 1.12), able to provide results that are not inferior to the Planoscan procedure if used for eyes with a low incidence of aberrations, and that are certainly better in aberrated or nonsymmetrical eyes. The procedure is certainly more and longer investigated than a preestablished procedure, such as that of Planoscan, and the evaluation of acquired data requires an experienced refractive surgeon. Furthermore, as we have seen, in spherical corrections of more than 4 D, one does not note a significant difference in the capacity to induce spherical aberrations compared to Planoscan. Thus, the two procedures are not different in corrective predictability of the spherical component (a predictability index of 0.95 for Planoscan vs 0.956 for Zyoptix). Consequently, based on these evaluations, we believe that the wavefront-guided PRK procedure should be elective for 10% to 12% of eyes for first treatment and for 50% to 60% of eyes for retreatments (and practically all cases of retreatment with transparent cornea). In cases of first myopic treatments with cylindrical defects of less than 1.5 D, it would be preferable, and more predictable, to chose the optimization of the treatment, using the tissue saving with adjustment of K average or tissue saving with aspherical optimization options, taking advantage of the tissue saving capacity for enlarging the optical areas or aspherical ablation, both individually or together, with the aim of minimizing the quantity of spherical aberrations generated by the modifications of profile necessary for correcting spherical defects.

The option of tissue saving is therefore a procedure in which optimization of ablation produced by mean K adjustment in the Munnerlynn formula makes it possible to improve ablative precision by better adaptation of the angle of impact of the laser in paracentral regions (Caporossi, Proceedings of National Congress "Società Italiana Laser in Oftalmologia," 1993) leading to more precise ablation produced by the most appropriate tissue removal. Adaptation of the quantity of tissue ablated to the mean radius of curvature[34-36] is the main factor leading to greater predictability with respect to Zyoptix WF and Planoscan (index of predictability 0.98 vs 0.96 and 0.95, respectively, in a consecutive series of 94 personal cases with follow-up greater than 24 months) and the possibility of 24% greater tissue sparing (range 20% to 30%) than with Planoscan. The Zyoptix TS system therefore sets a new ablative standard for the Bausch & Lomb platform and can implement the FDA-approved results of Planoscan.

The Zyoptix aspheric procedure has the same objectives as the TS system and also the objective of inducing limited primary spherical aberration in the central 4.5 mm of the cornea by removing tissue using an algorithm having radius of curvature as a (aspherical) variable. Although the model seems valid in theory, in clinical practice the choice of the point on which to center the ablation turns out to be critical.[37-39] In fact, if a lens with a constant (spherical) radius of curvature is slightly decentered (by <0.1 to 0.2 mm), in the corneal plane the optical geometry of the system does not change significantly. On the other hand, if a lens with a variable radius of curvature is similarly decentered, there are much more significant optical effects (primary effects[40] on low order aberration and above all secondary effects on paracentral[41] third, fifth, and other aberrations) that devastate the optical performance of the system. These theoretical aspects therefore suggest that this aspherical ablation profile requires further training of pupillographic-eye tracking systems and better defined indications before it can be proposed as a standard and safely used to correct high myopic defects.

References

1. Munnerlyn CR, Koons SJ, Marshall J. Photorefractive keratectomy: a technique for laser refractive surgery. *J Cataract Refract Surg.* 1988;14(1):46-52.
2. O'Donnell CB, Kemner J, O'Donnell FE Jr. Ablation smoothness as a function of excimer laser delivery system. *J Cataract Refract Surg.* 1996;22(6):682-685.
3. Krueger RR, Seiler T, Gruchman T, Mrochen M, Berlin MS. Stress wave amplitudes during laser surgery of the cornea. *Ophthalmology.* 2001;108(6):1070-1074.
4. Hanna KD, Chastang JC, Asfar L, Samson J, Pouliquen Y, Waring GO 3rd. Scanning slit delivery system. *J Cataract Refract Surg.* 1989;15(4):390-396.
5. Seiler T, Bende T, Wollensak J, Trokel S. Excimer laser keratectomy for correction of astigmatism. *Am J Ophthalmol.* 1988;105(2):117-124.
6. Lubatschowski H, Kermani O, Welling H, Ertmer W. A scanning and rotating slit arF excimer laser delivery system for refractive surgery. *J Refract Surg.* 1998;14(2 Suppl):S186-S191.
7. MacRae SM, Williams DR. Wavefront guided ablation. *Am J Ophthalmol.* 2001;132(6):915-919.
8. Manns F, Ho A, Parel JM, Culbertson W. Ablation profiles for wavefront-guided correction of myopia and primary spherical aberration. *J Cataract Refract Surg.* 2002;28(5):766-774.
9. Rusin D, Hall PB, Nichol RC, Marlow DR, Richards AM, Myers ST. Adaptive optics imaging of the CLASS gravitational lens system B1359+154 with the Canada-France-Hawaii telescope. *Astrophys J.* 2000;533(2):L89-L92.
10. Roorda A. Adaptive optics ophthalmoscopy. *J Refract Surg.* 2000;16(5):S602-S607.
11. Zhang DY, Justis N, Lien V, Berdichevsky Y, Lo YH. High-performance fluidic adaptive lenses. *Appl Opt.* 2004;43(4):783-787.
12. Mrochen M, Kaemmerer M, Seiler T. Wavefront-guided laser in situ keratomileusis: early results in three eyes. *J Refract Surg.* 2000;16(2):116-121.
13. Cosar CB, Saltuk G, Sener AB. Wavefront-guided laser in situ keratomileusis with the Bausch & Lomb Zyoptix system. *J Refract Surg.* 2004;20(1):35-39.
14. Nuijts RM, Nabar VA, Hament WJ, Eggink FA. Wavefront-guided versus standard laser in situ keratomileusis to correct low to moderate myopia. *J Cataract Refract Surg.* 2002;28(11):1907-1913.
15. Auffarth GU, Wang L, Völcker HE. Keratoconus evaluation using the Orbscan Topography System. *J Cataract Refract Surg.* 2000;26:222-228.
16. Rao SN, Raviv T, Majmudar PA, Epstein RJ. Role of Orbscan II in the screening Keratoconus suspects before refractive corneal surgery. *Ophthalmology.* 2002;109:1642-1646.
17. Fakhry A, Artola A, Belda JI, Ayala MJ, Alio JL. Comparison of corneal pachymetry using ultrasound and Orbscan II. *J Cataract Refract Surg.* 2002;28:248-252.
18. Thibos LN, Hong X. Clinical applications of the Shack-Hartmann aberrometer. *Optom Vis Sci.* 1999;76(12):817-825.
19. Rozenblium IZ, Kivaev AA, Korniushina TA, Abugova TD. Aberrometry in the diagnosis of eye diseases. *Oftalmol Zh.* 1990;(8):474-479.
20. Hament WJ, Nabar VA, Nuijts RM. Repeatability and validity of Zywave aberrometer measurements. *J Cataract Refract Surg.* 2002;28(12):2135-2141.
21. Zernike F. Polynomyal calculation to describe light aberrations. *Experientia.* 1953;9(12):473-474.
22. Schwiegerling J, Greivenkamp JE, Miller JM. Representation of videokeratoscopic height data with Zernike polynomials. *J Opt Soc Am A Opt Image Sci Vis.* 1995;12(10):2105-2113.
23. Kim TI, Yang SJ, Tchah H. Bilateral comparison of wavefront-guided vs conventional laser in situ keratomileusis with Bausch and Lomb Zyoptix. *J Refract Surg.* 2004;20(5):432-438.
24. Cosar CB, Saltuk G, Sener AB. Wavefront-guided laser in situ keratomileusis with the Bausch & Lomb Zyoptix system. *J Refract Surg.* 2004;20(1):35-39.
25. Chang AW, Tsang AC, Contreras JE, Huynh PD, Calvano CJ, Crnic-Rein TC, Thall EH. Corneal tissue ablation depth and the Munnerlyn formula. *J Cataract Refract Surg.* 2003;29(6):1204-1210.
26. Marcos S, Cano D, Barbero S. Increase in corneal asphericity after standard laser in situ keratomileusis for myopia is not inherent to the Munnerlyn algorithm. *J Refract Surg.* 2003;19(5):S592-S596.
27. Kanjani N, Jacob S, Agarwal A, et al. Wavefront- and topography-guided ablation in myopic eyes using Zyoptix. *J Cataract Refract Surg.* 2004;30(2):398-402.
28. Kim H, Joo CK. Visual quality after wavefront-guided LASIK for myopia. *J Korean Med Sci.* 2005;20(5):860-865.
29. Lee DH, Oh JR, Reinstein DZ. Conservation of corneal tissue with wavefront-guided laser in situ keratomileusis. *J Cataract Refract Surg.* 2005;31(6):1153-1158.
30. Kohnen T, Buhren J, Kuhne C, Mirshahi A. Wavefront-guided

LASIK with the Zyoptix 3.1 system for the correction of myopia and compound myopic astigmatism with 1-year follow-up: clinical outcome and change in higher order aberrations. *Ophthalmology.* 2004;111(12):2175-2185.
31. Wachler BS, Hiatt JA. Understanding pre-market approval and labeling differences of two leading customized ablation platforms: a call for reform at the FDA. *J Refract Surg.* 2004;20(5):S588-S692.
32. Pop M, Payette Y. Correlation of wavefront data and corneal asphericity with contrast sensitivity after laser in situ keratomileusis for myopia. *J Refract Surg.* 2004;20(5 Suppl):S678-S684.
33. Yoon G, McRae S, Williams DR, Cox IG. Causes of spherical aberration induced by laser refractive surgery. *J Cataract Refract Surg.* 2005;31(1):127-135.
34. Mrochen M, Seiler T. Influence of corneal curvature on calculation of ablation patterns used in photorefractive laser surgery. *J Refract Surg.* 2001;17(5):S584-S587.
35. Taneri S, Zieske JD, Azar DT. Evolution, techniques, clinical outcomes, and pathophysiology of LASEK: review of the literature. *Surv Ophthalmol.* 2005;50(5):502-504.
36. Roberts C. Biomechanics of the cornea and wavefront-guided laser refractive surgery. *J Refract Surg.* 2002;18(5):S589-S592.
37. Bueeler M, Mrochen M, Seiler T. Maximum permissible lateral decentration in aberration-sensing and wavefront-guided corneal ablation. *J Cataract Refract Surg.* 2003;29(2):257-263.
38. Fea AM, Sciandra L, Annetta F, Musso M, Dal Vecchio M, Grignolo FM. Cyclotorsional eye movements during a simulated PRK procedure. *Eye.* 2005;July.
39. Wang Z, Yang B, Huang XH, Huang GF, Qiu P, Chen JQ. The influence of pupil center shift on wavefront-guided laser in situ keratomileusis. *Zhonghua Yan Ke Za Zhi.* 2005;41(1):24-26.
40. MacRae SM, Williams DR. Wavefront guided ablation. *Am J Ophthalmol.* 2001;132(6):915-919.
41. Kremer I, Bahar I, Hirsh A, Levinger S. Clinical outcome of wavefront-guided laser in situ keratomileusis in eyes with moderate to high myopia with thin corneas. *J Cataract Refract Surg.* 2005;31(7):1366-1371.

CHAPTER 23

NO ALCOHOL LASEK VS PRK: A COMPARATIVE STUDY

Leopoldo Spadea, MD; Arianna Fiasca, MD

Refractive surgery using the 193-nm argon fluoride excimer laser has become a reasonably predictable, effective, and safe method to treat low to moderate myopia, hyperopia, and astigmatism.[1] However, photorefractive keratectomy (PRK) requires an epithelial debridement and has three disadvantages:

* Postoperative pain, which can be severe
* Temporary loss of corneal transparency ("corneal haze")
* Slow visual rehabilitation[2]

Laser in situ keratomileusis (LASIK) avoids these disadvantages by using an intrastromal ablation,[3] but it presents some corneal flap-related complications, such as flap wrinkling, dry eye, night halos, epithelial ingrowths, iatrogenic keratectasia, and diffuse lamellar keratitis (DLK).[4]

Laser-assisted subepithelial keratectomy, or LASEK, is a modified PRK technique that was introduced by Camellin in 1999.[5] This technique is based on creating a large epithelial flap after the application of an alcohol solution, ablating the stroma, and then repositioning the epithelial flap. The epithelial trephination is performed with a special microtrephine that creates a hinge of 90 degrees at the 12-o'clock position. The 80-μm calibrated blade for the 8.0-mm optic zone is used for the myopic treatment, and the 90-μm calibrated blade for the 9.0-mm optic zone is used for the hyperopic treatment. The pre-cut must be dried in order to highlight it. A cone slightly wider than the trephine and with a watertight double hinge must be used to allow the penetration of the alcoholic solution inside the pre-cut and to prevent conjunctival contamination. Subsequently, some drops of a 20% alcohol solution are instilled by a little pear-shaped container with a round needle. The alcohol solution is left for 30 seconds, then it must be carefully dried and abundantly irrigated with balanced salt solution (BSS). The appearance of a light epithelial edema after a few seconds is the first sign that the epithelium flap is detached. The epithelial flap is gently gathered at the 12-o'clock position with little movements perpendicular to the edge.

Alcohol delamination of the corneal epithelium before LASEK or PRK consistently results in a very smooth cleavage at the level between the lamina lucida and the lamina densa of the basement membrane, where integrin β4 interacts with lamina 5 to form hemidesmosomes.[6] It leaves behind a very smooth surfaces, which is ideal for PRK. It also allows for an intact epithelial flap to be lifted as a sheet from the corneal surface and hence is ideally suited for LASEK.[7] At this time, a standard PRK is performed, the flap is repositioned, and a soft contact lens is applied. Local therapy and follow-up are performed in the same method as after PRK. Since no lamellar flap is created, LASEK may retain the biomechanical stability shown with PRK and therefore can be an alternative to LASIK in cases where the corneal thickness is reduced too much.

The suggested advantages of LASEK over PRK are no more than faster corneal epithelial,[8,9] healing, lower discomfort, lower pain, early better visual acuity postoperatively, and decreased haze. The corneal epithelial healing and the visual rehabilitation are fast when the flap is not damaged during the procedure and when it is composed of vital epithelial cells. In this case, the epithelial healing takes place from the central cornea to the limbus and back again. Therefore, the visual rehabilitation time after LASEK is not faster than after LASIK one. The re-epithelialization defect never happened in the follow-up after LASIK.[10]

The presence of pain and its degree in postoperative follow-up after LASEK is controversial and some authors do not attest to the superiority of LASEK vs PRK.[11]

It is known that consequential events take place during the recovery process after PRK that can be causes of haze.[12,13] The epithelial flap prevents the release of cytokines and growth factor and that reduced apoptosis of anterior stromal keratocytes, decreased synthesis of collagens,[14] moreover like a mechanical barrier protects the surface of stroma from tears.[15]

Some works have been published in the past few years that declared LASEK an effective and safe procedure in the surgical correction of low and moderate myopia.[8,16,17] Comparative works about LASEK and PRK are few and have shown conflicting evidences.[18-20] The suggested advantages of LASEK over PRK are the consequence of the vitality of the epithelial flap during its repositioning. The use of alcohol, a cytotoxic agent, to detach the epithelial cells from the Bowman's membrane is probably a crucial factor in the dampened wound response in LASEK vs PRK.[21] The alcohol has multiplicity of toxic effect mechanisms, but the predominant mode of action appears to derive from enzymatic protein coagulation and denaturation. Consequently, the cell function is lost. An electron microscopy study on human cornea showed the loss of the cell membrane permeability and the increase of the intracellular esterase activity, disruptions, irregularities, discontinuities and duplications of basement membrane and autophagic vacuoles in basal epithelial cells. The exposure of the human cornea to ethanol reduces the number of vital epithelial cells rapidly[12] and increases cell death in a dose- and time-dependent manner.[22]

Usually the corneal epithelium is strongly attached to the stroma and therefore the use of a diluted ethanol solution is necessary to perform an epithelial flap. Nevertheless, in 4.6% of eyes this link is less strong and is possible to perform a no-alcohol LASEK.

In one study,[23] the effectiveness and safety of LASEK with mechanical deepithelialization without the use alcohol solution after long follow-up were evaluated, and the results with no alcohol standard PRK for the treatment of low and moderate myopia were compared.

Fifty eyes of 39 myopic patients were enrolled in the study and stratified in two groups. The first group had a no-alcohol LASEK procedure: 25 eyes (18 patients), 10 males and 8 females, mean age 37.7 years (±7.0), range 27 to 48 years, the mean myopia preoperative was -3.87 D (±2.61 D), range -1.0 to -7.75 D. In this group, the preoperative mean value of the UCVA was 0.33 (±0.28) and of the BCVA was 1 (± 0), the mean K_1 and K_2 were respectively 44.62 D and 45.34 D, the mean corneal pachymetry was 512 μm (±26.8), the preoperative mean endothelial microscopy was 2010 cells/mm^3 (±178), and the mean pupillometry was 6.4 mm (±0.6).

The second group had PRK with mechanical deepithelialization: 25 eyes (18 patients), 10 males and 8 females, mean age 35.4 years (±6.89), range from 24 to 48 years, the mean myopia preoperative was -3.9 D (± 2.06 D), range from -1.0 to -6.5 D. In this group the preoperative mean value of the UCVA was 0.34 (±0.28) and of the BCVA was 0.98 (±0.06), the mean K_1 and K_2 were respectively 44.89 D and 46.24 D, the mean corneal pachymetry was 514 μm (±28.5), the preoperative mean endothelial microscopy was 2023 cells/mm^3 (±183), and the mean pupillometry was 6.3 mm (±0.7). The mean ablation depth was 78.5 μm (±27.3) in LASEK and 78.8 μm (±23.6) in PRK.

There was no statistically significant difference between the two groups for age (p=0.27), optic zone (p=0.2), ablation depth (p=0.96), UCVA (p=0.9), BCVA (p=0.1), or spherical equivalent (p=0.87).

Surgical Techniques

A Mel 70 excimer laser (Carl Zeiss, Meditec, Jena, Germany) set at 193 nm, 35 Hz frequency, and 180 mJ/cm^2 fluency with a 0.25-μm ablation rate was used. The laser uses a 1.8-mm diameter flying spot with a Gaussian profile. To extract smoke or particles in the air without creating a draft, removing all obstacles on the path to the laser beam, a CCA (cone for controlled atmosphere) has been added to the laser. An active eyetracking system was used.

In PRK technique, after topical anesthesia (oxybuprocaine 0.4%), mechanical deepithelialization and photoablation on a dry cornea was performed. The mean optical zone diameter, corresponding to the diameter intended for the treatment area, was 6.92 mm ± 0.23 mm with a transition zone of 1.8 mm. An active eye-tracking system, oriented to an iron ring put on the limbus, constantly monitored the central position of the treatment. After the photoablation, a soft contact lens was applied and topical antibiotic (ofloxacin 3%) and artificial tears were given until the epithelial healing was complete. Topical corticosteroid (butyrate clobetasone 0.1%) drops were administrated for at least 1 month, then the drops were tapered and titrated depending on the corneal haze and refractive outcome.

In our personal LASEK technique, after topical anesthesia (oxybuprocaine 0.4%), pre-incision of the corneal epithelium was performed to circumscribe the flap area with a marker 9.0-mm diameter. We do not use an alcohol solution performing the procedure in patients with a light adhesion of the whole epithelial surface. The epithelium was then lifted and an intact flap was carried out with a smooth spatula. The epithelial flap was gently gathered at the 12-o'clock position. At this time we performed the photoablation; the optical zone diameter mean was 6.83 mm ± 0.38 mm. After laser ablation, the stromal surface was irrigated with topical antibiotic (ofloxacin 3%) and artificial tears, then after repositioning the epithelial flap, a soft contact lens was applied to the eye. Topical corticosteroids were administrated (like PRK cases).

In both groups the soft contact lens was removed after 5 days post refractive surgery. The follow-up was performed after 5 and 15 days; 1, 3, and 6 months; and 1 and 2 years.

The PC software program Primit (Version 3.03, 1994, McGraw-Hill, Italy) was used for statistical analysis (Student t-test).

Results

The epithelial defect was completely healed in the LASEK group after a mean time of 5.04 days (±2.31) (Figure 23-1) and after a mean time of 6.09 days (±2.25) in the PRK group. This difference was not statistically significant (p>0.01).

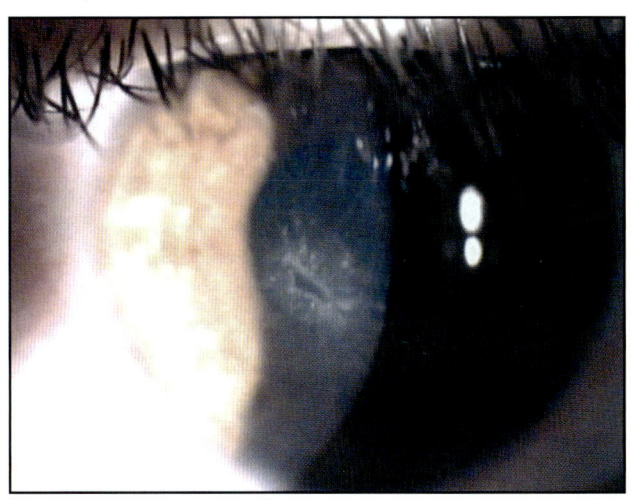

Figure 23-1. Re-epithelialization defect at VI day after LASEK after removed CL.

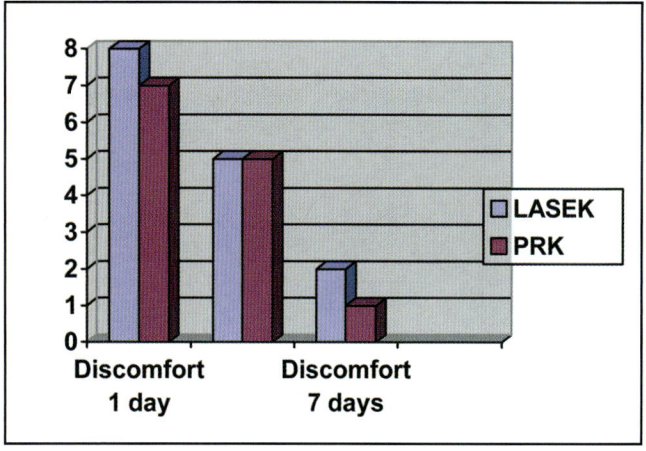

Figure 23-2. The presence of discomfort in the first week follow-up after LASEK and PRK.

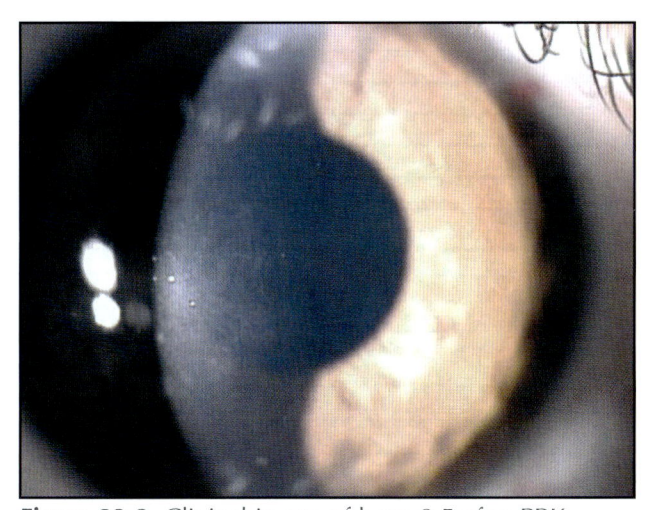

Figure 23-3. Clinical image of haze 0.5 after PRK.

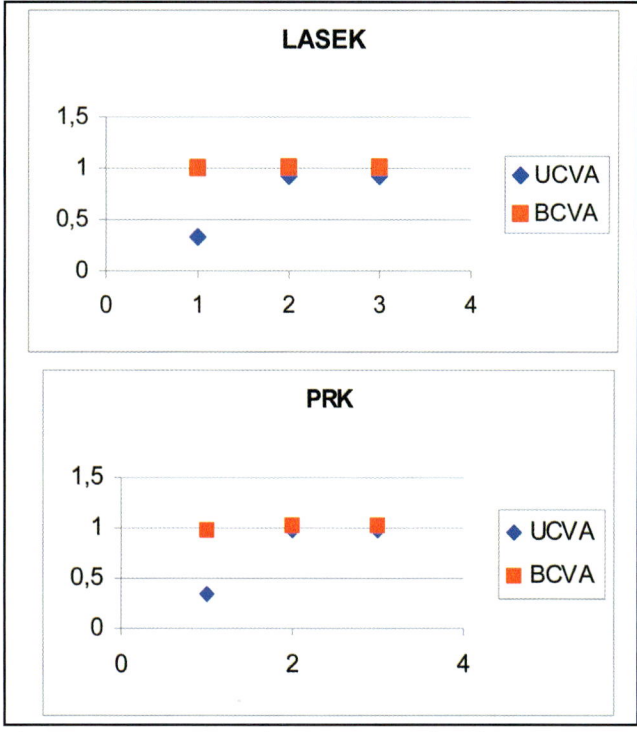

Figure 23-4. UCVA and BCVA 3 months after LASEK and PRK.

In the PRK group, discomfort was reported in 12 eyes (52%) after 1 day postoperative; in the LASEK group, at the same step, 14 eyes (56%) reported discomfort. This difference was not statistically significant (p>0.01) (Figure 23-2). After a follow-up of 2 years, the presence of haze ≤1 (0-5) was 2 eyes (8%) in the LASEK group and 3 eyes (12%) (p>0.01) in the PRK group (Figure 23-3). In the LASEK group at 1 month follow-up, the mean UCVA was 0.92 (±0.15) and the mean BCVA was 1.01 (±0.10). In the PRK group after 1 month follow-up the mean UCVA was 0.97 (±0.18) and the BCVA was 1.02 (±0.12) (Figure 23-4). No statistically significant difference was shown of the postoperative UCVA (p=0.31) and BCVA (p=0.75) between the two groups (Table 23-1). These results were unchanged at 24 months follow-up (Figures 23-5 through 23-10).

After 2 years of follow-up, the mean refraction of within ±0.5 D was measured in 68% (17 eyes) in the LASEK group and in 72% (18 eyes) in the PRK group, ±1.0 D in 88% (22 eyes LASEK) and 92% (23 eyes PRK), and ±2.0 D in 100% in both groups (Table 23-2). There was no statistically significant difference. The mean residual spherical equivalent was +0.27 D (±0.79) in the LASEK group and +0.54 D (±0.89) in the PRK group, also the difference about the spherical equivalent was not statistically significant (p=0.28) (Figures 23-11 and 23-12). The mean refractive astigmatism outcome vs time is shown in Figures 23-13 through 23-16.

Conclusion

In our study, the long-term result showed a good recovery in terms of UCVA, BCVA, and spherical equivalent reduction in both groups. We suppose that this result depended on the absence of an alcohol debridement. In our treatment, in fact, we obtain a mechanical delamination of the epithelial flap in LASEK or a mechanical deepithelialization in PRK.

Table 23-1. Paired Student T-Test

	6 Months	12 Months	24 Months
UCVA	P=0.24	P=0.20	P=0.15
BCVA	P=1	P=1	P=1
SE	P=0.43	P=0.09	P=0.12
CYL	P=0.45	P=0.60	P=0.60

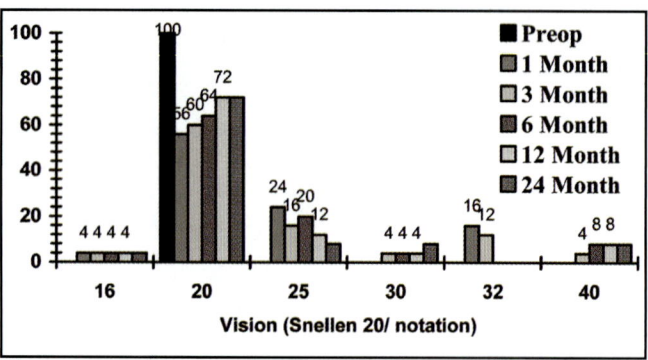

Figure 23-5. The preoperative BSCVA and the postoperative UCVA after LASEK.

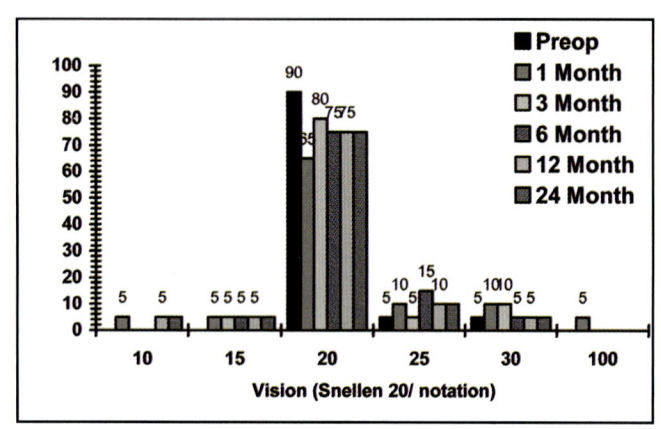

Figure 23-6. The preoperative BSCVA and the postoperative UCVA after PRK.

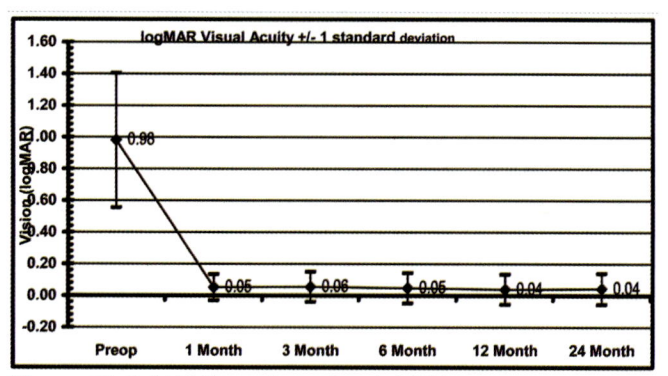

Figure 23-7. UCVA vs time after LASEK.

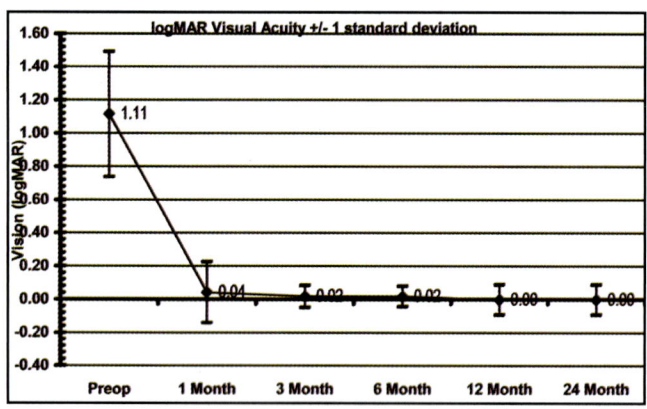

Figure 23-8. UCVA vs time after PRK.

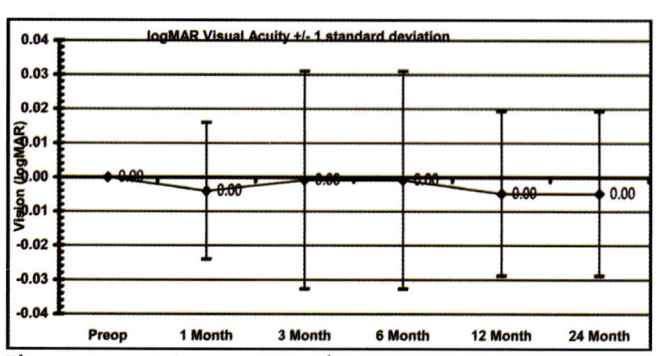

Figure 23-9. BCVA vs time after LASEK.

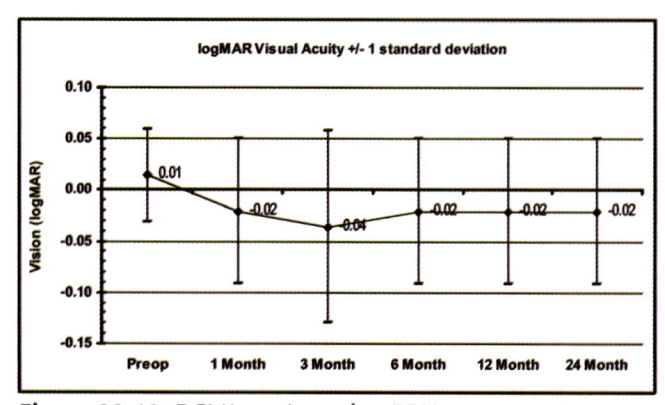

Figure 23-10. BCVA vs time after PRK.

Table 23-2. The Mean Spherical Equivalent After 24 Months Follow-Up

Spherical Equivalent	LASEK	PRK
+/-0.5 D	68%	70%
+/-1 D	88%	90%
+/-2 D	100%	100%

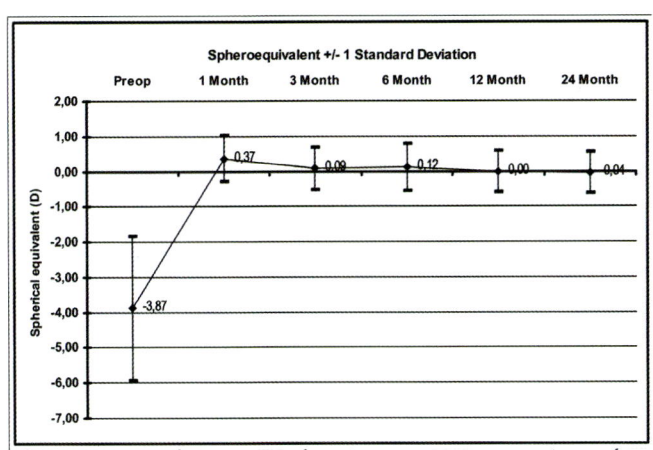

Figure 23-11. The mean refractive outcome over time after LASEK.

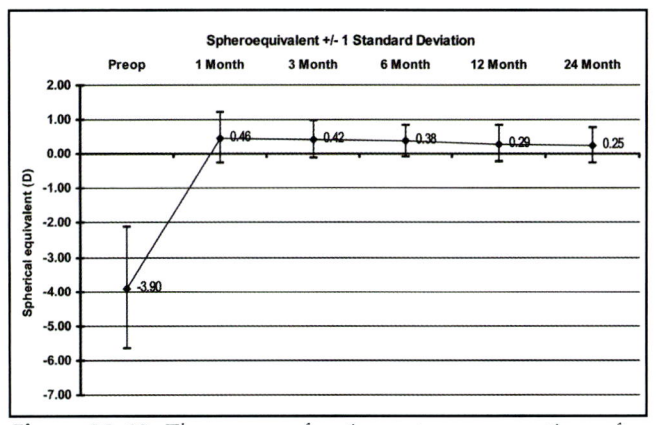

Figure 23-12. The mean refractive outcome over time after PRK.

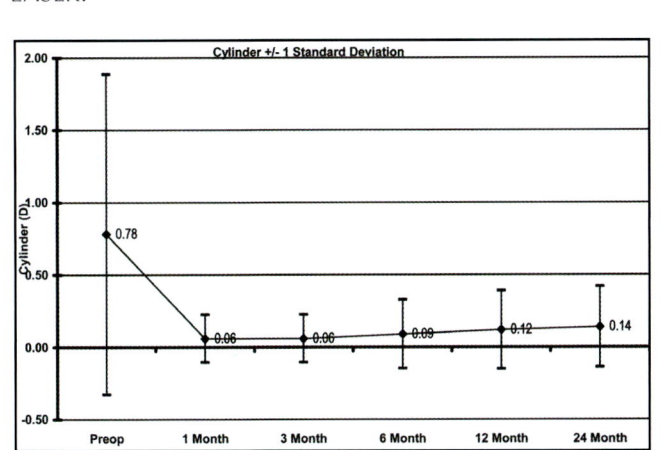

Figure 23-13. The mean astigmatic outcome over time after LASEK.

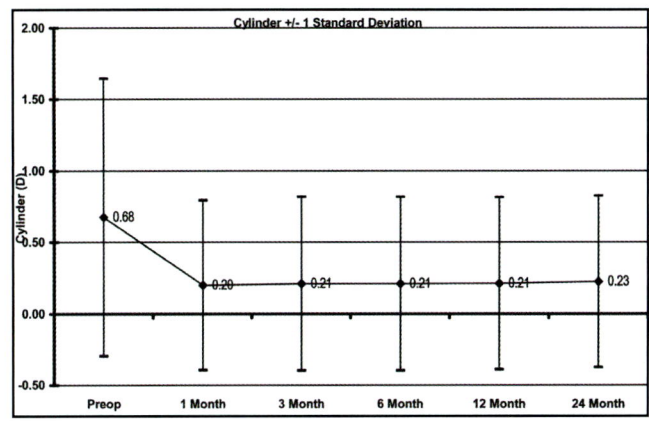

Figure 23-14. The mean astigmatic outcome over time after PRK.

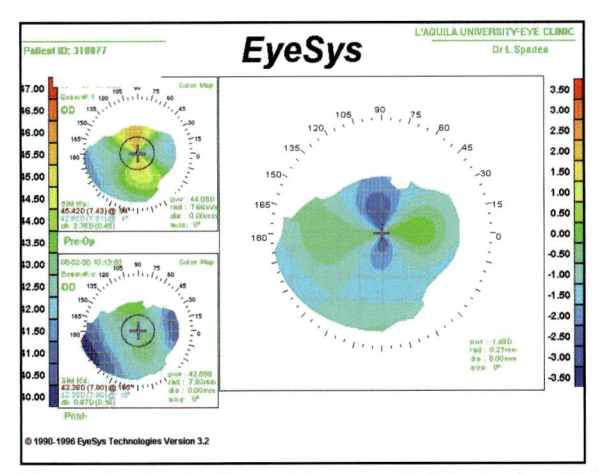

Figure 23-15. Differential map (right): Male, 32 years old; highlights the improved profile obtained from before (manifest refraction: –2sf=-2.75 cyl 5 degrees; visual acuity: 20/20) (top left) and at 24-months follow-up after LASEK (bottom left) (manifest refraction: plano; visual acuity: 20/20).

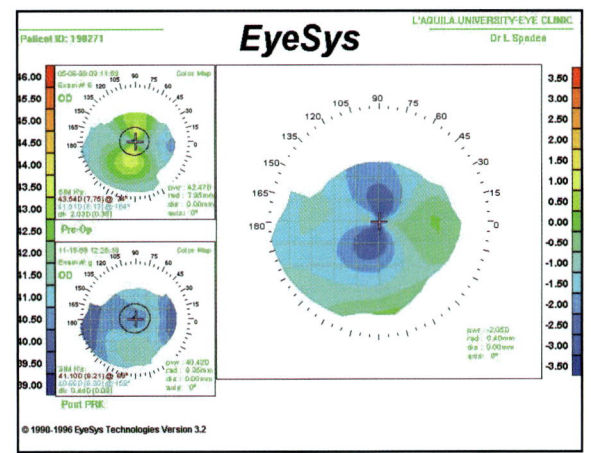

Figure 23-16. Differential map (right): Male, 29 years old; highlights the improved profile obtained from before (manifest refraction: –1sf=-2 cyl 180 degrees; visual acuity: 20/20) (top left) and at 24-months follow-up after PRK (bottom left) (manifest refraction: plano; visual acuity: 20/20).

There was not a statistically significant difference between the two groups. It seems to confirm that LASEK without a chemically altered epithelial flap does not show significant difference from standard PRK. The LASEK technique without alcohol deepithelialization is an effective and safe procedure for low and moderate myopia such as PRK. Therefore, the absence of a statistical difference between the two techniques in our experience could be caused by an insufficient group of patients. Further studies are necessary to confirm these results.

References

1. Trokel SL, Srinivasan R, Braren B. Excimer laser surgery of the cornea. *Am J Ophthalmol.* 1983;96:710-715.
2. American Academy of Ophthalmology. Excimer laser photorefractive keratectomy for myopia and astigmatism. Ophthalmic procedure assessment. *Ophthalmology.* 1999;106:422-437.
3. Hersh PS, Brint SF, Maloney RK. Photorefractive keratectomy versus laser in situ keratomileusis for moderate to high myopia: a randomized prospective study. *Ophthalmology.* 1998;105:1512-1522.
4. Wang Z, Chen J, Yang B. Posterior corneal surface of topographic changes after laser in situ keratomileusis are related to residual corneal bed thickness. *Ophthalmlogy.* 1999;106:406-410.
5. Camellin M. LASEK may offer the advantages of both LASIK and PRK. *Ocular Surgery News, International Edition.* 1999; March.
6. Espana EM, Grueterich M, Mateo A, et al. Cleavage of corneal basement components by ethanol exposure in laser assisted subepithelial keratectomy. *J Cataract Refract Surg.* 2003;29:1192-1197.
7. Browning AC, Shah S, Dua HS, Maharajan SV, Gray T, Bragheeth MA. Alcohol debridement of the corneal epithelium in PRK and LASEK: an electron myscroscopic study. *Invest Ophthalmol Vis Sci.* 2003;44:510-513.
8. Lee JB, Seong GJ, Lee JH, et al. Comparison of laser epithelial keratomileusis and photorefractive keratectomy for low to moderate myopia. *J Cataract and Refract Surg.* 2001;27:565-570.
9. Rouweyha RM, Chuang AZ, Yee RW. Laser assisted epithelial keratomileusis—outcomes in high myopia. ARVO abstract 3221. *Invest Ophthalmol Vis Sci.* 2001;42(4):S599.
10. Camellin M. Laser epithelial keratomileusis for myopia. *J Refract Surg.* 2004;20(5 Suppl):S693-S698.
11. Chalita MR, Tekwani NH, Krueger RR. Laser epithelial keratomileusis: outcome of initial cases performed by an experienced surgeon. *J Refract Surg.* 2003;19:412-415.
12. Sandwig KU, Kravik K, Haaskjold E, Blika S. Laser epithelial wound healing of the rat cornea after excimer laser ablation. *Acta Ophthalmol Scand.* 1997;75:115-119.
13. Balestrazzi E, De Molfetta V, Spadea L, et al. Excimer laser photorefractive keratectomy: histological, immunohimical and ultrastructural study in human corneas. *Ital J Ophth.* 1992;VI/2:95-100.
14. Wilson SE. Keratocyte apoptosis in refractive surgery. *CLAO.* 1998;24:181-185.
15. Zhao J, Nagasaky T, Maurice DM. Role of tears in keratocyte loss after epithelial removal in mouse cornea. *Invest Ophthalmol Vis Sci.* 2001;42:1743-1749.
16. Lee JB, Choe CM, Seong GJ, Gong HY, Kim EK. Laser subepithelial keratomileusis for low to moderate myopia: 6 months follow-up. *Jpn J Ophthalmol.* 2002;46:299-304.
17. Taneri S, Feit R, Azar DT. Safety, efficacy, and stability indices of LASEK correction in moderate myopia and astigmatism. *J Cataract Refract Surg.* 2004;30(10):2130-2137.
18. Feit R, Taneri S, Azar DT, Chen CC, Ang RT. LASEK results. *Ophthalmol Clin North Am.* 2003;16(1):127-35, viii.
19. Hashemi H, Fotouhi A, Foudazi H, Sadeghi N, Payvar S. Prospective, randomized, paired comparison of laser epithelial keratomileusisand photorefractive keratectomy for myopia less than −6.50 diopters. *J Refract Surg.* 2004;20(3):217-222.
20. Litwak S, Zadok D, Garcia-de Quevedo V, Robledo N, Chayer AS. Laser-assisted subepithelial keratectomy versus photorefractive keratectomy for the correction of myopia. *J Cataract Refract Surg.* 2002; 28:1330-1333.
21. Gabler B, von Mohrenfels CW, Dreiss AK, Marshall J, Lohmann CP. Vitality of epithelial cells after alcohol exposure during laser assisted subepithelial keratectomy flap preparation. *J Cataract Refact Surg.* 2002;28:1841-1846.
22. Chen C, Chang JH, Lee JB, Javier J, Azar DT. Human corneal epithelial cell viability and morphology after dilute alcohol exposure. *Invest Ophthalmol Vis Sci.* 2002;43:2593-2602.
23. Spadea L. No alcohol LASEK vs PRK: a comparative study. *Refractive onLine.* 2003;Sept:11-13.

CHAPTER 24

In Vivo Confocal Microscopy
Clinical Relevance in Refractive Surgery and in Epithelial Flap-Based Surface Ablation Techniques

Leonardo Mastropasqua, MD; Mario Nubile, MD; Manuela Lanzini, MD

Introduction

The understanding of cellular and tissutal events that take place in the dynamic of corneal physiology and pathology has always been a challenge for clinicians and researchers. It is known, in fact, that in almost all clinical conditions, the slit-lamp biomicroscopic evidence (which should be intended actually as a macroscopic observation) represents only the "epi-phenomenon" which resumes a complex pathway of biochemical, cellular, and tissutal modifications, which together mediates the real basis of the physiopathology of corneal processes, both in health and disease. Microscopic anatomical and functional observations have been limited, for several decades, to *ex vivo* in vitro investigations. A recent advance in this field of interest has been represented by the introduction in the clinical practice of instruments capable of performing a microscopic imaging analysis of the human corneal structure, *in vivo*, without significant invasiveness. This imaging diagnostic procedure, which was used initially for research purposes in the late 1980s, has been termed as "*in vivo* confocal microscopy of the cornea." One of the clinical fields in which *in vivo* confocal microscopy has been successfully applied, leading to a better comprehension of the tissutal microscopic response of the cornea to the surgical stress and damage, is represented by excimer laser refractive surgery. Initially, the aims of researchers, utilizing such a imaging technique in the evaluation of laser ablation effects induced in the corneal structure, were particularly focused on the possibility of investigation of the cell loss or damaging produced by the photoablation mediated by direct necrotic or indirect apoptotic mechanisms, of stromal wound healing phenomena (leading to the possibility of haze and regression which had a not negligible incidence, particularly with the old generation excimer lasers), and of surgically related nerve fiber loss and following nerve fiber regeneration processes. Recently, the increased knowledge and the standardization of confocal images interpretation have led to better understanding of the micro-anatomy, which has followed the technological advances and the work of researchers in clinical studies, opened a new window on the possibility of investigation of dynamic processes occurring within the corneal tissues, increasing the fields of application and the obtainable information from such exams. The capability of producing images at a cellular level of almost every corneal layer is principally based on the intrinsic transparency of corneal tissues. However, the *in vivo* imaging of cellular and a cellular components of the corneal structure derived by confocal microscopy suffers actually from a basic limitation: only a very small part of the entire cornea can be visualized at the same time, and precise topographic identification of the scanned area (particularly for noncentral cornea areas) is still to achieve. This means that although confocal microscopy gives us a great and novel view of microscopic processes occurring within the cornea, the clinical interpretation of confocal images should always come from the merging of the microscopic features with the clinical biomicroscopic ones, which although macroscopic, give generally a more complete picture of the entire cornea within its anatomical environment and relation to the rest of the eye.

Basic Principles of *In Vivo* Confocal Microscopy of the Cornea

The major limit affecting conventional light microscopic observation of the cornea is due to the fact that light is reflected by the tissues surrounding the point of observation. The increased magnification in ophthalmic slit lamp

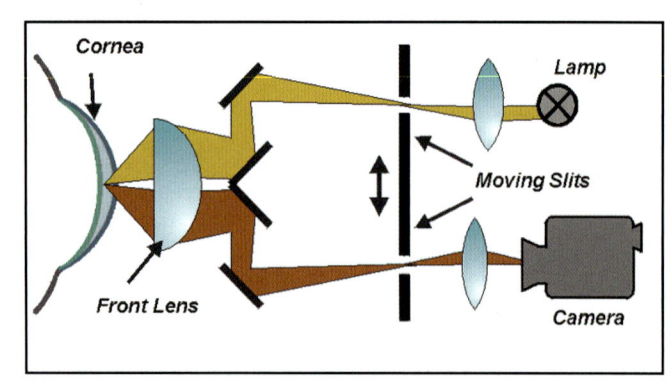

Figure 24-1. Diagrammatic representation of the optical principles of slit scanning confocal microscopy.

biomicroscopes, for example, leads to obscuration and reduction of the image contrast, and thus useful magnifications in this kind of ophthalmic clinical microscope cannot exceed 40 times with a resolution of approximately 20 µm. The clinical confocal microscope was invented in 1957 by Marvin Minsky[1] and since that time, particularly during the last decade, this instrument has undergone a rapid technological evolution, becoming a powerful diagnostic tool that allows clinicians to observe the living corneal tissue at a cellular level. It is based on the principle that both the illumination and the objective of the microscope are focused on the same point (sharing a common focal point), giving name to the method ("confocal" microscopy). This technological characteristic provides two main advantages compared to standard microscopes: enhancement of lateral (x,y) and axial (z) resolution, thanks to the elimination or reduction of unfocused information. Due to the fact that the cornea is generally a nearly transparent tissue, with minimal light absorption, the increase in axial resolution is responsible for the main advantage provided by confocal microscopy: the possibility to obtain optical sections of the entire corneal thickness producing high magnification (up to 1000 X, with dependence on the numerical aperture of the objective lens employed) "en face images" of the cornea (maintaining lateral and axial resolution within values comprised between 1 and 3 µm and 5 up to 10 µm, respectively). Different systems of confocal technology have been employed to develop the clinically available microscopes: 1) the tandem scanning confocal microscope (TSCM), which uses rotating Nipkow disk technology [2-4]; 2) the slit scanning confocal microscope (SSCM), based on oscillating slit aperture in an ophthalmic microscope configuration (Figure 24-1)[5-7]; and 3) the laser-scanning microscope (LSM), which instead of white-light illumination source uses the 670-nm wavelength of the beam emitted from a diode-laser.[8,9] Each of these technologies presents advantages and disadvantages, a discussion of which is beyond the scope of this chapter. However, the new confocal microscopes available and approved for clinical uses are based on a charge-coupled device (CCD) camera digital imaging technology, with real time acquisition of frames and automatically controlled focal plane of the objective through computerized motors (particularly the SSCM which presents

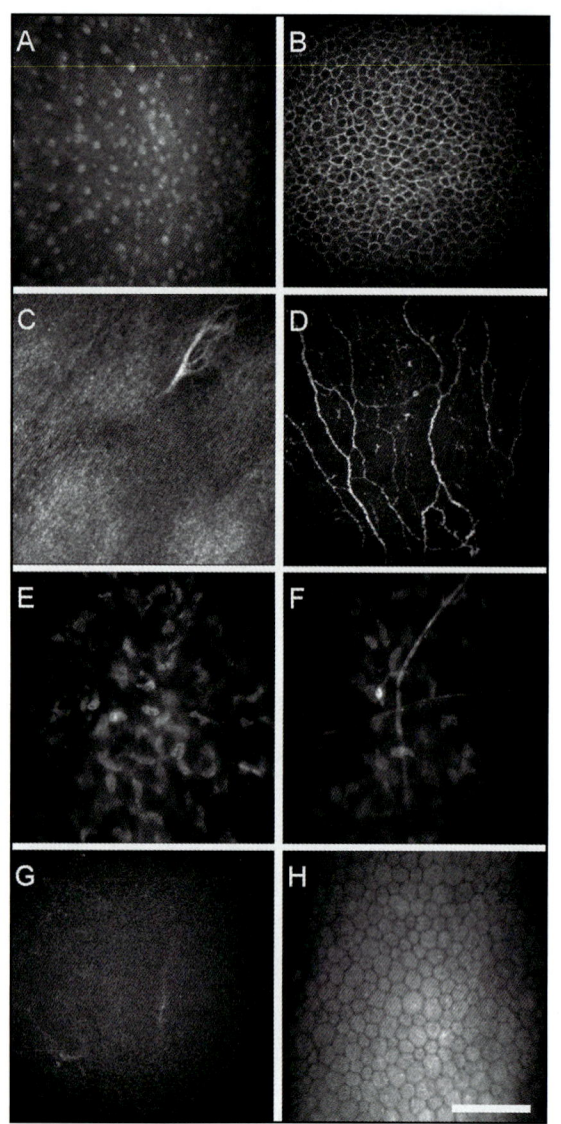

Figure 24-2. *In vivo* confocal microscopy of the central human cornea. Bar represents 100 µm. From top left to bottom right are shown: (A) Superficial epithelial cells. (B) basal epithelial cell layer. (C) Bowman's membrane with a perforating nerve fiber. (D) Subepithelial nerve plexus. (E) Anterior stroma with high density keratocyte nuclei. (F) Midstroma with deep nerve fibers. (G) Descemet's membrane appearing as an homogeneous grayish layer. (H) Endothelial cells.

all of these features). Current confocal instruments provide images of sufficient resolution to detect and visualize corneal cells, but not to resolve intracellular organelles.

Almost all anatomical corneal layers are clearly imaged by confocal microscopy: superficial epithelium, basal epithelium, Bowman's membrane, subepithelial nerve plexus, corneal stroma with resident keratocytes, deep nerve fibers, Descemet's membrane, and endothelium.[6,7,10-14] Figure 24-2 shows a composition of images illustrating confocal microscopic anatomy of the central human corneal layers. As

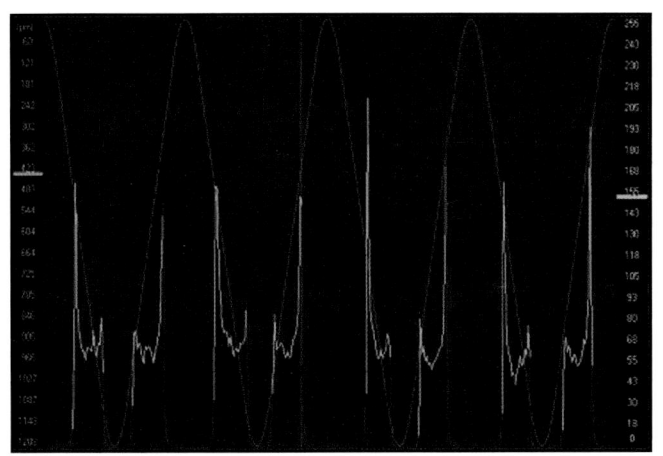

Figure 24-3. Z-scan function of the Confoscan SSCM. Multiple scans of normal central human cornea. Each curve represents a complete scan of the entire corneal thickness and is delimited by two peaks of reflectivity: the endothelial peak (highest) and the epithelial peak. The corneal stroma discloses lower reflectivity (greater in the subepithelial zone). The backscattered light of each point of a curve (corresponding to one captured image) is plotted in light reflectivity units (LRU) on the scale at the right side. The relative depth of each point/image is reported in the left side scale expressed in μm. Total corneal and sublayer thickness can be measured by using the dedicated software.

clearly visible by the example presented in Figure 24-2, *in vivo* confocal images are oriented parallel to the microscope objective and to the corneal surface, differently than histological specimens, that we are familiar with, which are sectioned perpendicular to the surface of the cornea, and thus the observer has to become familiar with the imaging in the coronal plane.

Confocal microscopes can be used to measure corneal thickness.[7,13-17] In the automated scanning of the cornea, each recorded image is characterized by its position on the z-axis of the cornea and its reflectivity. This is possible thanks to precise movements of the objective lens (or of its focus) in the z-axis, during which a computer registers the one-dimensional anteroposterior spatial position. A second feature, the integrated brightness in the middle area of the images, is calculated. A graphic showing the depth coordinate on the z-axis and the level of reflectivity on the y-axis can be elaborated (this is called the Z-scan graphic or profile) and can display the absolute depth (ie, distance between the starting point of the scan and the actual image along the sagittal anteroposterior line) where each image was captured (Figure 24-3). The brightness of the Z-scan depends on the mean level of reflectivity of each corneal layer. Transparent layers present low reflectivity (thus a low mean brightness on the intensity profile), while opaque layers disclose a high reflectivity. With reference to a normal transparent cornea, it is clearly visible that the corneal layers have an intrinsically different reflectivity. The endothelium shows the highest reflectivity while the rear stroma the lowest. The epithelium has intermediate values. This explains the morphology of the Z-scan curves that typically present, in normal corneas, on the intensity profile, a high endothelial peak, followed by a reduction of the reflectivity toward the anterior layers, and a middle-level superficial epithelial peak. The movements of the eye and the ocular blood pulse, presently, limits the precise determination of corneal thickness. However, confocal microscopy through focusing (CMTF) on the TSCM,[15] and the recent advance of Z-ring use, along with the reduction of image separation to a value lower than 10 μm which has been developed for the fourth-generation SSCM, provides good repeatability. The main advantage of this technology is represented by the fact that dedicated software allows the examiner to visualize the image corresponding to each point located on the Z-graphic and to determine the distance of two points of interest chosen within the curve, thus permitting the determination of partial thickness and corneal sublayer measurements (ie, epithelial thickness, residual stromal thickness after excimer laser ablation, flap thickness, interface depth in laser-assisted in situ keratomileusis (LASIK) and lamellar keratoplasty, and so on). Another useful function provided by a Z-scan graphic derived by a confocal scan of the cornea is the possibility of objective measurement of corneal transparency. The backscattered light measured in light reflectance units is correlated with the degree of corneal opacity, with obvious dependence to the illumination level used for the scan. So it is possible to evaluate with moderate precision and repeatability[18] processes affecting corneal transparency, such as stromal wound healing and corneal haze following surface ablations.

Confocal Microscopy in Excimer Laser Refractive Surgery

In the past decade, excimer laser surgical procedures for the treatment of ametropias gained significant success in the field of ophthalmic refractive surgery. In fact, the main evolution that completely changed the approach to refractive correction, based on the modification of the corneal shape, happened thanks to the development of the excimer laser, which is able to sculpt the cornea with microscopic accuracy.[19]

LASIK, photorefractive keratectomy (PRK), and, among the surface ablation procedures, the more recent laser-assisted subepithelial keratectomy (LASEK) and Epi-LASIK represent the most currently and successfully used evolving corneal laser surgical interventions for the correction of myopia. Recent surveys of trends among the US members of the International Society of Refractive Surgery[20] and of the American Society of Cataract and Refractive Surgeons[21] evidenced that although LASIK is the leading surgical procedure for myopia, the surface ablation techniques show a clear tendency of increment and increasing preferences with particular reference to LASEK.[21] On the other hand, in several European countries, PRK is more commonly used than LASIK, and similarly the new surface ablation techniques with epithelial flap are rapidly growing.

A review of the literature shows that the majority of refractive surgery publications are principally focused on the evaluation of clinical outcomes with lower emphasis on the physiopathology of corneal response to the ablation and wound healing.

Correct preoperative screening, absence of contraindications, choice of the more suitable technique for a specific patient, kind of laser technology, and type of surgical procedure, as well as the postoperative therapeutic management, represent critical steps for the outcome of this kind of surgery. However, some of the most important factors influencing the final results in treated corneas are strongly linked to the postoperative wound healing and response corneal processes occurring after the excimer laser ablation, intended to furnish the desired surface corneal profile in order to correct the visual defect.[22] It is known that the ablation induces a corneal response due to the stimulation of inflammation, tissue remodeling, and wound healing in the complex of living tissues that compose the anterior corneal anatomy.

As explained in the other parts of this book, although based on the same principle of excimer laser removal of corneal stromal tissue, there are critical differences among the LASIK surgical procedure and the so-called "surface ablation techniques." In LASIK, after having created a subtle superficial corneal flap (generally 130 to 160 μm thick), contains the epithelium, the Bowman's membrane, and the most anterior stroma, with a microkeratome, the stroma of the exposed corneal bed is then photoablated with the excimer laser to create the desired refractive shape, and then the flap is simply repositioned on the cornea, thanks to the spontaneous adhesion of the flap onto the stromal bed. The PRK procedure is based on the ablation of the anterior part of the cornea, the superficial subepithelial stroma, after mechanical or chemical removal of the epithelial layer. Surface ablation techniques with epithelial flap (LASEK and Epi-LASIK) are based on the sparing (and not removal) of the epithelial layer, in order to combine favorable features of both LASIK and PRK to improve the risk/benefit ratio. In the LASEK technique, diluted alcohol is used to loosen the epithelial adhesion to the underlying tissues to create the flap, while with Epi-LASIK, specialized epithelial microkeratomes are used to cut the epithelial flap without the aid of chemical alcoholic action, as explained in other chapters. The photoablation is performed onto the exposed stroma, moving aside the epithelium as a hinged sheet which is then repositioned onto the ablated surface, in both procedures.

Confocal Microscopy and PRK

After refractive excimer laser photoablation of the corneal surface, epithelial and stromal wound healing represent fundamental processes influencing the final morphological and refractive outcome of treated corneas. The role of inflammatory response, keratocyte functions, collagen lamellae organization, stromal rethickening, and collagen fiber production gives an important contribution to that complex phenomenon defined as stromal healing.[22]

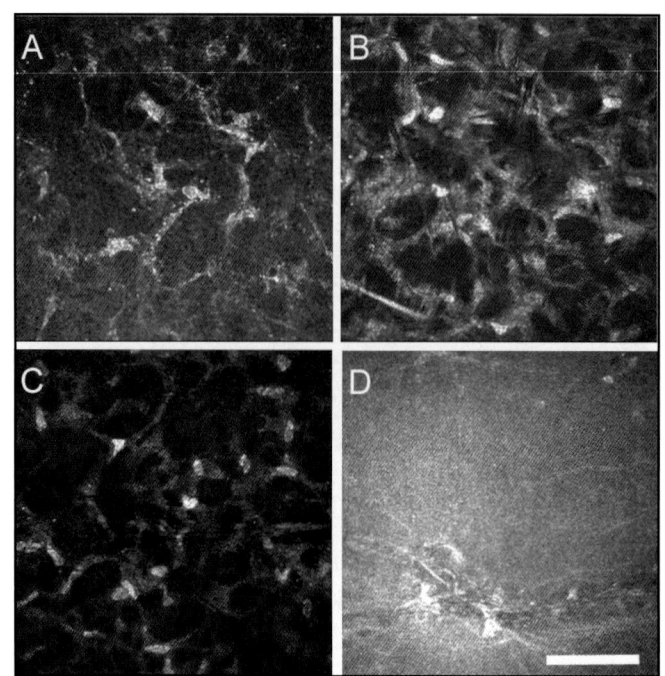

Figure 24-4. IVCM images of central cornea after PRK. (A) most anterior stroma 2 hours after PRK evidencing necrotic/apoptotic cells, alteration of the ECM transparency and markedly reduced cell density at the level of the exposed stromal bed. (B) Activation of keratocytes with myofibroblast activity characterized by reflective nuclei and spindle-shaped cytoplasmic processes with granular structure, starting ECM remodelling 7 days after surgery. (C) Anterior stroma 2 months after surgery evidencing initial reduction of keratocyte activation with regaining of ECM transparency. (D) Pseudo-Bowman's membrane regenerated at 1 year after PRK shows irregularity and increased light scattering in comparison with normal Bowman's layer. Bar represents 100 μm.

Confocal microscopy has been widely used to evaluate the human corneal microscopic changes after PRK,[23-34] confirming most of the wound healing processes observed in animals using *ex vivo* histology.

Postoperatively, the laser ablation induces the formation of reduced density cell layer in the anterior stroma at the edge of the photoablation,[28] caused by surgically induced keratocyte death,[35] and it is probable that this kind of cell death occurs by apoptosis or programmed cell death.[14,22] This kind of cell loss lasts for a few days, but necrosis plays a role contributing to cell death within 24 hours after surgical injury.[36] Confocal microscopy enables the visualization of such stromal cellular alterations soon after surgery, at the level of the exposed stromal bed, near the limit of photoablation[37] (Figure 24-4A). The following wound healing processes are then mediated by activated keratocytes that lead to increased collagen deposition, and it has been proposed that the extent of surgically induced keratocyte apoptosis, keratocyte proliferation, and activation with myofibroblast functions regulate the postoperative wound healing and the scar tissue formation.[38]

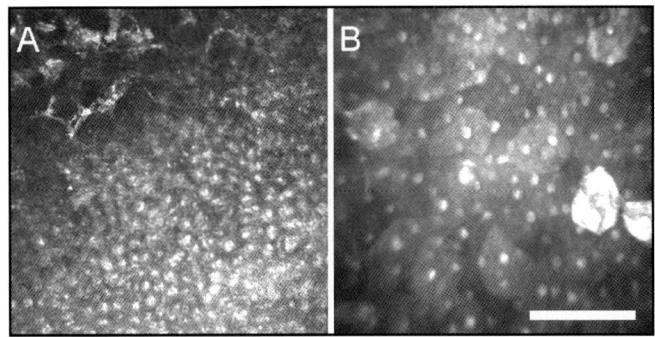

Figure 24-5. Confocal images of epithelial recovery after PRK. (A) Edge of the epithelial front moving toward the central cornea to close the epithelial wound: note the exposed stroma where the epithelium is absent (the image was obtained with correct alignment avoiding oblique sections which may produce artefacts). (B) Large immature surface epithelial cells 4 days after PRK. Bar represents 100 μm.

Proliferation and activation of keratocytes lining the apoptotic zone, during the first postoperative weeks, is a well-documented phenomenon, by using confocal microscopy, occurring after PRK,[14,22,25,28,31] as shown in Figure 24-4B. Activation of keratocyte and deposition of new extracellular matrix (ECM) can be imaged soon after the ablation, as early as 1 week following the treatment. Normal-appearing keratocytes start to replace the population of activated cells and myofibroblasts (Figure 24-4C) during the subsequent months (generally between 1 and 3 months) after surgery, but the time onset, duration, speed, and magnitude of this process is highly variable among individuals, as well as an individual's wound healing tendency (eg, "strong healers" vs "weak healers").[22,39] During this phase, the ECM regains transparency (see Figure 24-4C) and the wound healing process decreases slowly, showing generally a steady state at 1 year after surgery. However, persistent alterations, remnants of the previous surgical lesions, and wound activity may be seen microscopically even years after surgery, demonstrating that a real *"restitutio ad integrum"* does not occur.[14,22,27,34] These permanent tissutal changes that can be evidenced by in vivo confocal microscopic (IVCM) analysis briefly consist in: a) formation of a thin layer of subepithelial scar tissue (often transparent at slit-lamp biomicroscopy), deposited at the epithelial stromal interface strictly adjacent to the pseudoregenerated Bowman's membrane,[13,14,25,27] as shown in Figure 24-4D; and b) incomplete restoration of keratocyte density in the anterior stroma compared to the high density levels present in the preoperative stroma.[14] A recent report evaluating *ex vivo* long-term histopathological and confocal microscopic features, after different refractive surgical procedures, confirmed the finding of hypercellular fibrotic stromal scar, present as net-like pattern of subepithelial haze, as a late persistent structural alteration after PRK.[24] Confocal microscopy is also helpful in the evaluation of wound healing anomalies, such as the genesis of corneal haze, allowing a better comprehension of the clinical stage, the responsible mechanisms and dynamics of cellular and acellular components generating the alteration of stromal transparency.[18,23,28,29] One of the major advantages of IVCM in the study of haze after excimer laser ablation is the opportunity to objectively and quantitatively evaluate, with follow-up over time, reflectivity and thickness of the hazy anterior stromal layers that produce a measurable peak on the intensity profile by using CMTF or Z-scans graphics (previously explained at the beginning of this chapter).

IVCM morphology of the regeneration of corneal epithelium after PRK (and in general, after every surface ablation technique) is to date poorly understood, due to the intrinsic difficulties in obtaining reliable scans and images of the peripheral epithelial front (Figure 24-5A), progressing to cover the nonepithelized area, and due to the use of bandage contact lenses. A better analysis can be performed for the newly formed epithelium, after re-epithelialization is achieved.[14,26] The newly healed epithelial cells appear generally immature, larger in size than normal (Figure 24-5B), disposed into a thinner epithelium formed by two or three layers; the complete restoration to normal epithelial morphology and thickness takes about 6 weeks.[22] Changes from physiological epithelial thickness after ablations which variate the corneal profile, leading often to long-term epithelial hyperplasia, can be measured by IVCM,[15] through CMTF or Z-Scan function. Epithelial hyperplasia presents clinical effects that affect the expected corneal asphericity values and corneal-related spherical aberration.[40] It has been shown by histological studies that one of the three major types of persistent changes in corneal structure following laser ablations is an epithelial modification, resulting in hypertrophic changes or hyperplasia of the epithelium over the surface of the treated cornea. Confocal microscopy is able to identify these changes mainly using quantitative measurements of epithelial thickness,[24] but the combination of both layer analysis and three-dimensional confocal microscopic reconstruction may provide excellent results *in vivo* in the future.

A brief summary of the features that can be investigated by IVCM after PRK is presented in Table 24-1. The description of nerve fiber regeneration, inflammation, and other complications occurring after PRK is beyond the scope of this chapter, and it is extensively treated in other publications.[6,14,18,26,28-30]

Confocal Microscopy and LASIK

LASIK has gained great popularity among refractive surgeons because it presents, compared to PRK, less postoperative pain, a faster recovery of vision, and lower incidence of haze and regression. Most of these features can be understood considering the microscopic physiopathological processes and wound healing that occur after this procedure. Although LASIK is based on excimer laser ablation of the corneal stroma, similar to PRK, with the difference being the ablation located in a deeper corneal site (on the exposed stromal

Table 24-1. Summary of the Features That Can Be Investigated by IVCM After PRK

Summary of the main parameters in the postoperative evaluation following PRK given by slit lamp and confocal microscopy examination for the different corneal layers involved. The main limit (see the first paragraph of this chapter) of IVCM is represented by the small field of analysis. IVCM should always be a complementary exam in the clinical practice. Note: Features of uncommon wound healing processes and infrequent complications are not mentioned.

Corneal layer	Slit-lamp biomicroscopy	IVCM
Epithelium	Reepithelialization, epithelial transparency, epithelial defects, delay in epithelial healing	Epithelial cell density, cell size, features of maturity, epithelial thickness
Subepithelial nerve plexus	Barely visible	Nerve fiber regeneration, density
Pseudo-Bowman's membrane	Transparency, regularity	Reflectivity, microscopic structure of pseudo-Bowman's regeneration, permanent alteration
Stroma	Transparency, haze, infiltrates	Objective reflectivity, thickness measurements, keratocyte death, activation of keratocytes, cell density, ECM morphology, wound healing, haze structure, thickness, and reflectivity

bed under the created epithelial-stromal flap), IVCM as well as histopathologic investigations showed a clearly different behavior of the corneal response with respect to PRK.[14,24,41-50] In LASIK, the stromal cascade of processes that characterize wound healing appeared identical to that of PRK in animal models studied with histopathologic methods.[13] However, another important difference in inducing tissutal response is given by the fact that in the LASIK technique the extent of epithelial injury is limited at the site of the flap margin, while in PRK the complete removal of the epithelium covering the ablation zone is performed. It is known that the simple scraping of the corneal epithelium as well as PRK, induces cellular apoptotic death of the subepithelial stromal keratocytes,[36] which, as explained in the previous paragraph, represent the trigger for the following cascade of events, and thus the wound healing in LASIK appears confined mainly in the stroma lining the flap interface. This interface can easily be imaged by IVCM,[6,7,13,14,37,43,45,48-50] and two main advantages in the understanding of the postsurgical status of the cornea are provided by the confocal technique:

* Imaging of the stromal microscopic structure and wound healing of the interface and adjacent stromal layers
* Flap thickness, interface depth, and residual stromal thickness measurement through CMTF or Z-scan function

IVCM morphology of the flap-stromal interface induced by LASIK is characterized by an evident discontinuity of the cellular architecture of the stroma. The interface is generally imaged microscopically as a poorly cellulated layer within the anterior stroma, with a variable amount of reflective debris and particles,[49,50] clearly distinguishable from the other corneal layers, as shown in Figure 24-6. These particles, which may appear with low or high reflectivity,[49] disappear only for a certain amount in the late period after surgery, and it has been proposed that these features could represent plastic particles that are generated during microkeratome oscillation and are deposited at the interface during LASIK.[50] Other studies suggest that the high-reflectivity particles, which remain constant over time, may be due to fine nonorganic debris arising from the surgical instruments, and that the other category of low-reflectivity dots may represent cell-degradation products or other organic material.[49] Another apparently constant feature at the LASIK flap interface which has been confirmed by IVCM is the lower cellular activity and stromal remodeling, with respect to surface ablations wound sites, found both in the early and late postoperative periods.[24,41,46,48,51] It has been shown that "acellular zones" are present on both sides of the interface and appear thicker when observed in the first days after surgery, whereas keratocyte cells are visible closer to the interface in the following weeks.[43] The keratocyte-free layers probably represent zone undergoing apoptosis or necrosis, but when compared with PRK ablations, LASIK causes lower magnitude of cell death and subsequent keratocyte proliferation, activation, and myofibroblast activity.[14,52] However, processes of keratocyte activity and new scar-type ECM formation at the interface level occur also in LASIK, although to a lesser extent,[14,43] but even though rarely the wound healing processes can be strongly active after LASIK, causing a stromal opacity termed as haze, similar to that of PRK.[53] These observations may be responsible for the reduced keratocyte density which is found in the flap, interface (see Figures 24-6A and 24-6B), and anterior retroablation layers.

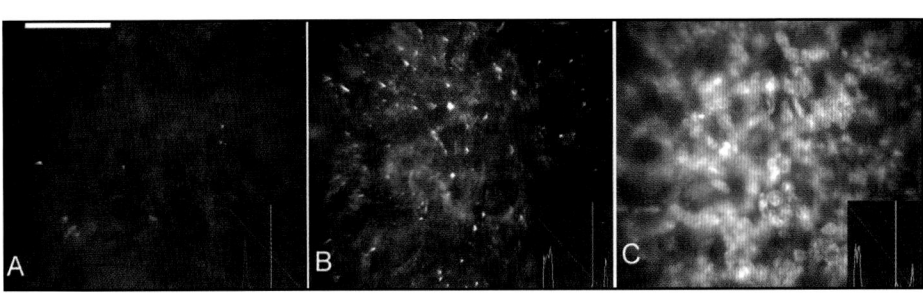

Figure 24-6. IVCM images of LASIK interfaces. Full-thickness Z-scan graphic is shown for each image. (A) Normal interface 2 year after LASIK with low keratocyte density and ECM microfolding. The interface is identified on the Z-scan curve at the point with lowest reflectivity (green line). (B) Interface evidencing diffuse high reflective particles and reduced transparency, in apparently acellular layer. The high reflectivity of the interface is evident in the Z-scan curve as a spike (green line). (C) Globular cell infiltration within the interface in DLK. A reflectivity spike is produced on the Z-scan curve (green line). Interface depth, flap, and residual stroma thickness can be measured as the distance of the interface from the epithelial and stromal peaks. Bar represents 100 μm.

This cellular decrement is significant in comparison with preoperative values and seems to be persistent for over 1 to 3 years after surgery and is probably permanent.[43,51,54] The clinical relevance of lack of keratocyte density restoration after LASIK is currently under investigation. A great cellular activity within the flap interface is observed in a typical complication of LASIK surgery, diffuse lamellar keratitis (DLK). DLK represents a sterile inflammation of unclear origin, probably related to multiple factors,[14,47,55] which may occur during the first week after surgery, frequently associated with epithelial defects,[56] and which can be successfully treated by topical steroids. IVCM allows the identification of ovoid or globular cells, which are probably leukocytes, accumulated within the interface during the clinical course of DLK (as shown in Figure 24-6C). However, IVCM does not identify types of inflammatory cells or distinguish these objects from some form of keratocytes. It has been shown in histological studies that a certain amount of leukocytes normally appear in the wound site soon after the ablation also in PRK,[14,36,52,57,58] but IVCM generally fails to evidence this kind of cells. It is possible that the resolution capacity of confocal microscopes may not be adequate in identifying leukocytes among a variable population of keratocytes, cell fragments, and apoptotic cells, as in normal early postoperative stromal wound healing layers after excimer ablations, but inflammatory cells may become visible when they reach a certain density per field, with lower presence of keratocytes, as in DLK at the interface site (see Figure 24-6C). The new generation SSCM and the LSM furnish a greater resolution and may improve detection of different kinds of nonresident stromal and epithelial cells, such as leukocytes and dendritic cells.

As explained previously, IVCM, by means of CMTF and Z-scan function, allows determination of corneal sublayer thickness. The importance of such measurements is related to the clinical relevance of determining flap and residual stromal bed thickness after LASIK, as the thickness of stromal bed under the flap is critical for keratectasia and epithelial thickness, which is often increased due to hyperplasia after LASIK with possible refractive effects. Figures 24-6A through 24-6C show Z-Scan graphics of post-LASIK corneas in which interface is displayed in the image. The distance of the interface layer from the endothelial or epithelial peak represents the residual stromal bed and flap thickness, respectively.

A brief description of the advantages of confocal microscopy examination over conventional biomicroscopy after LASIK is presented in Table 24-2.

The *In Vivo* Microscopic Evaluation of Epi-LASIK and LASEK

Two different excimer laser surface ablation techniques have been developed in the past few years, combining favorable elements of both PRK and LASIK. These two laser procedures are called LASEK and Epi-LASIK. Surgical techniques and clinical aspects are discussed in specific chapters of this book. In both methods the presence of an epithelial flap, instead of simply removing the epithelium, makes the techniques different from PRK. The main problem was to develop a reproducible technique able to standardize the creation of an intact epithelial flap. In LASEK, instead of removing the epithelium as in PRK, the biological effect of diluted alcohol solution is used to loosen the epithelial layer adhesion to the underlying corneal tissues.[59,60] In the Epi-LASIK technique, the epithelial flap is created mechanically by means of special devices, derived from microkeratomes used to obtain LASIK flaps, called epithelial microkeratomes, which allows separation of the epithelial flap.[61-63] The rationale for creating an epithelial flap is combining favorable elements of PRK (avoiding LASIK flap-related complications such as free cap, incomplete cut, epithelial ingrowth, flap melt, DLK, and corneal ectasia) and of LASIK (including benefits of low haze risk, low postoperative pain, and quick visual recovery). The main goal expected, for presence of the epithelial flap (mechanical or alcoholic) repositioned onto the photoablated corneal surface, is principally related to the theoretical properties of the flap, which may act as a biological bandage (similarly to amniotic membrane in ocular surface pathologies), providing an intact basement membrane for protection of the underlying exposed stromal bed.[59,64] The first stages of wound healing after surface excimer laser refractive procedures (PRK, LASEK, and Epi-LASIK) are mediated by epithelial migration (covering

Table 24-2. Advantages of Confocal Microscopy Examination Over Conventional Biomicroscopy After LASIK

Summary of the main parameters in the postoperative evaluation following LASIK given by slit lamp and confocal microscopy examination for the different corneal layers involved. Note: Features of complications other than epithelial ingrowth, DLK, flap striae and interface fluid are not mentioned. See also Table 24-1 legend.

Corneal layer	Slit-lamp biomicroscopy	IVCM
Epithelium	Epithelial transparency, epithelial defects, epithelial ingrowth	Epithelial cell density, cell size, epithelial thickness, micromorphology of epithelial ingrowth
Subepithelial nerve plexus	Barely visible	Nerve fiber regeneration, density
Flap stroma	Transparency, regularity, folds and striae	Thickness, cellularity, ECM morphology, Bowman's and stromal layer microfolds, keratocyte density and activation
Interface	Transparency, regularity, epithelial ingrowth, DLK, interface fluid	Depth, reflectivity, cellularity, wound healing, debris, inflammatory cell density in DLK, interface fluid thickness, epithelial ingrowth morphology
Residual stromal bed	Transparency, regularity	Objective reflectivity, thickness measurements, wound healing, cell density, ECM morphology

the wound area), epithelial hyperplasia (maturation), and initial superficial stromal events (explained in the paragraph of this chapter dedicated to PRK). It is well known that the epithelial dynamics, in surface refractive surgery, are strictly connected to the underlying stromal phenomena, influencing keratocyte activity at a cellular and biochemical level.[22] Cytokine induction stimulated by damaged epithelial cells can contribute to the process of keratocyte apoptosis, which subsequently leads to keratocyte activation near the area of cell death, and following migration and fibroblast transformation repopulating the wound area.[35,36] This means that the preservation of epithelial viability and integrity during surface ablations may be useful to achieve uneventful wound healing and clinical recovery.[59] Haze is an expression of both irregular ECM production by myofibroblasts and activated keratocytes, and is also produced by the high reflectivity of anterior stromal accumulation of cells themselves.[28-31] Moreover, haze appears related to the depth of surgical injury, and wounds that remove epithelial basement membrane as well as Bowman's membrane (eg, PRK) produce greater myofibroblast activity than surgical excimer wounds that spare these two important layers (eg, LASIK).[59] Ablation techniques with epithelial flap, although ablating the Bowman's layer, should maintain a relatively intact epithelial basement membrane patching the wounded stroma (at least during the first postoperative 48 to 72 hours) before a new epithelium is generated. This mechanism, based on the role of the epithelial flap on the cascade of epithelial-stromal interactions in wound healing (epithelial/ablation injury, apoptosis/cell death, keratocyte activation/myofibroblast, ECM deposition), represents one of the main possible advantages of epithelial flap techniques. However, to date, there is no clear evidence in scientific literature that LASEK/Epi-LASIK present significant lower incidence of haze or better corneal transparency at long term. Moreover, it is not completely understood if differences in re-epithelialization quality, epithelial maturation, and related early postoperative symptoms, such as pain, between PRK and epithelial flap-based surface ablation techniques may be objectively identified.

IVCM examination, in LASEK[37,65] and Epi-LASIK postoperative follow-up, provides two main advantages in the *in vivo* investigation of the corneal morphology after surgery:

* Imaging at a cellular level of epithelial flap and new corneal epithelial morphology (in the early postoperative period)
* Subepithelial stromal cellular activity and wound healing, including objective measurement of anterior stromal reflectivity and cell density

Confocal microscopic images of LASEK epithelial flap are shown in Figure 24-7. Superficial epithelial layer may present, soon after the ablation, barely distinguishable cell borders and highly reflective debris on its surface (see Figure 24-7A) probably due to alcoholic cell damage. The flap basal epithelial cell layer (see Figures 24-7B and 7C) generally appears intact (but microscopic breaks of the flap can be observed), however, an overall increase of basal epithelial layer reflectivity (with respect to normal nondetached basal layers in healthy corneas) appears as a typical feature. Focal areas of epithelial lesions may also be identified. Thus, IVCM examination in

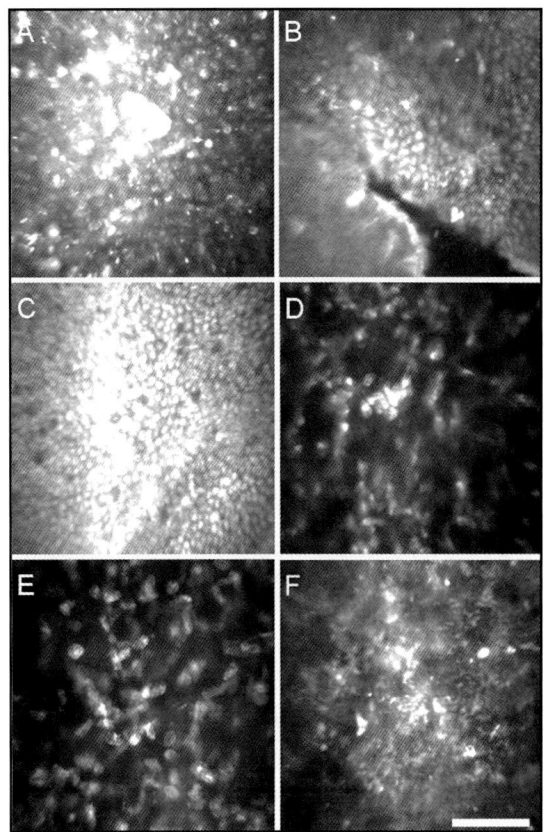

Figure 24-7. IVCM images after LASEK (20% alcohol solution applied for 25 seconds). (A) Superficial epithelial layer of the flap 2 hours after surgery: marked cellular alterations and high reflective debris. (B) Basal epithelial layer of the flap 2 hours after surgery: nonhomogeneous reflectivity of basal cells and evident microscopic break of the flap. (C) Basal epithelial cell layer of the flap 2 hours after surgery: note the high reflectivity and the integrity of the flap. (D and E) Globular cells within the anterior stroma underlying the flap 24 and 48 hours after ablation, respectively. (F) Absence of globular cell infiltration beneath the flap 24 hours after LASEK. Bar represents 100 μm.

standard LASEK techniques[37,65] allowed the identification of a certain amount of flap cell damage soon after the surgical procedure, although the clinical appearance may show intact, transparent, and well-adherent epithelial flap. These lesions may be due to surgical manipulation of the flap after epithelial detachment, effect of alcoholization, or a combination of both. It has been shown by histopathological immunofluorescence staining that the cleavage plane of the ethanol-induced corneal epithelial flap is located between the lamina lucida and the lamina densa of the basement membrane, and thus ethanol acts on the corneal epithelium-basement membrane complex by splitting the basement membrane without affecting the anchoring of the membrane to the Bowman's layer, which is ablated by the laser beam.[60] It has also been reported that the conventional concentrations and duration of alcohol treatment (20%, 25 seconds) produce varying morphologic changes in the basement membrane zone by electron microscopy, and varying viability in standard tissue culture conditions, with a dose- and time-dependent effect of alcohol on epithelial cells.[66] These features may be consistent with epithelial alterations of in situ flap morphology soon after surgery, which can be imaged *in vivo* by confocal microscopy. The presence of globular cells between 1 and 3 days after LASEK (see Figures 24-7D and 24-7E), which probably represents inflammatory cells, is another finding that distinguishes early wound healing phases in the most anterior stroma of LASEK from uneventful PRK features. These infiltrating cells appear morphologically different from resting keratocyte nuclei and activated keratocyte cell bodies, similar to ovoid cells observable within the LASIK interface during DLK (see Figure 24-6C). Thus, it is possible to hypothesize that leukocyte infiltration may occur in the anterior stroma underlying the flap due to inflammation induction promoted by necrotic or damaged epithelial cells of the flap, which are directly in contact with the wounded stroma, without the interposition of an intact basal membrane and Bowman's layer. In some cases, this inflammatory infiltration does not occur at the same follow-up period, and the anterior stromal changes appear similar to that of PRK (see Figure 24-7F). This variable behavior may be related to variable damaging, and consequent inflammation induction, of flap epithelial cells occurring during surgical manipulation and ethanol exposure of the LASEK flap. However, these findings, suggested from data obtained in our studies, need to be confirmed by further studies.[37,65]

IVCM images of Epi-LASIK epithelial flaps are shown in Figures 24-8 through 24-10. To date, IVCM investigations of Epi-LASIK flap are not reported yet in the scientific literature, and the following findings (personal, unpublished data) need to be confirmed by further controlled studies. Surface epithelial cells may present a certain degree of cell lesions, represented by partial disappearance of cell nuclei, focal cytoplasmic granular inclusions, alteration of reflectivity, and features of focal cell death (see Figures 24-8A and 24-8B). Basal and intermediate epithelial cell layer of the Epi-LASIK flap disclose generally a lower level of cell damaging (see Figures 24-8C and 24-8D). Basal epithelial cell layer may present variable signs of cell damaging and reflectivity (see Figures 24-9A and 24-9B). When basal cell reflectivity results increased, a thin layer of fluid accumulation between the basal lamina and the underlying stromal bed is often visible (see Figure 24-9C). IVCM findings of Epi-LASIK flap immediately after surgery suggest the hypothesis that epithelial cell integrity is more preserved than in LASEK flaps. These preliminary results are in agreement with a previous histopathologic study of light and electron microscopy which showed that the manual excision of epithelial disks (Epi-LASIK) is less invasive to epithelial integrity than LASEK using either alcohol concentration.[62]

In both techniques, the epithelial cells of the flap do not persist attached to the corneal surface, but undergo a pro-

Figure 24-8. IVCM images of Epi-LASIK flap 3 hours after surgery. (A and B) Superficial epithelial cell layer evidencing focal alterations and disappearance of cell nuclei; cell borders are preserved. (C) Basal epithelial layer of the flap appears almost intact. (D) Minor alterations are visible for intermediate cell layer. Bar represents 100 µm.

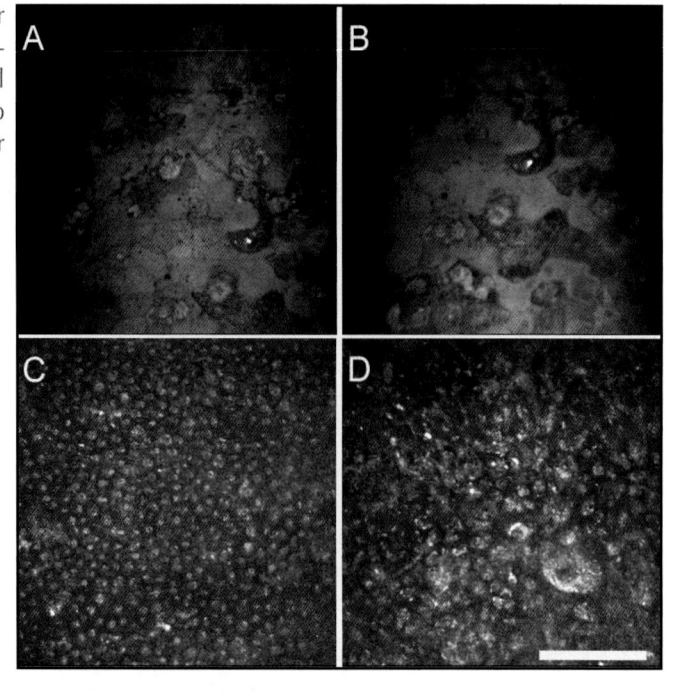

Figure 24-9. IVCM images of Epi-LASIK flap 3 hours after surgery. (A) Basal epithelium with low reflectivity but with focal cell disruption. (B) Basal epithelium with preserved integrity evidencing high reflectivity. (C) Fluid and cells accumulated beneath the basal lamina of the flap in the same patient as B. Bar represents 100 µm.

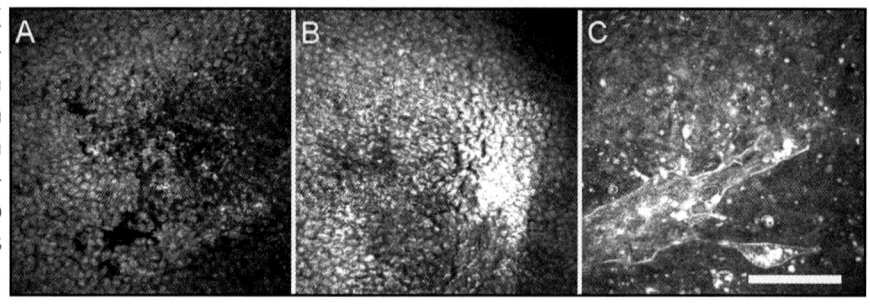

gressive degradation, and a new corneal epithelium, with its own basal lamina, is regenerated by transient amplifying cells and limbal stem cells, sliding beneath the flap. IVCM clearly shows the degradation of cells within the surgical epithelial flap and allows the imaging of new cells providing re-epithelialization of the corneal surface (Figures 24-10A through 10D). Epithelial closure time in epithelial flap-based procedures did not differ from PRK in clinical studies and thus it is not proven that the presence of an epithelial flap may lead to faster epithelial recovery.[59,61,64] Confocal microscopic initial signs of flap degradation are visible beginning from 24 hours after surgery (shown in Figure 24-10 for Epi-LASIK), and remnants of the flap may be observed up to 5 days after surgery, when epithelial closure is generally complete.

Anterior stromal reaction, in the early phase after Epi-LASIK, appears similar to that of PRK and LASEK (findings are reported in Figure 24-11). Immediately after the ablation, a superficial stromal layer presenting reduced cell density and a fragment of necrotic/apoptotic keratocytes is visible under the flap (see Figure 24-11A). In the following hours, repopulation of this layer by activated keratocytes and globular cells occurs similarly to the other surface techniques (see Figure 24-11B). The presence of ovoid cells (possibly inflammatory cells, among keratocytes) seems to be less recognizable than LASEK, and it is possible to hypothesize that this may be due to lower inflammation induction thanks to a better preservation of flap cells and basal membrane integrity in mechanical epithelial separation. However, during the subsequent phase of wound healing, the features are not different from the other surface procedures: activated keratocytes repopulate the anterior stroma during the first weeks after surgery with variable presence of myofibroblast morphology and ECM production (see Figures 24-11C and 24-11D).

A brief description of the features that can be shown by IVCM after epithelial flap-based surface ablation techniques is reported in Table 24-3.

Although microscopic early findings at the level of epithelial layers may present differences among the three surface ablation techniques (PRK, LASEK, Epi-LASIK), mainly concerning epithelial flap integrity and adhesion (for flap-based procedures), apoptosis and inflammation induction into the anterior stroma, we found no differences in the morphological parameters (reflectivity, thickness, cell density, and cell morphology) 1 month after surgery, when epithelial recovering is completed[65] (Figure 24-12).

Additional studies of the biochemical and histopathologic mechanisms of the healing response and further application of IVCM in the evaluation of epithelial, nerve fiber layer, and stromal dynamics occurring after surface excimer refractive ablations based on epithelial flaps, in a randomized compara-

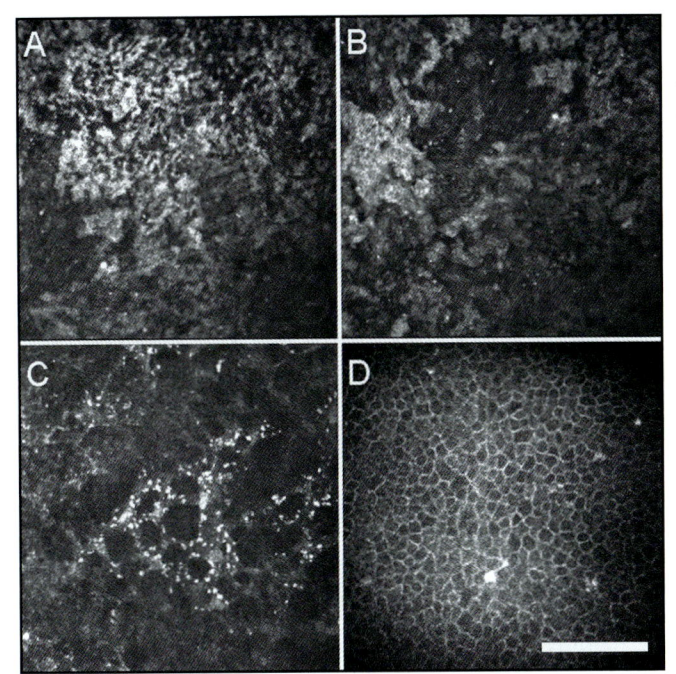

Figure 24-10. IVCM images of Epi-LASIK flap at different times after surgery. (A) At 24 hours after ablation initial signs of flap cell disruption are visible. (B) Basal cells appeared disgregating at 48 hours after surgery. (C) Remnant of the Epi-LASIK flap 5 days after surgery: there are no distinguishable epithelial cells. (D) Newly formed basal epithelial cell layer 5 days after Epi-LASIK. Bar represents 100 µm.

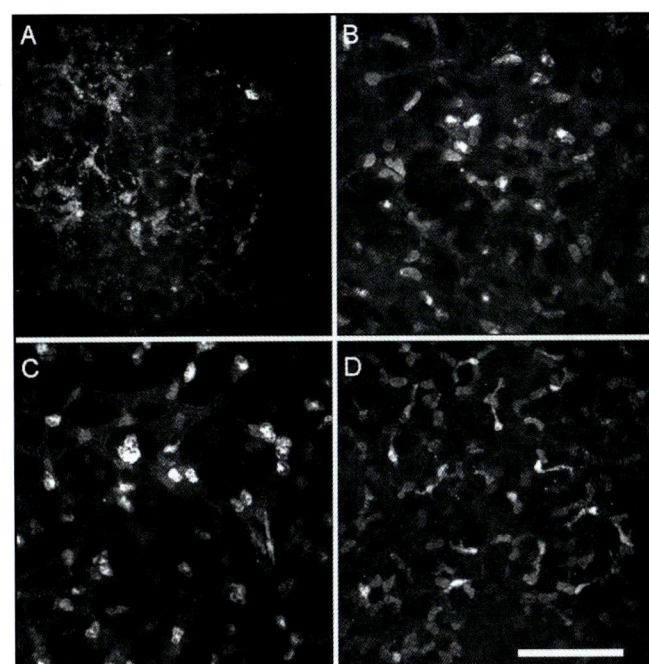

Figure 24-11. IVCM images of Epi-LASIK anterior stroma at different times after surgery. (A) Most anterior stroma 2 hours after procedure evidencing necrotic/apoptotic cells, alteration of the ECM transparency, and markedly reduced cell density at the level of the exposed stromal bed. (B) Activation of keratocytes with reflective nuclei and repopulating the anterior stromal wound 2 days after surgery. (C) Anterior stromal keratocytes with evident cytoplasm 2 weeks after surgery. (D) Anterior stromal keratocytes at 3 months after surgery losing the "activated morphology" and increasing in density. Bar represents 100 µm.

Table 24-3. Description of Features Shown by IVCM After Epithelial Flap-Based Surface Ablation Techniques

Summary of the main parameters in the postoperative evaluation following LASEK/Epi-LASIK furnished by slit lamp and confocal microscopy examination for the different corneal layers involved. Note: features of uncommon wound healing processes and unfrequent complications are not mentioned. See also Table 24-1 and 24-2 legends.

Corneal layer	Slit-lamp biomicroscopy	IVCM
Epithelium	Flap integrity, location, folding, transparency, adhesion	Microscopic imaging of flap cells, flap integrity, focal areas of damaging, interface fluid, flap reflectivity, re-epithelialization quality and maturity
Subepithelial nerve plexus	Barely visible	Nerve fiber regeneration, density
Pseudo-Bowman's membrane	Transparency, regularity	Reflectivity, microscopic structure of pseudo-Bowman's regeneration, permanent alterations
Stroma	Transparency, haze, infiltrates	Objective reflectivity, thickness measurements, keratocyte death, activation of keratocytes, cell density, inflammatory cells, ECM morphology, wound healing, haze structure, thickness, and reflectivity

tive fashion, could lead to the comprehension of problems which to date are still unclear: where the real advantages of epithelial flap, if any, play a role in corneal wound healing and clinical outcomes.

References

1. Minsky M. Memoir on inventing the confocal scanning microscope. *Scanning*. 1988;10:128-138.
2. Petrán M, Hadravsky M, Egger MD, et al. Tandem-scanning reflected-light microscope. *J Opt Soc Am*. 1968;58:661-664.
3. Jester JV, Cavanagh HD, Lemp MA. Confocal microscopy imaging of the living eye with tandem scanning confocal microscopy. In: Masters BR, ed. *Noninvasive Diagnostic Techniques in Ophthalmology*. New York, NY: Springer Verlag; 1990:172-188.
4. Lemp MA, Dilly PN, Boyde A. Tandem scanning (confocal) microscopy of the full thickness cornea. *Cornea*. 1986;4:205.
5. Wiegand W, Thaer AA, Kroll P, et al. Optical sectioning of the cornea with a new confocal *in vivo* slit-scanning videomicroscope. *Ophthalmology*. 1995;102:56-575.
6. Mastropasqua L, Nubile M. *In Vivo Confocal Microscopy of the Cornea*. Thorofare, NJ: SLACK Incorporated; 2002.
7. Kaufman SC, Musch DC, Belin MW, et al. Confocal microscopy: a report by the American Academy of Ophthalmology. *Ophthalmology*. 2004;111(7):1306.
8. Stave J, Zinser G, Grummer G, et al. Modified Heidelberg retinal tomograph HRT. Initial results of *in vivo* presentation of corneal structures. *Ophthalmologe*. 2002;99(4):276-280.
9. Leduc C, Dupas B, Ott-Benoist AC, et al. Advantages of the *in vivo* HRT2 corneal confocal microscope for investigation of the ocular surface epithelia. *J Fr Ophthalmol*. 2004;27:978-986.
10. .omii S, Kinoshita S. Observations of human corneal epithelium by tandem scanning confocal microscope. *Scanning*. 1994;16:305-306.
11. Patel S, McLaren J, Hodge D, et al. Normal human keratocyte density and corneal thickness measurement by using confocal microscopy *in vivo*. *Invest Ophthalmol Vis Sci*. 2001;42:333-339.
12. Chiou AG, Kaufman SC, Beuerman RW, et al. Differential diagnosis of linear corneal images on confocal microscopy. *Cornea*. 1999;18:63-66.
13. Jalbert I, Stapleton F, Papas E, et al. *In vivo* confocal microscopy of the human cornea. *Br J Ophthalmol*. 2003;87:225-236.
14. Tervo T, Moilanen J. *In vivo* confocal microscopy for evaluation of wound healing following corneal refractive surgery. *Prog Ret Eye Res*. 2003;22:339-358.
15. Li HF, Petroll WM, Møller-Pedersen T, et al. Epithelial and corneal thickness measurements by *in vivo* confocal microscopy through focusing (CMTF). *Curr Eye Res*. 1997;16:214-221.
16. McLaren JW, Nau CB, Erie JC, et al. Corneal thickness measurement by confocal microscopy, ultrasound, and scanning slit methods. *Am J Ophthalmol*. 2004;137(6):1011-1020.
17. Patel S, McLaren J, Hodge D, et al. Normal human keratocyte density and corneal thickness measurement by using confocal microscopy *in vivo*. *Invest Ophthalmol Vis Sci*. 2001;108(1):112-120.
18. Møller-Pedersen T, Vogel M, Li HF, et al. Quantification of stromal thinning, epithelial thickness, and corneal haze after photorefractive keratectomy using *in vivo* confocal microscopy. *Ophthalmology*. 1997;104:360-368.
19. Trokel SL, Srinivasan R, Braren B. Excimer laser surgery of the cornea. *Am J Ophthalmol*. 1983;96:710-715.
20. Duffey RG, Leaming D. US trends in refractive surgery: 2002 ISRS survey. *J Refract Surg*. 2003;19:357-363.
21. Leaming DV. Practice styles and preferences of ASCRS members–2003 survey. *J Cataract Refract Surg*. 2004;30(4):892-900.
22. Fagerholm P. Wound healing after photorefractive keratectomy. *J Cataract Refract Surg*. 2000;26(3):432-447.

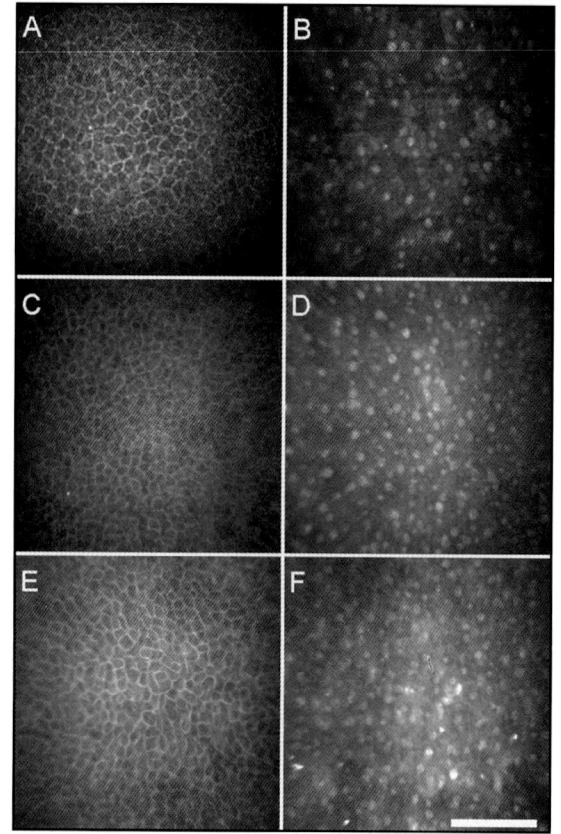

Figure 24-12. IVCM basal and superficial epithelial morphology 1 month after PRK (A and B), LASEK (C and D), and Epi-LASIK (E and F).

23. Corbett MC, Prydal JI, Verma S, et al. An *in vivo* investigation of the structures responsible for corneal haze after photorefractive keratectomy and their effect on visual function. *Ophthalmology*. 1996;103:1366-1380.
24. Dawson DG, Edelhauser HF, Grossniklaus HE. Long term histopathologic findings in human corneal wounds after refractive surgical procedures. *Am J Ophthalmol*. 2005;139:168-178.
25. Frueh BE, Cadez R, Böhnke M. *In vivo* confocal microscopy after photorefractive keratectomy in humans. *Arch Ophthalmol*. 1998;116:1425-1431.
26. Linna T, Tervo T. Real-time confocal microscopic observations on human corneal nerves and wound healing after excimer laser photorefractive keratectomy. *Curr Eye Res*. 1997;16:640-649.
27. Böhnke M, Thaer A, Schipper I. Confocal microscopy reveals persisting stromal changes after myopic photorefractive keratectomy in zero haze corneas. *Br J Ophthalmol*. 1998;82:1393-1400.
28. Moller-Pedersen T, Li HF, Petroll WM, et al. Confocal microscopic characterization of wound repair after photorefractive keratectomy. *Invest Ophthalmol Vis Sci*. 1998;39(3):487-501.
29. Moller-Pedersen T, Cavanagh HD, Petroll WM, et al. Stromal wound healing explains refractive instability and haze development after photorefractive keratectomy: a 1-year confocal microscopic study. *Ophthalmology*. 2000;107:1235-1245.
30. Lee YG, Chen WYW, Petroll WM, et al. Corneal haze after photorefractive keratectomy using different epithelial removal techniques. *Ophthalmology*. 2001;108:112-120.
31. Moller-Pedersen T. Keratocyte reflectivity and corneal haze. *Exp Eye Res*. 2004;78(3):553-560.
32. Erie JC, Hodge DO, Bourne WM. Confocal microscopy evaluation of stromal ablation depth after myopic laser in situ keratomileusis and photorefractive keratectomy. *J Cataract Refract Surg*. 2004;30(2):321-325.

33. Erie JC, Patel SV, McLaren JW, et al. Keratocyte density in the human cornea after photorefractive keratectomy. *Arch Ophthalmol.* 2003;121(6):770-776.
34. Moilanen JA, Vesaluoma MH, Muller LJ, et al. Long term corneal morphology after PRK by *in vivo* confocal microscopy. *Invest Ophthalmol Vis Sci.* 2003;44(3):1064-1069.
35. Wilson SE, He Y-G, Weng J, et al. Epithelial injury induces keratocyte apoptosis: hypothesized role for the interleukin-1 system in the modulation of corneal tissue organization and wound healing. *Exp Eye Res.* 1996;62:325-337.
36. Helena MC, Baerveldt F, Kim WJ, et al. Keratocyte apoptosis after corneal surgery. *Invest Ophthalmol Vis Sci.* 1998;39:273-276.
37. Mastropasqua L, Nubile M, Carpineto P, et al. *In vivo* investigation of corneal response after PRK, LASEK and LASIK excimer laser surgey by means of confocal microscopy. In: Midena E, ed. *Myopia and Related Diseases.* New York, NY: Ophthalmic Communication Society Inc; 2005:432-442.
38. Moller-Pedersen T, Cavanagh HD, Petroll WM, et al. Neutralizing antibody to TGFbeta modulates stromal fibrosis but not regression of photoablative effect following PRK. *Curr Eye Res.* 1998;17(7):736-747.
39. Durrie DS, Lesher MP, Cavanaugh TB. Classification of variable clinical response after photorefractive keratectomy for myopia. *J Refract Surg.* 1995;11(5):341-347.
40. Gatinel D, Malet J, Hoang-Xuan T, et al. Analysis of customized corneal ablations: theoretical limitations of increasing negative asphericity. *Invest Ophthalmol Vis Sci.* 2002;43(4):941-948.
41. Ivarsen A, Moller-Pedersen T. LASIK induces minimal regrowth and no haze development in rabbit corneas. *Curr Eye Res.* 2005;30(5):363-373.
42. Linna TU, Vesaluoma MH, Pérez-Santonja JJ, et al. Effect of myopic LASIK on corneal sensitivity and morphology of subbasal nerves. *Invest Ophthalmol Vis Sci.* 2000;41:393-397.
43. Vesaluoma MH, Petroll WM, Perez-Santonja JJ, et al. Laser in situ keratomileusis flap margin: wound healing and complications imaged by *in vivo* confocal microscopy. *Am J Ophthalmol.* 2000;130:564-573.
44. Gokmen F, Jester JV, Petroll WM, et al. *In vivo* confocal microscopy through-focusing to measure corneal flap thickness after laser in situ keratomileusis. *J Cataract Refract Surg.* 2002;28:962-970.
45. Erie JC, Patel SV, McLaren JW, et al. Effect of myopic laser in situ keratomileusis on epithelial and stromal thickness. *Ophthalmology.* 2002;109:1447-1452.
46. Ivarsen A, Laurberg T, Moller-Pedersen T. Role of keratocyte loss on corneal wound repair after LASIK. *Invest Ophthalmol Vis Sci.* 2004;45(10):3499-3506.
47. De Rojas Silva MV, Diez-Feijoo E, Rodriguez-Ares MT, et al. Confocal microscopy of stage 4 diffuse lamellar keratitis with spontaneous resolution. *J Refract Surg.* 2004;20(4):391-396.
48. Vesaluoma M, Pérez-Santonja J, Petroll WM, et al. Corneal stromal changes induced by myopic LASIK. *Invest Ophthalmol Vis Sci.* 2000;41:369-376.
49. Perez-Gomez I, Efron N. Confocal microscopic evaluation of particles at the corneal flap interface after myopic in situ keratomileusis. *J Cataract Refract Surg.* 2003;29:1373-1377.
50. Ivarsen A, Thogersen J, Keiding SR, et al. Plastic particles at the LASIK interface. *Ophthalmology.* 2004;111:18-23.
51. Erie JC, Nau CB, McLaren JW, et al. Long-term keratocyte deficits in the corneal stroma after LASIK. *Ophthalmology.* 2004;111:1356-1361.
52. Mohan RR, Hutcheon AEK, Choi R, et al. Apoptosis, necrosis, proliferation, and myofibroblast generation in the stroma following LASIK and PRK. *Exp Eye Res.* 2003;76(1):71-87.
53. Buhren J, Kohnen T. Stromal haze after laser in situ keratomileusis. Clinical and confocal microscopy findings. *J Cataract Refract Surg.* 2003;29:1318-1726.
54. Mitooka K, Ramirez M, Maguire LJ, et al. Keratocyte density of central human cornea after laser in situ keratomileusis. *Am J Ophthalmol.* 2002;133:307-314.
55. Johnson JD, Harissi-Dagher M, Pineda R, et al. Diffuse lamellar keratitis: incidence, associations, outcomes, and a new classification system. *J Cataract Refract Surg.* 2001;27:1560-1566.
56. Moilanen J, Holopainen J, Helinto M, et al. Keratocyte activation and inflammation in diffuse lamellar keratitis after formation of an epithelial defect. *J Cataract Refract Surg.* 2004;30:341–349.
57. Jester JV, Petroll WM, Cavanagh HD. Corneal stromal wound healing in refractive surgery: the role of myofibroblasts. *Prog Retin Eye Res.* 1999;18:311-356.
58. Wilson SE, Mohan RR, Ambrosio R, et al. The corneal wound healing response: cytokinemediated interaction of the epithelium, stroma, and infammatory cells. *Prog Retin Eye Res.* 2001;20:625-637.
59. Taneri S, Zieske JD, Azar DT. Evolution, techniques, clinical outcomes and pathophysiology of LASEK: review of the literature. *Surv Ophthalmol.* 2004;49:576-602.
60. Espana EM, Grueterich M, Mateo A, et al. Cleavage of corneal basament membrane components by ethanol exposure in laser-assisted subepithelial keratectomy. *J Cataract Refract Surg.* 2003;29(6):1192-1197.
61. Pallikaris IG, Kalyvianaki MI, Katsanevaki VJ, et al. Epi-LASIK: preliminary clinical results of an alternative surface ablation procedure. *J Cataract Refract Surg.* 2005;31(5):879-885.
62. Pallikaris IG, Naoumidi II, Kalyvianaki MI, et al. Epi-LASIK: comparative histological evaluation of mechanical and alcohol assisted epithelial separation. *J Cataract Refract Surg.* 2003;29(8):1496-1501.
63. Pallikaris IG, Katsanevaki VJ, Kalyvianaki MI, et al. Advances in subepithelial excimer refractive surgery techniques: Epi-LASIK. *Curr Opin Ophthalmol.* 2003;14(4):207-212.
64. Lee JB, Seong GJ, Lee JH, et al. Comparison of laser epithelial keratomileusis and photorefractive keratectomy for low to moderate myopia. *J Cataract Refract Surg.* 2001;27:565-570.
65. Nubile M, Lanzini M, Costantino O, et al. Comparison of early and middle-term microscopic morphological corneal response after PRK, LASEK and alcohol-free LASEK. *Ophthalmic Res.* 2004;36(S1):83.
66. Chen CC, Chang JH, Lee JB, et al. Human corneal epithelial cell viability and morphology after dilute alcohol exposure. *Invest Ophthalmol Vis Sci.* 2002;43:2593-2602.

CHAPTER 25

CORNEAL WOUND HEALING RESPONSE IN LASEK

*Marcelo V. Netto, MD; Rajiv R. Mohan, PhD;
Renato Ambrósio Jr, MD; Steven E. Wilson, MD*

Introduction

The refractive surgery field has undergone substantial development during the past few years, as refractive surgical procedures have become the most commonly performed surgeries in medicine. Remarkable effort has gone into refining the excimer laser for use in refractive surgery. Technological improvements on the laser platforms, including accurate delivery systems, eye-trackers, and more precise algorithms, have allowed smoother aspheric ablations. More recently, customized corneal treatments, linking the excimer laser with an individual's wavefront information, have emerged with the promise of creating a better optical system.

Greater clinical experience with several refractive surgical techniques has led to better and more predictable results after refractive surgery. However, factors such as corneal wound healing and biomechanical responses continue to influence the outcomes of all refractive surgical procedures.

Biological diversity in the corneal wound healing responses is of particular relevance to the outcomes of keratorefractive surgical procedures. Wound healing is a major determinant of the efficacy and safety of these procedures. Thus, complications such as overcorrection, undercorrection, and corneal stromal opacity are, in large part, related to corneal wound healing.

Many studies have been performed to elucidate the major steps involved in the corneal wound healing cascade with the aim of preventing complications and improving the outcomes of refractive surgery. This chapter will review the main processes involved in corneal wound healing and compare the response in laser-assisted subepithelial keratomileusis (LASEK) to those noted with other keratorefractive techniques.

Corneal Wound Healing After Refractive Surgery: A Brief Overview of the Component Processes

The corneal wound healing response is a remarkably complex cascade that is initiated by epithelial injury.[1-3] The response after corneal injury involves epithelial cells, keratocytes, bone marrow-derived cells, corneal nerves, the lacrimal glands, the tear film, and possibly cell types that are yet to be identified.[4-6] Interactions between these cells and tear film orchestrate the corneal wound healing response and contribute to the maintenance and restoration of the corneal structure and function.[7] Many different cytokines, chemokines, growth factors, and receptors participate directly in this process.[8]

An epithelial injury initiating the corneal wound healing response can be caused by a microkeratome blade, alcohol exposure, mechanical scrape, or any other trauma. This initial insult results in the release of many cytokines, including interleukin (IL)-1, tumor necrosis factor ALPHA (TNF), epidermal growth factor (EGF), platelet derived growth factor (PDGF), and production of collagenases and metalloproteinases.[1,2,9-13] Among all mediators, IL-1 ALPHA appears to play a special role in initiating the stromal response as a "master regulatory" cytokine.[14-16]

Mediators produced by stromal cells are also extremely important in regulating epithelial healing and immune cell infiltration. Examples of cytokines produced by keratocytes and lacrimal glands to modulate epithelial proliferation, migration, and differentiation include hepatocyte growth factor (HGF) and keratinocyte growth factor (KGF).[11,17]

Following injury, there is a breakdown of epithelial barrier function and damage to the epithelial basement membrane that allows cytokines to reach the stroma and bind their receptors on keratocyte cells.[8,18] Receptor activation triggers the wound healing cascade and orchestrates a variety of biological responses,[7,9,18,19] including keratocyte apoptosis, proliferation and differentiation of corneal fibroblasts, generation of myofibroblasts, collagen gel contraction, and production of extracellular matrix (ECM) materials.[20,21]

In the earliest observable stromal alteration, keratocyte cells adjacent to the site of injury respond by undergoing apoptosis.[20,22] The apparent disappearance of keratocytes after epithelial injury has been described since 1968.[9] However, in 1992, it was demonstrated that the early disappearance of keratocytes that follows epithelial injury is mediated by apoptosis or programmed cell death.[22,23] Keratocyte apoptosis in response to epithelial injury has been noted in several species, including rabbits, rats, mice, chickens, monkeys, and humans.[24-26]

Apoptosis is a genetically driven mechanism of cell death that occurs without significant release of lysosomal enzymes or other intracellular components that could damage the surrounding tissues or cells. It can be detected immediately after an epithelial injury by transmission electron microscopy (TEM).[9] The TUNEL assay (TdT-mediated dUTP nick end labeling) is a immunofluorescent method that detects individual cells that are undergoing apoptosis by labeling the ends of the highly degrading DNA with the polymerase terminal deoxyribonucleotidyl transferase (TdT). The TUNEL assay shows a peak in keratocyte apoptosis at approximately 4 hours after the epithelial injury to the cornea and stromal cell apoptosis typically persists for 1 week.[9,20,27-30] Initially, all of the cells in the anterior stroma undergoing apoptosis are keratocytes, but by 12 to 24 hours the apoptotic cells likely include corneal fibroblasts and bone-derived immune cells.

As the wound healing response continues, an increasing proportion of dying cells in the stroma undergo necrosis.[31] Necrosis is characterized by loss of plasma membrane integrity, cell swelling and lysis, random degradation of DNA, and a subsequent inflammatory response.[32]

During the first 4 to 24 hours after injury, IL-1 and TNF ALPHA released from injured epithelium stimulate keratocytes and corneal fibroblasts to produce chemokines such as granulocyte colony stimulating factor (G-CSF), neutrophil-activating peptide (ENA-78), monocyte-derived neutrophil chemotactic factor (MDNCF), and monocyte chemotactic activating factor (MCAF). These chemokines attract inflammatory cells such as macrophages/monocytes, T cells, and polymorphonuclear cells into the stroma from the limbal vessels and the tear film.[21,31,33-35] One function of these cells is to engulf apoptotic bodies, cellular organelles, and other cellular debris.[7] However, it has also been hypothesized that some of these inflammatory cells (macrophages) make more specific contributions to the wound healing response, perhaps by undergoing transition to another cell type that participates in stromal remodeling.[36] Thus, the same cytokines and bone marrow-derived cells that participate in the differentiation of monocytes into osteoclasts in bone are also expressed in the corneal stroma.[36]

Residual keratocytes in the posterior and peripheral stroma, depending on the injury, begin to proliferate approximately 12 hours after the initial injury and are thought to give rise to activated keratocytes, myofibroblasts, and mature keratocytes that repopulate the depleted stroma.[3,31]

Beginning 1 to 2 weeks after injury, depending on the extent and type of injury, cells called myofibroblasts may appear in the stroma immediately beneath the epithelium.[31] These cells are presumably derived from proliferating keratocytes influenced by TGFβ derived from corneal epithelial cells.[13,37-40] The integrity and normal function of the basement membrane appears to be an important determinate of the amount of epithelial cell-derived TGFβ that gains access to the stroma and, therefore, whether myofibroblasts are generated.[40] An important characteristic of these cells is decreased transparency related to diminished corneal crystallin production compared to keratocytes.[41] Generation of myofibroblasts results in variable levels of corneal haze.[41] These cells can be identified by using immunohistochemical methods to detect specific markers, such as alpha smooth muscle actin (αSMA).

In the weeks to months following injury, corneal cellularity and function slowly return toward normalcy in eyes that have refractive surgical procedures.[21] Keratocyte apoptosis, necrosis, and proliferation diminish markedly approximately 1 week after surgery[31] and regeneration of the basement membrane correlates with loss of the fibrotic phenotype.[39]

The disappearance of most immune cells from the cornea is probably mediated by apoptosis. (Netto, Mohan, Perez, and Wilson, unpublished data, 2004). However, some components of this normalization process may require months to years, depending on the type of surgery. For example, in cases of severe haze associated with myofibroblast generation, the myofibroblast cells disappear over several years—either by late apoptosis or transdifferentiation back to keratocytes or both. This process is accompanied by remodeling of disorganized stromal collagen and ECM components, resulting in clearing of the stromal scar.

Biological variations in the cellular responses occur with different surgical techniques and even in the eyes of different patients who have the same procedure. The intensity and duration of these events are directly responsible for the postoperative outcomes and many complications following refractive surgical procedures.

Corneal Wound Healing After Surface Ablation and Lamellar Procedures

Clinical outcomes after surface ablation and lamellar procedures are, to a significant extent, dependent on the corneal wound healing response. Depending on the level of attempted correction, the corneal wound healing response and the

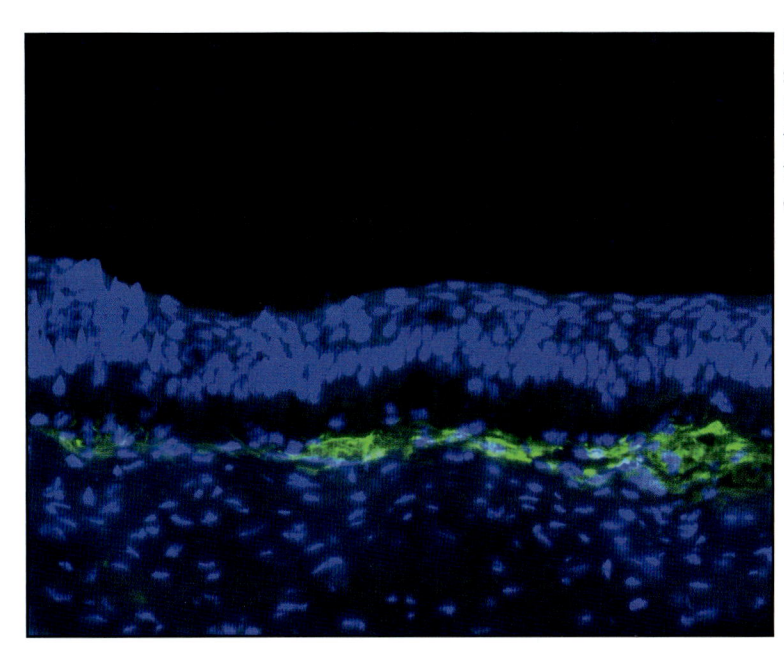

Figure 25-1. Immunohistochemistry to detect alpha smooth muscle actin-expressing myofibroblasts (arrows) beneath the epithelium in a rabbit eye that had severe surface irregularity introduced at the stromal surface during PRK for 4.5 D myopia compared to a normal 4.5-D PRK.

stimulus for the fibrotic response are usually stronger after surface ablation techniques, most likely as a consequence of disrupting the basement membrane overlying the central cornea and abnormalities in regeneration of the basement membrane that can occur when there is surface irregularity following the ablation (Netto, Mohan, and Wilson, unpublished data, 2004).[39,42] There are also fundamental differences in the location and intensity of the wound healing events following PRK and LASIK.

Many wound healing experimental studies have been performed with animal models.[43-45] Mohan et al[31] analyzed qualitative and quantitative differences in the cellular responses in the corneal stroma after PRK and LASIK in rabbits. In this study, keratocyte apoptosis, keratocyte proliferation, and myofibroblast generation were significantly greater in the high PRK eyes compared to the high LASIK eyes (9.0-D corrections for myopia). In LASIK, keratocyte apoptosis and keratocyte proliferation occur directly above and below the lamellar interface. Conversely, in PRK, keratocyte apoptosis occurs in the superficial stroma and keratocyte proliferation occurs in the posterior and peripheral stroma outlying the area where apoptosis occurs following epithelial injury. Interestingly, there was no myofibroblast generation in the central cornea in eyes that had high LASIK in contrast to eyes that had high PRK, which is in agreement with minimal central haze formation following normal LASIK procedures in humans.[31] The creation of a flap during LASIK maintains a zone of normal cornea between the epithelium and the stroma and retains a normal basement membrane, diminishing cytokine-mediated interactions between stromal cells and the overlying epithelium. At the flap margins, however, there is direct contact between the stromal tissue and injured epithelium and the basement membrane.[46] As a result, the healing response is much higher in the periphery of the cornea, as can be observed clinically by noting the circumferential scar at the edge of the flap. In the center of the cornea, however, the intact basement membrane and uninjured epithelium results in minimal stromal cell activation and little tendency toward myofibroblast generation in normal cases.[47-49]

In PRK, the removal of the epithelial basement membrane and Bowman's layer at the time of the ablation leaves the anterior stroma directly exposed to the effects of cytokines and growth factors released by the epithelial cells and present in the tears. Mohan et al[31] also showed greater intensity of keratocyte apoptosis, keratocyte proliferation, and myofibroblast generation after PRK for high corrections in contrast to PRK for low corrections. These results correlate with the clinical findings of higher incidence of regression and haze formation after PRK for high myopia than low myopia, with approximately 6.0 D of correction for myopia being a transition point between clinically significant differences such as increased risk of haze.[50-52]

Additionally, it has been observed clinically by Paolo Vinciguerra and Dan Epstein that smoother excimer laser ablations are associated with less haze. Results of recent experiments have demonstrated the importance of the stromal bed irregularity in corneal haze formation. (Netto, Mohan, and Wilson, unpublished data, 2004). Results in animal models have demonstrated a remarkable correlation between postoperative excimer laser-induced stromal bed irregularity and the level of haze formation (Figure 25-1). The mechanism involved in myofibroblast generation and haze formation in eyes with stromal bed irregularity seem to involve defective basement membrane regeneration and function and the increased cytokine-mediated communication between epithelial cells and cells in the anterior stroma.

Corneal Wound Healing After LASEK

LASEK is a modification of the PRK technique that involves creation of an epithelial flap after the application of dilute alcohol solution. The flap is repositioned after laser ablation of the underlying stroma. The main clinical advantages of LASEK that have been reported are less postoperative pain and haze formation.[53]

Few studies have analyzed the wound healing response involved in LASEK, primarily due to technical difficulties in reproducing this technique in animal models. The epithelial flap in LASEK could serve as a mechanical barrier that protects the stroma from the direct exposure to epithelial and tear growth factors. Such an effect could depend on whether the basement membrane remains attached to the epithelial flap or is damaged during lifting of the flap. Lee et al[54] reported a lower TGFβ1 release into the tear fluid in the early postoperative days following LASEK in comparison to PRK. Theoretically, decreased release of TGFβ1 might result in lower stimulus for a fibrotic healing response, including less myofibroblast generation and reduced haze formation. However, clinical results verifying corneal haze formation after LASEK published in the literature are contradictory.[55,56]

Keratocytes Apoptosis After LASEK

A study performed in rabbits suggested that fewer keratocytes undergo apoptosis after LASEK compared to PRK.[57] Whether a decrease in keratocyte apoptosis would lead to decreased keratocyte mitosis and/or myofibroblast generation remains uncertain in the absence of pharmacological mediators to inhibit keratocyte apoptosis and establish with certainty whether any interrelationship is present between these stromal wound healing events. In other words, the question remains whether a decrease in the early keratocyte apoptosis response results in a decrease in later wound healing events such as myofibroblast generation. These investigators also observed that the peak of apoptosis occurred significantly later after LASEK compared to PRK.[57] Chicken or pig eyes may provide better models to study wound healing in LASEK.[58]

Epithelial Viability in LASEK

Viability of the epithelium following surgery is likely a critical factor determining increased efficacy of LASEK relative to PRK. If the epithelial cells in the flap do not remain viable, then dead cells and cellular debris may provide a mechanical barrier for epithelial healing, possibly resulting in delayed epithelial healing and visual recovery in comparison to simple PRK. In vitro studies with epithelial monolayers have demonstrated that cell death varies with different alcohol concentrations and exposure times.[59] These studies have shown that alcohol concentrations in excess of 25% markedly reduce epithelial cell viability.[59] Thus, alcohol concentration and exposure time are both important factors determining epithelial viability. A 20% ethanol concentration with an exposure time less than 30 seconds appears to be appropriate to have a significant chance of the epithelium remaining viable after LASEK.[60,61] Other factors, such as the type of alcohol, dilution vehicle, and temperature of the solution, may also play important roles. None of the studies published to date have established the percentage of viable basal epithelial cells retained following LASEK with a particular alcohol concentration and exposure time. Studies such as this, in the chicken model, for example, could be helpful in guiding clinical treatments in humans. Another critical determinant of epithelial viability is whether the epithelium of the LASEK flap remains attached to the underlying basement membrane. When epithelial cells are displaced from their basement membrane, they tend to undergo apoptosis.[61,62] Therefore, if the basement membrane remains with the stroma and is subsequently ablated, the epithelial flap is unlikely to remain viable.[63-65] Clearly, when the basement membrane is damaged or removed in a particular LASEK procedure, the cytokine- and growth factor-mediated interactions between the epithelium and the underlying stromal cells will be very different, and this may affect the clinical outcome of the procedure—including accuracy of the correction, haze, and other outcome measures. Some have proposed that, viable or not, the temporary epithelial bandage may be beneficial in modulating wound healing and decreasing discomfort,[66] but support for this hypothesis is limited. Published studies in animal models of refractive surgical procedures suggest that reducing damage to epithelial cells results in decreased release of epithelium-derived factors that promote keratocyte apoptosis and inflammatory cell influx.[10,11,18,36]

Vinciguerra[53] developed the "butterfly" LASEK technique to retain the connection and communication between limbal stem cells and the epithelial flap to improve viability of the epithelium. In the "butterfly" LASEK technique, epithelial flaps are formed peripherally from a paracentral linear de-epithelialization,[53] rather than from a peripheral trephination used in the classic LASEK technique.

Immunofluorescence studies have been performed to determine the anatomic cleavage plane relative to the epithelium after LASEK. Espana et al,[67] monitored laminin 5, integrins (β4 and β6), and collagen VII in cadaver eyes and patients who had surface ablation refractive surgery. The epithelial adhesion complex includes hemidesmosomes that adhere to the anchoring network in the superficial stroma. These hemidesmosomes have inner and outer plaques, with the outer plaque containing α6β4 integrin. The anchoring network is composed by anchoring filaments (laminin 5), anchoring fibrils (collagen VII) and anchoring plaque (collagen IV). Espana and coworkers[67] found that patches of laminin 5 and α6β4 integrin remain attached to the epithelial flap following LASEK. In contrast, linear staining with collagen VII was observed in the stromal bed in this study. Thus, the cleavage plane of the ethanol-induced corneal epithelial flap in most eyes appeared to be located between the lamina lucida and the lamina densa of the basement membrane, where integrin β (4) interacts with laminin 5 to form hemidesmosomes.[67]

Ethanol weakens the adhesions of the basal epithelial cells to the anterior stroma. However, there are individual variations in epithelial-stromal adhesions between the corneas of normal patients that have important effects on the efficacy of

LASEK. These variations are the likely cause in the variability of the technique in different eyes and lead to inconsistencies in the ethanol exposure time required for the epithelial flap creation in a particular patient. These variations, in turn, result in differences in stromal dehydration during ablation from cornea to cornea that may affect the outcome of the procedure. This could result in more difficulty in generating reliable nomograms compared to PRK and LASIK and may result in higher rates of undercorrections or overcorrections, although clinical data testing this hypothesis are lacking.

Epi-LASIK as an Alternative to LASEK

More recently, Epi-LASIK microkeratomes have been introduced as an alternative method for creating epithelial flaps without ethanol exposure.[68] There are several instruments available or under development for Epi-LASIK. The typical device incorporates a suction ring and a blunt oscillating blade that is designed to rapidly separate the epithelium from the underlying stroma. Pallikaris et al[69] first described the Epi-LASIK technique and hoped that the basement membrane and its attachments to the epithelium would be preserved after flap creation. Even with this technique, microfocal damage to the lamina densa of the basement membrane has been noted.[69] It appears likely that there will be variations in the location of the cleavage plane from eye to eye, with it being above the basement membrane in some eyes and below in others. This in turn would lead to differences in wound healing described for LASEK in the prior sections of this chapter. The timing of the Epi-LASIK procedure would seem to be an advantage, but further studies are needed to examine the viability and function of the epithelium and basement membrane in animal models and the clinical outcomes, including discomfort, rate of visual recovery, and rate of significant haze formation, compared with PRK.

Conclusions

The corneal wound healing response following LASEK is a complex series of events that play a major role in clinical outcomes. Further studies are needed to fully characterize the possible benefits of LASEK over PRK and other refractive procedures.

Acknowledgments

Supported in part by an unrestricted grant from Research to Prevent Blindness, New York, NY, and US Public Health Service grant EY 10056 from the National Eye Institute, National Institutes of Health, Bethesda, MD.

The authors have no proprietary or financial interest in relation to this manuscript.

References

1. Mohan RR, Liang Q, Kim WJ, et al. Apoptosis in the cornea: further characterization of Fas/Fas ligand system. *Exp Eye Res.* 1997;65:575-589.
2. Mohan RR, Kim WJ, Mohan RR, Chen L, Wilson SE. Bone morphogenic proteins 2 and 4 and their receptors in the adult human cornea. *Invest Ophthalmol Vis Sci.* 1998;39:2626-2636.
3. Zieske JD, Guimaraes SR, Hutcheon AE. Kinetics of keratocyte proliferation in response to epithelial debridement. *Exp Eye Res.* 2001;72:33-39.
4. Wilson SE, Mohan RR, Mohan RR, et al. The corneal wound healing response: cytokine-mediated interaction of the epithelium, stroma, and inflammatory cells. *Prog Retin Eye Res.* 2001;20:625-637.
5. Wilson SE, Mohan RR, Hong JW, Lee JS, Choi R, Mohan RR. The wound healing response after laser in situ keratomileusis and photorefractive keratectomy: elusive control of biological variability and effect on custom laser vision correction. *Arch Ophthalmol.* 2001;119:889-896.
6. Wilson SE. Role of apoptosis in wound healing in the cornea. *Cornea.* 2000;19(3 Suppl):S7-12.
7. Wilson SE, Netto M, Ambrosio R Jr. Corneal cells: chatty in development, homeostasis, wound healing, and disease. *Am J Ophthalmol.* 2003;136:530-536.
8. Wilson SE, Liu JJ. Stromal-epithelial interactions in the cornea. *Prog Retin Eye Res.* 1999;18:293-309.
9. Wilson SE, He YG, Weng J, Li Q, et al. Epithelial injury induces keratocyte apoptosis: hypothesized role for the interleukin-1 system in the modulation of corneal tissue organization and wound healing. *Exp Eye Res.* 1996;62:325-327.
10. Mohan RR, Mohan RR, Kim WJ, Wilson SE. Modulation of TNF-alpha-induced apoptosis in corneal fibroblasts by transcription factor NF-kb. *Invest Ophthalmol Vis Sci.* 2000;41:1327-1334.
11. Wilson SE, Chen L, Mohan RR, Liang Q, Liu J. Expression of HGF, KGF, EGF and receptor messenger RNAs following corneal epithelial wounding. *Exp Eye Res.* 1999;68:377-397.
12. Tuominen IS, Tervo TM, Teppo AM, et al. Human tear fluid PDGF-BB, TNF-alpha and TGF-beta1 vs corneal haze and regeneration of corneal epithelium and subbasal nerve plexus after PRK. *Exp Eye Res.* 2001;72:631-641.
13. Jester JV, Huang J, Petroll WM, Cavanagh HD. TGFbeta induced myofibroblast differentiation of rabbit keratocytes requires synergistic TGFbeta, PDGF and integrin signaling. *Exp Eye Res.* 2002;75:645-657.
14. West-Mays JA, Sadow PM, Tobin TW, et al. Repair phenotype in corneal fibroblasts is controlled by an interleukin-1 alpha autocrine feedback loop. *Invest Ophthalmol Vis Sci.* 1997;38:1367-1379.
15. Strissel KJ, Rinehart WB, Fini ME. Regulation of paracrine cytokine balance controlling collagenase synthesis by corneal cells. *Invest Ophthalmol Vis Sci.* 1997;38:546-552.
16. Fini ME, Strissel KJ, Girard MT, Mays JW, Rinehart WB. Interleukin 1 alpha mediates collagenase synthesis stimulated by phorbol 12-myristate 13-acetate. *J Biol Chem.* 1994;269:11291-11298.
17. Tervo T, Vesaluoma M, Bennett GL, et al. Tear hepatocyte growth factor (HGF) availability increases markedly after excimer laser surface ablation. *Exp Eye Res..* 1997;64:501-504.
18. Wilson SE, Mohan RR, Mohan RR, et al. The corneal wound healing response: cytokine-mediated interaction of the epithelium, stroma, and inflammatory cells. *Prog Retin Eye Res.* 2001;20:625-637.
19. Mohan RR, Mohan RR, Kim WJ, Wilson SE. Modulation of TNF-alpha-induced apoptosis in corneal fibroblasts by transcription factor NF-kb. *Invest Ophthalmol Vis Sci.* 2000;41:1327-13236.
20. Helena MC, Baerveldt F, Kim W-J, Wilson SE. Keratocyte apoptosis after corneal surgery. *Invest Ophthalmol Vis Sci.* 1998;39:276-283.
21. Wilson SE. Analysis of the keratocyte apoptosis, keratocyte proliferation, and myofibroblast transformation responses after photorefractive keratectomy and laser in situ keratomileusis. *Trans Am Ophthalmol Soc.* 2002;100:411-433.

22. Wilson SE, Kim WJ. Keratocyte apoptosis: implications on corneal wound healing, tissue organization, and disease. Invest *Ophthalmol Vis Sci.* 1998;39:220-226.
23. Dohlman CH, Gasset AR, Rose J. the effect of the absence of corneal epithelium or endothelium on stromal keratocytes. *Invest Ophthalmol Vis Sci.* 1968;7:520-526.
24. Ambrósio R Jr, Kalina R, Mohan RR, et al. Early wound healing response to epithelial scrape injury in the human cornea. Association for Research in Vision and Ophthalmology (ARVO) Annual Meeting, Program No. 4206 (May 2002).
25. Campos M, Szerenyi K, Lee M, McDonnell JM, Lopez PF, McDonnell PJ. Keratocyte loss after corneal deepithelialization in primates and rabbits. *Arch Ophthalmol.* 1994;112:254-260.
26. Lee JB, Javier JA, Chang JH, Chen CC, Kato T, Azar DT. Confocal and electron microscopic studies of laser subepithelial keratomileusis (LASEK) in the white leghorn chick eye. *Arch Ophthalmol.* 2002;120:1700-1706.
27. Gao J, Gelber-Schwalb TA, Addeo JV, Stern ME. Apoptosis in the rabbit cornea after photorefractive keratectomy. *Cornea.* 1997;16:200-208.
28. Gavrieli Y, Sherman Y, Ben-Sasson SA. Identification of programmed cell death in situ via specific labeling of nuclear DNA fragmentation. *J Cell Biol.* 1992;119:493-501.
29. Lovelace CIP, Zhang J, Vanek PG, Collier B. Detecting apoptotic cells in situ. *Biomed Prod.* 1996;21:76-77.
30. Wijsman JH, Jonker RR, Keijzer R, Van de Cees DJH. A new method to detect apoptosis in paraffin sections: in situ end-labeling of fragmented DNA. *J Histochem Cytochem.* 1993;41:7-12.
31. Mohan RR, Hutcheon AE, Choi R, et al. Apoptosis, necrosis, proliferation, and myofibroblast generation in the stroma following LASIK and PRK. *Exp Eye Res.* 2003;76:71-87.
32. Graf B, Pouliquen Y, Frouin MA, De Montaut F. The phenomena of reabsorption in the course of cicatrization of experimental wounds of the cornea (ultrastructural study). *Exp Eye Res.* 1972;13:24-32.
33. O'Brien T, Li Q, Ashraf MF, Matteson DM, Stark WJ, Chan CC. Inflammatory response in the early stages of wound healing after excimer laser keratectomy. *Arch Ophthalmol.* 1998;116:1470-1474.
34. Hong JW, Liu JJ, Lee JS, et al. Proinflammatory chemokine induction in keratocytes and inflammatory cell infiltration into the cornea. *Invest Ophthalmol Vis Sci.* 2001;42:2795-803.
35. Ramirez-Florez S, Maurice DM. Inflammatory cells, refractive regression, and haze after excimer laser PRK. *J Refract Surg.* 1996;12:370-381.
36. Wilson SE, Mohan RR, Netto MV, et al. RANK, RANK-L, OPG, M-CSF expression in stromal cells during corneal wound healing. *Invest Ophthalmol Vis Sci.* 2004;45:2201-2211.
37. Folger PA, Zekaria D, Grotendorst G, Masur SK. Transforming growth factor-beta-stimulated connective tissue growth factor expression during corneal myofibroblast differentiation. *Invest Ophthalmol Vis Sci.* 2001;42:2534-2541.
38. Jester JV, Huang J, Barry-Lane PA, Kao WW, Petrol WM, Cavanagh HD. Transforming growth factor (beta)-mediated corneal myofibroblast differentiation requires actin and fibronectin assembly. *Invest Ophthalmol Vis Sci.* 1999;40:1959-1967.
39. Maltseva O, Folger P, Zekaria D, Petridou S, Masur SK. Fibroblast growth factor reversal of the corneal myofibroblast phenotype. *Invest Ophthalmol Vis Sci.* 2001;42:2490-495.
40. Stramer BM, Zieske JD, Jung JC, Austin JS, Fini ME. Molecular mechanisms controlling the fibrotic repair phenotype in cornea: implications for surgical outcomes. *Invest Ophthalmol Vis Sci.* 2003;44:4237-4246.
41. Jester JV, Moller-Pedersen T, Huang J, et al. The cellular basis of corneal transparency: evidence for corneal crystallins. *J Cell Sci.* 1999;112:613-622.
42. Nakamura K, Kurosaka D, Bissen-Miyajima H, Tsubota K. Intact corneal epithelium is essential for the prevention of stromal haze after laser assisted in situ keratomileusis. *Br J Ophthalmol.* 2001;85:209-213.
43. Miyamoto T, Saika S, Yamanaka A, Kawashima Y, Suzuki Y, Ohnishi Y. Wound healing in rabbit corneas after photorefractive keratectomy and laser in situ keratomileusis. *J Cataract Refract Surg.* 2003;29:153-158.
44. Wachtlin J, Langenbeck K, Schrunder S, Zhang EP, Hoffmann F. Immunohistology of corneal wound healing after photorefractive keratectomy and laser in situ keratomileusis. *J Refract Surg.* 1999;15:451-458.
45. Park CK, Kim JH. Comparison of wound healing after photorefractive keratectomy and laser in situ keratomileusis in rabbits. *J Cataract Refract Surg.* 1999;25:842-850.
46. Ivarsen A, Laurberg T, Moller-Pedersen T. Characterisation of corneal fibrotic wound repair at the LASIK flap margin. *Br J Ophthalmol.* 2003;87:1272-1278.
47. Soubrane G, Jerdan J, Karpouzas I, et al. Binding of basic fibroblast growth factor to normal and neovascularized rabbit cornea. *Invest Ophthalmol Vis Sci.* 1990;31:323-333.
48. Kim WJ, Mohan RR, Mohan RR, Wilson SE. Effect of PDGF, IL-1alpha, and BMP2/4 on corneal fibroblast chemotaxis: expression of the platelet-derived growth factor system in the cornea. *Invest Ophthalmol Vis Sci.* 1999;40:1364-1372.
49. Zieske JD, Mason VS, Wasson ME, et al. Basement membrane assembly and differentiation of cultured corneal cells: importance of culture environment and endothelial cell interaction. *Exp Cell Res.* 1994;214:621-633.
50. Kim JH, Sah WJ, Park CK, Hahn TW, Kim MS. Myopic regression after photorefractive keratectomy. *Ophthalmic Surg Lasers.* 1996;27(S):435-439.
51. Williams DK. Multizone photorefractive keratectomy for high and very high myopia: long-term results. *J Cataract Refract Surg.* 1997;23:1034-1041.
52. Moller-Pedersen T, Cavanagh HD, Petroll WM, Jester JV. Neutralizing antibody to TGF beta modulates stromal fibrosis but not regression of photoablative effect following PRK. *Curr Eye Res.* 1998;17:736-747.
53. Vinciguerra P, Camesasca FI, Randazzo A. One-year results of butterfly laser epithelial keratomileusis. *J Refract Surg.* 2003;19:S223-226.
54. Lee JB, Choe CM, Kim HS, Seo KY, Seong GJ, Kim EK. Comparison of TGF-beta1 in tears following laser subepithelial keratomileusis and photorefractive keratectomy. *J Refract Surg.* 2002;18:130-134.
55. Litwak S, Zadok D, Garcia-de Quevedo V, Robledo N, Chayet AS. Laser-assisted subepithelial keratectomy versus photorefractive keratectomy for the correction of myopia. A prospective comparative study. *J Cataract Refract Surg.* 2002;28:1330-1333.
56. Lee JB, Seong GJ, Lee JH, Seo KY, Lee YG, Kim EK. Comparison of laser epithelial keratomileusis and photorefractive keratectomy for low to moderate myopia. *J Cataract Refract Surg.* 2001;27:565-570.
57. Laube T, Wissing S, Theiss C, Brockmann C, Steuhl KP, Meller D. Decreased keratocyte death after laser-assisted subepithelaial keratectomy and photorefractive keratectomy in rabbits. *J Cataract Refract Surg.* 2004;30:1998-2004.
58. Lee JB, Javier JA, Chang JH, Chen CC, Kato T, Azar DT. Confocal and electron micoscopic studies of laser subepithelial keratomileusis (LASEK) in the white leghorn chick eye. *Arch Ophthalmol.* 2002;120:1700-1706.
59. Chen CC, Chang JH, Lee JB, Javier J, Azar DT. Human corneal epithelial cell viability and morphology after dilute alcohol exposure. *Invest Ophthalmol Vis Sci.* 2002;43:2593-2602.
60. Kim SY, Sah WJ, Lim YW, Hahn TW. Twenty percent alcohol toxicity on rabbit corneal epithelial cells: electron microscopic study. *Cornea.* 2002;21:388-92.
61. Wadsworth SJ, Freyer AM, Corteling RL, Hall IP. Biosynthesized matrix provides a key role for survival signaling in bronchial epithelial cells. *Am J Physiol Lung Cell Mol Physiol.* 2004;286:L596-603.
62. Fouquet S, Lugo-Martinez VH, Faussat AM, et al. Early loss of E-cadherin from cell-cell contacts is involved in the onset of Anoikis in enterocytes. *J Biol Chem.* 2004;279:43061-43069.
63. Suzuki K, Saito J, Yanai R, et al. Cell-matrix and cell-cell interactions during corneal epithelial wound healing. *Prog Retin Eye Res.* 2003;22:113-133.

64. Suzuki K, Tanaka T, Enoki M, Nishida T. Coordinated reassembly of the basement membrane and junctional proteins during corneal epithelial wound healing. *Invest Ophthalmol Vis Sci.* 2000;41:2495-2500.
65. Kurpakus MA, Daneshvar C, Davenport J, Kim A. Human corneal epithelial cell adhesion to laminins. *Curr Eye Res.* 1999;19:106-114.
66. Song IK, Joo CK. Morphological and functional changes in the rat cornea with an ethanol-mediated epithelial flap. *Invest Ophthalmol Vis Sci.* 2004;45:423-428.
67. Espana EM, Grueterich M, Mateo A, et al. Cleavage of corneal basement membrane components by ethanol exposure in laser-assisted subepithelial keratectomy. *J Cataract Refract Surg.* 2003;29:1192-1197.
68. Pallikaris IG, Katsanevaki VJ, Kalyvianaki MI, Naoumidi II. Advances in subepithelial excimer refractive surgery techniques: Epi-LASIK. *Curr Opin Ophthalmol.* 2003;14:207-212.
69. Pallikaris IG, Naoumidi II, Kalyvianaki MI, Katsanevaki VJ. Epi-LASIK: comparative histological evaluation of mechanical and alcohol-assisted epithelial separation. *J Cataract Refract Surg.* 2003;29:1496-1501.

SECTION V
Management of Complications

CHAPTER 26

PHOTOREFRACTIVE KERATECTOMY
COMPLICATIONS DURING THE EPITHELIAL AND STROMAL HEALING PHASES

*Aldo Caporossi, MD; Marco Lazzarotto, MD;
Tomaso Caporossi, MD; Stefano Baiocchi, MD, PhD*

After surface keratectomy performed with an excimer laser (PRK), a process of corneal healing follows that includes two important phases: that of epithelial healing and that of stromal healing.

In this chapter, we will discuss the complications that may occur during epithelial healing, from diagnosis to therapy, and possible strategies to prevent their onset.

These complications principally include pain and postoperative inflammation, linked to tissual injury during surgery and to the absence of the corneal epithelium, delays in re-epithelialization, and infective keratitis. The latter two are rare events that may, however, evolve into serious complications that are difficult to manage. For this reason, early diagnosis and correct management of their course can avoid possible medical-legal consequences.

Postoperative Pain and Control of Inflammation

The possible appearance of pain after PRK typically starts 1 to 2 hours after surgery. It is of an acute type with a sudden onset and is associated to a clinical situation comprising photophobia, tearing, conjunctive hyperemia, and palpebral edema of a variable extent. It is present in 10% to 15% of patients after surgery and is more frequent in young patients and in bilateral treatments. Its duration is variable, but generally takes a few hours to disappear. Patients usually complain of itching, slight burning or foreign body sensation, photophobia, and blepharospasm.

Corneal epithelial tissue is the most highly enervated tissue in the body: anatomically there are a sub/basal-epithelial nerve plexus and a deep stromal nerve plexus, which originate from long ciliar nerves, of trigeminal pertinence. There is also a sympathetic component, which originates from the superior cervical ganglia. The spatial distribution of nerve fiber is higher in the central corneal region and along the horizontal meridian, and it diminishes at the periphery. These fibers carry stimuli from the aspecific polymodal receptors, which respond to mechanical thermal or chemical stimuli and from specialized receptors in the transduction of only mechanical stimuli. The first are type C, which have a low velocity of conduction and are responsible for the transmission of late, dull, and deep pain; the second are of the A-delta type, rapidly conducted and assigned to transport immediate and acute pain stimuli.

Almost complete removal of the corneal epithelium before photoablative treatment and further tissue removal by excimer laser leave the nerve residues uncovered and directly exposed to mechanical action of friction induced by ocular or palpebral movement. In addition, the algogenic action of the substances that mediate postoperative inflammation must be mentioned.

It is evident from this that the treatment of postoperative pain can act on three fundamental points:
* A reduction in the sensitivity of the receptor system
* A reduction in mechanical stimulation of the cornea
* Direct pharmacological action to control inflammation and pain

Obviously, pharmacological action to accelerate the epithelial healing process will also contribute to reducing the pain over time; we will discuss this last point more thoroughly in the chapter dedicated to delays in re-epithelialization.

In order to obtain a reduction in receptor sensitivity, techniques that cool the corneal tissue have been proposed, using a cold balanced salt solution or metallic cylinders cooled to a low temperature (4° C) to be placed on the corneal tissue (cooling PRK).[1,2] The physical action of cold permits almost

Table 26-1. MEDIATORS OF PAIN

Prostaglandins
Leukotrienes
Serotonin
Bradykinin
Histamine
Kalium
P substance

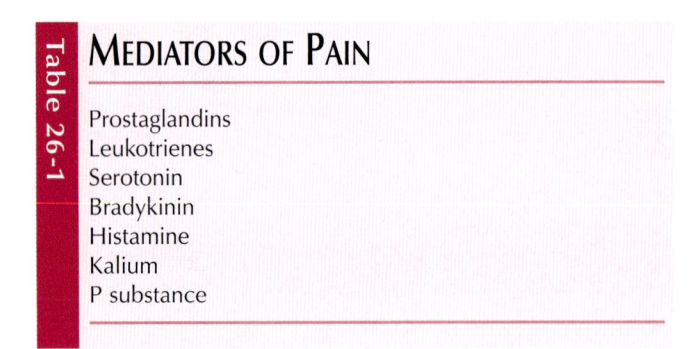

Table 26-2. NSAID OPHTHALMIC SOLUTIONS

Indomethacin
Suprofen
Flurbiprofen
Ketorolac
Diclofenac

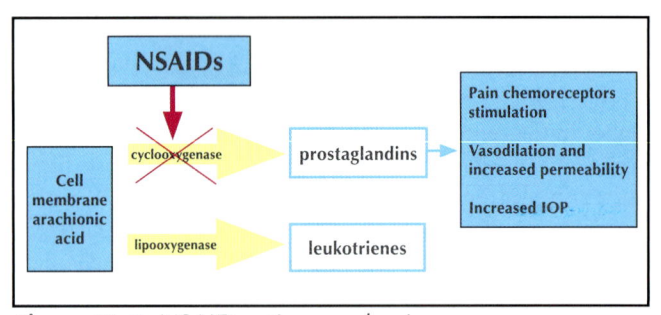

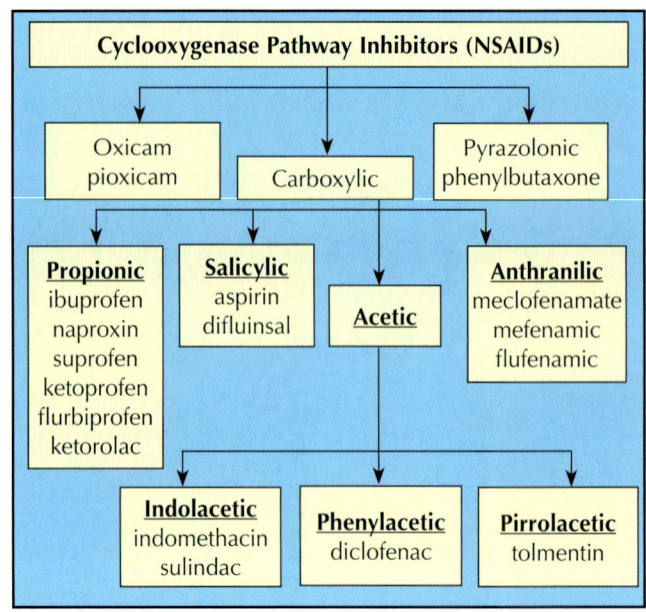

Figure 26-1. Main chemical categories of NSAIDs and derivatives.

Figure 26-2. NSAID action mechanism.

complete local analgesia and inhibition of the inflammation process; the transience in time of the hypothermal effect, however, invalidates these indisputable advantages.

Application, at the end of surgery, of a permanent, highly hydrophilic, corneal lens has an important effect on the reduction of mechanical stimulation. It also accelerates and regularizes the process of epithelial recovery.[3] Postoperative comfort of patients to whom a corneal lens has been applied is clearly higher than that of patients treated with a semicompressive bandage with ocular gauze; this also provokes an increase in the temperature of the conjunctiva favoring bacterial proliferation and, in case of bilateral treatment, prevents patients from attending to normal activities.

Pharmacological control of pain goes hand in hand with the control of inflammation. Some chemical mediators of pain (Table 26-1), such as prostaglandins and leukotrienes, which originate from lipids of the cell membrane, also play an important role as modulators of the inflammation process. Other mediators, such as serotonin, bradykinin, and histamine, derive from plasma or from blood cells because of the altered permeability and dilatation of vessels induced by inflammation.

Topical use of nonsteroidal anti-inflammatory drugs (NSAIDs) has been proven to obtain a good analgesic effect after PRK.[4-7] This category of drugs includes numerous chemical categories (Figure 26-1) of which only five substances are currently used for topical treatment (Table 26-2). NSAIDs perform an inhibiting action on the production of substances that mediate postoperative inflammation by acting on the cyclooxygenase pathway (Figure 26-2). Only diclofenac is thought to have an indirect action inhibiting the synthesis of leukotrienes by moving arachidonic acid in the triglyceride pool.

In our experience, a systemic administration of NSAIDs with a peaked analgesic effect (eg, ketorolac tromethamine) or of a centrally acting analgesic (paracetamol) has been useful, particularly if administered immediately after surgery. Triptans may represent a new approach for the control of severe pain.[8]

Systemic use offers advantages of longer term pharmacological action and avoids the toxic effects that topical NSAIDs, and, above all, excipients and preservatives possibly present in the preparation, may have on the epithelium. For this reason, topical preservative-free formulations are preferable.

Administration of topical anesthetics (eg, tetracaine or bupivacaine) must be avoided, even if limited to a short period. Beuerman has shown on rabbit cornea that a sensorial denervation considerably slows the process of epithelial healing. Furthermore, anesthetics exert a notable direct toxic effect on the epithelium and the risk of a toxic corneal abuse pathology should not be underestimated.

Inflammation is activated by different pathways (Figure 26-3): therefore, it is correct to assume that substances that act by blocking diverse pathways of activation also have an effect on the control of pain. For this reason, the pharmacology industry has recently turned its attention to attempting to neutralize high reactivity oxidant substances (-OH, H_2O_2,

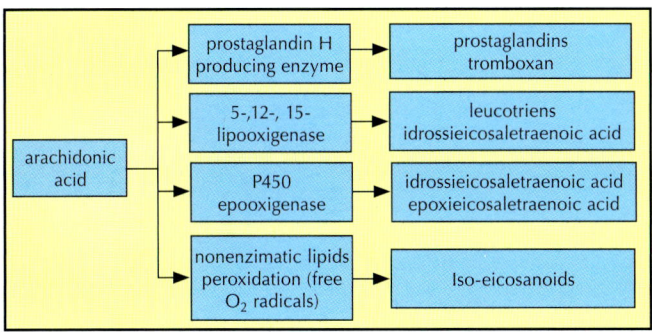

Figure 26-3. Various inflammation activation pathways.

Table 26-3

HAZE INCIDENCE IN LATE RE-EPITHELIALIZED EYES

820 Eyes (1997-1999)

2.25% (18): re-epithelielization time >15 days

77.7& (14/18) +++ at 1 to 3 months

22.2% (4/18): haze ≥ ++ at 12 months

27.8% (5/18): refractive error at 12 months > -0.75

1867 Eyes (2003)

0.16% (3/1867): reepithelialization time > 15 days
1.8% (33/1867): haze > + at 12 months

O_2, and organic peroxides) produced during the interaction of ultraviolet light with corneal tissue and the consequent toxic effects on the phospholipids in the cellular membrane. In addition to the well-known antioxidant effects of some vitamins (A, E), other recently developed substances with a high affinity for H_2O_2, such as cytochrome-c peroxidases, can help the physiological corneal antioxidant systems (eg, the glutathione system) and have an important and selective action against pain and postoperative inflammation. These, however, need broader clinical experimentation to demonstrate their usefulness.

Delay in Re-epithelialization

Obtaining fast re-epithelialization after PRK surgery is an important objective to pursue for numerous reasons: faster functional recovery, less time spent in a protected environment, and a reduction of discomfort translate into higher patient satisfaction. Furthermore, less neoformation of collagen (haze) occurs: late re-epithelialization involves a higher incidence of haze and myopic regression. Our data show that when re-epithelialization takes longer than 15 days, there is an incidence of 2+ haze or higher 12 months after surgery equal to 22% of this population, compared to an incidence of 1.8% of 1+ haze 1 year after surgery in a total of 1867 eyes that underwent surgery in 2003 (Table 26-3).

The corneal epithelium serves a dual function: that of a barrier, with mechanical and refractive properties, due to the high difference in the index of refraction existing between air and the tear film.

The cells are joined by tight-junctions (zonula occludens) and form a highly resistant semipermeable membrane that protects the cornea from pathogenic germs and supports palpebral friction. The epithelial basal cells are anchored to the underlying Bowman's membrane by high-resistance filamentous structures defined hemidesmosomes.

The basal cells meet with frequent mitosis, particularly at the limbus, and a movement of centripetal cellular migration is associated with cellular migration and differentiation in the apical direction. Thoft and Friend illustrated this epithelial dynamic balance in 1993 with the x-y-z theory, which presumes a balance between the quantity of epithelial cells lost in exfoliation (Z) and their substitution through new cells that come from the basal layer (X) and the limbus (Y). In normal conditions, a complete turnover of the corneal epithelium occurs in about 2 weeks.

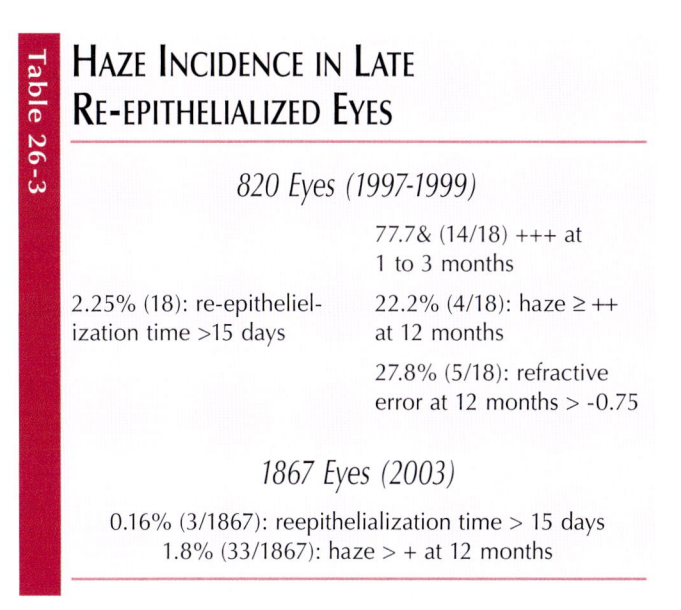

In the case of epithelial lesion, the processes of mitosis, migration, and cellular adhesion undergo strong acceleration. The presence of a complete Bowman's membrane permits rapid formation of the hemidesmosomial junctions; however, about 4 to 6 weeks are necessary for the complete *ad integrum* restitution of the junction complexes where the Bowman's membrane is missing.

In 1986, Crosson outlined the epithelial healing process on rabbit cornea, distinguishing two main phases that occur after a period of latency of about 8 hours, during which time hypertrophy of the basal epithelial cells with the accumulation of material necessary for cellular migration and replication occurs. The phase of linear healing lasts for about 48 to 72 hours and is characterized by centripetal migration and monostratified proliferation of the basal epithelial cells with formation of intercellular and, between cells and stroma, focal points of adhesion. The phase of adhesion and epithelial pluristratifications lasts about 6 weeks.

The speed of repair of the corneal epithelium assumes an even more important role in light of the current trend in refractive surgery whereby broader optical zones are treated. The first excimer lasers created optical zones of 4 to 5 mm, without transition zones, while more recent systems for personalized surgery are able to create treatment zones of more than 10 mm, including the transition zone. The de-epithelialized corneal area is thus quadrupled, with an inevitable increase in time necessary for epithelial recovery.

The development of lasers (from wide flat-top beams to flying-spot beams, initially flat-top and then with Gaussian profile) (Figures 26-4 and 26-5) and a smoothing procedure[9-12] performed at the end of surgery has been shown to obtain a reduction in the re-epithelialization time (Table 26-4). In fact, a smoother and more homogeneous ablated surface favors the advancement of the epithelial fronts.

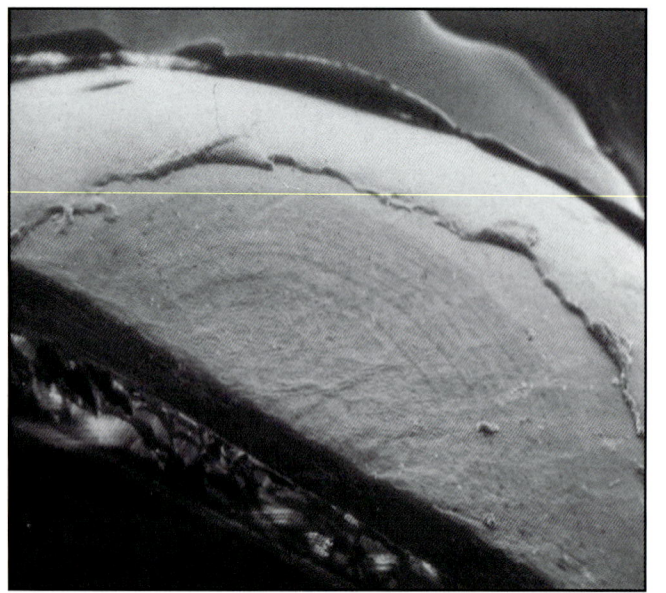

Figure 26-4. SEM appearance of a corneal surface treated with a broad beam (Summit UV200) laser for myopia: a steep ablation profile is clearly visible on the surface.

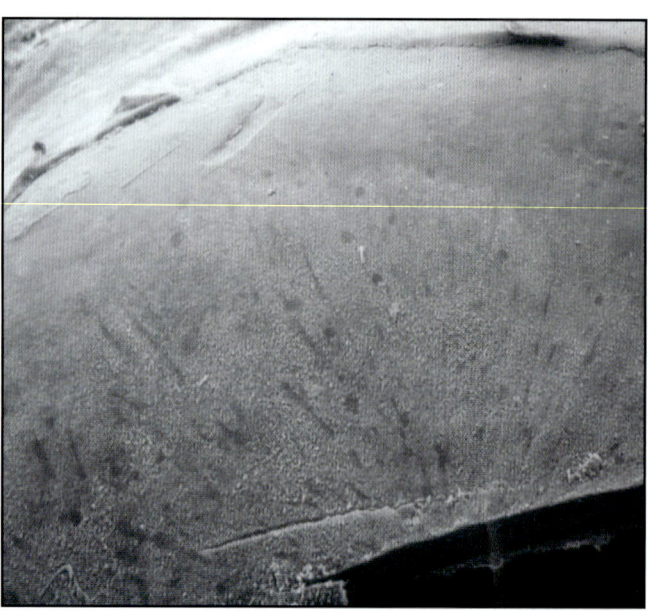

Figure 26-5. SEM appearance of a corneal surface treated with a flying spot (Bausch & Lomb 217c) laser for myopia: a very uneven ablation surface was obtained.

Table 26-4. SMOOTHING AFTER PRK vs PRK: OUTCOME ANALYSIS IN A GROUP OF PATIENTS

	PRK	PRK and Smoothing
Patients	40	40
Eyes	40	40
Mean Age	31.3 ± 5.98 (22/48)	31.3 ± 5.98 (22/48)
Refraction (SE)	-4.33 ± 1.88 (0.5/7.0)	-4.17 ± 1.82 (0.38/7.0)
Male/Female	7/13	8/12
Re-epithelialized Area (%): 1st day	38	45
Totally Re-epithelialized Eyes (%): 3rd day	82.5 (33/40)	90 (36/40)
Totally Re-epithelialized Eyes (%): 7th day	100	100

The use of a high hydrophilic therapeutic corneal lens at the end of the procedure has also been demonstrated to be able to significantly reduce the re-epithelialization period: 3 to 4 days are currently necessary for a complete recovery, compared to 6 to 7 days with the use of semicompressive bandage for an equal area of deepithelialization (Table 26-5).

A small percentage of eyes (5% in our experience) need 7 days to complete the re-epithelialization that proceeds slowly but progressively.

Therefore, we can define a delay in re-epithelialization as those cases in which one notes a total arrest in the progression of epithelial fronts or which take more than 7 days.

There are numerous pharmacological principles accredited with re-epithelialization activity (Table 26-6). Among these, growth factors are the most effective but also the most expensive, as well as being more sensitizing and difficult to find. Our clinical experience with epithelial growth factor (EGF)[13,14] after PRK (Table 26-7) has demonstrated, with gauze bandage, a reduction in the re-epithelialization time equal to 18%, but has not supplied a significant statistic outcome due to the small number of eyes studied. These, however, have reached a significant number in other clinical situations that involve broader epithelial recovery. In our opinion, further experimental development of these is therefore to be hoped for.

Among the other pharmacological principles of which we have direct experience, polydeoxyribonucleotides act by the *salvage* pathway (recovery of preformed nucleotides for the synthesis of nucleic acids) as an alternative to the traditional metabolic pathways in "ex novo" synthesis.

In the case of late re-epithelialization, when a complete stasis of growth of the epithelial fronts occurs with a contact lens, it is often useful to suspend its use: this may lead to a revival of the process of epithelial recovery, probably via neurogena.

In these cases, it is also advantageous to combat the inflammation process concomitantly with a topical steroid therapy, which prevents massive keratocyte activation that may result in alterations to corneal transparency. It should, however, be administered with extreme caution subjecting

Table 26-5. CLINICAL EXPERIENCE WITH DIFFERENT LASERS AT THE DEPARTMENT OF OPHTHALMOLOGICAL AND NEUROSURGICAL SCIENCES, UNIVERSITY OF SIENA

Laser	Healing Time	De-epithelialized Area (Radius)	Optical/Transition Zone
Summit Eximed UV 200 (gauze)	2.75 days	55 (r=5.5)	OZ
VISX 20/20 V 3.1 (gauze)	5.82 days	201 (r=8)	OZ
Bausch & Lomb 217 – Planoscan (gauze)	6.54 days	380 (r=11)	OZ + TZ
Bausch & Lomb 217 – Planoscan (contact lens)	4.18 days	380 (r=11)	OZ + TZ
Bausch & Lomb 217 – Zyoptix (contact lens)	3.52 days	380 (r=11)	OZ + TZ

Table 26-6. SOME SUBSTANCES THAT STIMULATE CORNEAL RE-EPITHELIALIZATION

Xanthopterin
Fibronectin
Vitamins A & E
Amino acids
Growth factors
Citocrome-c peroxidase
Polydeoxyribonucleotide

Table 26-7. CLINICAL EXPERIENCE WITH EGF AFTER PRK AT THE DEPARTMENT OF OPHTHALMOLOGICAL AND NEUROSURGICAL SCIENCES, UNIVERSITY OF SIENA

		Eyes	Time (Days)	
Post-epikeratophakia	EGF	8	3.38 ($P<0.01$)	-36%
	Controls	24	5.42	
Post-epikeratoplasty	EGF	6	2.83 ($P<0.01$)	-40%
	Controls	18	4.72	
Post-PRK	EGF	10	2.1 ($P=0.08$)	-19%
	Controls	10	2.6	

the patient to frequent examinations to monitor the evolution of the situation.

Infective Keratitis

Immediately after laser ablation, the center of the anterior corneal surface is completely de-epithelialized, without the Bowman's membrane and with the formerly ablate stroma directly in contact with the tear film and with the posterior surface of the therapeutic corneal lens, which has been routinely fitted after surgery since the mid-1990s. A period of 3 to 4 days is required to obtain complete re-epithelialization, and this means that an important mechanical barrier against implant and proliferation of bacteria is missing during this period. Corneal infection after PRK is a rare event and, in literature, only a few dozen cases have been reported. Nevertheless, the differing incidence in the various case studies analyzed certainly makes it a very dreadful complication, strongly dependent on prophylactic measures that are not always taken (Table 26-8).

As previously stated, the absence of the epithelial barrier is a very important risk factor regarding infection, but this is not the only risk. The permanent presence of a contact lens, qualitatively and quantitatively altered secretion of the tear film, as well as, when prescribed, a pharmacological regime

Table 26-8. INCIDENCE OF INFECTIVE KERATITIS POST-PRK

1/120	Gimbel
1/300	Arshinoff
1/800	Caporossi 1991 to 1995 (gauze)
1/930	Hersch 1998
1/5000	Caporossi 2000 to 2005 (therapeutic contact lens)

Table 26-9. MAIN INFECTIVE MICRO-ORGANISMS AFTER PRK

+++	Gram + (staphylococci, streptococci)
+--	Gram –
Rare	Mycetes

Table 26-10. CLINICAL SYMPTOMATOLOGY OF INFECTIVE KERATITIS

Symptoms	Signs
Pain	Blepharospasm
Photophobia	Eyelid edema
Visual acuity reduction	Purulent secretion
	Conjunctival hyperemia/edema
	Perikeratic hyperemia
	Corneal infiltrate or ulcer
	Tyndall/flare
	Hypopion
	Iris hyperemia/edema

including topical steroids, may favor an infective complication. Finally, it must be remembered that the patient him- or herself plays a fundamental role in such situations and may considerably influence the risk of developing a corneal infection during the postoperative phase soon after surgery. In fact, Gram-positive pathogen bacteria, such as staphylococcus, which often populate the palpebral and periocular skin, are those most frequently isolated in cultures of samples taken (Table 26-9). Avoiding touching the eyes, hygienic cleansing of the hands before medication, remaining at home, and complying with time periods and methods of medication are behavioral norms that the patient must scrupulously observe in order to minimize the risk of infection.

Finally, the surgical environment and observance of the commonplace norms of asepsis that surgeons must demand and maintain should not be neglected.

In our opinion, the choice of the postoperative therapeutic regime also plays an important role in the prevention of infections.

The topical antibiotic prophylaxis of choice should have two principal characteristics: a broad spectrum of action and an effective activity against Gram-positive bacteria. It should also have a minimal toxic effect on the corneal epithelium in formation. Fluoroquinolones are the drugs that best respond to these needs. Chloramphenicol also appears to be a good therapeutic choice due to its broad spectrum of action and its scarce resistance, particularly in the formulation associated with vitamin A. Aminoglycosides, due to their inhibitory effect on epithelial regrowth and betalactamics, due to the possibility of resistance on the part of some Gram-positive and scarce efficacy for Gram-negative, are less indicated.

The clinical symptomatology of infective keratitis is broadly variable and depends upon both etiological agents and the period of time of the appearance of infection (Table 26-10). However, it requires hospitalization due to the seriousness of the possible complications. The most appropriate therapy to be followed can be determined by an antibiotic sensitivity test carried out on cultures of corneal samples taken.

Differential diagnosis must consider sterile infiltrates that can sometimes be observed under the contact lens, but that, however, do not have an evolutional tendency (but instead a tendency to regression), are clearly delimited and do not give a perikeratic reaction. The anatomical and functional results of uncomplicated cases depend upon their extent and the possible involvement of the central cornea; in fact, it determines the excavation of the corneal tissue that could result in the production of leukoma or of an area of superficial irregularity that could reduce the better visual acuity corrected with spectacles.

The invalidating functional results of infective keratitis may necessitate further phototherapeutic regularization treatment (PTK) in order to obtain isorefractivity of the corneal surface.

Complications of the Stromal Healing Phase: Haze

Haze indicates increased corneal reflectivity (scattering of light) observable by biomicroscopy and induced by the subepithelial deposit of newly produced collagen and extracellular matrix in response to tissue removal.

During the normal postoperative course of PRK, it is constantly present in slight cases. It is clinically characterized by gradual appearance, 2 to 3 weeks after laser treatment, by a limited duration (1 to 2 months), and can easily be observed by biomicroscopy.

Modern patterns of corneal ablation, characterized by very smooth profiles without steps/inclines/slopes and integrated with transition zones, have considerably limited the entity of its clinical occurrence.

Currently, haze is rarely a postoperative complication (ie, evolving in elevated gradations) and is limited to treatment

Table 26-11. Treatment Limits Currently in Use at the Department of Ophthalmological and Neurosurgical Sciences, University of Siena*

	Planoscan	Zyoptix
Myopia	-9.0 D	-7.0 D
Astigmatism (-)	-4.0 D	-6.0 D
Astigmatism (+)	+3.0 D	+4.0 D
Hyperopia	+2.5 D	+3.5 D

*Stromal residual bed not less than 400 μm

Table 26-13. Haze Grading

Grade	Description
0	Completely clear cornea
0.5	Trace haze, seen with careful oblique illumination with slit-lamp biomicroscopy
1	More prominent haze, not interfering with visability of line iris details
2	Mild obscuration of iris details
3	Moderate obscuration of the iris and lens
4	Completely opaque stroma in the area of ablation

Adapted from Fantes et al. Wound healing after excimer laser keratomileusis (PRK) in monkeys. *Arch Ophthalmol.* 1990;108:665-675.

Table 26-12. Haze Stimulating Factors

High treatments
Small optical zone
Absence of transition zone
Delay in reepithelialization
Low compliance to therapy
UV exposure
Local or systemic inflammation
Age
Hormonal factors

---

of high visual defects with respect to reasonably contained values of treatment (Table 26-11) and in association with an adequate topical corticosteroid therapy.

Histologically, it corresponds initially to a subepithelial corneal area that is particularly rich in hydrophilic hyaluronan, which is gradually replaced by proteoglycans and immature collagen tissue produced by activated keratocytes and by epithelial cells.[15-17] The newly formed stroma then starts a process of reorganization to restore corneal transparency. Studies using a confocal microscope on animal models have shown an initial numerical reduction in stromal keratocytes mediated by cellular apoptosis that involves the stroma underlying ablation up to 200 μm and a successive repopulation of the area with activated keratocytes that appear hypertrophic, hyperplastic, and highly reflective. However, on human corneas, the apoptosis-mediated numerical reduction of keratocytes that precede their activation has not been convincingly demonstrated. A transformation in the myofibroblastic sense of keratocytes mediated by transforming growth factor-β (TGFβ) was hypothesized for those rare cases of particularly pronounced haze that result in corneal scars.

There is a well-known series of various natural factors that are able to stimulate haze in the postoperative period of PRK (Table 26-12); rarely, also in the absence of such factors, hyperresponsive subjects, defined as "aggressive responders,"[18] produce abnormal reparative processes independently of the value of treatment.

Various types of scales, based on biomicroscopy, can be used for its clinical gradation (Table 26-13). Recently, gradations based on light reflectivity by confocal microscopy have been proposed: they offer the advantage of being objective but are difficult to apply in routine clinical practice and are limited only to research.

We previously outlined the importance of carrying out a therapy based on topical corticosteroids that can control or even suppress postoperative keratocyte activation; it must therefore be protracted with a scaled modality for a sufficiently long period of time to avoid the appearance of haze when therapy is suspended (4 or 5 months). Topical steroids with a low capacity of penetration in the anterior chamber (such as fluorometholone, clobetasone, etc) are the drugs of choice for efficacy and a low incidence of collateral effects.

Interocular pressure (IOP) increasing to over 21 mmHg occurs, in our experience, in 3.8% of eyes treated for 5 months (eg, myopic treatments of more than 6.0 D) and is always controllable with the addition of local therapy as well as being reversible upon suspension of steroid therapy.

Haze typically has a limited influence on visual acuity and a tendency toward spontaneous disappearance, but when it is present at an elevated degree it may induce a regression of the refractive result obtained. Furthermore, when asymmetrical forms occur, it can induce the appearance of irregular astigmatisms and/or pseudodecentralizations that can be observed with computerized videokeratography.

Exceptionally, late onset haze may occur years after surgery, always in a secondary form (eg, after pathology of the posterior segment[19] or ocular surgery or even autoimmune collagen disorders).

Total control of stromal healing is currently impossible; it would be useful in the treatment of high-entity visual defects and for the current personalized methods of ablation (wavefront-guided treatments) that also aim to correct high order aberrations. Furthermore, it would also permit us to bring the rare cases of patients with abnormal reparative responses within normal parameters.

References

1. Niizuma T, Ito S, Hayashi M, Futemma M, Utsumi T, Ohashi K. Cooling the cornea to prevent side effects of photorefractive keratectomy. *J Refract Corneal Surg.* 1994;10(2 Suppl):S262-266.
2. Kitazawa Y, Maekawa E, Sasaki S, et al. Cooling effect on excimer laser photorefractive keratectomy. *J Cataract Refract Surg.* 1999;25(10):1349-1355.
3. Caporossi A, Baiocchi S, Frezzotti P, Sforzi C, Lazzarotto M. *Patching Versus Soft Contact Lenses Bondage After PRK: Comparison of Anatomic and Functional Results.* XII Congress of the European Society of Ophthalmology, Stockholm, June 27-July 1 1999, Abstract book p. 185 (P13 0012).
4. Sher NA, Frantz JM, Talley A, et al. Topical diclofenac in the treatment of ocular pain after excimer photorefractive keratectomy. *Refract Corneal Surg.* 1993;9(6):425-436.
5. Arshinoff S, D'Addario D, Sadler C, Bilotta R, Johnson TM. Use of topical nonsteroidal anti-inflammatory drugs in excimer laser photorefractive keratectomy. *J Cataract Refract Surg.* 1994;20(Suppl):S216-222.
6. Price FW Jr, Price MO, Zeh W, Dobbins K. Pain reduction after laser in situ keratomileusis with ketorolac tromethamine ophthalmic solution 0.5%: a randomized, double-masked, placebo-controlled trial. *J Refract Surg.* 2002;18(2):140-144.
7. Goes F, Richard C, Trinquand C. Comparative study of two non-steroidal anti-inflammatory eyedrops, 0.1% indomethacin versus 0.1% diclofenac in pain control post photorefractive keratectomy. *Bull Soc Belge Ophthalmol.* 1997;267:11-19.
8. May A, Gamulescu MA, Bogdahn U, Lohmann CP. Intractable eye pain: indication for triptans. *Cephalalgia.* 2002;22(3):195-196.
9. Fagerholm P. Phototherapeutic keratectomy: 12 years of experience. *Acta Ophthalmol Scand.* 2003;81(1):19-32.
10. Vinciguerra P, Azzolini M, Airaghi P, Radice P, De Molfetta V. Effect of decreasing surface and interface irregularities after photorefractive keratectomy and laser in situ keratomileusis on optical and functional outcomes. *J Refract Surg.* 1998;14(2 Suppl): S199-S203.
11. Vinciguerra P, Torres I, Camesasca FI. Applications of confocal microscopy in refractive surgery. *J Refract Surg.* 2002;18(3 Suppl): S378-S381.
12. Serrao S, Lombardo M, Mondini F. Photorefractive keratectomy with and without smoothing: a bilateral study. *J Refract Surg.* 2003;19(1):58-64.
13. Caporossi A, et al. Epidermal growth factor in topical treatment following epikeratoplasty. *Ophthalmologica.* 1992;205:121-124.
14. Caporossi A, et al. *Nostra esperienza con l'epidermal growth factor nella patologia corneale.* XXVII Congress of Società Oftalmologica Meridionale proceedings. Palermo 4-6 June 1993. Ed. Tipografica–Bari.
15. Fitzsimmons T, Fagerholm P, Harfstrand A, Schenholm M. Hyaluronic acid in the rabbit cornea after excimer laser superficial keratectomy. *Invest Ophthalmol Vis Sci.* 1992;33:3011-3016.
16. Weber B, Fagerholm P. Presence and distribution of hyaluronan in human corneas after phototherapeutic keratectomy. *Acta Ophthalmol Scand.* 1998;76:146-148.
17. Caporossi A, Baiocchi S, Manetti C, Frezzotti R, Alessandrini C, Losi M. *Excimer laser photokeratectomy: clinical and hystopathological aspects in the human corneas.* S.I.L.O. meeting, Cortina d'Ampezzo, Belluno, Italy, 16-18 Jan 1992, Acts Volume, pg. 267-284.
18. Durrie DS, Lesher MP, Cavanaugh TB. Classification of variable clinical response after photorefractive keratectomy for myopia. *J Refract Surg.* 1995;11:341-347.
19. Tosi GM, Baiocchi S, Caporossi T. Late corneal haze following retinal detachment surgery forty-two months after PRK. *J Cataract Refract Surg.* 2004;30(5):1124-1126.

CHAPTER 27

REDUCING THE RISK FOR POST-LASIK ECTASIA

Daniel Epstein, MD, PhD; Paolo Vinciguerra, MD

When laser in situ keratomileusis (LASIK) first appeared on the corneal refractive surgery scene, many surgeons expressed concern about the risk for postoperative ectasia. The main reason for this concern was the fact that the creation of the stromal flap—the hallmark of the procedure—causes a drastic change in the normal cornea's biomechanics, possibly weakening its structure and making it more susceptible to developing ectasia. Predictions of the expected incidence of post-LASIK ectasia ranged up to 5% of all LASIK procedures, raising the spectrum of the need for tens of thousands of penetrating keratoplasties (PKPs).[1-4]

Fortunately, an ectasia epidemic did not materialize. Although hard numbers are impossible to come by (because there are no reliable registries for ectasia cases), it is generally estimated that less than 0.1% of all LASIK eyes develop ectasia. Nevertheless, ectasia remains one of the most serious complications of LASIK and is all the more troubling because it remains unclear which eyes are likely to develop the complication.

Originally, it was assumed that two specific scenarios are most likely to explain the development of postoperative ectasia: 1) eyes in which too much tissue is ablated by the excimer laser, leaving a remaining stromal bed of less than 250 μm; and 2) eyes with a missed keratoconus or a missed early keratoconus. However, as reports of ectasia began to trickle into the refractive surgery literature, it became evident that even without thin stromal beds or keratoconus, ectasia did develop. Such eyes typically had normal preoperative central corneal thickness and topography and only low to medium corrections (ie, moderate amounts of stromal ablation). Why a normal eye that had, for example, undergone a 2.0-D treatment of myopia should end up with an ectasia remains unclear. Equally confusing is the observation that eyes with a residual stromal bed of less than 250 μm (remnants of the early days of LASIK) have not, as a rule, developed ectasia.

Evolution of a Hypothesis

In view of these contradictory findings, an attempt was made to analyze possible major factors that could predispose for ectasia. Theoretically, some eyes may have a genetic predisposition for ectasia. While there is no specific data on this theory, and no preoperative exams that can exclude such a factor, this possibility has to be kept in mind when faced with an inexplicable ectasia case (eg, normal cornea, low correction).

A thin preoperative cornea may be a risk factor. A thin cornea means that less stroma is available for treatment and that a larger percentage of the total available stroma is ablated even when moderate refractive errors are corrected. It is interesting that there is a general acceptance in the refractive surgery community that corneas thinner than 500 μm should not be subjected to LASIK.

The prerequisite of preserving a residual stromal bed of at least 250 μm after LASIK is a consequence of this reasoning around corneal thickness. But the 250-μm limit is, in fact, a historic guideline that has its roots in the original (nonlaser) keratomileusis era. It has never been clinically proven.

A further factor that may enter into the elusive ectasia equation is the uncertainty of the actual flap thickness. The vast majority of the LASIK flaps that have been performed around the world have been done with manual keratomy. Keratomes have improved vastly over the past decade, but the accuracy of flap thickness is still a problem. It has repeatedly been shown that the standard deviation (SD) of flap thickness can vary up to 30 μm, even in modern keratomes.[5] This means that a surgeon aiming at a 180-μm flap may in fact obtain a 210-μm or a 150-μm flap. When working with a corneal thickness that is borderline (ie, around 500 μm), a 210-μm flap may well undermine the aim of preserving a 250-

µm residual stromal bed. The newly-introduced femtosecond laser can cut thinner flaps (around 100 µm) and do so more accurately (lower SD) than manual keratomes, but it is too early to state with certainty that normal eyes treated with the femtosecond laser are immune to developing ectasia.

If a cornea has an unevenly distributed thickness preoperatively that goes unnoticed because a pachymetry map had not been obtained, a LASIK procedure may disturb the normal biomechanical structure of the cornea more than in a cornea with an evenly distributed thickness. Abnormal thickness gradients may even be unknown precursors of keratoconus. Corneal thickness beyond central pachymetry may play a role in ectasia.

Another aspect to be considered is the ablation rate variability of the excimer laser used. Once the ablation settings are punched in and the laser procedure is initiated, the surgeon cannot monitor inconsistencies in the ablation rate during the course of the operation. A possibly, uneven treatment may predispose for ectasia.

In addition, a simple error in preoperative pachymetry may also lead to an excessively thin postoperative cornea. If a procedure is calculated on the basis of inaccurate pachymetry (and because it appears that most surgeons do not perform intraoperative pachymetry), it is possible to unknowingly breach the 500- and 250-µm guidelines.

All of the previous considerations may play a role in the evolution of ectasia. We simply lack prospective, controlled studies to prove any or all of these points. And the hitherto low incidence of ectasia makes it very difficult to gather enough cases to prove one hypothesis or another. The refractive surgeon is thus faced with the fact that aside from preoperative pachymetry and early keratoconus or obvious keratoconus findings, there are no established criteria for preselecting corneas that may be at risk for developing post-LASIK ectasia.

Learning From Keratoconus

Starting with the assumption that keratoconus may well be the best ready-made model in nature to understand the development of corneal ectasia, we attempted to find a feature common to all (or most) keratoconus eyes that could also be used to identify at-risk eyes that appear normal in standard preoperative work-ups.[6-9] With the advent of instruments able to supply pachymetry maps (the Orbscan [Bausch & Lomb, Rochester, NY] has been available for a number of years, the Pentacam [Oculus, Lynnwood, Wash] is a relative newcomer), we found a tool that made it possible to identify just such a feature.

By analyzing a large number of Orbscan keratoconus maps and comparing them with maps of normal corneas, we observed that the pachymetry map provided well-defined and distinct differences between these 2 categories of eyes.

Normal corneas typically exhibited the following characteristics in pachymetry maps:

* The thinnest point is located centrally
* The thinnest point does not correspond to the steepest site
* Corneal thickness at the thinnest point is normal
* There is a symmetric pattern of distribution of thickness values throughout the cornea
* There is a normal gradient of thickness values from the corneal center to the periphery

In contrast, keratoconus eyes clearly deviated from the normal pachymetry map pattern described above. We, therefore, reasoned that it might be wise to exclude any eye from LASIK surgery if one or more of these 5 characteristics does not correspond to the findings expected in a normal cornea.

Accordingly, a checklist was set up to screen all LASIK candidates from the at-risk-for-ectasia perspective. In essence, this list represents the opposite of the features seen in the pachymetry map of normal corneas. Thus, the following findings should alert the refractive surgeon to question the suitability of a given eye for a LASIK procedure:

* The thinnest point is eccentric (ie, not central)
* The thinnest point *does* correspond to the steepest site
* Corneal thickness at the thinnest point is *not* normal
* There is an asymmetric pattern of distribution of thickness values throughout the cornea
* There is an abnormal gradient of thickness values from corneal center to the periphery

In the course of screening potential candidates for LASIK, the refractive surgeon must anticipate that from time to time, a cornea with a perfectly normal topography may eventually develop a post-LASIK ectasia. Corneal ectasia being one of the worst and most feared of LASIK complications, it is comforting to establish that a pachymetry map can provide useful data, above and beyond topography maps, to alert the surgeon to a possible at-risk-for-ectasia case. The working hypothesis presented here suggests that the pachymetry map may identify suspect corneas that otherwise would be missed in routine screening. Although "suspect" does not necessarily mean "ectasia-prone," there is sufficient uncertainty about why ectasia develops to warrant extreme caution when approaching a LASIK candidate with a "suspect" pachymetry map.

Proving the hypothesis and nailing down the definitive proof is extraordinarily difficult not only because of the dearth of ectasia cases, but also because in our experience most ectasia patients cannot provide a preoperative pachymetry map. The next section of this chapter will provide the basic evidence for our hypothesis, and the following segment will provide clinical examples supporting the hypothesis.[10-18]

Pachymetry Maps

Figure 27-1 presents an example of a normal astigmatic cornea. Note the symmetric pattern of thickness values. The thinnest point is central and measures 589 µm. Figure 27-2 is

Reducing the Risk for Post-LASIK Ectasia 239

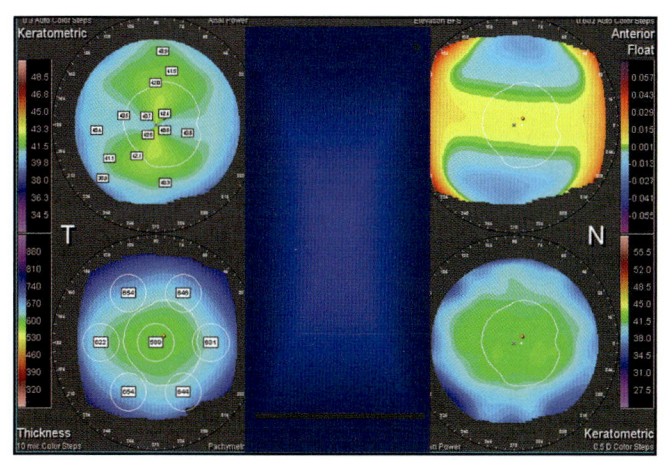

Figure 27-1. Normal astigmatic cornea. Note symmetric pachymetry (lower left). The thinnest point is central and measures 589 μm.

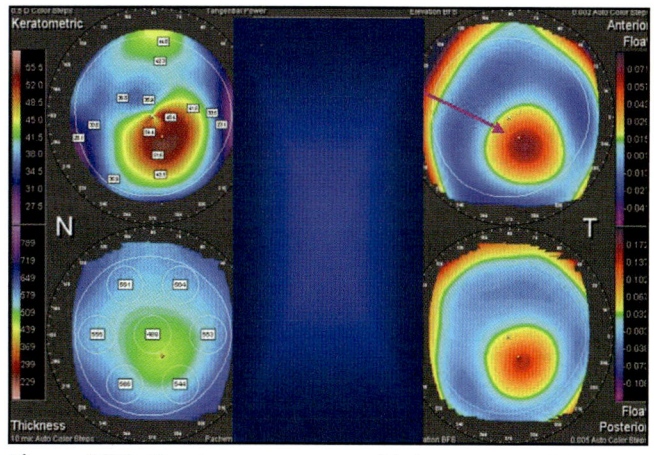

Figure 27-2. Keratoconus cornea. Note asymmetric pattern of thickness (lower left). The K-value is >48.0 D. The thinnest point (462 μm) is decentered and corresponds to the steepest site.

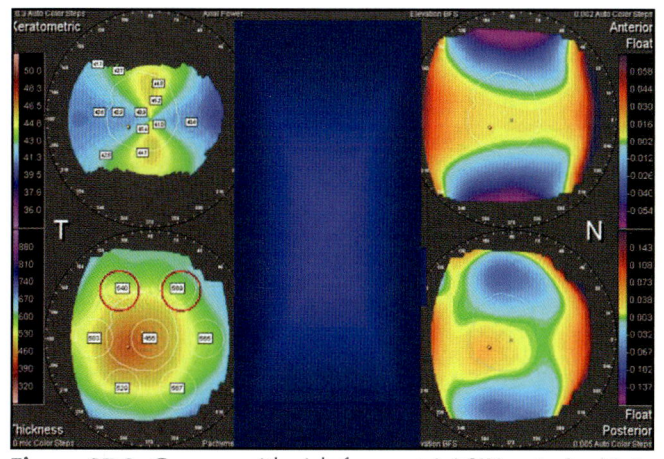

Figure 27-3. Cornea with risk for post-LASIK ectasia. Note asymmetric pattern of thickness (lower left). The thinnest point (426 μm) is eccentric.

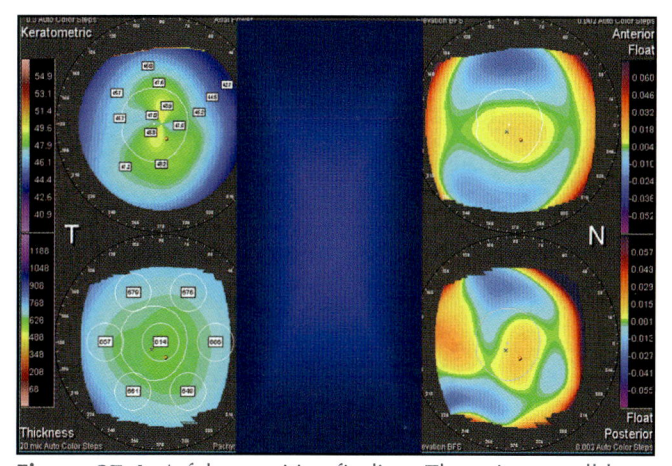

Figure 27-4. A false-positive finding. There is a small bow tie and a K-value of 48.0 D. But the pachymetry (lower left) is symmetric, and the thinnest point (607 μm!) is fairly central.

an example of a keratoconus. Note the asymmetric pattern of thickness values. The thinnest point (462 μm) is decentered, and corresponds to the steepest site. A possible risk for ectasia is seen in Figure 27-3. There is an asymmetric pattern of corneal thickness values. The thinnest point (426 μm) is eccentric. The axial and altitudinal maps are normal. Figure 27-4 illustrates a false-positive finding. Other data suggest a pathological cornea, but the pachymetry map clearly shows a symmetric pattern. The thinnest point is fairly central, and has a normal thickness (607 μm). A false-negative finding is demonstrated in Figure 27-5. Note the completely normal axial topography map. Yet, the asymmetric pachymetry map and eccentric thinnest point (484 μm) make this a suspect cornea. Figure 27-6 presents warpage caused by contact lens wear. The axial topography map is reminiscent of keratoconus, but the pachymetry map absolves this patient, displaying a symmetric pattern and a thinnest point that is central and shows normal thickness (575 μm).

Clinical Examples

CASE 1

Preoperative spherical equivalent (SE) refraction was -8.75 D OD and -5.87 D OS.

Preoperative pachymetry registered at 511 and 505 μm, respectively.

The preoperative pachymetry map OD shows that the thinnest point (515 μm) is slightly decentered. Considering that a correction of almost 9.0 D was performed, it can be argued that a central corneal thickness of slightly over 500 microns is cutting it close. The pachymetry map also shows asymmetry (Figure 27-7).

Ectasia was documented OD 3 years postoperatively (Figure 27-8). A PKP had to be performed.

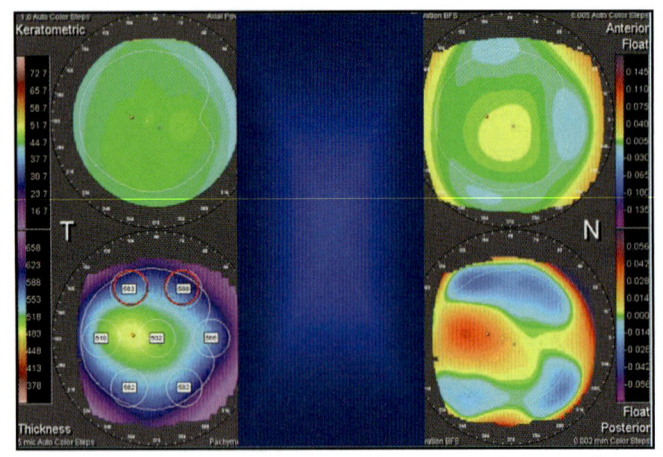

Figure 27-5. A false-negative finding. Note the completely normal axial topography (upper left). But the asymmetric pachymetry (lower left) and the eccentric thinnest point (484 μm) make this a suspect cornea.

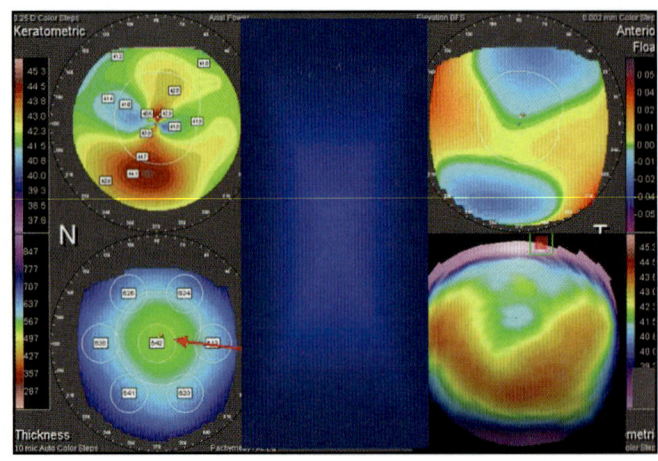

Figure 27-6. Warpage caused by contact lens wear. The axial topography (upper left) is reminiscent of keratoconus, but the pachymetry map (lower left) shows a symmetric pattern, and the thinnest point is normal (575 μm) and central.

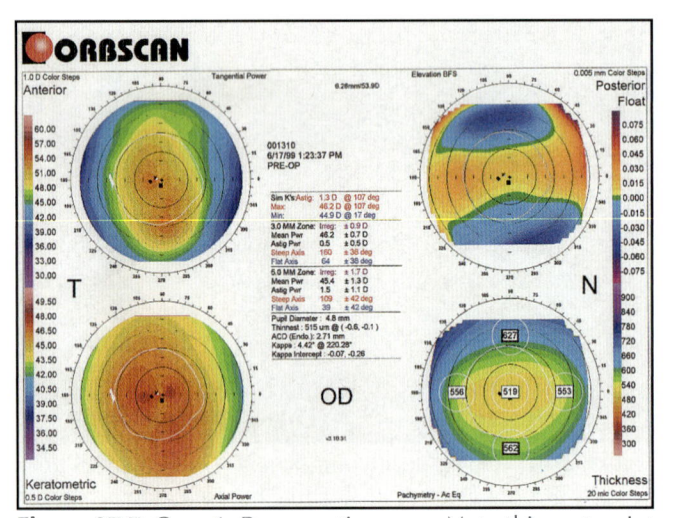

Figure 27-7. Case 1. Preoperative map. Note thinnest point (515 μm) is slightly decentered and the pachymetry map (lower right) is asymmetric.

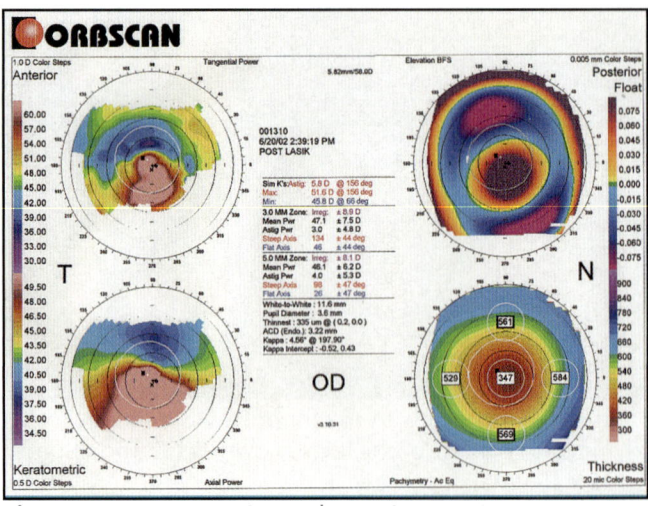

Figure 27-8. Case 1. Corneal ectasia seen 3 years postoperatively.

Case 2

Preoperative SE was -6.63 D OD and -7.0 D OS. Preoperative pachymetry measured 524 and 517 μm, respectively.

The preoperative pachymetry map OS shows that the thinnest point (520 μm) is slightly decentered. The map also shows asymmetry (Figure 27-9).

Ectasia was documented OS 3 years postoperatively (Figure 27-10). A PKP had to be performed.

Conclusion

The pachymetry map appears to identify suspect corneas that otherwise would be missed in routine screening. Suspect corneas resemble keratoconus corneas, and may be at higher risk for developing ectasia. In view of the dearth of reliable criteria (other than keratoconus and abnormal corneal thickness), the pachymetry map data may reduce the odds of inadvertently performing LASIK on potentially pathological, ectasia-prone corneas.

Acknowledgment

We wish to thank Dr. C. N. Moshegov, MB, BS, FRACO, FRACS, Gordon, NSW, Australia, for providing the two clinical cases presented here.

References

1. Binder PS. Ectasia after laser in situ keratomileusis. *J Cataract Refract Surg.* 2003;29(12):2419-2429.
2. Chiang RK, Park AJ, Rapuano CJ, Cohen EJ. Bilateral keratoconus after LASIK in a keratoconus patient. *Eye Contact Lens.* 2003;29(2):90-92.

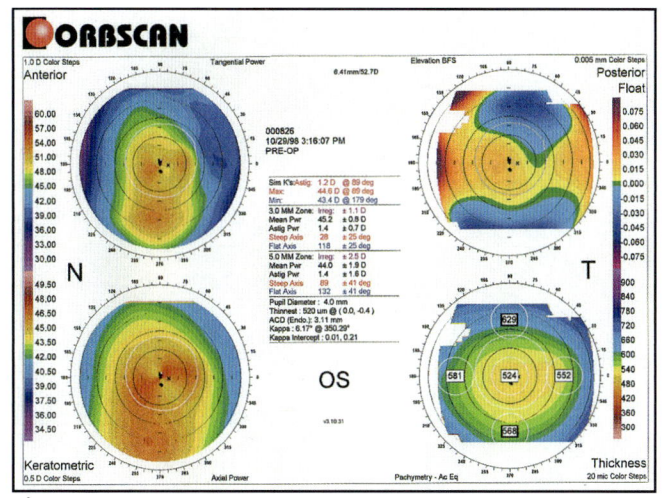

Figure 27-9. Case 2. Preoperative map. Note asymmetry in the pachymetry map (lower right). The thinnest point (520 µm) is slightly decentered.

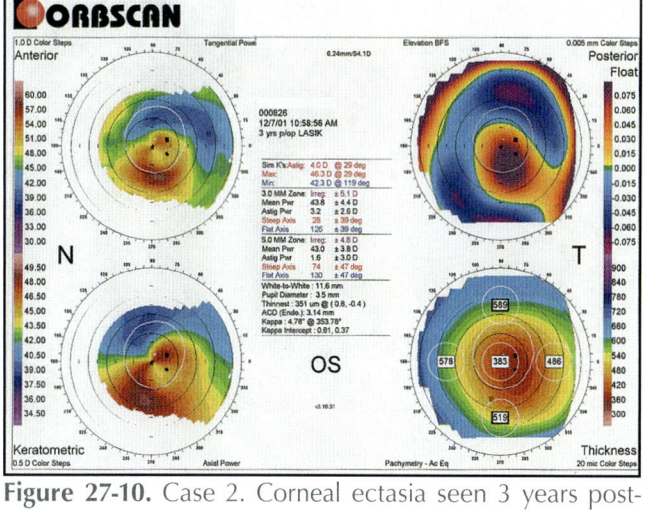

Figure 27-10. Case 2. Corneal ectasia seen 3 years postoperatively.

3. Dupps WJ Jr. Biomechanical modeling of corneal ectasia. *J Refract Surg.* 2005;21(2):186-190.
4. Faraj HG, Gatinel D, Chastang PJ, Hoang-Xuan T. Corneal ectasia after LASIK. *J Cataract Refract Surg.* 2003;29(1):220.
5. Flanagan GW, Binder PS. Precision of flap measurements for laser in situ keratomileusis in 4428 eyes. *J Refract Surg.* 2003;19(2):113-123.
6. Fogla R, Padmanabhan P. Bilateral keratectasia after unilateral laser in situ keratomileusis. *J Cataract Refract Surg.* 2004;30(10):2033-2034.
7. Jory W. Corneal ectasia after LASIK. *J Refract Surg.* 2004;20(3):286.
8. Kamiya K, Oshika T. Corneal forward shift after excimer laser keratorefractive surgery. *Semin Ophthalmol.* 2003;18(1):17-22.
9. Lifshitz T, Levy J, Klemperer I, Levinger S. Late bilateral keratectasia after LASIK in a low myopic patient. *J Refract Surg.* 2005;21(5):494-496.
10. Mitchell GL, Cruickshanks KJ, Schanzlin DJ. Characteristics of corneal ectasia after LASIK for myopia. *Cornea.* 2004;23(5):447-457.
11. Miyata K, Tokunaga T, Nakahara M, et al. Residual bed thickness and corneal forward shift after laser in situ keratomileusis. *J Cataract Refract Surg.* 2004;30(5):1067-1072.
12. Piccoli PM, Gomes AA, Piccoli FV. Corneal ectasia detected 32 months after LASIK for correction of myopia and asymmetric astigmatism. *J Cataract Refract Surg.* 2003;29(6):1222-1225.
13. Rad AS, Jabbarvand M, Saifi N. Progressive keratectasia after laser in situ keratomileusis. *J Refract Surg.* 2004;20(5 Suppl):S718-722.
14. Randleman JB, Russell B, Ward MA, Thompson KP, Stulting RD. Risk factors and prognosis for corneal ectasia after LASIK. *Ophthalmology.* 2003;110(2):267-275.
15. Seitz B, Rozsival P, Feuermannova A, et al. Penetrating keratoplasty for iatrogenic keratoconus after repeat myopic laser in situ keratomileusis: histologic findings and literature review. *J Cataract Refract Surg.* 2003;29(11):2217-2224.
16. Seiler T. Iatrogenic corneal ectasia after LASIK—is the end in sight? *Klin Monatsbl Augenheilkd.* 2005;222(5):429.
17. Teichmann KD. Bilateral keratectasia after laser in situ keratomileusis. *J Cataract Refract Surg.* 2004;30(11):2257-2258.
18. Twa MD, Nichols JJ, Joslin CE, et al. Bilateral keratectasia after unilateral laser in situ keratomileusis: a retrospective diagnosis of ectatic corneal disorder. *J Cataract Refract Surg.* 2003;29(10):2015-2018.

CHAPTER 28

Diagnosis of Decentered Treatment

Paolo Vinciguerra, MD; Alessandro Randazzo, MD

Introduction

One of the worst complications after refractive surgery is decentration of the ablation area. Decentration is often the cause of patient dissatisfaction due to visual acuity reduction, glare, halos, and monocular diplopia in the most severe cases. Functional deficits are obviously dependant on the amount of decentration. Decentration is a function of the extent of treated refractive defect, degree of astigmatism,[1] and optical zone (OZ) used.[2] Not all decentration causes functional deficits. Decentration up to 1 mm (0.8% to 15% of myopic photorefractive keratectomy [PRK][1-3]) does not appear to cause any significant loss of either uncorrected visual acuity (UCVA) or best corrected visual acuity (BCVA). The introduction of eye-tracking technologies in refractive surgery has considerably reduced the percentage of decentration, although it has not eliminated it altogether.[4-8]

Diagnosis of Decentration

We still need to understand how to assess ablations that are actually decentered. The confusion arises initially from the belief that the ablation diameter should correspond exactly to the optical zone useful for vision; however, not all ablation profiles are equally effective in ensuring a satisfactory level of correction. In theory, the OZ useful to vision should coincide with the laser setting, while the transition zone (TZ) should join the OZ to the nontreated cornea. In actual fact, not all lasers' ablation profiles provide the same refractive effectiveness. In some of them, the OZ resulting from ablation is larger than the setting; in others, due to the significant difference in curvature radius between the treated and the nontreated area, the final OZ is smaller than treatment settings. In effect, with the diopter power correction and the diameter of OZ used being equal, if the ablation and transition profiles are different, the tangential map will show an OZ different in size. The final result will therefore be determined by a higher diopter gradient in treatment. Diopter gradient means the curvature difference in diopters between two adjacent corneal zones, measured using a tangential topographic algorithm. A high diopter gradient causes primary and secondary spherical aberration.

High spherical aberration will reduce the functionally useful OZ and increase the refractive effect of decentration. Therefore, the refractive effect of decentration will not depend only on the amount of decentration but should also be seen in connection with the degree of spherical aberration. Ideally, the ablation profile should generate a new aspherical prolate surface larger than the pupil diameter. Because this is not always possible, the operator is often forced to compromise between two options. The first option is to use an OZ combined with a TZ touching the limbus; the second is a wide OZ and a narrow TZ. In the latter case, the difference in curvature between the treated and nontreated area will be concentrated in a small space, generating a high diopter gradient (ie, high spherical aberration) and, as a result, will shrink the functionally useful OZ. From the point of view of refractive quality, therefore, it is more useful to have an average-sized OZ with a wide, even TZ, rather than a wider OZ with a short TZ because the functionally useful OZ will be larger. The technical assessment of decentration is often based on ablation profile analysis in axial map. This algorithm determines the refractive impact of a change in shape but not the zone curvature. Also, because it is based on a spherical approximation, the axial map will show a spherical cornea, not a prolate cornea, as ideal. Using a wavefront map is a more appropriate way to determine OZ size and quality. However, even this method is not infallible in measuring decentration.

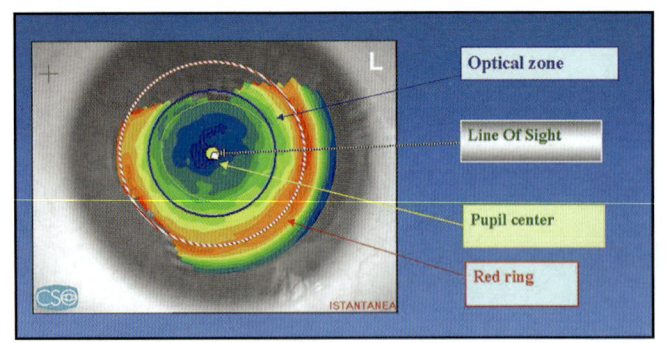

Figure 28-1. Tangential map of well-centered myopic ablation.

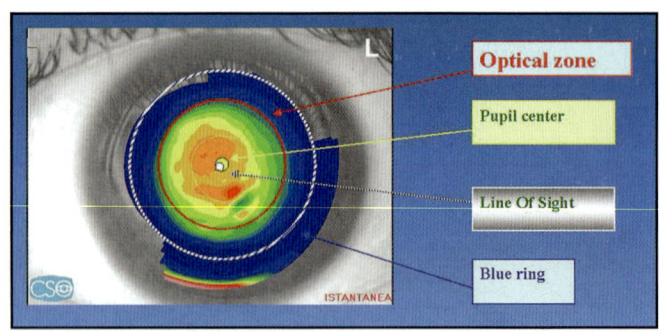

Figure 28-2. Tangential map of well-centered hyperopic ablation.

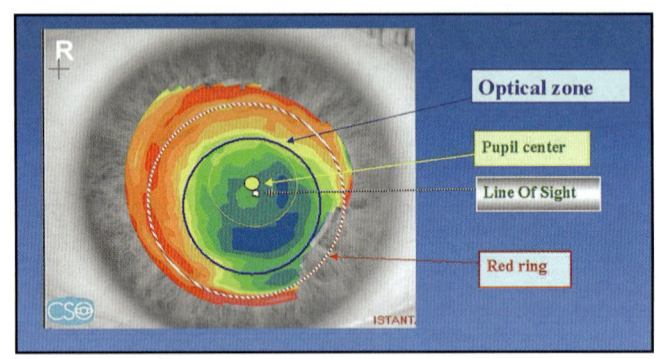

Figure 28-3. Decentered myopic treatment.

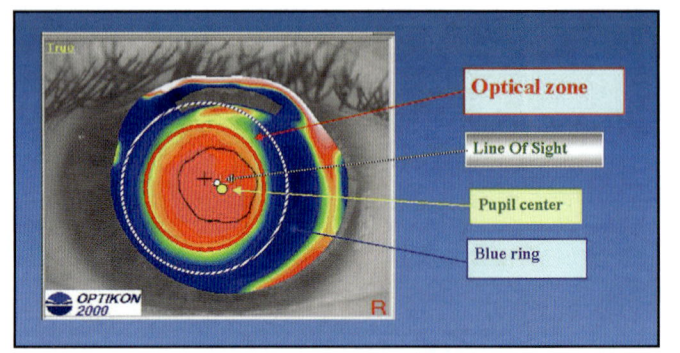

Figure 28-4. Decentered hyperopic treatment.

In effect, in this type of map, decentration appears as coma. On the other hand, coma can also be generated by ectasia, focal scarring, or internal coma (due to the natural lens, the retina, high-order astigmatism, etc). When decentration is suspected, an elevation map can be useful to identify ectasias or central islands. Comparing these data with a pachymetry map, it will be possible to distinguish an ectasia from a central island because in ectasia, the area with the highest degree of curvature is also the thinnest, while in a central island, it is the thickest. Conversely, the actual determination of centration as a geometric effect of ablation is seen in a tangential map. The most reliable and repeatable method to evaluate the real ablation profile is to determine the position of the ablation edge through topography. The ablation edge is the least affected by the repair processes because of the smaller amount of tissue removed (and, therefore, lower repair response) and is the site with the highest curvature variation. In a tangential map, the ablation edge is shown in warm colors (red-yellow) for myopic treatments (Figure 28-1) and in cold colors (blue-green-purple) in hyperopic treatments (Figure 28-2). The position of this red-blue ring (R-BR) can be related to the pupil center or, even better, to the line of sight (LOS).

The tangential map correctly highlights the edge and the ablation area, the curvature change between the treated and the untreated area with a R-BR that outlines exactly the edge of the ablation area and its centration on the pupil or the LOS. Characteristics of the ablation edge to be measured are the width, centration and diopter gradient relative to the pupil center or LOS, and distance from the pupil edge. Thus, a treatment is well centered when both the topography-generated R-BR and the ablated area are centered on the pupil, or the LOS (see Figures 28-1 and 28-2). On the basis of the above, a diagnosis of decentration is unequivocal when both the R-BR and the ablated area are decentered relative to the pupil center or the LOS (Figures 28-3 and 28-4).

This paradigm is essential because the cases most frequently reported as decentrations are, in fact, wrongly diagnosed as such. When the tangential map shows a decentered OZ, but an R-BR that is centered relative to the pupil center or LOS, the diagnosis should be one of pseudodecentration rather than decentration. We will, therefore, have pseudodecentration in the presence of uneven distribution of the corneal dioptric gradient (nasal pupil, astigmatism correction in one meridian, central island), focal scarring, or high corneal dioptric gradient.

Therefore, a paracentral island in the axial map may simulate a decentered treatment (Figure 28-5). Small repair process alterations with OZ haze may change the central corneal power, simulating a decentration in the axial map (Figure 28-6). This also occurs in high corneal diopter gradient in high myopic treatment (Figure 28-7). However, if these cases are analyzed through the tangential map and the ablation area and R-RB are correlated to the pupil center and LOS, the final diagnosis should be one of pseudodecentration (see Figures 28-5, 28-6, and 28-7).

Therefore, for a postrefractive surgery diagnosis of decentration or pseudodecentration to be correct, it is necessary to examine on the tangential map the correlation between the ablation area and R-BR relative to the pupil center or LOS, as shown in Figure 28-8. On the basis of the above, we collaborated with CSO (Florence, Italy) to develop a software

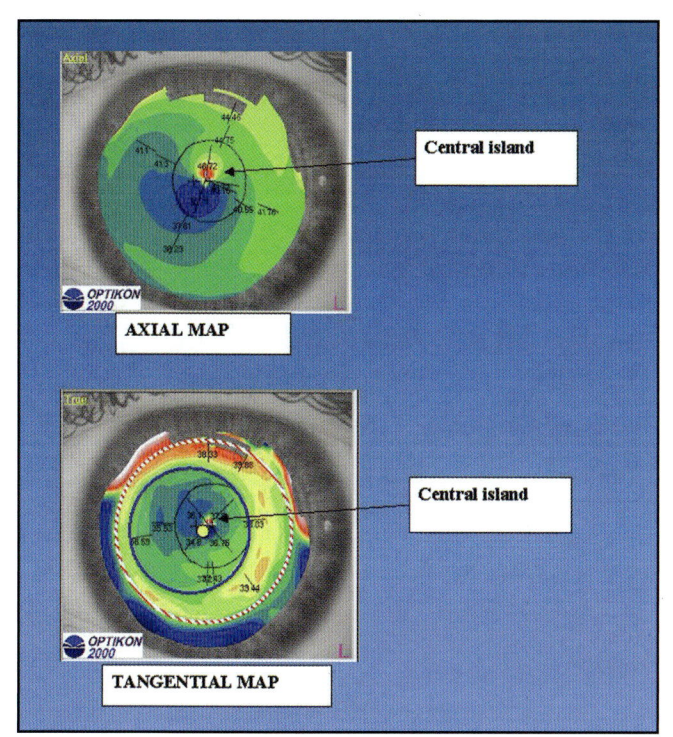

Figure 28-5. Pseudodecentered treatment due to a central Island (optical zone decentered; red ring centered relative to a pupil center).

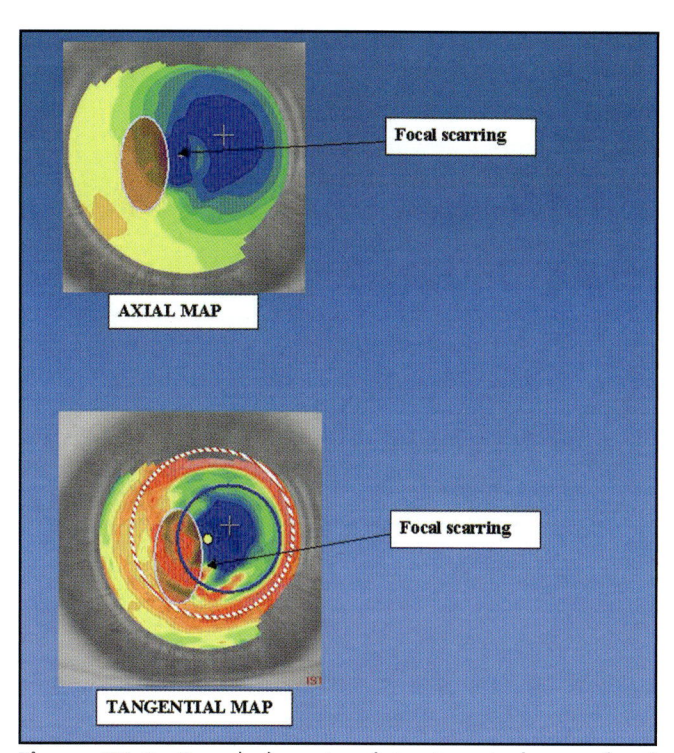

Figure 28-6. Pseudodecentered treatment due to focal scarring (optical zone decentered; red ring centered relative to a pupil center).

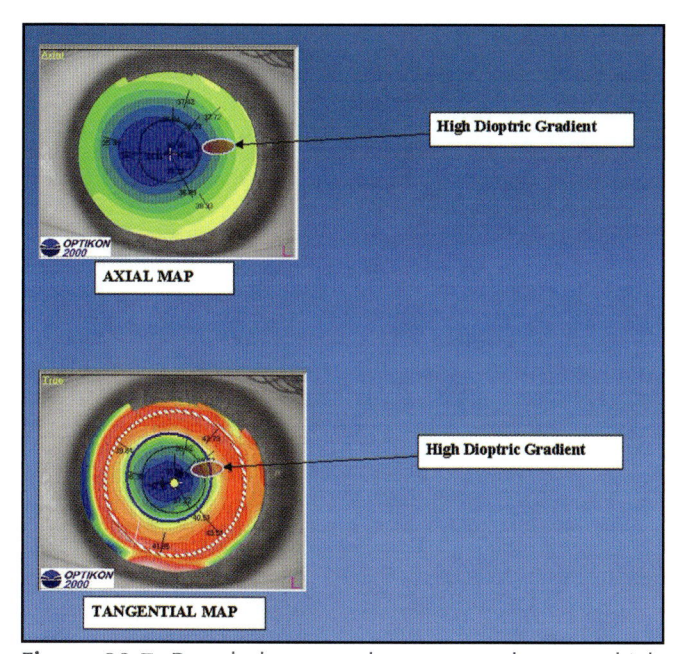

Figure 28-7. Pseudodecentered treatment due to a high dioptric gradient in elevated myopic treatment (optical zone decentered; red ring centered relative to a pupil center).

Treatment PRK/LASIK	Decentered	Pseudo-decentered
Optical zone	Decentered	Decentered
RedBlue-Ring	Decentered	Centered

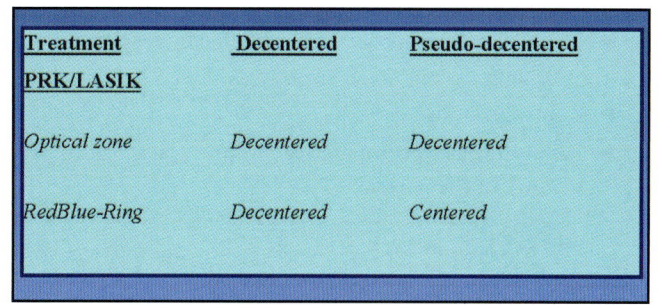

Figure 28-8. Decentered vs pseudodecentered treatment relative to pupil center or LOS.

Causes of Decentration

Several causes may lead to pseudodecentration:

INTRAOPERATIVE CAUSES

* Incomplete epithelial removes (PRK)
* Focal moisture causing laser masking (PRK/LASIK)
* Bad microkeratome cut (LASIK)
* Decentered cut (LASIK)
* Malpositioned flap protection, with projection of fluid toward the corneal center (the effects are more serious in hyperopic treatments because it falls exactly onto the ablation area) (LASIK)
* Ocular tilting (PRK/LASIK)

application of the analysis and measurement of ablation area centration (Figures 28-9 and 28-10). Using this software, it is possible to measure in millimeters the exact x- and y-axis distance of the ablation area decentration relative to the pupil and the corneal top, as well as the size of the OZ.

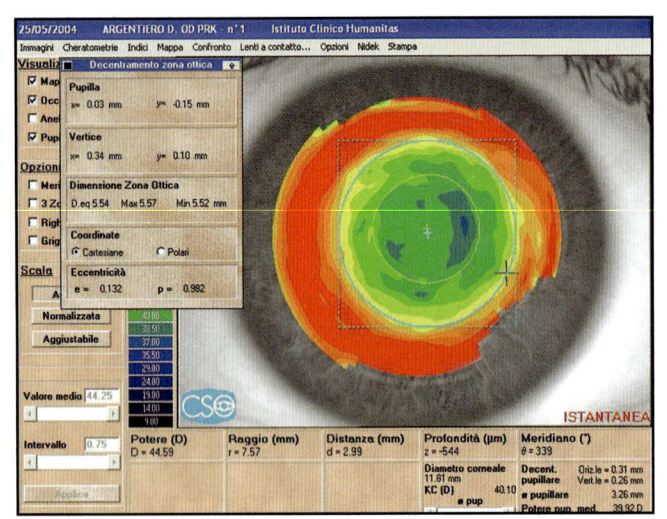

Figure 28-9. Decentration software analysis of well-centered treatment.

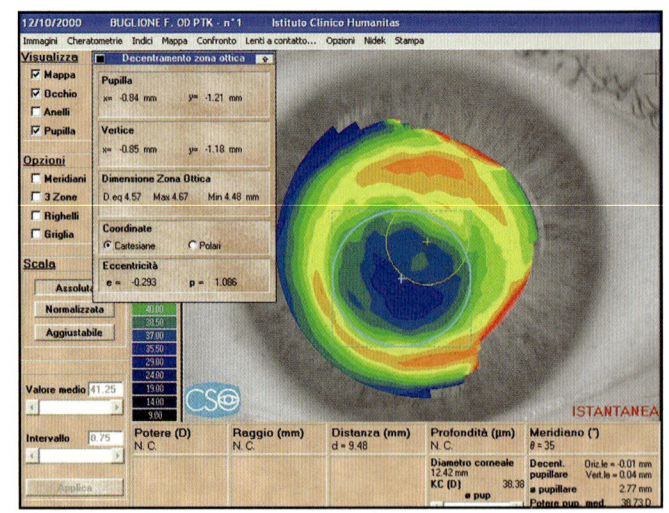

Figure 28-10. Decentration software analysis of myopic decentered treatment.

* Mistracking due to progressive stroma opacization during the ablation, resulting in loss of tracker (PRK/LASIK)
* Flap striae or malpositioning (LASIK)

Postoperative Causes

* Abnormal repair processes (epithelial hyperplasia, focal scarring)
* Central islands
* Late ectasias (postoperative failure starts more frequently in the periphery)

Conclusions

Only an accurate topographic analysis can prevent incorrect decentration diagnoses, which often mislead surgeons into performing a second procedure with the risk of making the initial situation worse. In fact, out of 148 cases referred to our center with decentration diagnoses, only 5 (3.4%) were actually decentered treatments; 28 were irregular ablation areas, 107 had a high diopter gradient, and 8 were central islands. An analysis of the cases referred to us showed that only a small number of treatments are actually decentered, while the other cases can often be improved with a surface PTK to eliminate the scar.

References

1. Schwartz-Goldstein BH, Hersh PS. Corneal topography of phase III excimer laser photorefractive Keratectomy. Optical zone centration analysis. Summit Photorefractive Keratectomy Topography Study Group. *Ophthalmology*. 1995;102:951-962.
2. Kim WJ, Chung ES, Lee JH. Effect of optic zone size on the outcome of photorefractive keratectomy for myopia. *J Cataract Refract Surg*. 1996;22;1434-1438.
3. Hersh ps, Shah SI, Geiger D, Holladay JT, Corneal Optical irregularity after excimer laser photorefractive keratectomy. Summit Photorefractive Keratectomy Topography Study Group. *J Cataract Refract Surg*. 1996;22:197-204.
4. Mc Donald MB, Carr JD, Frantz JM, et al. Laser in situ keratomileusis for myopia up to -11 diopters with up to -5 diopters of astigmatism with the Summit autonomous LADAR Vision excimer laser system. *Ophthalmology*. 2001;108:1695-1703.
5. Tsai YY, Tseng SH, Lin JM. Comparison of ablation centration in initial and retreatment active eye-tracker-assisted laser in situ keratomileusis and the effect on visual outcome. *J Cataract Refract Surg*. 2004;30(7):1521-1525.
6. Giaconi JA, Manche EE. Ablation centration in laser in situ keratomileusis for hyperopia: comparison of VISX S3 ActiveTrak and VISX S2. *J Refract Surg*. 2003;19(6):629-635.
7. Pineros OE. Tracker-assisted versus manual ablation zone centration in laser in situ keratomileusis for myopia and astigmatism. *J Refract Surg*. 2002;18(1):37-42.
8. Tsay YY, Lin JM. Ablation centration after active eye-tracker-assisted photorefractive keratectomy and laser in situ keratomileusis. *J Cataract Refract Surg*. 2000;26(1):28-34.

CHAPTER 29

THE USE OF MITOMYCIN C IN SURFACE ABLATION

Francesco Carones, MD

In Europe, unlike the United States, excimer laser photorefractive keratectomy (PRK) has been the predominant refractive surgical procedure for years. Subepithelial fibrosis with wound healing is a major complication of PRK. Its clinical appearance at slit-lamp examination consists of opacity that is variable in density and commonly referred to as haze. Haze can be very mild, not inducing any visual impairment, and usually tends to regress spontaneously with time. In the majority of cases, haze is simply reported by the ophthalmologist during postoperative examinations, while the patient does not convey any visual problems.

Haze formation represents the abnormal wound healing response to ultraviolet (UV) corneal tissue ablation and is characterized by stromal reaction, keratocyte activation, collagen, and amorphous material deposition. Certain circumstances tend to amplify both haze density and chance of appearance. Among them, the amount of intended correction is probably the most important: the higher the correction, the worse the haze.[1-4] But other factors like UV exposure, delayed reepithelialization, and irregular surface ablation are also implicated in haze formation. Dense haze may significantly reduce best spectacle-corrected visual acuity (BSCVA), induce regression; induce irregular astigmatism; and provoke visual symptoms such as blurred vision, haloes, glare, and ghost images.

Treatment of severe haze involves the use of topical pharmaceuticals. Corticosteroids produced some controversial results and are frequently ineffective.[1,2] The second category of drugs employed is antimetabolites, of which mitomycin C (MMC), 5 fluorouracil, and thio-pepa[1] are those experimented with the most. Haze can be removed by a second laser ablation in a therapeutic fashion, but this approach is also often ineffective because laser ablation generated the haze in the first place.

MMC is a systemic chemotherapeutic agent. It is commonly used topically after glaucoma surgery, after pterygium excision, in the treatment of conjunctival and corneal intraepithelial neoplasia, and in the treatment of ocular pemphigoid. It is used because of its long-term, possibly permanent, cytostatic effect on tissue. More specifically, its use after PRK is intended to inhibit subepithelial fibrosis as the result of an abnormal activation or proliferation of stromal keratocytes following laser ablation.[2] This use was originally proposed by Talamo and associates on an experimental model.[2] Haze reduction following MMC administration was also documented by Xu and associates in rabbit eyes.[2] Recently, Majmudar and coworkers reported a successful series of eyes treated using a 0.02% (0.2 mg/ml) MMC solution, to remove haze after PRK and radial keratotomy.[2]

The peculiar action of MMC on the corneal tissue allows two possible applications in the field of laser surface ablation. It can be used therapeutically in those eyes already exposed to surface ablation that present significant haze, or it can be used in a prophylactic fashion to avoid haze formation in those treatments at risk.

Mitomycin C for the Treatment of Haze

The rationale to this therapy is the removal of haze by any method (eg, excimer laser PTK, mechanical scraping) and the application of MMC to inhibit further haze formation. Because, I had excellent results with manual scraping, my surgical approach is described in the following section.

The corneal epithelium is removed using a 20%-diluted alcohol solution, applied topically by filling the barrel of a 9.0-mm Hoffer marking trephine. The alcohol is removed by

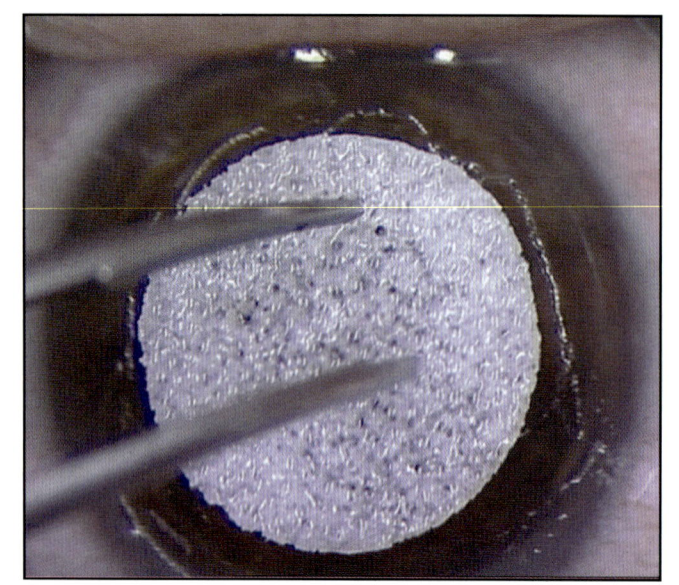

Figure 29-1. The image shows the delivery system, a circular sponge soaked with MMC.

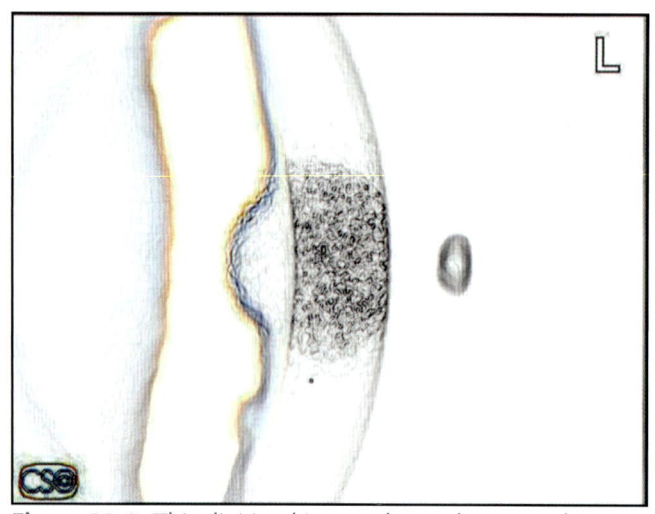

Figure 29-3. This digitized image shows the stromal irregularity resulting from haze in the left eye.

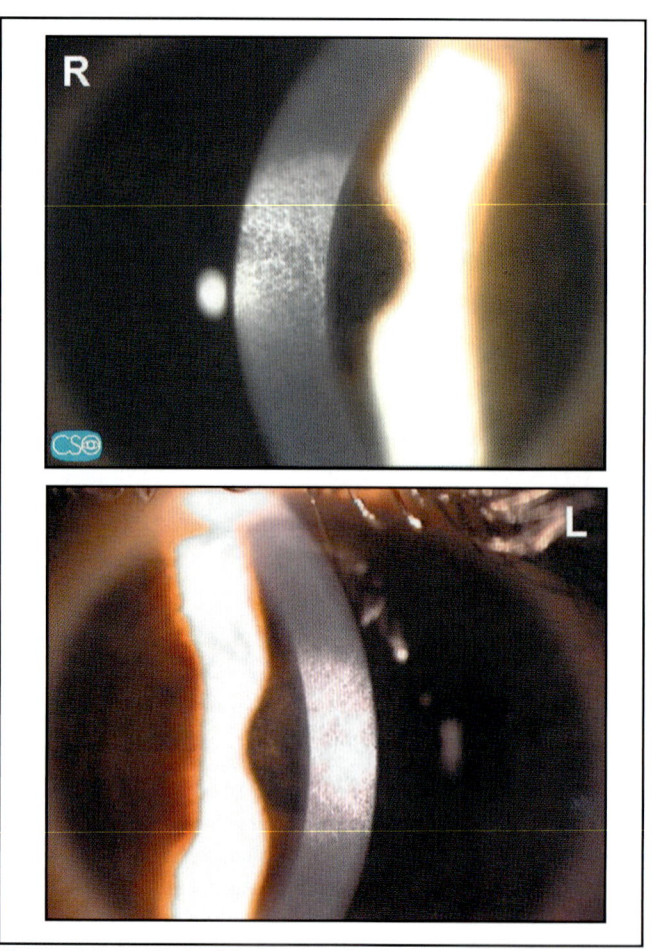

Figure 29-2. Clinical images of both corneas of the patient described in the text, before the treatment. Note the density of the haze.

Merocel microsponges, and the epithelium is gently removed with Merocel (Medtronic, Jacksonville, Fla) surgical microsponges. Once the epithelium is removed, using a Desmarres sharp blade, I scrape the stromal surface quite vigorously in an attempt to remove as much newly-generated tissue as possible. This process is complete when no material is visible on the sharp edge of the blade. At this point, the stromal surface should look much more transparent than before scraping (slit-lamp examination is mandatory at this aim) and much more regular and smooth. Immediately after scraping, a circular Merocel microsponge soaked with a 0.02% (0.2 mg/ml) MMC solution is placed on top of the stromal surface (Figure 29-1). This must be left in place for 2 minutes. The surface is then irrigated copiously with 20 cc balanced salt solution (BSS) to remove all MMC particles and remnants.

Obviously, the scar can also be removed using the excimer laser in a therapeutic fashion, where the choice is upon the surgeon's personal experience. In this case, the surgeon may consider programming either a plano correction or a refractive procedure, depending on the refraction. It is important to notice that with all approaches, there will be some unpredictable refractive change due to the removal of fibrotic tissue, thus, the programmed refractive change should be conservative.

Postoperatively, a bandage contact lens is applied to both eyes and left in place until reepithelialization is complete (usually 4 days). During this period, antibiotic drops and nonsteroidal anti-inflammatory drops are applied 4 times per day, together with artificial tears. The patient is also prescribed oral narcotics as needed for pain. Once the bandage contact lens is removed, topical fluorometholone drops are applied 3 times per day for 2 weeks and then for twice a day for 2 weeks. Artificial tears are administered as needed thereafter.

The results of this therapy are very positive. My personal series involves more than 80 treated eyes with a follow-up exceeding 7 years, and the results are overlapping to those we published previously.[2]

Figures 29-2 to 29-5 show a case story of both eyes of the same patient who underwent PRK for -12.0 D correction in

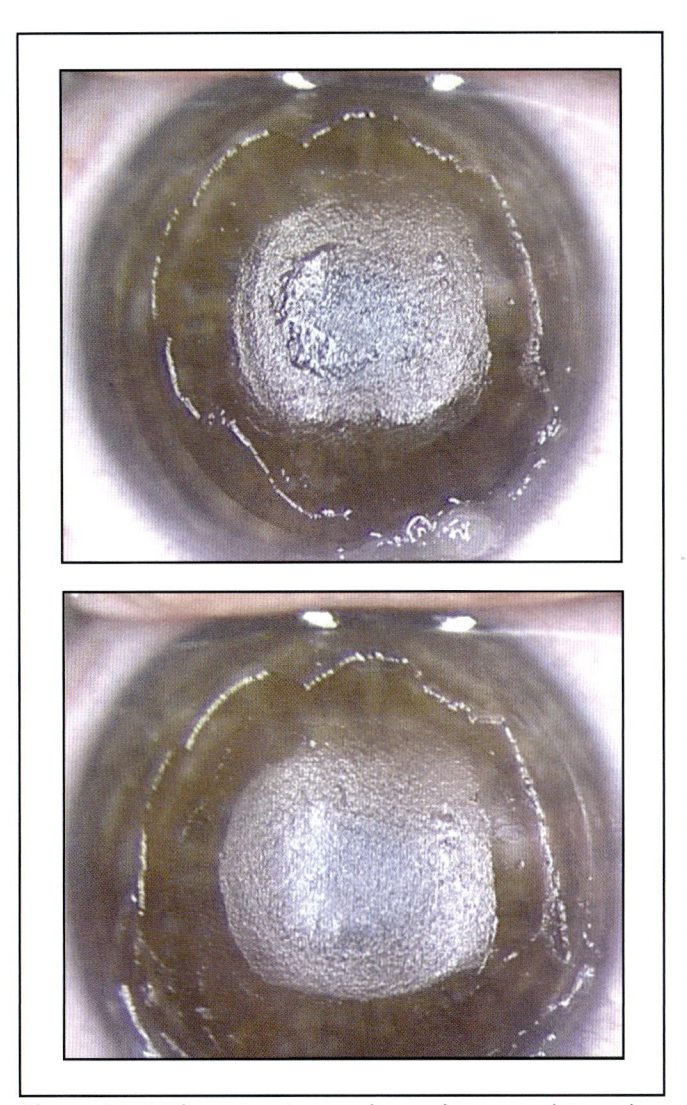

Figure 29-4. The upper image shows the stromal irregularity due to the scarring process, before scraping. The lower image shows the gained regularity after scraping.

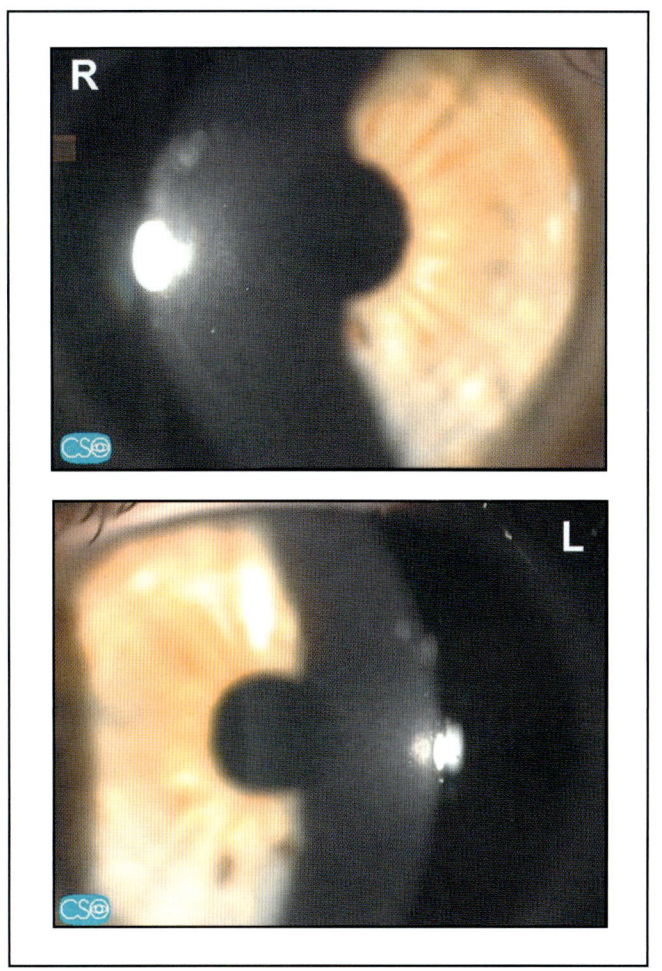

Figure 29-5. Clinical images of the cornea of both eyes of the patient described in the text, 7 years after treatment. There is no haze trace.

the year 1996 and had this therapy 2 years later (1998). The patient was on a lamellar keratoplasty waiting list at another center. In both eyes, the opacity was so dense that it obscured iris details visualization at slit-lamp examination, and the irregularity generated by the scarring was so severe that it determined a very high irregular astigmatism at corneal topography. In both eyes, best spectacle-corrected visual acuity was 20/40 (preoperative BCVA was referred to be 20/16) with -4.75 D in the right eye and -4.5 D in the left eye, while uncorrected visual acuity was 20/800 in both eyes. Haze was reported to appear 1 year after surgery, immediately following a long vacation that the patient took during the summer, in a country with high UV exposure. Uncorrected and best spectacle-corrected visual acuities before haze onset were reported to be 20/16 in both eyes with plano refraction. Immediately after the appearance of haze, both eyes were treated for 6 months with a high-dosage topical corticosteroid eyedrops therapy (dexametazone 4id) that was ineffective in reducing haze and reversing myopic regression. One month after treatment, both corneas were completely transparent with no haze at all. In both eyes, uncorrected and best spectacle-corrected visual acuities were 20/20 with +0.25 D refraction. Corneal topography revealed a quite regular surface with no irregular astigmatism. These findings did not change over a 7-year follow-up period (see Figure 29-5). Corneal transparency was maintained and haze did not recur; uncorrected and best spectacle-corrected visual acuities as well as refraction remained stable. No long-term toxic effects, such as corneal melting and endothelial changes, were noticed.

This case presentation exemplifies the average results achievable with MMC used to avoid further haze formation once the scar is removed.[2-4] Corneal transparency, once restituted, is maintained over time in the vast majority of the cases. Regression of the induced correction is a common finding when haze occurs. The graph presented in Figure 29-6 shows the change in refraction toward the original achieved correction that commonly follows the therapy, thus suggesting that one be very conservative when programming the laser to correct any residual refractive error at the time of haze removal. Figure 29-7 presents the change in best spectacle-corrected visual acuity before and after the treatment,

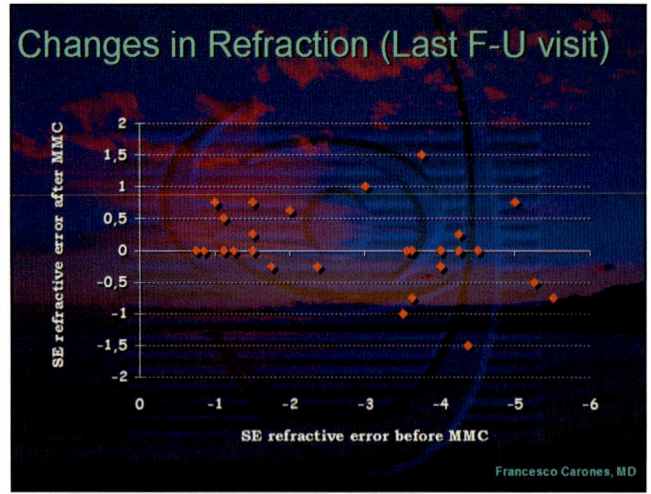

Figure 29-6. This graph shows changes in refraction after scraping and MMC application, with a significant recovery in the myopic shift associated with haze formation.

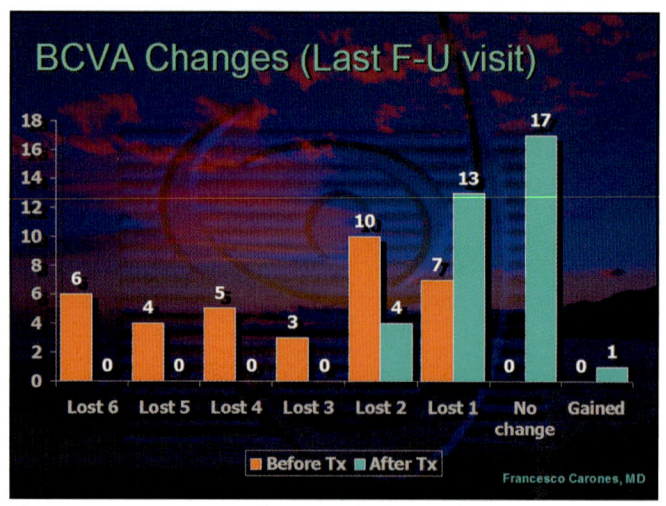

Figure 29-7. BCVA changes before after scraping and MMC administration, with reference to baseline (pre-PRK) values. Note the significant gain after treatment.

compared to the preoperative (pre-PRK) status. The gain is significant in most of the cases and may mean avoiding more invasive procedures like penetrating keratoplasty. Recurrence of haze is quite rare and in all cases milder than the original onset. Literature suggests a recurrence of haze in around 5% to 10% of cases; in these cases, a second approach may be advisable. Also, this therapeutic approach is more likely to be successful when applied to recent scars; recent-onset haze is more easily removed and recurrence is even less frequent.

MMC has some potential side effects and complications, as discussed in the following section. There is the question as to what stage this therapy should be considered or, in other words, when the surgeon has to take the risk of potential (very rare) side effects and complications and proceed with the treatment, as opposed to waiting for natural haze disappearance using conventional (steroid) therapy. My indication to MMC therapy is for eyes in which haze compromises best spectacle-corrected visual acuity and/or induces severe quality of vision disturbances and previous steroids therapy was unsuccessful. In these cases, I like to proceed to scraping and MMC application, if the patient agrees.

Mitomycin C for Prophylactic Use to Avoid Haze Formation

In all cases of surface ablation at risk of haze formation, MMC may be applied prophylactically to avoid complications. Indications include high volumes of ablated tissue (high attempted corrections, generically speaking) and surface ablation enhancements: ablation on the top of a previous LASIK flap, either for enhancement purposes or to manage a flap complication[2-4] (aborted, buttonhole, irregular), ablation over previous refractive (radial keratotomy) or therapeutic corneal surgery (penetrating keratoplasty), and keloid formers.

MMC is delivered in the same manner as for therapeutic purposes; after the ablation, a 0.2 mg/ml (0.02%) soaked microsponge is positioned over the corneal stroma. The original protocol consisted of a 2-minute application time. Today, in order to reduce the risk of potential side effects and complications, several investigators propose shorter application times according to individual nomograms that are based upon attempted correction and ablation depth (1 minute, 30 seconds, 12 seconds). The reported results are as good as longer application times. Once the microsponge is removed, it is suggested that the doctor thoroughly wash the corneal surface and the entire conjunctival sac in order to remove all MMC remnants. Postoperative care should be carried out in the same way as for conventional surface ablation; there are no contraindications to the use of a bandage contact lens or to the replacement of the epithelial layer in a LASEK or epi-LASIK fashion. Steroids and lubricants should be administered according to individual protocols and experience.

Results are astonishing,[2-5] as MMC does not interfere with reepithelialization or early wound healing period. Haze rates are extremely low, whenever present, also for high corrections and ablation depths. Particularly, all complicated cases, such as complicated LASIK flaps, RK, and PKP treatments, do behave as virgin eyes. The accuracy of the procedure is reported as much higher than for surface ablation without the use of MMC, with lower standard deviations. All the published series report a marked trend to overcorrection (in the range 10% to 15%, according to the laser used and individual nomograms), thus suggesting a programmed undercorrection when using MMC.

The potential use of MMC appears of particular interest for those eyes with limited stromal thickness, in which LASIK is contraindicated. These eyes may benefit from the great accuracy of MMC prophylactic therapy and the application of wide ablation.

I believe that MMC can be used prophylactically for applications in all complicated eyes (complicated LASIK flaps, surface ablation in eyes after RK and PKP, PRK enhancements, etc). In all these cases, particular care must be used when removing the epithelium so as to not induce any keratocyte activation or tissue damage. My personal protocol involves the use of the routine concentration of MMC (0.2 mg/ml) for a 2-minute application. Virgin eyes are another matter. I use MMC for an attempted ablation depth of 80 μm or more. I always use the same concentration (0.2 mg/ml), while the application time goes for 30 seconds for ablation depth up to 100 μm, and 1 minute for higher ablation depth.

Safety Issues

The major criticism of MMC use after laser refractive surgery refers to the potential side effects and complications associated with its long-term cytostatic action on tissues when applied in a topic fashion on the corneal stroma. Several authors reported corneoscleral melt after MMC application after pterygium excision.[2-4] Also, the long-term integrity of the endothelial layer is supposed to be at risk.

It is worth mentioning that all reports citing corneoscleral melting differ in content regarding the approach used after refractive surgery. First, the concentration of MMC was reported to be higher, and for application times longer than the 2-minute maximum time, it is currently performed when MMC is applied on the corneal stroma. Second, the previous melting reports always involve the conjunctivoscleral district, which is substantially different from the cornea in tissue structure, vascularization, and origin.

So far, it is estimated that more than 100,000 procedures worldwide have been performed with the use of MMC, and there are no reports of corneal melting or endothelium toxicity over an 8-year follow-up period. However, MMC must be used with caution in order to minimize these potential risks. The concentration must be 0.2 mg/ml because higher concentrations determined the previously reported complications while lower concentrations are therapeutically not effective. The application time should never exceed 2 minutes; current studies are evaluating the efficacy at shorter application times. After MMC application, the corneal surface and the entire conjunctival sac should be washed thoroughly using BSS in order to avoid the interaction of MMC both with the epithelial stem cells and the conjunctiva. The use of MMC according to these rules has proven safe and effective.

References

1. McCarthy CA, Aldred GF, Taylor HR. Comparison of results of excimer laser correction of all degrees of myopia at 12 months postoperatively. *Am J Ophthalmol*. 1996;121:372-383.
2. Krueger RR, Talamo JH, McDonald MB, et al. Clinical analysis of excimer laser photorefractive keratectomy using a multiple zone technique for severe myopia. *Am J Ophthalmol*. 1995;119:263-274.
3. Sher NA, Hardten DR, Fundingsland B, et al. 193-nm excimer photorefractive keratectomy in high myopia. *Ophthalmology*. 1994;101:1575-1582.
4. Carson CA, Taylor HR. Excimer laser treatment for high and extreme myopia. *Arch Ophthalmol*. 1995;113:431-436.
5. Gartry D, Kerr Muir MG, Lohmann CP, Marshall J. The effect of topical corticosteroids on refractive outcome and corneal haze after photorefractive keratectomy. *Arch Ophthalmol*. 1992;110:944-952.
6. Carones F, Brancato R, Venturi E, et al. Efficacy of corticosteroids in reversing regression after myopic photorefractive keratectomy. *Refract Corneal Surg*. 1993; 9(suppl):S52-S56.
7. Penno EA, Braun DA, Kamal A, et al. Topical thiopepa treatment for recurrent corneal haze after photorefractive keratectomy. *J Cataract Refract Surg*. 2003;29:1537-1542.
8. Shipper I, Suppelt C, Gebbers JO. Mitomycin C reduces scar formation after excimer laser (193 nm) photorefractive keratectomy in rabbits. *Eye*. 1997;11:649-655.
9. Talamo JH, Gollamudi S, Green RW, et al. Modulation of corneal wound healing after excimer laser keratomileusis using topical mitomycin C and steroids. *Arch Ophthalmol*. 1991;109:1141-1146.
10. Xu H, Liu S, Xia X, et al. Mitomycin C reduces haze formation in rabbits after excimer laser photorefractive keratectomy. *J Refract Surg*. 2001;17:342-349.
11. Majmudar P, Forstrot L, Dennis R, et al. Topical mitomycin-C for subepithelial fibrosis after refractive corneal surgery. *Ophthalmology*. 2000;107:89-94.
12. Vigo L, Scandola E, Carones F. Scraping and mitomycin C to treat haze and regression after photorefractive keratectomy for myopia. *J Refract Surg*. 2003;19(4):449-454.
13. Porges Y, Ben-Haim O, Hirsh A, et al. Phototherapeutic keratectomy with mitomycin C for corneal haze following photorefractive keratectomy for myopia. *J Refract Surg*. 2003;19:40-43.
14. Winkler von Mohrenfelds C, Hermann W, Gabler B, et al. Topical mitomycin C for the prophylaxis of recurrent haze after excimer laser photorefractive keratectomy. *Klin Monatsbl Augenheilkd*. 2001;218:763-767.
15. Raviv T, Majmudar PA, Dennis RF, et al. Mitomycin-C for post-PRK corneal haze. *J Cataract Refract Surg*. 2000;26:1105-1106.
16. Weisenthal RW, Salz J, Sugar A, et al. Photorefractive keratectomy for treatment of flap complications in laser is situ keratomileusis. *Cornea*. 2003;22:399-404.
17. Lane HA, Swale JA, Majmudar PA. Prophylactic use of mitomycin-c in the management of a buttonholed LASIK flap. *J Cataract Refract Surg*. 2003;29:390-392.
18. Muller LT, Candal EM, Epstein RJ, Dennis RF, Majmudar PA. Transepithelial phototherapeutic keratectomy/photorefractive keratectomy with adjunctive mitomycin-C for complicated LASIK flaps. *J Cataract Refract Surg*. 2005;31(2):291-296.
19. Carones F, Vigo L, Scandola E, Vacchini L. Evaluation of the prophylactic use of mitomycin-C to inhibit haze formation after photorefractive keratectomy. *J Cataract Refract Surg*. 2002;28(12):2088-2095.
20. Lacayo GO, Majmudar PA. How and when to use mitomycin-C in refractive surgery. *Curr Opin Ophthalmol*. 2005;16(4):256-259.
21. Gambato C, Ghirlando A, Moretto E, Busato F, Midena E. Mitomycin C modulation of corneal wound healing after photorefractive keratectomy in highly myopic eyes. *Ophthalmology*. 2005;112(2):208-218.
22. Hashemi H, Taheri SM, Fotouhi A, Kheiltash A. Evaluation of the prophylactic use of mitomycin-C to inhibit haze formation after photorefractive keratectomy in high myopia: a prospective clinical study. *BMC Ophthalmol*. 2004;4(1):12.
23. Rubinfeld RS, Pfister RR, Stein RM, et al. Serious complications of topical mitomycin-C after pterygium surgery. *Ophthalmology*. 1992; 99:1647-1654.
24. Fujitani A, Hayasaka S, Shibuya Y, Noda S. Corneoscleral ulceration and corneal perforation after pterygium excision and topical mitomycin C therapy. *Ophthalmologica*. 1993;207:162-164.
25. Dougherty PJ, Hardten DR, Lindstrom RL. Corneoscleral melt after pterygium surgery using a single intraoperative application of mitomycin-C. *Cornea*. 1996;15:537-540.

SECTION VI

PHOTOTHERAPEUTIC KERATECTOMY: MAKING POSSIBLE THE IMPOSSIBLE

CHAPTER 30

Custom Phototherapeutic Keratectomy With Intraoperative Topography

Paolo Vinciguerra, MD; Fabrizio I. Camesasca, MD

Introduction

Phototherapeutic keratectomy (PTK) represents an interesting application of excimer laser, and it has progressively proved to be an interesting alternative to penetrating or lamellar keratoplasty.[1-8] Due to its high ablation precision, the excimer laser is now an ideal tool for focal removal of corneal irregularities.

However, until recently, PTK has remained a rather craftsman-like treatment, due to the use of normal ablations, focal ablations, and smoothing with masking fluid. The unpredictability of the procedure has always hindered its wide acceptance and common use by refractive surgeons.[9] The introduction of custom ablation initially spurred new enthusiasm for PTK performed on the basis of aberrometrical data. However, custom ablation did not confirm these expectations, since the results were not encouraging. Total aberrometric measurement, however, is performed through a limited pupillary diameter, and thus optimization of the corneal surface with this approach leaves large portions of peripheral cornea untouched, together with their irregularities, with consequent incomplete treatment and possible regression. It must also be remembered that when substantial stromal opacities are present, aberrometry becomes totally unreliable.

Most aberrometers provide information based on hundreds of points, while a topographer evaluates corneas on the basis of 20,000 points. Due to this problem and overlap of points, it is sometimes difficult to define the effective light deviation with aberrometers.

Careful consideration of the actual situation of eyes undergoing PTK sheds some light on this failure. Usually, PTK eyes have very irregular surfaces resulting from ulcers, trauma, or previous decentered treatments, and the epithelium plays a primary role in smoothing the surface. Once the epithelium is removed, the actual stromal corneal surface may be significantly different from the topographical situation observed when the epithelium was present. The same situation may be present in laser-assisted in situ keratomileusis (LASIK) in which the flap concurs with the epithelium in covering macro- and microirregularities of the stromal interface. Based on this observation, we decided to develop a system for intraoperative, topography-based aberrometry that starting from the real stromal situation, would provide the custom ablation software with a more reliable source for analysis and development of a treatment aimed at reducing irregularities on the largest possible corneal surface as well as treating residual refractive defects.

Because this approach applies photorefractive keratectomy (PRK) features and customization to the classical PTK technique, we suggested custom phototherapeutic keratectomy (CPK) as a new name for this technique.

Custom Phototherapeutic Keratectomy Technique and Clinical Results

In a recent study, we evaluated eyes expected to undergo CPK.[10] All patients signed an informed consent and received information about the only possible alternative, which was penetrating or lamellar keratoplasty in all cases.

Table 30-1 lists possible indications for CPK. The usual selection criteria are listed in Table 30-2. Preoperatively, all patients must undergo a full ophthalmologic examination, with determination of refractive defects under cycloplegia, pupillometry, endothelial cell counts, corneal topography using either a Keratron Scout (Optikon 2000, Rome, Italy) or a CSO (Florence, Italy) topographer.

Table 30-1. POSSIBLE INDICATIONS FOR PHOTOTHERAPEUTIC KERATECTOMY

Ocular Disease

1. Superficial stromal dystrophies and degenerations
2. Recurrent erosions
3. Corneal leucomas following trauma, surgery, or infection
4. Corneal neovascularization

Following Refractive Surgery

1. PRK
   - Corneal irregularities and/or opacities after photorefractive ablation
   - Central islands
   - Small optical zones
   - Decentered treatments
2. LASIK
   - Decentered treatments
   - Corneal irregularities and/or opacities after photorefractive ablation
   - Interface opacities
   - Small optical zones
   - Compensation of corneal irregularities caused by loss of stromal tissue
   - Preparation of a regular corneal stromal bed for a future lamellar graft, when the residual stromal thickness is insufficient to provide adequate corneal resistance
   - Regularization of corneal surface after partial or total loss of flap

Table 30-2. SELECTION CRITERIA

General

1. No known systemic, metabolic, or collagen disease
2. Unrealistic expectations by the patient

Corneal

1. Insufficient corneal thickness
2. Ectasic disease (pellucid degeneration, Mooren's ulcer, Terrien's degeneration)
3. Reduced endothelial cell counts
4. Superficial flap cut
5. Active keratitis

Ocular

1. Increased intraocular pressure
2. Tear deficiency

After topical anesthesia by two applications of oxybuprocaine chlorhydrate eye drops, the patient is prepared and draped, and a lid speculum applied. The epithelium is removed manually, and after instillation of a drop of masking fluid (hyaluronic acid 0.4% [Laservis, Chemedica, Munchen, Germany]), immediate intraoperative topography is performed using either a Keratron Scout or a CSO topographer. Topography-based corneal aberrometry can then be calculated.

We perform CPK with the NIDEK EC 5000 excimer laser (NIDEK, Gamagori, Japan), based on analysis by the surgeon of corneal aberrometric data with the Final Fit ablation software, featuring the Custom Ablation Transition Zone (CATZ) software (NIDEK). Ablation includes an aspherical component for treatment of spherical defects (radially symmetric aberrations), a toric component for treatment of astigmatism (linearly symmetric aberrations), and a flying spot component for treatment of high-order aberrations (irregular components) (see Figure 18-1). The transition zone features a diameter of 10 mm.

After the ablation, smoothing is performed to remove corneal microirregularities of a size lower than the spot size (0.89 mm) and the ablation height (0.25 µm) and to achieve a regular stromal bed, as similar as possible to the physiological Bowman's layer. Smoothing is performed by applying a hyaluronic acid masking fluid (Laservis), continuously distributed over the corneal surface with a special spatula (Buratto's spatula [ASICO, Westmont, Ill]). The smoothing diameter measures 10 mm, thus involving the entire corneal diameter and preventing a hyperopic shift. To avoid overheating the tissue, the frequency has to be set at 10 Hz and the ablation at 30 µm. During the smoothing phase, masking fluid is continuously added and evenly distributed with the spatula in order to keep a thin layer of fluid and avoid the formation of dry areas. Due to the protective action of the masking fluid, the actual ablation is only 8 µm.[11,12]

Intraoperative topography can then be repeated and topography-based corneal aberrometric data again transferred to the Final Fit ablation software, processed by the surgeon, and applied for ablation. Smoothing always follows

Table 30-3. CAUSES OF CORNEAL OPACITIES AND/OR IRREGULARITIES IN 35 HIGHLY ABERRATED EYES REQUIRING PHOTOTHERAPEUTIC KERATECTOMY

Cause	Number of Eyes
Opacity and/or irregularity following myopic PRK	12
Opacity and/or irregularity following hyperopic PRK	6
Decentered PRK	2
Opacity and/or irregularity following LASIK	1
Opacity and/or irregularity following PK	2
Opacity and/or irregularity following herpetic keratitis or corneal ulcers	4
Post-traumatic scar	2
Recurring corneal erosions	1
Stromal dystrophy (Groenouw's, Reis-Bückler's)	4
Band keratophaty	1

Table 30-4. DEMOGRAPHICAL DATA OF THE STUDY EYES

Eyes	52
Patients	50
Sex	42.0% women (n=21), 58.0% men (n=29)
Mean age	44 years
Age range	25 to 87 years

an ablation. This cycle is repeated until the surgeon obtains the planned morphological or refractive target, unless the corneal thickness safety limit of 250 µm is reached. Finally, a protective contact lens is placed in position.

Postoperatively, the patient must be monitored daily until complete corneal reepithelialization and then undergo a full ophthalmologic examination with corneal topography at days 30, 90, and 180.

We reported on 52 eyes in 50 patients.[10] Table 30-3 lists the causes of corneal opacities and/or irregularities in the study eyes. Table 30-4 gives demographic and refractive data. Pre- and postoperative refraction at follow-up intervals is shown in Table 30-5. Corneal haze was graded according to Epstein, and mean preoperative haze was 1.7 ± 1.4 in eyes with previous refractive surgery.[13] Mean preoperative pachymetry, as measured by Orbscan (Bausch & Lomb) was 399.5 ± 127.1 µm. Stability, indicating the change achieved in refraction over time, is presented in Figure 30-1. Figure 30-2 shows best spectacle-corrected visual acuity (BSCVA) at the different time intervals.

Mean preoperative SE refraction was -1.13 ± 3.33 D ranging from -9.25 D to +10.0 D. No eye reached 20/15 BSCVA, and only 59% could see 20/30 BSCVA. At final examination, at 12 months, mean SE refraction was -0.38 ± 4.11 D, ranging from -11.0 D to +6.0 D. Eighty-eight percent of eyes reached 20/30 or better BSCVA, and 25% had 20/15 or better BSCVA. Safety of the procedure, showing lines of visual acuity gained, unchanged, or lost, is presented in Figure 30-3. Figure 30-4 shows the corneal topography of an eye with post-PRK narrow optical zone before (left) and after (right) epithelium removal. The differential map is shown below. Figures 30-5 through 30-17 show several other clinical cases.

Custom Phototherapeutic Keratectomy: Indications and Strategy

The aim of CPK is to re-establish corneal surface transparency and curvature regularity, therefore avoiding more invasive and complicated surgery, such as penetrating keratoplasty (PK). Application of this technique requires adequate residual corneal thickness, appropriate excimer laser ablation diameter, and proper equipment for intraoperative control.

A cornerstone of CPK is the concept that corneal regularity is more important than its transparency. Often, when choosing cases with the above-mentioned indications, the opposite happens, and more importance is given to minimal stromal opacities than to irregularities. The concept can be explained better with an everyday life example: a window pane is transparent, and raindrops on it are transparent too. However, a window pane covered with raindrops, even if transparent, does not permit good vision quality because of its lack of uniformity. On the contrary, sunglasses are not totally transparent, yet they permit good vision quality because of their regularity. A clinical example of this phenomenon is provided by keratoconus eyes with reduced visual acuity where the regularity of curvature is significantly altered.

It has been proven that irregularities of the ablated corneal surface play an important role in enhancing collagen deposition and therefore variation from the planned refractive result.[14,15] On the contrary, a smooth ablated surface induces a lower reparatory response, leading to less haze formation and unpredictability of refractive result.[16,17]

At present, the data source for custom ablation may be based on topography-corneal aberrometry or on aberrometric measurement of corneal and intraocular aberrations, determined through the pupil-total aberrometry.

There are several arguments in favor of topography-based CPK. Corneal aberrometry treatments enable handling not only of highly aberrated eyes, where total aberrometry is unreliable, but also of eyes with marked loss of stromal

Table 30-5. Pre- and Postoperative Refraction at the Different Follow-Up Intervals

Time	Eyes	Mean Sphere ± SD (D)	Range, Sphere (D)	Mean Cylinder ± SD (D)	Range, Cylinder (D)	Mean SE ± SD (D)	Range, SE (D)
Preoperative	52	-0.51 ± 3.43	-6.00 to +13.00	-1.24 ± 1.59	-6.75 to +1.00	-1.13 ± 3.33	-9.25 to +10.00
1 month	43	-0.10 ± 2.90	-9.50 to +6.00	-0.95 ± 1.44	-8.25 to 0.00	-0.57 ± 3.11	-12.50 to +4.00
3 months	31	+0.32 ± 3.10	-6.00 to +5.50	-0.79 ± 0.99	-3.50 to +0.00	-0.07 ± 3.02	-7.25 to +5.00
6 months	20	-0.35 ± 3.59	-8.50 to +6.00	-0.71 ± 1.25	-5.50 to +0.00	-0.71 ± 3.85	-11.25 to +5.25
12 months	16	-0.20 ± 3.72	-7.75 to +6.00	-1.16 ± 1.68	-6.25 to +0.00	-0.38 ± 4.11	-11.00 to +6.00

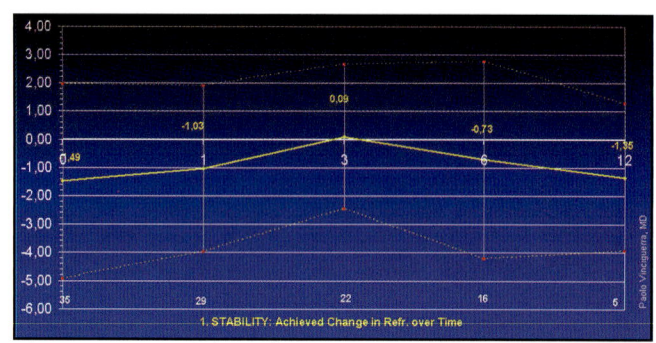

Figure 30-1. Stability of refractive defect.

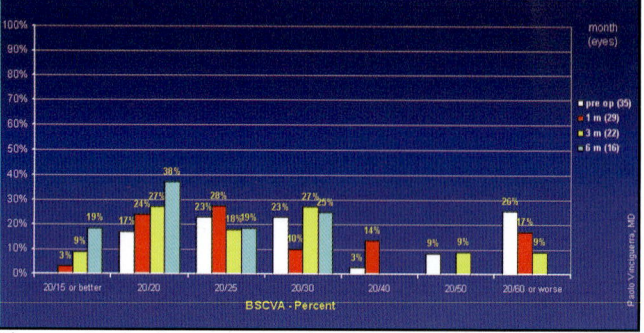

Figure 30-2. Percentage of BSCVA at the various time intervals.

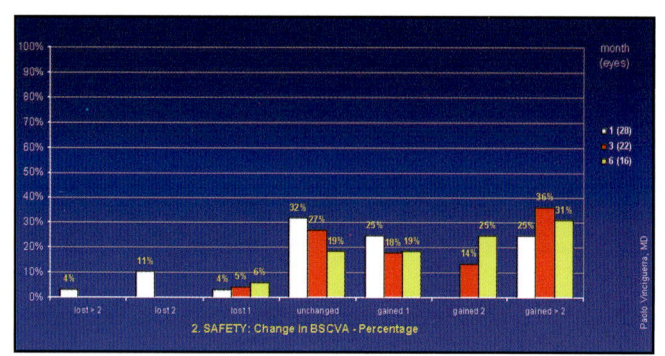

Figure 30-3. Safety of PTK. Percentage of change in BSCVA.

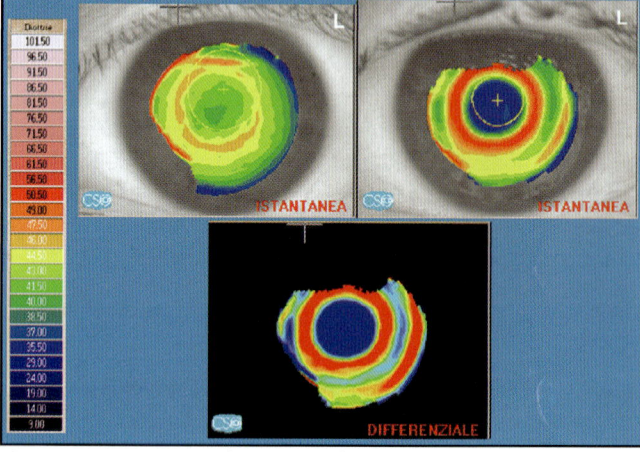

Figure 30-4. Corneal topography of an eye with post-PRK narrow optical zone before (left) and after (right) epithelium removal. Differential map is shown below.

transparency, where aberrometric determination would be almost impossible. Corneal aberrometry treatments can be performed on a corneal area wider than any total aberrometry-based one, involving up to 10 mm in diameter. Furthermore, surface analysis is based on a much larger number of points (22,000 in topography vs 90 to 1500 in aberrometry).

It is our belief that each single CPK case can be properly evaluated only after epithelium removal, establishing the number of corneal irregularities and residual corneal thickness without the corrective action of the epithelium. Corneal epithelium stratification is less pronounced on stromal "peaks," while it tends to be marked in "valleys," in order to make the corneal surface as regular as possible while masking the real amount of irregularity. Once the real stromal surface is visible, a case may appear profoundly different. If the residual stromal thickness appears limited, the surgeon must decide whether to continue the treatment, abort it, or achieve only limited regularization of the corneal surface.

When based on preoperative, epithelial surface analysis, corneal aberrometry-based CPK may lead to unreliable results because the surface on which the treatment was calculated—the epithelium—is not the one on which it will

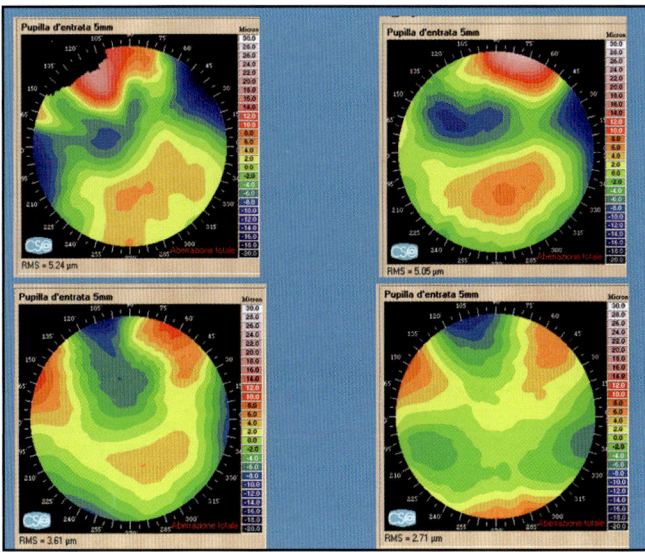

Figure 30-5. Intraoperative corneal aberrometry, with a 5-mm pupil, of a highly aberrated eye during, left to right, top to bottom, successive custom PTK phases.

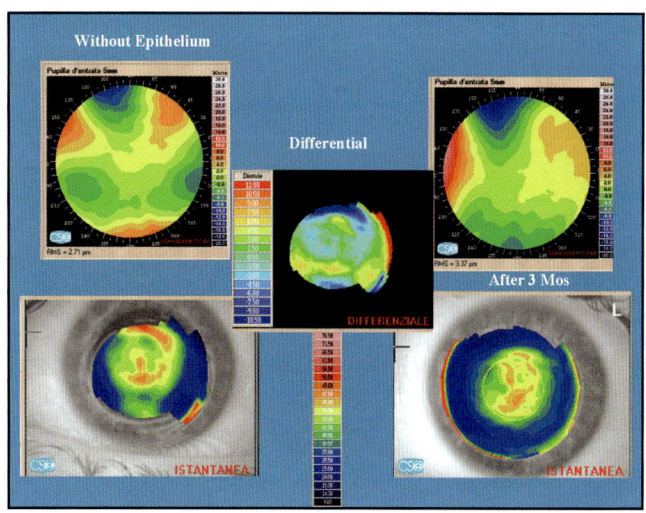

Figure 30-6. Same eye as in Figure 30-5, comparison between corneal aberrometry and topography at the end of PTK procedure, thus without epithelium, and 3 months postoperatively. Note how the situation at the end of surgery accurately reflects the future topography and aberrometry at 3 months.

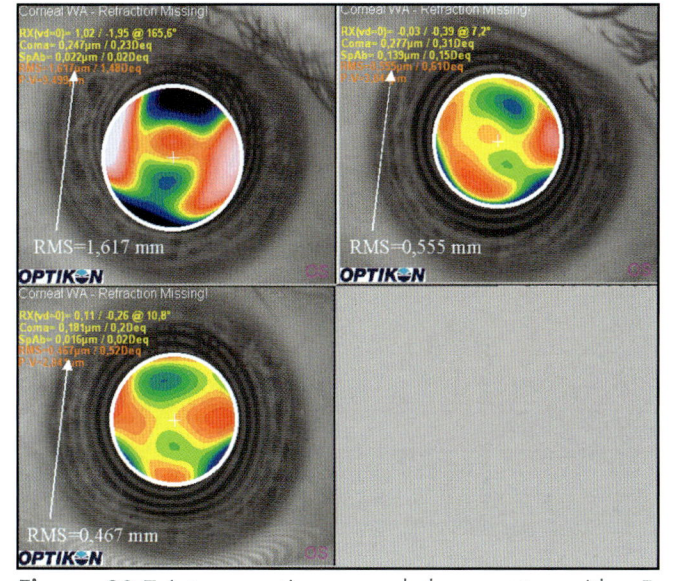

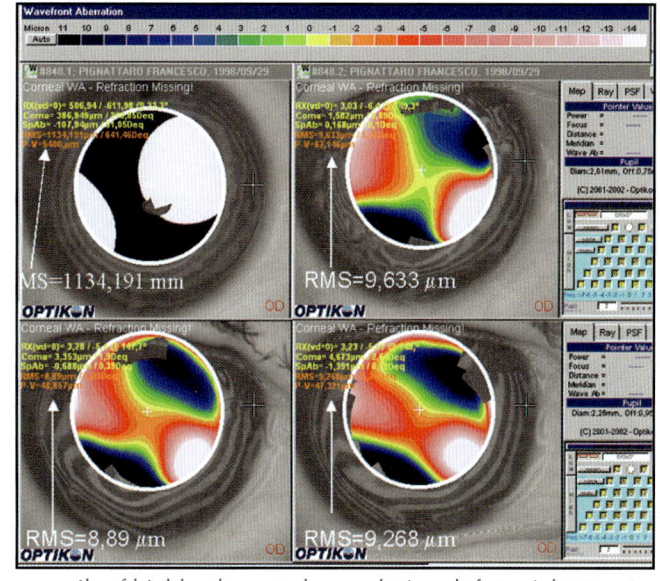

Figures 30-7. Intraoperative corneal aberrometry, with a 5-mm pupil, of highly aberrated eyes during, left to right, top to bottom, successive custom PTK phases. Note progressive decrease of aberrations as well as of total RMS.

be actually performed—the stroma. Intraoperative, epithelium-free analysis of the corneal wavefront provides more reliable information for an accurate treatment. Acquisition of intraoperative topography-based corneal aberrometry is thus a critical step because an imprecise aberrometry could provide misleading information.

A revolutionary approach to the problem of unpredictability has been introduced by Cynthia Roberts with the concept of corneal biomechanical response to laser ablation.[18] The concept is based on the anatomical lamellar structure of the corneal stroma and on its tensile strength, central severing of lamellae due to creation of a new refractive surface by excimer laser tissue removal causes elastic contraction of the remaining peripheral lamellae, with consequent corneal curvature variation. This consists of an increase in the peripheral corneal curvature and thickness and central flattening, leading to refractive change just where the curvature was carefully modified to achieve a planned power (see Chapter 6).

The introduction of custom ablation, using the approach described herein based on intraoperative topography applied to the Final Fit software, offers an important opportunity for planned treatment even in cases with very thin corneas. The Final Fit software permits deselection of the ablation components for high-order aberrations, astigmatism, and sphere. If there is enough tissue available, all the components may be treated, otherwise high-order aberrations (ie, coma) will be

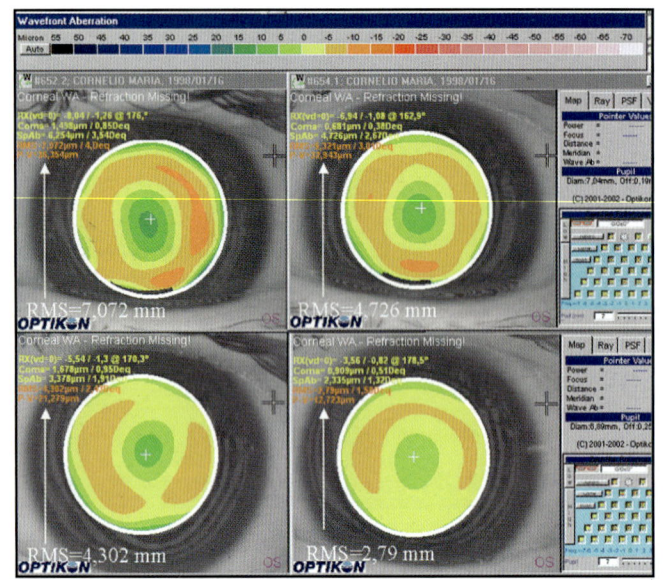

Figure 30-8. Intraoperative corneal aberrometry of an highly aberrated eye with a marked central loss of substance following a corneal ulcer during, left to right, top to bottom, successive custom PTK phases. Note progressive decrease of aberrations as well as of total RMS.

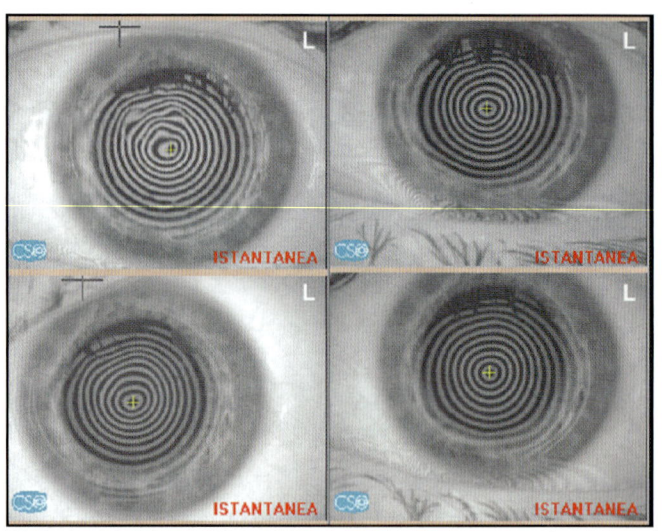

Figure 30-9. Postulcerative scar in a contact lens wearer. Keratoscopy in several consecutive intraoperative PTK phases. Keratoscopy is essential for the comprehension of the actual corneal curvature.

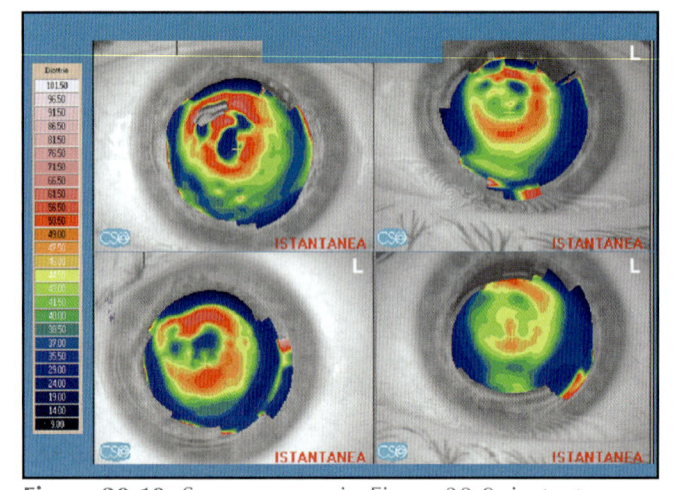

Figure 30-10. Same case as in Figure 30-9, instantaneous topography of several consecutive intraoperative PTK phases. Without keratoscopy, PTK could induce in treatment of false elevations or depressions. Final refractive results detailed in text show how wide PTK and smoothing do not induce worrisome hyperopia.

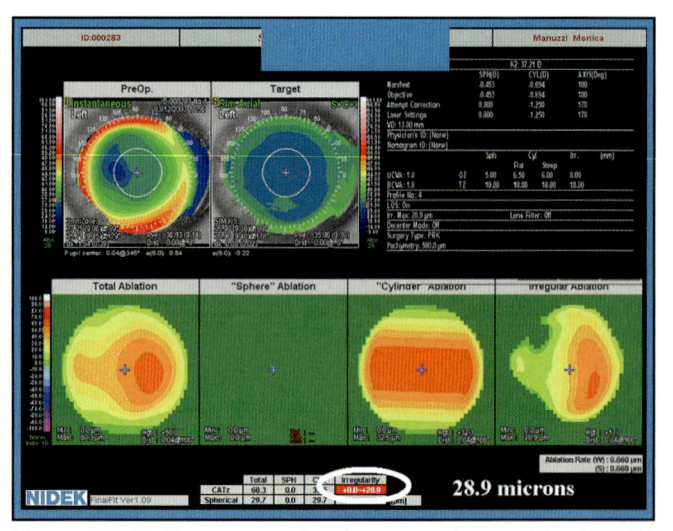

Figure 30-11. Treatment of a decentered case. The NIDEK Final Fit software shows the target map (axial, upper right), achieved through irregular ablation of 28.9 μm.

ablated first, then the astigmatic component, and, if enough tissue is left, the spherical component will be ablated too. The NIDEK Final Fit software features several alternatives for a custom treatment. Presently, two of the most interesting are those based on corneal aberrometry and the superficial wavefront.

Smoothing with masking fluid is another important step (see Chapter 8).[19,20] Lamination of the masking fluid with a special spatula is essential and can be performed with two methods. A fast, to-and-fro motion on the stromal surface permits homogeneous lamination of the masking fluid. Conversely, slow and unidirectional motion with final lifting of the spatula will induce thinning of the fluid. In the first phase of smoothing, when large irregularities may be present, lamination must be thin, to allow the irregularity "peaks" to emerge and be selectively ablated, while protecting the lower corneal areas ("valleys"). The surface will rapidly improve, as highlighted by intraoperative keratoscopy. Usually, CPK ablation does not subtract more than 50 μm of corneal stroma.

Elimination of refractive defects may also be considered during treatment of corneal opacities and/or irregularities following PRK, LASIK, or PK, when sufficient stromal thickness is available. Otherwise, the treatment must aim to resolve only irregularities that cause high-order aberrations. Often residual haze will disappear spontaneously with time. It must be remembered that ablation of stromal opacities may

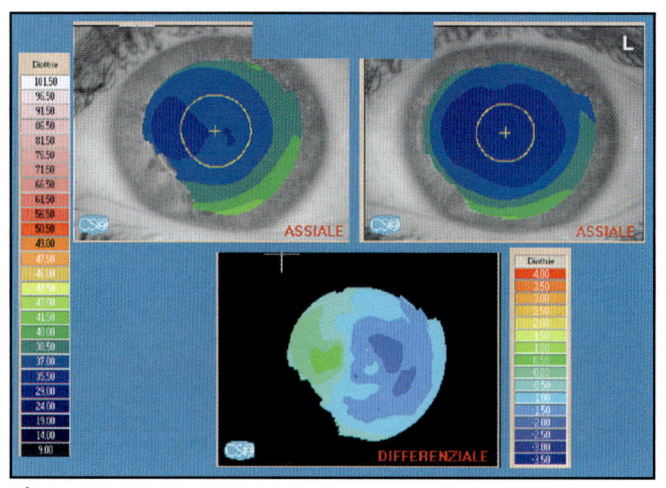

Figure 30-12. Same eye as in Figure 30-11. Postoperative axial map (upper right) shows achievement of planned result, with recentration of treatment.

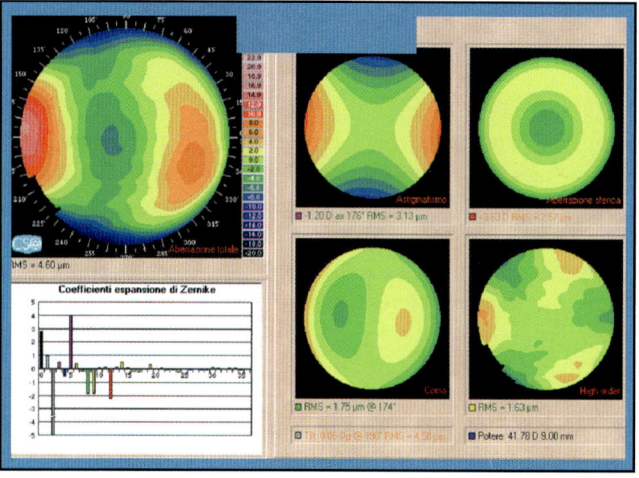

Figure 30-13. Same eye as in Figure 30-11. Preoperative aberrometric map.

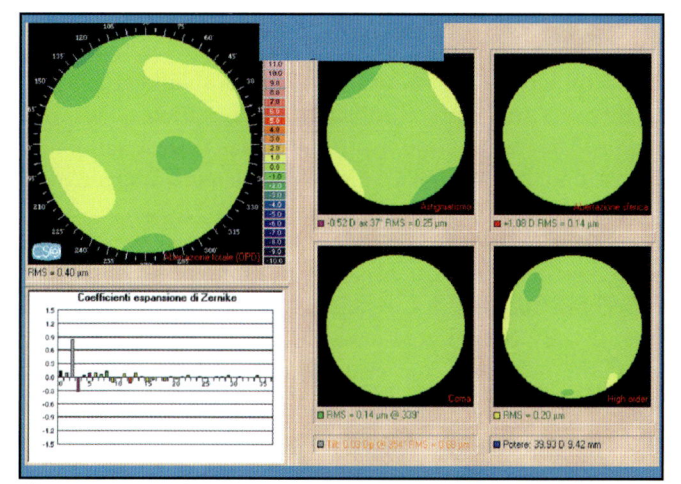

Figure 30-14. Same eye as in Figure 30-11. Postoperative aberrometric map.

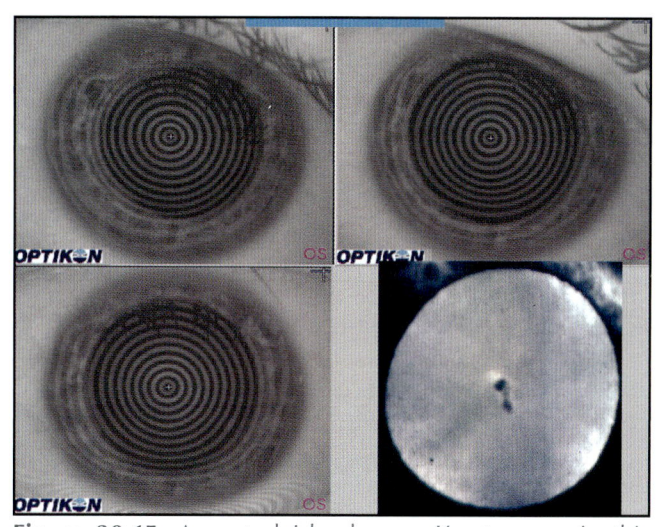

Figure 30-15. A central island case. Keratoscopy in this case looks almost normal, while the Scheimpflug image shows a diffractive change in the center of the cornea.

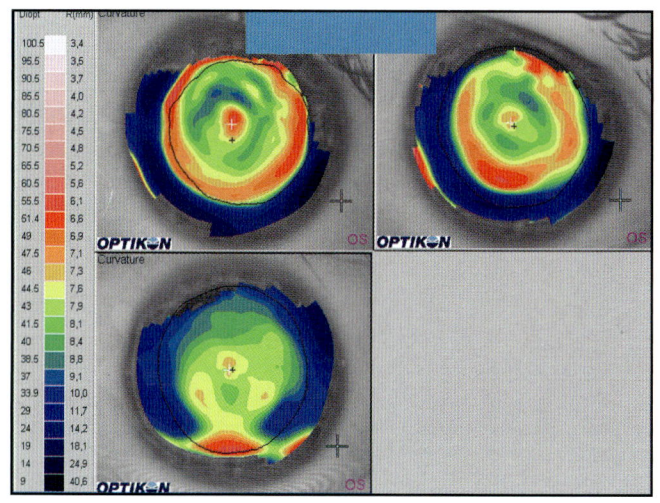

Figure 30-16. Same eye as in Figure 30-15. Instantaneous maps of consecutive PTK intraoperative phases.

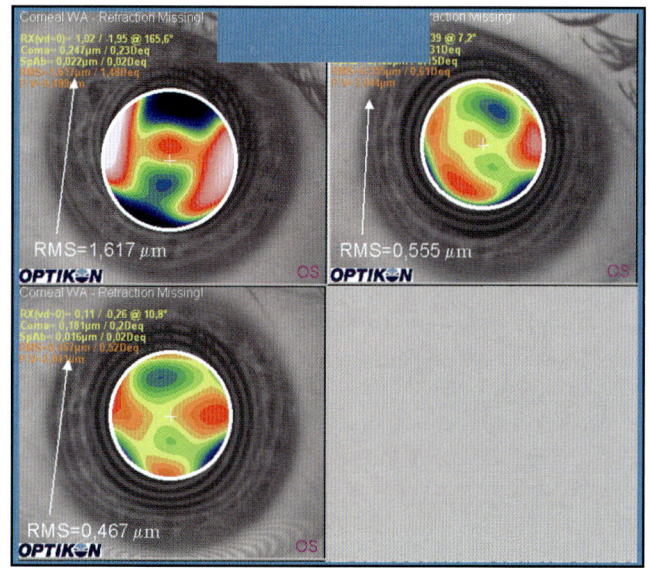

Figure 30-17. Same eye as in Figure 30-15. Wavefront maps of consecutive PTK intraoperative phase. Note: how HO RMS progressively decreases.

have taken place at different rates, thus a cautious approach, together with several intraoperative evaluations, is mandatory.

Decentered PRK eyes present marked differences when examined with or without epithelium. An important concept, which applies to other types of PTK also, is that the single correction of high-order aberrations induces a new cylindrical component. This must be carefully evaluated by the surgeon, a simple task with the Final Fit software, which offers the theoretical resulting surface after ablation. This new cylinder must be taken into account before correcting the other two components: the cylinder initially defined and the spheric defect (see Chapter 18).

Patients operated for opacity and/or irregularity following herpetic keratitis must take antiviral drugs before and after surgery to prevent the possibility of a relapse. Frequently, high hyperopic defects are observed in eyes suffering the after-effects of corneal ulcers due to the lack of stromal tissue caused by ulceration, with sudden variations of curvature in the surrounding tissue.

Epithelium removal in eyes with post-traumatic scars may reveal epithelium-filled wound gaps that require scraping to reactivate the inflammatory process and suturing to make the wound lips coalesce permanently. CPK will then be performed as second-step surgery months later. Scar tissue has a different ablation rate than normal cornea and, in our experience, multistep custom CPK proves to be an effective tool to achieve a final homogeneously regular stromal surface.

Eyes with recurring corneal erosions very often present significant stromal substance defects once the epithelium is removed. These defects cause high-order aberrations.

Corneal dystrophies, such as Groenouw's or Reis-Bückler's, will show a subepithelial membrane that will require surgical removal. The CPK phase will target elimination of high-order aberrations first.

Eyes with band keratopathy present subepithelial deposits that may or may not be bound by ethylenediaminetetraacetic acid (EDTA). In both cases, CPK permits effective removal of opacities and irregularities. EDTA-bound deposits, once removed, show a highly irregular, punctate stroma with higher frequency of extensive postoperative haze.

In our experience, amino acid supplement in these CPK eyes proves to be particularly helpful in accelerating the epithelial healing process.[21] The application of an amniotic membrane was necessary in only 1 case of our series to obtain stable and complete epithelialization.

One of the well-known problems of PTK has been the induction of hyperopia.[9] PTK ablation should maintain the initial corneal curvature, thus the hyperopic shift may appear hard to explain.

An ablation regular in depth like that induced by CPK theoretically induces a hyperopic shift if we assume that the junction between treated and untreated cornea is a sharp, vertical step. Actually, this step is smoothed by epithelial hyperplasia and collagen deposition, creating a slope that generates a negative lens shape. Hyperopic shift quantity is directly related to ablation depth and inversely proportional to ablation diameter. According to Munnerlyn's law, to obtain refractive correction of 1.0 D with a 10-mm wide ablation, a 30-μm deep ablation is necessary, while with 3 mm of width only 3 μm are required. The adoption of a masking agent during the CPK part of the procedure, as well as the wide, 10-mm application of the excimer laser, in our experience, solves this problem.[15,17,22-24]

The main difficulty in CPK can be summarized by the following question: "When to stop?"

How can surgeons judge that a positive result of the treatment has been attained and thus decide to end surgery? Parameters usually considered were achievement of homogeneous, and thus regular, stromal thickness; regular intraoperative keratoscopic rings; corneal transparency; and intraoperative visual acuity, which is influenced by possible undesired residual astigmatic or hyperopic refractive defects.[9]

Often the optimal surgical target is quite ambitious and thus not completely achievable. An experienced surgeon will understand the limits of each case and stop in time, when the appropriately planned goals have been achieved. The ideal target should be complete correction of the refractive defect and elimination of all aberrations. Priority should be given to quality of vision, with elimination of aberrations. This may require leaving a residual of ametropia. Perfect refraction with residual aberrations, which will constantly impede good vision, will be less tolerated by the patient. Finally, the duration of the procedure is also important. An excessively long procedure will lead to corneal hydration, with consequent unreliable aberrometric readings and a different ablation rate. In very complicated cases, it may thus be advisable to abort the procedure and evaluate a second procedure once the situation has been stabilized in the following months.

Conclusions

Custom CPK based on intraoperative topography-derived wavefront is a surgical procedure aimed at treating eyes that would otherwise benefit only from PK. Unlike PK, the risks of the procedure are limited (ie, endothelial damage is limited). The procedure does not preclude future treatment with PK or lamellar keratoplasty. Visual acuity can always be improved. Topography-derived wavefront also permits treatment of eyes with severe opacity or high aberration. Ultrasound-guided PTK is discussed in Chapter 36.

References

1. Serdarevic O, Darrell RW, Krueger RR, Trokel SL. Excimer laser therapy for experimental candida keratitis. *Am J Ophthalmol.* 1985;99:534-533.
2. Fagerholm P, Fitzsimmons TD, Orndahl M, Ohman L, Tengroth B. Phototherapeutic keratectomy: long-term results in 166 eyes. *Refract Corneal Surg.* 1993;9(Suppl):76-81.
3. Forster W, Grewe S, Atzier U, Lunecke C, Busse H. Phototherapeutic keratectomy in corneal diseases. *Refract Corneal Surg.* 1993;9(Suppl):85-90.
4. Gottsch JD, Gilbert ML, Goodmann DF, Sulewsky ME, Dick JD, Stark WJ. Excimer laser ablative treatment of microbial keratitis. *Ophthalmology.* 1991;98(2):146-149.

5. Hersh PS, Spinak A, Garrana R, Mayers M. Phototherapeutic keratectomy: strategies and results in 12 eyes. *Refract Corneal Surg.* 1993; 9(Suppl):90-95.
6. Vinciguerra P, Sborgia M, Airaghi P, Bailo G, De Molfetta V. La cheratectomia fototerapeutica (PTK) come alternativa alla cheratoplastica. *Atti Soc Oftalm Lombarda.* 1994;49:439-442.
7. Wu WCS, Stark WJ, Green WR. Corneal wound healing in excimer laser keratectomy. *Arch Ophthalmol.* 1991;109:1426-1432.
8. Vinciguerra P, Prussiani A. Fotocheratotomia terapeutica (PTK). In: *Chirurgia Refrattiva: Principi e Tecniche.* Asti, Italy: Fabiano; 2000: 439-462.
9. Dogru M, Chikako K, Yamanaka A. Refractive changes after excimer laser phototerapeutic keratectomy. *J Cataract Refract Surg.* 2001;27:686-692.
10. Vinciguerra P, Camesasca FI. Custom phototherapeutic keratectomy with intraoperative topography. *J Refract Surg.* 2004;20:S555-S563.
11. Huang D, Tang M, Shekhar R. Mathematical model of corneal surface smoothing after refractive surgery. *Am J Ophthalmol.* 2003;135:267-278.
12. Balestrazzi E, De Molfetta V, Spadea L, et al. Histological, immunoistochemical, and ultrastructural findings in human corneas after photorefractive keratectomy. *J Refract Surg.* 1995;11:181-187.
13. Epstein D, Fagerholm P, Hamberg-Nyström H, Tengroth B. Twenty-four-month follow-up of excimer laser photorefractive keratectomy for myopia. Refractive and visual acuity results. *Ophthalmology.* 1994; 101:1558-1564.
14. Vinciguerra P, Azzolini M, Radice P, et al. A method for examining surface and interface irregularities after photorefractive keratectomy and laser in situ keratomileusis: predictor of optical and functional outcomes. *J Refract Surg.* 1998;14:S204-S206.
15. Vinciguerra P, Azzolini M, Airaghi P, et al. Effect of decreasing surface and interface irregularities after photorefractive keratectomy and laser in situ keratomileusis on optical and functional outcomes. *J Refract Surg.* 1998;14:S199-S203.
16. Vinciguerra P, Camesasca FI. Butterfly laser epithelial keratomileusis for myopia. *J Refract Surg.* 2002;18:S371-S373.
17. Vinciguerra P, Camesasca FI, Randazzo A. One-year results of butterfly laser epithelial keratomileusis. *J Refract Surg.* 2003;19:S223-S226.
18. Roberts C. Biomechanics of the cornea and wavefront-guided laser refractive surgery. *J Refract Surg.* 2002;18:S589-S592.
19. Kornhehl EW, Steinert RF, Puliafito CA. A comparative study of masking fluids for excimer laser phototherapeutic keratectomy. *Arch Ophthalmol.* 1991;109(6):860-863.
20. Vinciguerra P, Cro M, Giuffrida S, Airaghi P, De Molfetta V. A new strategy in excimer laser PTK: use of hyaluronic acid solution as masking fluid. *Inv Ophthalmol Vis Sci.* 1994;35(4):1300.
21. Vinciguerra P, Camesasca FI, Ponzin D. Use of amino acids in refractive surgery. *J Refract Surg.* 2002;18(Suppl):130-133.
22. Vinciguerra P, Camesasca FI, Urso R. Reduction of spherical aberration with the Nidek NAVEX customized ablation system. *J Refract Surg.* 2003;19:S195-S201.
23. Vinciguerra P, Torres I, Camesasca FI. Applications of confocal microscopy in refractive surgery. *J Refract Surg.* 2002;18:S378-S381.
24. Vinciguerra P, Camesasca FI. Treatment of hyperopia: a new ablation profile to reduce corneal eccentricity. *J Refract Surg.* 2002;18:S315-S317.

Long-Term Follow-Up of Ultrathin Corneas After Surface Retreatment With Photoptherapeutic Keratectomy

*Paolo Vinciguerra, MD; Maria Ingrid Torres Munoz, MD;
Fabrizio I. Camesasca, MD; Fabio Grizzi, PhD; Cynthia Roberts, PhD*

Introduction

Corneal surgery protocols have often recommended that total corneal thickness at the end of a procedure should be greater than 300 µm, so that the residual stroma is resistant enough not to incur keratectasia. According to this protocol, eyes with total corneal thickness below 400 µm are to be considered at risk of ectasia. This is why patients with corneal disorders causing poor vision and featuring low pachymetric values have been so far treated with perforating or lamellar keratoplasty, which was seen as the only possible therapeutic option.

The idea to study patients with thin corneas was suggested by examinations on a group of patients submitted to PTK surgery. These patients had been selected as extreme cases, with very thin corneas at the start, but on the other hand the only possible alternative to improve their situation was to perform a corneal transplant. As a therapeutic alternative in some of these cases, we had suggested the photoptherapeutic keratectomy (PTK) technique with masking fluid, which helps regularize the corneal surface, and therefore improves their vision without reducing the cornea thickness further in the thinner spots.

We evaluated PTK as an effective treatment alternative for patients with complications following previous photorefractive keratectomy (PRK) and featuring very thin corneas. Improved visual acuity as well as long-term corneal stability offered by PTK was studied.

Photoptherapeutic Keratectomy on Thin Corneas

In a recent study, we retrospectively evaluated a group of patients that underwent PTK between June 1998 and October 2000.[1] We included PRK patients with postoperative complications that determined low best spectacle-corrected visual acuity ([BSCVA] 0.3 or less). The sole therapeutic alternative to the corneal disorders selected for this study was corneal transplant. These patients had very thin corneas, and they were offered PTK as an alternative to penetrating keratoplasty.

All the customarily recommended exclusion criteria for refractive surgery (ie, markedly asymmetric corneal curvature, unstable refractive defect, keratoconus, ongoing inflammatory disorders, collagen diseases, glaucoma, autoimmune diseases), as well as previous laser-assisted in situ keratomileusis (LASIK), were applied, as if patients were to undergo refractive surgery for the first time.

The study group consisted of 48 eyes of 32 patients. Demographic data are listed in Table 31-1. Causes of reduced visual acuity are listed in Table 31-2. Corneal haze was graded as severe according to Epstein.[2] Preoperatively, all patients underwent complete ophthalmologic examination, with determination of cycloplegic refraction, corneal topography with CSO topographer (Florence, Italy) or Keratron Scout topographer (Optikon 2000, Rome, Italy), and endothelial cell counts. Preoperative pachymetry was assessed with ultrasounds (SP 2000, Tomey, Nagoya, Japan) in all eyes, while Orbscan topography (Bausch & Lomb, Rochester, NY) was performed in 10 eyes. Preoperatively, central corneal ultrasound pachymetry was 390 ± 38 µm (mean ± SD), ranging between 290 and 444 µm. Arbitrarily, we decided that, for safety reasons, the difference between the preoperative pachymetry value and the estimated amount of microns necessary to PTK should not be less than 200 µm. All patients signed a specific informed consent.

The surgical technique was as follows:
* Local anesthesia using eye drops containing a combination of oxybuprocaine 0.4% and lidocaine 4%

Table 31-1. Demographic Data of the Study Eyes

48 eyes
32 patients (14 females, 18 males)
Age (mean ± SD): 37 ± 5.6 years
Endothelial cell counts: 2840 ± 342/mm^2

Table 31-2. Causes of Reduced Visual Acuity in the Study Eyes

Cause	Number of Eyes
Severe regression and haze	18
Decentration	12
Highly aberrated corneas	8
Small optical zone	10
Total	48

- Application of a Castroviejo-style speculum
- Mechanical removal of the epithelium with a Vinciguerra spatula (ASICO, Westmont, Ill)
- Intraoperative topography to identify in details all corneal unevenness to be treated, using a Keratron Scout topographer
- Application of masking fluid[3,4] (hyaluronic acid 0.4%, [Laservis, Chemedica, Munich, Germany]) and treatment with a NIDEK EC 5000 excimer laser (NIDEK, Gamagori, Japan). Ablation diameter was 10 mm and frequency was 10 Hz. To avoid overheating the tissue, the ablation was set at 30 µm. During the ablation, gentle lamination of the masking fluid was performed using a Buratto's spatula (ASICO). The masking fluid has the same surface tension as the corneal epithelium and the same ablation rate as the stroma. This enables uneven areas to emerge, helping to perform a selective ablation so as to level the surface. The masking fluid also has the shear rate of viscoelastic material, and it can be laminated thin or thick by changing the speed of the spatular motion; a slower passage creates a higher fluid thickness and vice versa (see Chapter 8)[3,4]
- After wetting the surface with masking fluid, intraoperative topography was repeated to monitor the results and identify any remaining irregularity
- Application of focal ablations on any residual unevenness identified through the topographic scan
- New smoothing of the corneal surface through ablation with masking fluid
- Each ablation step removed usually 10 to 20 µm in localized areas
- The smoothing phase removed 8 to 10 µm on the whole surface. Smoothing is always performed with a thick layer of protective masking fluid. To remove 8 to 10 µm, the set laser ablation is about 50 µm
- All these repeated ablation phases lead to prolonged corneal exposure to UV. Total final stromal corneal tissue removal (previous PRK + PTK) was 200 µm or more
- At the end of the procedure, application of a Protec therapeutic contact lens (CIBAVision Ophthalmics, Duluth, Ga) and medication using netilmicin eye, cyclopentolate hydrochloride, and tobramicin-dexamethasone drops

Postoperative treatment was as follows. Netilmicin eye drops were administered until epithelial regrowth. Afterward, fluorometholone acetate 0.1% eye drops were used for 15 days, and hyaluronic acid sodium salt 0.2% eye drops were used for the first 6 months. After PTK surgery, the patients were medicated from day 1 to day 4 postoperatively until regrowth of the epithelium (mean time: 3.2 days). Follow-up examinations were performed after 1, 3, 6, and 12 months. From 1 year onward, the patients were submitted to annual follow-up checkups. At years 1 and 5 postoperatively, the eyes underwent complete ophthalmologic examination, corneal topography, and ultrasound pachymetry.

We considered pachymetry and visual acuity at year 1 as efficacy parameters, and optical refraction, corneal curvature, and pachymetry as stability parameters at year 1 and year 5.

Corneal stability was also evaluated monitoring mean curvature in diopters over the entire central 3 mm as well as 5-mm corneal area, as measured with the CSO corneal topographer.

Statistical analysis with Student's t-test (using StatSoft, Tulsa, Okla) was performed comparing refractive and corneal curvature parameters at year 1 with those measured at the end of the entire follow-up period.

Out of the 48 study eyes, all were seen at year 1 postoperatively and 31 eyes (64.5%) at 5 years ± 2 months SD. No eye was left with less than 200 µm of final total thickness. Mean preoperative BSCVA was 0.2 ± 0.095 SD. Visual acuity and refraction at the different follow-up intervals are reported in Table 31-3.

Efficacy Parameters

At year 1, mean postoperative pachymetry value was 341 µm ± 40 (mean ± SD), ranging between 264 and 414 µm (Table 31-4). Mean BSCVA was 0.6 ± 0.072 SD.

Stability Parameters

To evaluate corneal biomechanical stability, we took three parameters into consideration variation from years 1 to 5:

Table 31-3. Visual Acuity and Refraction at the Different Follow-Up Intervals

Time Interval	Number of Eyes	BSCVA (mean ± SD)	Refraction, SE (D, mean ± SD)
Preoperative	48	0.2 ± 0.09	-2.53 ± 2.34
Year 1	48	0.6 ± 0.72	-2.15 ± 1.67
Year 5	31	0.7 ± 0.15	-2.33 ± 1.12

Table 31-4. Ultrasound Pachymetry Values at the Different Follow-Up Intervals

Time Interval	Number of Eyes	Pachymetry (microns, mean ± SD)	Range (microns)
Preoperative	48	390 ± 38	290 to 444
Year 1	48	341 ± 40	264 to 414
Year 5	31	339 ± 48	258 to 466

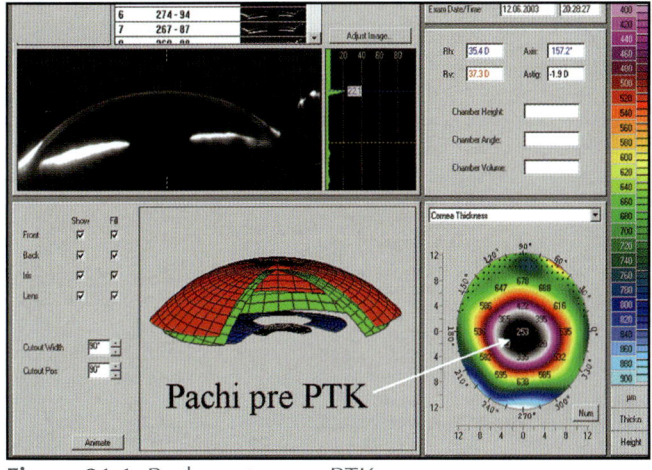

Figure 31-1. Pachymetry pre-PTK.

Figure 31-2. Two-year post-PTK pachymetry.

optical refraction, average topographic corneal curvature in the 3 and 5 mm central cornea, and pachymetry (Figures 31-1 through 31-3). We performed a statistical comparison of the values found at year 1 vs year 5. At the end of the follow-up period, there was an improvement of at least four Snellen lines in 100% of cases, and the mean postoperative BSCVA was 0.7 ± 0.15 SD.

The analysis of refractive parameters was divided into spherical correction, astigmatic correction, and astigmatism axis. Figure 31-4 shows spherical correction at year 1 vs year 5. No statistically significant differences were found between spherical correction at years 1 and 5 (p=0.93). The same was true for astigmatic correction and astigmatism axis.

No statistically significant changes emerged from a comparison between mean topography-derived corneal curvature values over the entire central 3 mm area at year 1 and year 5 (p=0.93) (Figure 31-5). Similarly, a comparison between the average corneal curvature values over the entire central 5 mm area at year 1 and year 5 (p=0.99) (Figure 31-6).

Figure 31-7A presents a post-myopic PRK patient with LE decentration, strong haze due to scarring, and an ultrathin cornea. This patient has undergone several surface procedures for the treatment of decentration and regression. Initial refraction was -9.0 -2.0 (180) and pre-PTK BSCVA was 0.2 with -0.75 -1.0 (175). Five years post-PTK, the situation is presented in Figure 31-7B and BSCVA was 0.9 with -0.5 (175).

Discussion

The aim of this study was to evaluate PTK as an effective treatment alternative for patients with complications following previous PRK and featuring very thin corneas. Improved

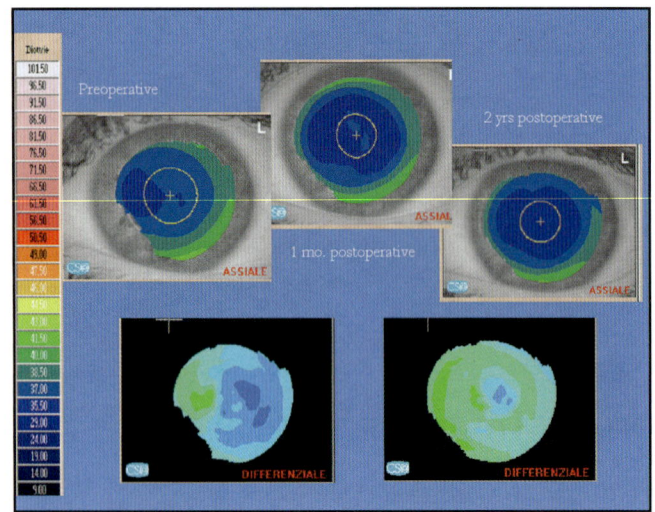

Figure 31-3. Same case as in Figures 31-1 and 31-2. Preoperative, 1-month, and 2-years postoperative topography, above. Differential map between preoperative and 1-month (below, left) and preoperative and 2-years maps (below, right).

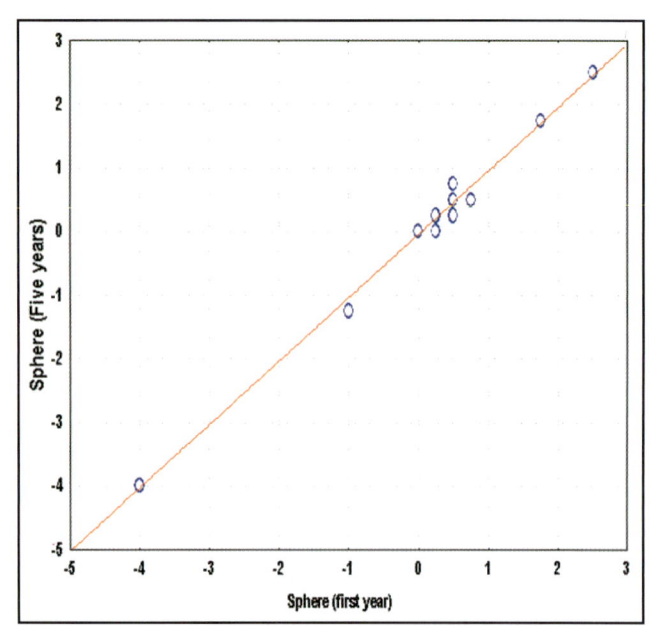

Figure 31-4. Spherical correction at year 1 vs year 5.

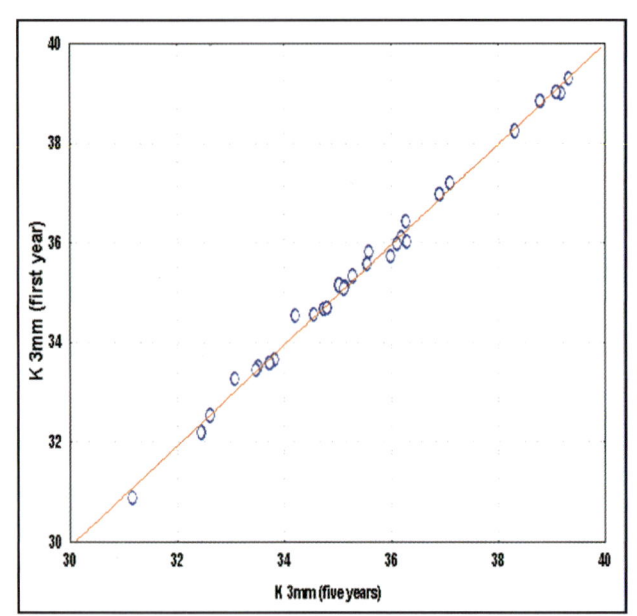

Figure 31-5. Comparison between mean topography-derived corneal curvature values over the entire central 3 mm area at year 1 and year 5.

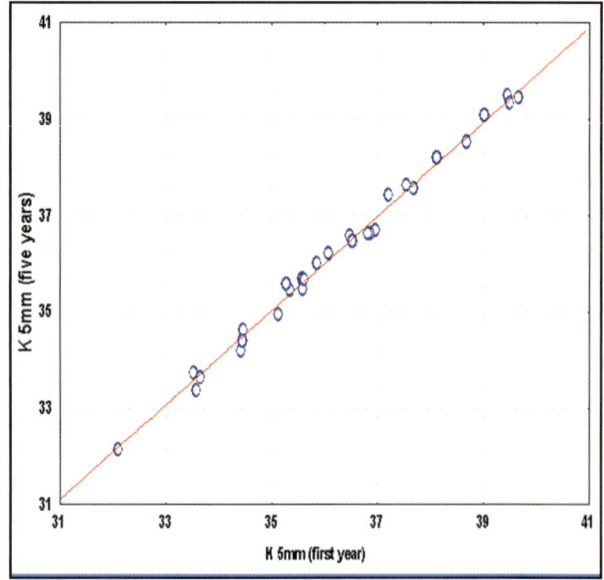

Figure 31-6. Comparison between mean topography-derived corneal curvature values over the entire central 5 mm area at year 1 and year 5.

visual acuity as well as long-term corneal stability offered by PTK was assessed.

A major problem concerning corneal thinning beyond certain values is the risk of inducing keratectasia. Corneal ectasia is generally recognized by several main clinical characteristics, such as progressive increase in corneal curvature compared with postoperative topography, progressive increase of myopia and/or astigmatism, and decrease of uncorrected visual acuity and best corrected visual acuity.[5-7]

The first cases of keratectasia after refractive surgery were described by Seiler et al in 1998,[5] following a laser-assisted in situ keratomileusis (LASIK) procedure for severe myopia. Since then, many authors have described cases of post-LASIK ectasia.[7-17] Several risk factors have been identified, such as the presence of forme fruste keratoconus, a post-LASIK residual stromal bed of less than 250 µm, and treatments for myopias exceeding -8.0 D. However, apart from potentially predisposing risk factors, keratectasia seems to be a postoperative complication much more frequently associated with LASIK technique than with PRK or PTK.[7,14-20]

Considering the long-term stability of corneal parameters found in our patients retreated with PTK despite low postoperative residual pachymetry, we asked ourselves why they did not show the occurrence of ectasia.

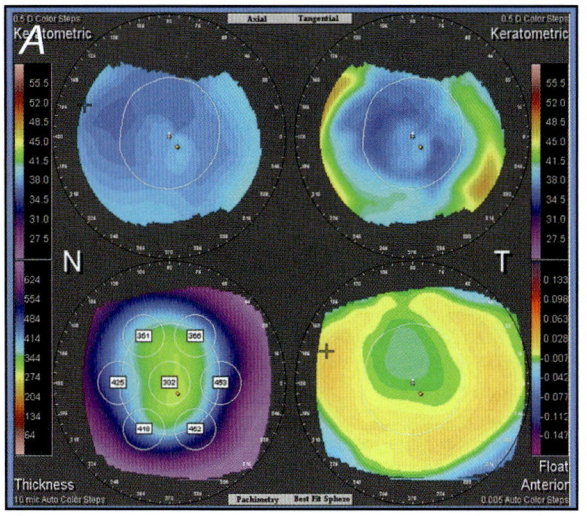

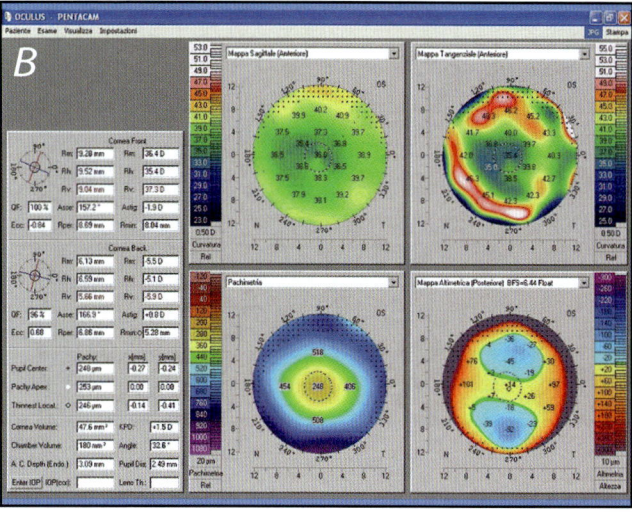

Figure 31-7. (A) Postmyopic PRK patient with LE decentration, strong haze due to scarring, and an ultrathin cornea. (B) Five years post-PTK situation.

We considered several factors. A primary factor is undoubtedly the cornea's biomechanical response, and a comparison between PTK and LASIK, the refractive procedure with the highest reported occurrence of ectasia, may be useful. After a surface retreatment, the residual thickness consists mostly of undamaged fibers. Conversely, after intrastromal surgery one-third or more of the stromal lamellae's thickness has been cut by the microkeratome, and this damage has been assumed to have a direct correlation with the loss of long-term biomechanical stability of the stroma. After the incision, the collagen lamellae loosen, producing a biomechanical response, investigated by some authors such as Cynthia Roberts that leads to a significant central flattening and peripheral corneal thickening, which also affects the procedure's refractive outcome (see Chapter 6).[21,22]

The lamellae incised by the microkeratome may endure tension differently. Some histological studies have even identified the fibers of the front half of the stroma as those responsible for maintaining biomechanical stability, and the incision of these lamellae might be directly involved in the cornea's loss of structural stability.[23]

According to our protocol, PTK, with an ablation diameter of at least 10 mm, spreads corneal thinning over virtually the entire corneal surface. Appropriate lamination of the masking fluid makes it thinner and exposes the most uneven curved corneal areas to excimer ablation. Repeated intraoperative topography monitors the results and identifies any remaining irregularity. Small, focal ablations can also be applied on any major residual unevenness identified through the topographic scan.

Therefore, PTK evens out the surface both centrally and peripherally. An interesting example is the retreatment of decentered or myopic eyes with severe regression and haze in which the most curved corneal areas are located in the periphery (corresponding to the "red ring" visible on topography map with instantaneous algorithm). As a result of PTK, tissue is removed in this peripheral portion, with thickness reduction distributed evenly over the entire cornea. The gradient of physiological corneal thickness from the center to the periphery is improved and rendered more similar to the pristine situation.

In our opinion, uniform thickness reduction over a wide zone may lead to more uniform stress distribution, with less chance of stress concentration in one single, thinner area with greater risk of ectasia. After a LASIK surgical procedure (ie, the microkeratome cuts the cornea with a maximum diameter of 8 to 9 mm), the subsequent refractive treatment must allow for the flap hinge, so that ultimately the ablation has a diameter of approximately 7 to 7.25 mm. In this way, the reduction in corneal thickness is not evenly distributed, but is concentrated in one area, further weakening its structure.

Thus, a more uniform, long-term stress distribution on the overall cornea due to more uniform thickness may contribute to long-term stability, as if the cornea behaved as a unit with similar elastic response from the center to the periphery. Comparing this situation with that of a tree, a deep, localized cut weakens the tree much more than a wide, uniform removal of wood on a large area, such as when creating a board (Figure 31-8). Similarly, an ultrathin cornea after a narrowly concentrated ablation may not be stable, while an ultrathin cornea with a wide ablation zone is, as shown by the results of this study on PTK, apparently stable.

Kazunori et al described a case of progressive keratectasia after PTK for the treatment of band keratopathy. The treatment zone was 66 mm with a transition zone of 0.7 mm, thus the ablation was not applied over the entire, 10-mm corneal surface. Furthermore, corneal transparency is not mentioned because scarring could contribute to an increase in frontal surface curvature.

We recommend evaluating pachymetry preoperatively and estimating the amount of tissue necessary to be removed with PTK in order to calculate safety residual corneal thickness values. Also, intraoperative corneal wetting with consequent edema may render pachymetry unreliable.

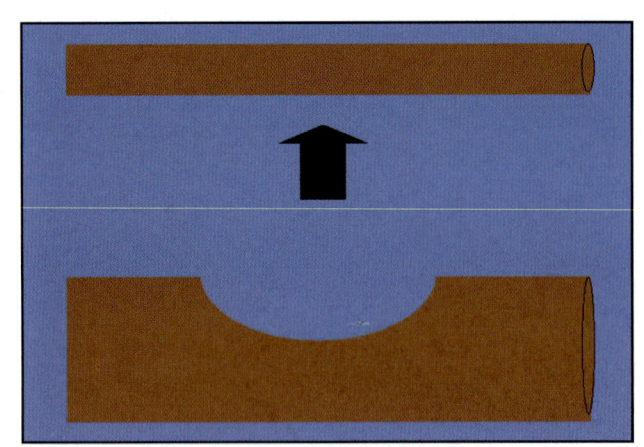

Figure 31-8. A deep, localized cut weakens a tree much more than the wide, uniform removal of wood on a large area, such as when creating a board.

Thorough comprehension of the role played by the epithelium is also mandatory, and intraoperative topography performed after epithelium removal may provide essential information to manage a case. For example, when a highly myopic eye has been treated with a narrow optical zone, the center-to-periphery corneal gradient is very high and induces a marked epithelial response with several layers of epithelium and increased collagen deposition. This leads to central corneal surface flattening and regression. PTK with ablation of the peripheral "red ring" reduces corneal curvature gradient, thus inducing less epithelial response with less structuring of cell layers and collagen deposition.

Our results with this study group, albeit small, led us to consider PTK retreatment a good therapeutic alternative that, in some cases, helps avoid a cornea transplant. In any case, this technique allows the maintenance of good thickness in the corneal periphery, ensuring the presence of a receiving bed sufficient to perform a perforating or lamellar keratoplasty afterward, if necessary.

An interesting speculation that deserves appropriate studies concerns PTK-generated prolonged corneal exposure to UV. This situation could partially reproduce that of collagen crosslinking with riboflavin/UVA, thus possibly inducing increased corneal mechanical resistance.[24]

References

1. Vinciguerra P, Munoz MI, Camesasca FI, Grizzi F, Roberts C. Long-term follow-up of ultrathin corneas after surface retreatment with phototherapeutic keratectomy. *J Cataract Refract Surg.* 2005;31:82-87.
2. Epstein D, Fagerholm P, Hamberg-Nyström H, Tengroth B. Twenty-four-month follow-up of excimer laser photorefractive keratectomy for myopia. Refractive and visual acuity results. *Ophthalmology.* 1994;101:1558-1564.
3. Vinciguerra P, Cro M, Giuffrida S, Airaghi P, De Molfetta V. A new strategy in excimer laser PTK: use of hyaluronic acid solution as masking fluid. *Inv Ophthalmol Vis Sci.* 1994;35(4):1300.
4. Kornhel EW, Steinert RF, Puliafito CA. A comparative study of masking fluids for excimer laser phototherapeutic keratectomy. *Arch Opthalmol.* 1991;109:860-863.
5. Seiler T, Quurke AW. Iatrogenic keratectasia after LASIK in a case of forme fruste keratoconus. *J Cataract Refract Surg.* 2000;24:1007-1009.
6. Seiler T, Koufala K, Richter G. Iatrogenic keratectasia after in situ keratomileusis. *J Refract Surg.* 1998;14:312-317.
7. Koch DD. The riddle of iatrogenic ectasia. *J Cataract Refract Surg.* 1999;25:453-454.
8. Joo C, Kim T. Corneal ectasia detected after in situ keratomileusis for correction of less than -12 diopters of myopia. *J Cataract Refract Surg.* 2000;26:292-295.
9. Mc Leod S, Kisla T, Caro N, McMahon T. Iatrogenic keratoconus: corneal ectasia following laser in situ keratomileusis for myopia. *Arch Ophthalmol.* 2000;118:282-284.
10. Schmitt-Bernard C, Lesage C, Arnaud B. Corneal ectasia induced by laser in situ keratomileusis in keratoconus. *J Refract Surg.* 2000;16:368-370.
11. Lafond G, Bazin, Lajoie C. Bilateral severe keratoconus after laser in situ keratomileusis in a patient with forme fruste keratoconus. *J Cataract Refract Surg.* 2001;27:1115-1118.
12. Pallikaris IG, Kymionis GD, Astyrakakis NI. Corneal ectasia induced by laser in situ keratomileusis in keratoconus. *J Cataract Refract Surg.* 2001;27:1796-1802.
13. Wang Z, Chen J, Yang B. Posterior corneal surface topographic changes after laser in situ keratomileusis are related to residual corneal bed thickness. *Ophthalmology.* 1999;106:406-410.
14. Rayan MS, Jaycock P, O'Brart D, et al. A long-term study of photorefractive keratectomy: 12-year follow-up. *Ophthalmology.* 2004;111:1813-1824.
15. Jabbur NS, Sakatani K, O'Brien T. Survey of complications and recommendations for management in dissatisfied patients seeking a consultation after refractive surgery. *J Cataract Refract Surg.* 2004;30:1867-1874.
16. Holland SP, Srivannaboon S, Reinstein DZ Avoiding serious corneal complications of laser assisted in situ keratomileusis and photorefractive keratectomy. *Ophthalmology.* 2000;107:640-652.
17. Dantas PE. Corneal ectasia after refractive surgery. *Ophthalmology.* 2001;108:834-835.
18. Kazunori M, Tetsuya T, Tomidokoro A, et al. Iatrogenic keratectasia after phototherapeutic keratectomy. *Br J Ophthalmol.* 2001;85:247-248.
19. Kamiya K, Oshika T. Corneal forward shift after excimer laser keratorefractive surgery. *Semin Ophthalmol.* 2003;18:17-22.
20. Kazunori M, Kazutaka K, Tetsuya T, et al. Time course of changes in corneal forward shift after excimer laser photorefractive keratectomy. *Arch Ophthalmol.* 2002;120:869-900.
21. Dupps WJ, Roberts C. Effect of acute biomechanical changes on corneal curvature after photokeratectomy. *J Refract Surg.* 2001;17:658-669.
22. Roberts C. Biomechanics of the cornea and wavefront-guided laser refractive surgery. *J Refract Surg.* 2002;18:S589-S592.
23. Muller LJ, Pels E, Vrensen GF. The specific architecture of the anterior stroma accounts for maintenance of corneal curvature. *J Refract Surg.* 2001;85:379-381.
24. Wollensak G, Wilsch M, Spoerl E, Seiler T. Collagen fiber diameter in rabbit cornea after collagen crosslinking by riboflavin/UVA. *Cornea.* 2004;23:432.

CHAPTER 32

NOMOGRAMS FOR SURFACE LASER CORRECTION

Guy M. Kezirian, MD, FACS

Accurate nomograms are essential for any laser correction procedure. Nomograms detect and compensate for the many influences that affect outcomes and can significantly improve refractive and visual outcomes. With valid nomograms and state-of-the-art laser technology, reoperations for refractive enhancements should be rare.

This is particularly true for surface ablation procedures. Surface ablation may lead to more predictable long-term visual outcomes and better results after wavefront-guided treatments[1,2] than similar procedures performed with LASIK. However, the various techniques used in surface correction procedures can affect ablation rates and refractive outcomes. Even with wavefront-guided procedures, the overall success of surface procedures depends on the ability to compensate for these differences in order to achieve accurate spherocylindrical outcomes. Accurate spherocylindrical outcomes, in turn, depend on accurate nomograms.

Nomograms for surface ablations introduce several different considerations than for LASIK procedures. Considerations include:

* *Ablation rates*: Bowman's layer may ablate at a different rate than the stroma, and this must be factored into nomograms to avoid undercorrections.[3] This effect is decreased as fluence levels increase, and many of the newer lasers use higher fluence levels. Nomograms can detect the impact of this effect and adjust for it.
* *Surface removal method*: Different methods for removing epithelium may alter stromal hydration and other properties, which may affect ablation rates.[4-8]
* *Healing*: Epithelial remodeling occurs at a higher rate after surface procedures than after LASIK and may alter the long-term refractive outcome.[9,10] The use of antimetabolites may alter this response[11-14] and induce nomogram differences. Nomograms must take this into consideration (Figure 32-1).
* *Biomechanical effects*: Biomechanical contraction of the flap may affect the refractive outcome after LASIK. This effect is avoided with surface ablation providing another reason why nomograms based on LASIK outcomes cannot be used for surface procedures.

Valid nomograms for surface treatment consider all these factors and compensate for them.

Refractive stability may occur later with surface procedures than with LASIK. Because nomograms depend on a known refractive endpoint, it is important to use data based on a stable postoperative refraction when creating nomograms. For myopia, the 3-month exam is probably adequate. While changes may occur beyond this time point, population statistics will likely be stable. For hyperopic procedures, the refractive endpoint may not occur for 6 months, or even 1 year following surgery. Only stable refractions should be entered into nomogram calculations.

The methodology for creating nomograms is simple in concept but can be complex in execution due to the larger number of calculations required and the many opportunities for mathematical errors. Today, computer software exists to facilitate the task of creating valid nomograms and to keep them current. However, it is important for the surgeon to understand these concepts in order to know how best to apply the information nomograms provide.

This chapter presents the concepts underlying nomogram development with special attention to factors that may affect outcomes after surface procedures.

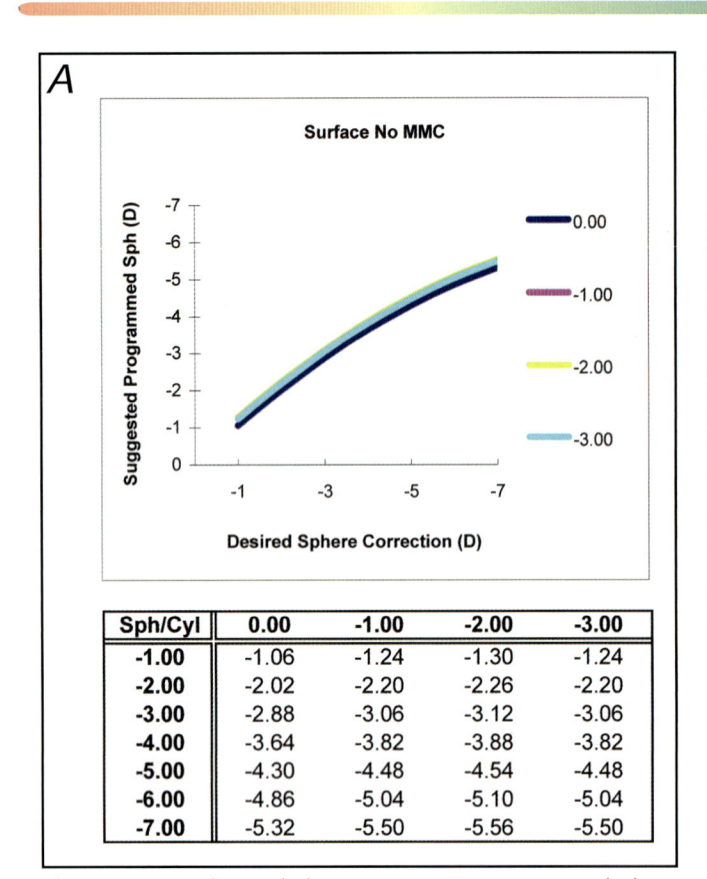

Figure 32-1. Plots of the nomogram recommended programmed amount for sphere vs the sphere and cylinder preoperative refraction amounts. All three nomograms in this figure were obtained from data from the same Allegretto laser at 6.5 mm optical zone, but for different procedures. (A) Nomogram plot and underlying data for surface treatments without mitomycin C. (MMC) (B) Nomogram for surface treatments with MMC. (C) LASIK nomogram. In all three plots, the sphere programmed amount is affected by the amount of concurrent cylinder treatment, a phenomenon known as "coupling." Note that differences are most pronounced in the higher treatment ranges and with higher cylinder amounts.

A — Surface No MMC

Sph/Cyl	0.00	-1.00	-2.00	-3.00
-1.00	-1.06	-1.24	-1.30	-1.24
-2.00	-2.02	-2.20	-2.26	-2.20
-3.00	-2.88	-3.06	-3.12	-3.06
-4.00	-3.64	-3.82	-3.88	-3.82
-5.00	-4.30	-4.48	-4.54	-4.48
-6.00	-4.86	-5.04	-5.10	-5.04
-7.00	-5.32	-5.50	-5.56	-5.50

B — Surface with MMC

Sph/Cyl	0.00	-1.00	-2.00	-3.00
-1.00	-1.00	-1.32	-1.52	-1.60
-2.00	-1.96	-2.23	-2.38	-2.41
-3.00	-2.88	-3.10	-3.20	-3.18
-4.00	-3.76	-3.93	-3.98	-3.91
-5.00	-4.60	-4.72	-4.72	-4.60
-6.00	-5.40	-5.47	-5.42	-5.25
-7.00	-6.16	-6.18	-6.08	-5.86

C — LASIK

Sph/Cyl	0.00	-1.00	-2.00	-3.00
-1.00	-1.05	-1.07	-1.09	-1.11
-2.00	-2.04	-2.04	-2.04	-2.04
-3.00	-2.97	-2.95	-2.93	-2.91
-4.00	-3.84	-3.80	-3.76	-3.72
-5.00	-4.65	-4.59	-4.53	-4.47
-6.00	-5.40	-5.32	-5.24	-5.16
-7.00	-6.09	-5.99	-5.89	-5.79

General Factors Improving the Accuracy of Laser Refractive Surgery

Nomograms have played a key role in improving refractive surgery results, but they are only one factor among many that have played a role.

Laser refractive surgery is very different today than it was 10 years ago. Today's procedures are far more accurate, they deliver better optics, and more information is available to guide surgeons in patient selection and management. The impact of these improvements is seen in better outcomes and in reduced reoperation rates for refractive modification (enhancements). With newer lasers, careful patient selection and state-of-the-art nomogram enhancement rates have been reduced to below 1% in many centers.

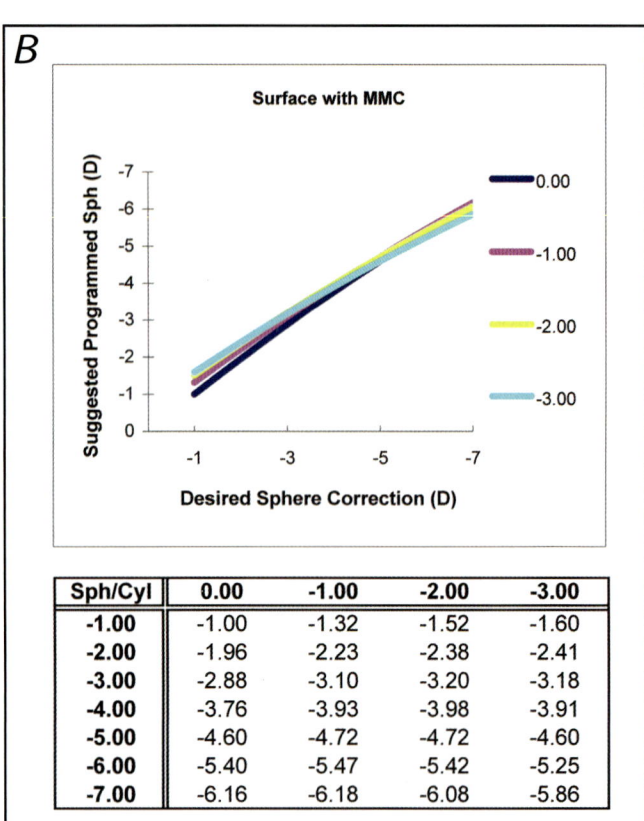

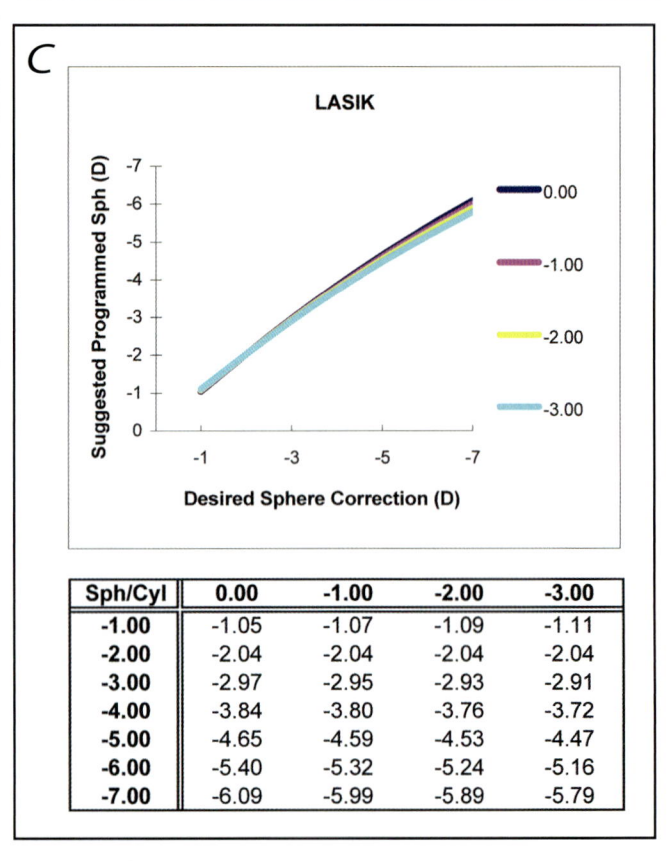

An important advance in recent years has been the availability of better preoperative diagnostic information through topography and aberrometry. Today, the manifest refraction is supplemented by topographic and wavefront data, allow-

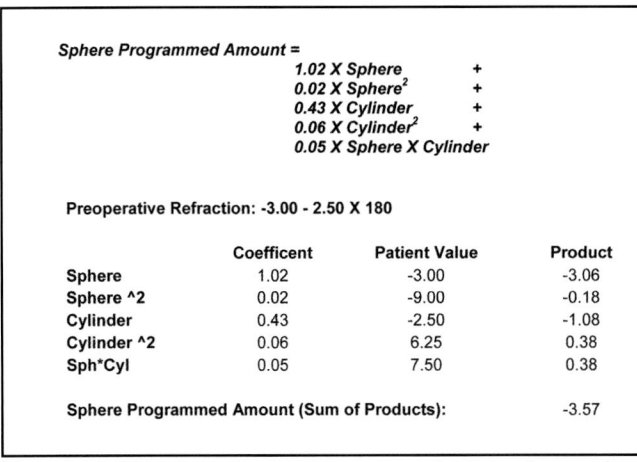

```
Sphere Programmed Amount =
                1.02 X Sphere      +
                0.02 X Sphere²     +
                0.43 X Cylinder    +
                0.06 X Cylinder²   +
                0.05 X Sphere X Cylinder

Preoperative Refraction: -3.00 - 2.50 X 180

                    Coefficent    Patient Value    Product
Sphere              1.02          -3.00            -3.06
Sphere ^2           0.02          -9.00            -0.18
Cylinder            0.43          -2.50            -1.08
Cylinder ^2         0.06           6.25             0.38
Sph*Cyl             0.05           7.50             0.38

Sphere Programmed Amount (Sum of Products):        -3.57
```

Figure 32-2. Nomograms are expressed in the form of an equation. Here, the sphere nomogram for surface treatment using MMC with an Allegretto laser (WaveLight Allegretto Wave, WaveLight Technologies, AG, Erlangen, Germany) and a 6.5-mm optical zone is presented. The equation appears at the top. It includes several expressions of the preoperative refraction and the nomogram coefficients for each variable. A sample calculation is provided at the bottom for an eye with the preoperative refraction shown. The nomogram calculation is performed by multiplying the coefficients times the patient's values. The suggested programmed amount for sphere is calculated as the sum of the products.

ing the surgeon to correlate information and to better design treatments. Aberrometers in particular provide independent confirmation of the manifest refraction, allowing the surgeon to verify the treatment amount prior to surgery.

Surface procedures have seen many advances in recent years. The epithelial healing response after surface procedures, sometimes referred to as surface remodeling, presented great challenges to early refractive surgeons.[15,16] Today's lasers provide smoother ablations,[17-20] resulting in less epithelial remodeling[21,22] and more predictable results. Early surgeons relied on topical steroids to control surface remodeling.[23] Today, better metabolic agents such as MMC can provide be used prophylactically to decrease regression.[11-14]

These advances provide surgeons with several techniques and procedures from which to choose when planning surgery. Unfortunately, this can decrease the refractive predictability of procedures by introducing new variables into surgery. Variations in surgical technique, medications, laser calibration, the laser room environment (temperature, humidity, and barometric pressure), patient variables, and many other factors can affect outcomes and must be understood to achieve predictable refractive results. This can only be done by modeling the effects of these variables using prior data and then applying the model when performing surgical planning.

Today, modeling of refractive results is done with nomograms, which can incorporate many variables to control for the various factors that influence outcomes. Because the factors that affect lasers and procedures may differ, the variables considered by specific nomograms may vary. The ability to detect and include significant variables is a key feature of modern nomograms and has led to significant improvements in nomogram predictability.

Nomogram Advances

Initial nomograms took the form of look-up tables printed on a sheet of paper. They provided adjustments based on spherocylindrical data and attempted to compensate for general over- or undercorrections by shifting the mean outcomes.[24] The result was a better mean outcome without much effect on overall predictability.

Modern nomograms are not look-up tables; they are multifactorial equations that consider different variables for each data set and suggest treatment amounts based on current information (Figure 32-2). Properly applied, nomograms can also provide likely outcome ranges to assist in setting the targeted amount (Figure 32-3).

Nomograms are not static, but instead change over time to factor for seasonal changes, aging optics, and modifications of surgical techniques. They separate data according to important attributes, such as the use of antimetabolites and the method for removing epithelium, and many other considerations. They model the sphere and cylinder components separately to detect and compensate for effects of cylinder treatments on sphere results and vice-versa (so-called "coupling," shown in Figure 32-1).

Software programs have been developed to create and maintain refractive surgery nomograms. These programs use dynamic algorithms to sense which variables are affecting outcomes and then create nomograms based on the findings. The result is that each surgeon may develop several different nomograms in order to accurately plan surgery for each treatment range (myopia, hyperopia), procedure (PRK, LASIK, and LASEK), ancillary equipment and techniques, (keratomes, MMC) and other factors. Some surgeons have a dozen or more nomograms for various procedures and treatment ranges, each providing surgical predictability well beyond what was obtainable with previous approaches.

Steps in Nomogram Development

Nomograms can be created using various approaches but key to all methods is regression analysis. Regression analysis is a mathematical process that describes the relationship between cause and effect. It can take several forms—linear, quadratic, simple, multiple, etc, and the result is an equation that puts the "dependent" variable on one side of the equation and the "independent" variables on the other.

The dependent variable used in most nomograms is the programmed amount for sphere or cylinder (each in its own equation because sphere and cylinder nomograms must be created separately). The independent variables include

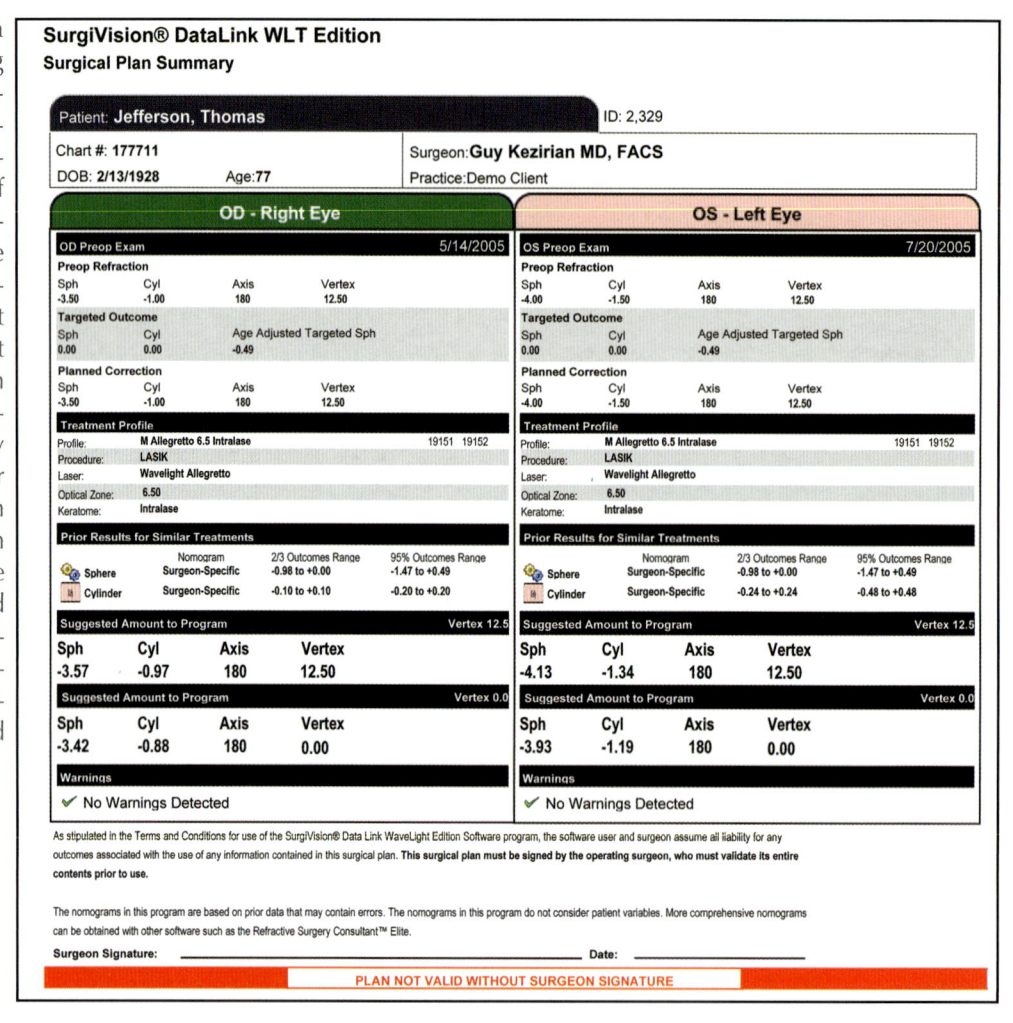

Figure 32-3. Example of a surgical plan obtained using a surgeon-specific nomogram. The predicted outcome range can be determined through analysis of prior results for similar treatments. Age adjustments are performed using this information to shift the target refraction in a direction that is less likely to result in an enhancement. Age adjustments typically target slightly more treatment in younger patients and less treatment in older patients. The surgeon can adjust the likely outcome range by altering the targeted refraction based on information about the patient's occupation and visual needs, further reducing the likelihood of enhancements.

refractive terms, patient variables, laser room temperature and humidity, and others depending on the factors that influenced outcomes.

Figure 32-4 lists the general steps that go into the development of valid nomograms. The process is conceptually straightforward, but in practice certain steps—such as calculating cylinder vectors, grouping data, repeating regressions to detect significant variables, and calculating trailing windows—can be tedious to perform and are usually left to computer software.

Nomograms identify and quantify the factors that influence outcomes. The outcome measured is the difference between the preoperative and postoperative refractions, also known as the "achieved" amount in attempted vs achieved scatterplots. To calculate this difference, it is necessary to define the preoperative and postoperative refractions.

When creating a nomogram for a procedure based on the manifest refraction, such as standard PRK, the manifest refraction should be used as the preoperative refraction. When creating nomograms for aberrometer-guided treatments, the aberrometer-calculate refraction should be used.

In most centers, agreement of the manifest and aberrometer refraction is used as a validation criterion when accepting wavefront images, so there is usually good agreement between these two measurements. Regardless, when creating a nomogram to guide the surgeon-adjustment of wavefront-based treatments, the aberrometer refraction should be used.

As seen in Figure 32-4, the first step in creating a nomogram is to validate and standardize the data. This includes a careful evaluation of the data for possible data entry errors such as sign and decimal errors, axis errors, incomplete data, and other errors.

Calculations of refractive data should only be done at the corneal plane, so it is necessary to vertex all refractions to zero.[25] Refractions should be converted to the same cylinder notation and outliers should be eliminated. Calculation of the attempted vs achieved results is performed separately for the sphere and cylinder components of the refraction, and must be done using vector analysis.

Once the data are standardized and the attempted vs achieved amounts have been calculated, they should be separated into groups to avoid combining dissimilar eyes in one nomogram. For example, data from different lasers (even if the lasers are the same model) should be separated, myopes should be separated from hyperopes, LASIK from PRK, etc. Commonly used attributes are listed in Figure 32-4. Proper data grouping is essential to producing valid nomograms and should be performed carefully.

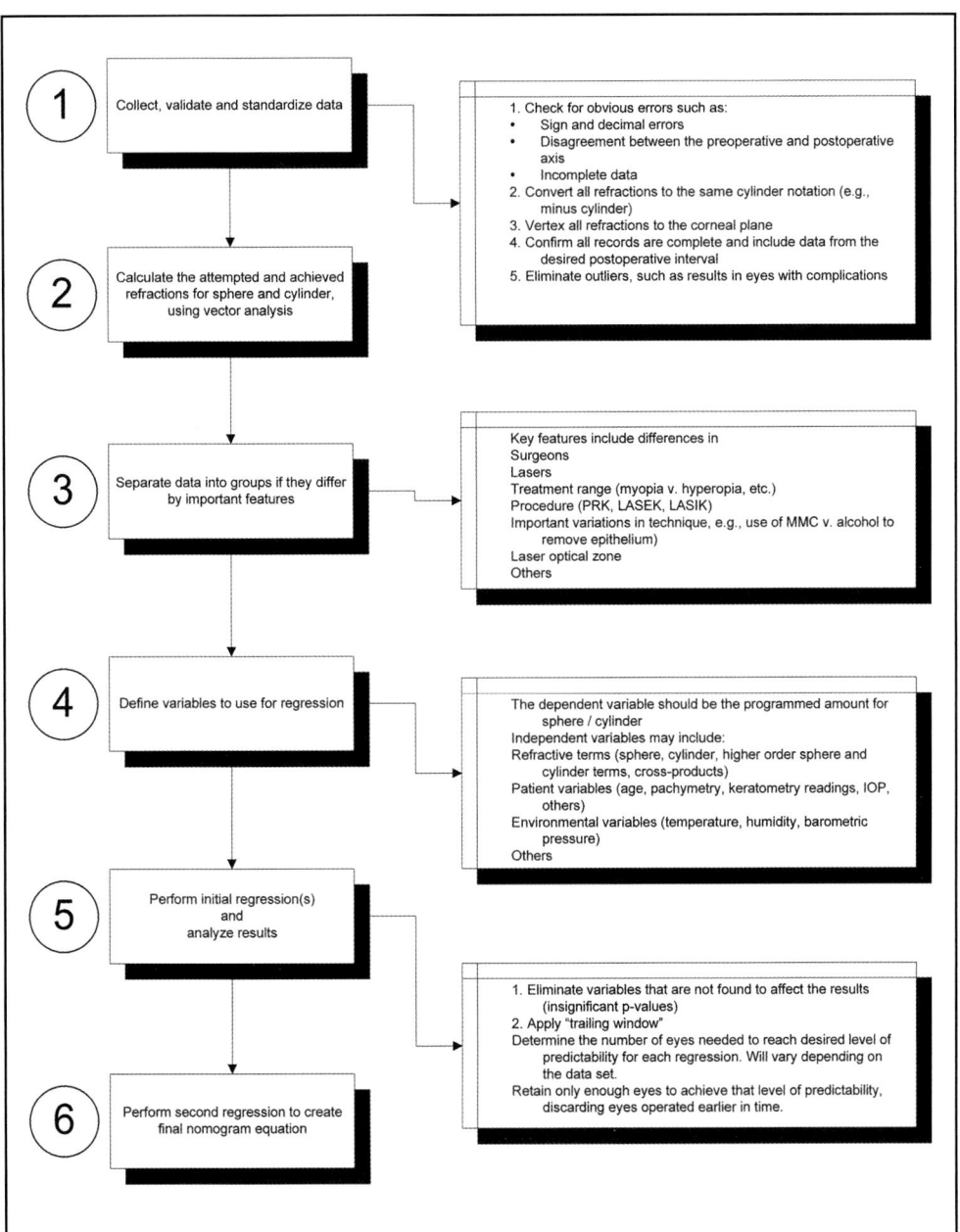

Figure 32-4. A summary of the general steps that go into the development of valid nomograms. Nomograms can be calculated manually but in practice the steps are automated using commercial software.

1. Collect, validate and standardize data
   1. Check for obvious errors such as:
      - Sign and decimal errors
      - Disagreement between the preoperative and postoperative axis
      - Incomplete data
   2. Convert all refractions to the same cylinder notation (e.g., minus cylinder)
   3. Vertex all refractions to the corneal plane
   4. Confirm all records are complete and include data from the desired postoperative interval
   5. Eliminate outliers, such as results in eyes with complications

2. Calculate the attempted and achieved refractions for sphere and cylinder, using vector analysis

3. Separate data into groups if they differ by important features
   - Key features include differences in
   - Surgeons
   - Lasers
   - Treatment range (myopia v. hyperopia, etc.)
   - Procedure (PRK, LASEK, LASIK)
   - Important variations in technique, e.g., use of MMC v. alcohol to remove epithelium
   - Laser optical zone
   - Others

4. Define variables to use for regression
   - The dependent variable should be the programmed amount for sphere / cylinder
   - Independent variables may include:
   - Refractive terms (sphere, cylinder, higher order sphere and cylinder terms, cross-products)
   - Patient variables (age, pachymetry, keratometry readings, IOP, others)
   - Environmental variables (temperature, humidity, barometric pressure)
   - Others

5. Perform initial regression(s) and analyze results
   1. Eliminate variables that are not found to affect the results (insignificant p-values)
   2. Apply "trailing window"
   Determine the number of eyes needed to reach desired level of predictability for each regression. Will vary depending on the data set.
   Retain only enough eyes to achieve that level of predictability, discarding eyes operated earlier in time.

6. Perform second regression to create final nomogram equation

Selection of the independent variables to include is a common source of confusion when creating nomograms. The goal is to include all the variables that significantly affect results and to exclude those that do not. The challenge is that the list varies from nomogram to nomogram, depending on the procedure, the laser, the surgeon, and many other factors.

All nomograms must include the achieved refractive result, expressed in sphere and cylinder components and calculated using vector analysis. Some nomograms express the refractive variables in various ways in an effort to bring out subtle influences. For example, the square and cube of the sphere and cylinder term may be incorporated, as well as reciprocals, cross-products, and other combinations. In most nomograms, the refractive terms describe most of the adjustments that are needed.

Other variables may include patient variables (eg, age, pachymetry readings, intraocular pressure [IOP], keratometry readings), laser room environmental variables, and increasingly, spherical aberration terms from the wavefront maps. The p-value for each variable is provided with the regression output and indicates whether or not the specific variables influenced outcomes. If not, the variable should be dropped from the list for that data set, and the regression repeated to produce the final nomogram.

Note that each data set will produce its own set of significant variables. This occurs because data generated from different treatment methods (eg, myopia vs hyperopia) are affected by different factors. As a result, the output from each regression must be evaluated separately in order to determine which variables apply.

Using Nomograms in Treatments Based on Aberrometer Measurements

Nomograms play a key role in planning refractive treatments, even when the treatment is based on information wavefront-measuring devices such as aberrometers. Importantly, they also provide critical information to assist in patient selection for aberrometer-based treatments.

Nomograms can be used to guide surgeon-adjustments of the treatment amount, but only if the nomogram has been based on the aberrometer refraction as described above. Using nomograms to guide surgeon adjustments results in far more accurate treatment adjustments than can be obtained by changing the treatment to match the manifest refraction because nomograms take into account factors such as coupling. Nomograms should be the primary source of information when deciding on the adjustments to the sphere and cylinder treatment amounts.

Most wavefront-guided systems limit the amount the surgeon can adjust the sphere and/or cylinder treatments. The limits prevent the use of inaccurate wavefront data. Suggested refractive adjustments that exceed system limits are an indication to convert to a standard treatment based on the manifest refraction, based on the assumption that gross errors in the sphere and/or cylinder indicate similar errors in the rest of the wavefront measurement.

Some systems do not permit the surgeon to modify the cylinder treatment amount at all. In these systems, the nomogram can be used to predict the likely cylinder outcome. For example, if the nomogram suggests treating less cylinder than the amount measured by the aberrometer, the surgeon can expect an overcorrection of the cylinder with induced astigmatism 90 degrees from the preoperative axis. Patients tolerate cylinder overcorrections poorly, so the role of the nomogram in these cases goes beyond adjusting the treatment amount and becomes a deciding factor in patient selection for aberrometer-based treatments.

Recently, algorithms have been developed to incorporate certain higher-order aberrations into the nomogram adjustments. The purpose is not to allow for adjustment of the higher-order aberrations but to improve the accuracy of the nomograms for sphere and cylinder. Commonly used terms include Z_4^0 (Z12) and Z_6^0 (Z24), both of which represent spherical aberration and are included in standard equations for calculation of refractions based on wavefront measurements.[26]

Monitoring Nomogram Effectiveness

Nomograms should be periodically evaluated for their effectiveness.

Opinions vary regarding which measures provide the best indication of nomogram effectiveness. Many argue that vision and refractive outcomes are the only objective measures. Others say that enhancement rates are more relevant because of the direct impact they have on patient satisfaction and on profits.

The objective measures, particularly refractive outcomes, are useful because they are direct measures of the effectiveness of nomograms in improving refractive predictability. However, objective results do not tell the whole story. For example, patients with plano spheroequivalent refractions may have significant astigmatism and poor vision. A 50-year-old patient with a +0.5 refraction will respond differently than a 20-year-old patient with the same refraction.

On the other hand, enhancement rates are significantly affected by subjective influences. Some surgeons offer enhancements to any patient with complaints, others reserve enhancements for refractive errors beyond a certain level. Over time, a surgeon's enhancement criteria may change.

Furthermore, enhancements tend to be a threshold phenomenon. Small errors are well tolerated, but at some point enhancements become more likely with incremental increases in residual refractive errors. For these reasons, enhancement rates serve only as indirect measures of nomogram effectiveness.

There may be a role for both approaches. Objective measures are useful to track predictability and may be of interest to surgeons, while enhancement rates may be of more interest to administrators because of their impact on patient flow and productivity.

Regardless of the metric used, it is very important to standardize the data sets in order to assure that comparisons are valid. A useful practice is to limit the analysis to eyes with preoperative refractions within a certain range such as 0 to 7.0 D spheroequivalent with 3.0 D or less astigmatism. Vision measurements should be based on eyes targeted for distance.

Enhancement rates should be calculated as the ratio of eyes operated for primary treatments vs those reoperated during a given time interval. Eyes undergoing reoperations for reasons other than refractive enhancement, such as haze removal or flap problems, should be excluded from the reoperation count. The rate should be calculated for a specific time interval, similar to the way that mortality rates are calculated in oncology. A typical measure is the "6-month enhancement rate," measured as the number of eyes undergoing refractive enhancement within 180 days from the primary treatment. Rates are often compiled on a quarterly basis.

Nomogram Implementation

The need for surgeon-specific nomograms for each procedure performed is well established. Nomograms vary widely among surgeons and lasers. Variations of ±15% for both sphere and cylinder adjustments are not uncommon from one center to another. In surface ablations, use of MMC can significantly affect nomogram adjustments as well, as was shown in Figure 32-1.

With current laser technology, 20/20 rates for low to moderate myopic treatments should be at 85% or above. Six-

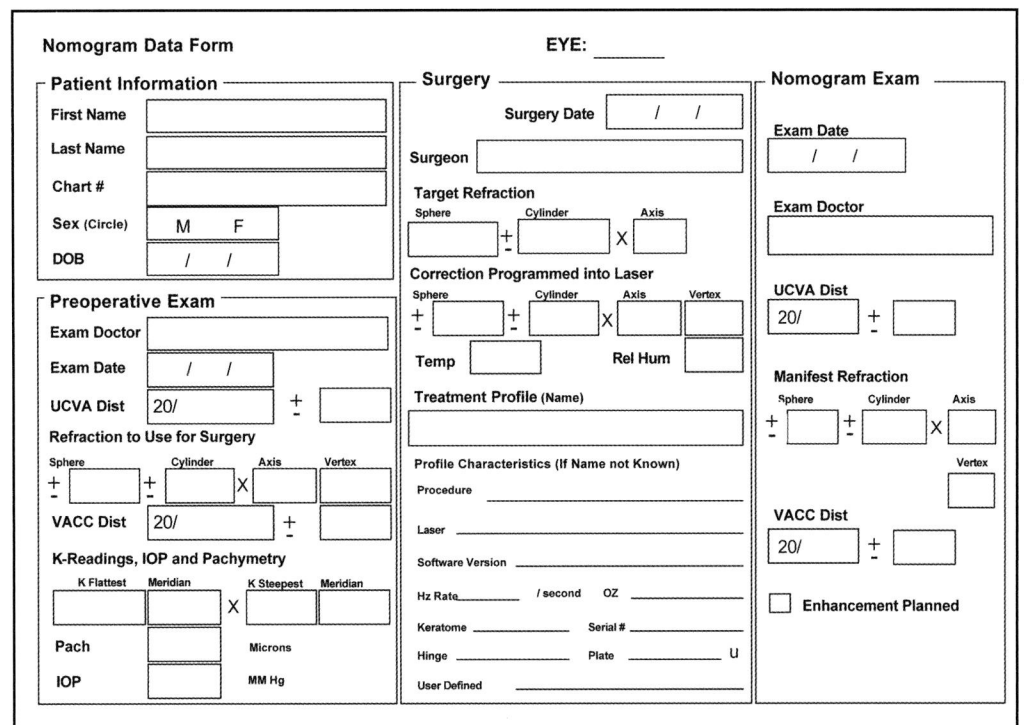

Figure 32-5. Sample data collection form listing the fields that are needed for development of nomograms and standard refractive outcomes.

month enhancement rates for eyes in this range should be rare, approximately 1%. Rates for other procedures such as hyperopia and higher levels of myopia should be commensurately low. In order to achieve these results, it is necessary to incorporate nomograms into the daily practice operations.

Valid nomograms depend on a steady flow of reliable data. Unless properly managed, this can place a significant data-entry burden on clinic personnel. With a little planning, however, the data collection process can be streamlined into the normal daily routine and with little impact on productivity.

An electronic link from the practice electronic medical record (EMR) system to the nomogram software is the easiest way to ensure the efficient transfer of data. If the practice does not have EMR, then paper forms can be used to capture data during the clinical examination for entry at weekly intervals. An example of such a form is provided in Figure 32-5. The information required for valid nomograms and outcomes analysis is not extensive; data from both eyes fits easily on one piece of paper.

In some clinics, postoperative refractions are not routinely performed in satisfied patients. This practice precludes development of valid nomograms; if the only postoperative refractive information available comes from the eyes with the worst outcomes, then the nomograms based on those data will not reflect the overall performance of the system. Data from eyes with excellent outcomes are needed as well.

Here is a pearl to ensure that accurate postoperative information is captured from all eyes: designate one postoperative examination the "nomogram visit." This practice alerts the entire staff—and the patient—to allot adequate time for the examination and to perform careful and complete examinations. As mentioned above, the 3-month exam is probably adequate for most myopic surface treatments. For hyperopic surface procedures, the refractive endpoint may not occur for 6 months, or even 1 year, following surgery. Only stable refractions should be entered into nomogram calculations.

Summary

Nomograms are necessary for every surgeon, every laser, and every procedure in laser refractive surgery. They can dramatically improve outcomes and lower enhancement rates.

Surface procedures present unique considerations to the development of valid nomograms, which must be based on stable postoperative refractions. Because refractions may not stabilize for 3 to 6 months following surface procedures, it can be challenging to obtain enough postoperative data to keep nomograms current.

The development of valid nomograms has become highly sophisticated and would not be practical without software tools. Nevertheless, it behooves the refractive surgeon to become familiar with the concepts underlying nomogram development in order to make the most effective use of them.

Nomograms offer many ancillary benefits in addition to improving surgical outcomes. They are sensitive indicators of laser stability and can be used by laser companies to monitor service needs. Nomogram data can also be used to develop quality assurance programs to monitor staff and technology performance. Marketing benefits and patient counseling are other potential uses of the information gathered in the course of nomogram development.

In the future, nomograms will become more integrated into equipment such as aberrometers, topographers, and lasers. Soon it will also be possible to link equipment directly to outcomes analysis programs. Such integration will permit surgeons and patients to anticipate the likely results of surgery before it is done and to use that information to select the right procedure for each eye. Vision simulation software will be used to demonstrate to the patient their likely outcomes with various procedures in order to assist them in selecting among different options. These applications will not be limited to laser refractive surgery but will extend to other procedures such as clear lens extractions and phakic IOLs.

References

1. Waheed S, Chalita MR, Xu M, Krueger RR. Flap-induced and laser-induced ocular aberrations in a two-step LASIK procedure. *J Refract Surg.* 2005;21(4):346-352.
2. Buzzonetti L, Iarossi G, Valente P, Volpi M, Petrocelli G, Scullica L. Comparison of wavefront aberration changes in the anterior corneal surface after laser-assisted subepithelial keratectomy and laser in situ keratomileusis: preliminary study. *J Cataract Refract Surg.* 2004;30(9):1929-1933.
3. Kriegerowski M, Bende T, Seiler T, Wollensak J. The ablation behavior of various corneal layers [Article in German]. *Fortschr Ophthalmol.* 1990;87(1):11-13.
4. Kim WS, Jo JM. Corneal hydration affects ablation during laser in situ keratomileusis surgery. *Cornea.* 2001;20(4):394-397.
5. Pallikaris IG, Ginis HS, Kounis GA, Anglos D, Papazoglou TG, Naoumidis LP. Corneal hydration monitored by laser-induced breakdown spectroscopy. *J Refract Surg.* 1998;14(6):655-660.
6. Oshika T, Klyce SD, Smolek MK, McDonald MB. Corneal hydration and central islands after excimer laser photorefractive keratectomy. *J Cataract Refract Surg.* 1998 Dec;24(12):1575-1580.
7. Dougherty PJ, Wellish KL, Maloney RK. Excimer laser ablation rate and corneal hydration. *Am J Ophthalmol.* 1994;118(2):169-176.
8. Pallikaris IG, Kalyvianaki MI, Katsanevaki VJ, Ginis HS. Epi-LASIK: preliminary clinical results of an alternative surface ablation procedure. *J Cataract Refract Surg.* 2005 May;31(5):879-885.
9. Wilson SE. Molecular cell biology for the refractive corneal surgeon: programmed cell death and wound healing. *J Refract Surg.* 1997;13(2):171-175.
10. Beuerman RW, McDonald MB, Shofner RS, Munnerlyn CR, Clapham TN, Salmeron B, Kaufman HE. Quantitative histological studies of primate corneas after excimer laser photorefractive keratectomy. *Arch Ophthalmol.* 1994;112(8):1103-1110.
11. Gambato C, Ghirlando A, Moretto E, Busato F, Midena E. Mitomycin C modulation of corneal wound healing after photorefractive keratectomy in highly myopic eyes. *Ophthalmology.* 2005;112(2):208-218; discussion 219.
12. Hashemi H, Taheri SM, Fotouhi A, Kheiltash A. Evaluation of the prophylactic use of mitomycin C to inhibit haze formation after photorefractive keratectomy in high myopia: a prospective clinical study. *BMC Ophthalmol.* 2004;4:12.
13. Carones F, Vigo L, Scandola E, Vacchini L. Evaluation of the prophylactic use of mitomycin C to inhibit haze formation after photorefractive keratectomy. *J Cataract Refract Surg.* 2002;28(12):2088-2095.
14. Schipper I, Suppelt C, Gebbers JO. Mitomycin C reduces scar formation after excimer laser (193 nm) photorefractive keratectomy in rabbits. *Eye.* 1997;11(Pt 5):649-655.
15. Durrie DS, Lesher MP, Cavanaugh TB. Classification of variable clinical response after photorefractive keratectomy for myopia. *J Refract Surg.* 1995;11(5):341-347.
16. Kim JH, Sah WJ, Kim MS, Lee YC, Park CK. Three-year results of photorefractive keratectomy for myopia. *J Refract Surg.* 1995;11(3 Suppl):S248-252.
17. Corbett MC, Verma S, O'Brart DP, Oliver KM, Heacock G, Marshall J. Effect of ablation profile on wound healing and visual performance 1 year after excimer laser photorefractive keratectomy. *Br J Ophthalmol.* 1996;80(3):224-234.
18. Doga AV, Shpak AA, Sugrobov VA. Smoothness of ablation on polymethylmethacrylate plates with four scanning excimer lasers. *J Refract Surg.* 2004;20(5 Suppl):S730-733.
19. Thomas JW, Mitra S, Chuang AZ, Yee RW. Electron microscopy of surface smoothness of porcine corneas and acrylic plates with four brands of excimer laser. *J Refract Surg.* 2003;19(6):623-628.
20. Argento C, Valenzuela G, Huck H, Cremona G, Cosentino MJ, Gale MF. Smoothness of ablation on acrylic by four different excimer lasers. *J Refract Surg.* 2001;17(1):43-45.
21. Serrao S, Lombardo M, Mondini F. Photorefractive keratectomy with and without smoothing: a bilateral study. *J Refract Surg.* 2003;19(1):58-64.
22. Huang D, Tang M, Shekhar R. Mathematical model of corneal surface smoothing after laser refractive surgery. *Am J Ophthalmol.* 2003;135(3):267-278.
23. Marques EF, Leite EB, Cunha-Vaz JG. Corticosteroids for reversal of myopic regression after photorefractive keratectomy. *J Refract Surg.* 1995;11(3 Suppl):S302-308.
24. Casebeer JC, Kezirian GM. Outcomes of spherocylinder treatments in the comprehensive refractive surgery LASIK study. *Semin Ophthalmol.* 1998;13(2):71-78.
25. Holladay JT, Moran JM, Kezirian GM. Analysis of aggregate surgically induced refractive change, prediction error, and intraocular astigmatism. *J Cataract Refract Surg.* 2001;27(1):61-79.
26. Atchison DA, Scott DH, Cox MJ. Mathematical treatment of ocular aberrations: a user's guide. In Lakshminarayanan V, ed. *Vision Science and its Applications: OSA Trends in Optics and Photonics Series* 2000;35:110-130.

SECTION VII

THE REFRACTIVE SURGERY PATIENT: AFTER SURGERY

CHAPTER 33

Cataract Extraction With Intraocular Lens Implant After Refractive Surgery

Paolo Vinciguerra, MD; Pietro Rosetta, MD; Nadia Incarnato, MD

The accuracy in determining the power of the intraocular lens (IOL) to be implanted depends on a correct evaluation of the axial length and of the corneal curvature power. The most reliable results can be achieved using a calculation formula that takes into account the measurement of the anterior chamber depth.

Axial Length Measurement

Approximately 50% of all refractive errors resulting from IOL implants are due to incorrect measurement of the axial length.[1] In acoustic biometry,[2] the traditional method in use since 1956, a probe applied by contact on the anterior corneal surface emits ultrasounds when passing through the acoustic barriers found along their way, send out echoes; the echoes' frequency helps calculate the axial length. Contact with the anterior corneal surface may cause surface trauma and has to be carried out in topical anesthesia[3]; visual axis determination is dependent on the correct alignment of the probe (Figure 33-1); the contact surface must be tangential to the corneal surface intersected by the visual axis, this is left to the operator's subjective judgment and is therefore subject to errors; a misalignment of 0.5 mm causes a postoperative refraction error of 1.4 D; the corneal applanation resulting from the probe's pressure (100 to 300 µm) and the interaction of this effect with the patient's anatomical characteristics will cause inter- and intraoperator measurements to be significantly variable[4,5] (Figure 33-2). An error of 100 µm corresponds to a postoperative refraction error of 0.28 D.[1,6]

Higher levels of accuracy and reliability in calculating the axial length can be achieved using interferometric biometry (Zeiss, Dublin, Calif) (Figure 33-3); this technique is a good alternative to traditional acoustic biometry.

Determination of the axial length is based on the interferometry of a λ 780-nm laser radiation with partial coherence light (PCI). A laser diode emits short-wavelength light that passes through a Michelson interferometer and splits into two rays (Figure 33-4). The two rays illuminate the eye and are both reflected by the cornea and retina through a semitransparent mirror. The light reflected by the cornea interferes with that reflected by the retina if the optical path of both rays is the same. The interference is captured by a photodetector. The instrument's resolution is 5 to 30 µm.[3,7-10] Optical biometry measures the distance between the light barriers represented by the anterior surface of the tear film and the pigmented retinal epithelium[11] since both the plexiform layer and the photoreceptor layer are transparent (the retinal nervous fiber layer is approximately 100 to 350 µm thick), whereas acoustic biometry measures the distance between the acoustic barriers constituted by the corneal surface and the inner limiting surface.

Additionally, through its luminous fixation aim, the optical biometer performs the biometric measurement on the visual axis, achieving accurate alignment independent of the operator; this is especially beneficial when a significant myopic staphyloma is present. In order to achieve fixation even with a high refractive defect (>6 D), the biometric exam can be carried out with the patient wearing glasses; because no contact with the corneal surface is required, this investigation is noninvasive, thus reducing the transmission of infections[9] from patient to patient and the risk of causing iatrogenic corneal lesions. Also, the use of a noncontact method eliminates the risk of inaccurate measurements due to indentations caused by the ultrasound probe's pressure on the corneal surface. Lastly, the value is not affected by defocused measurement aim (Table 33-1). The introduction of phacoemulsification and the need to reduce the extent

Figure 33-1. Ultrasonic probe: Alignment.

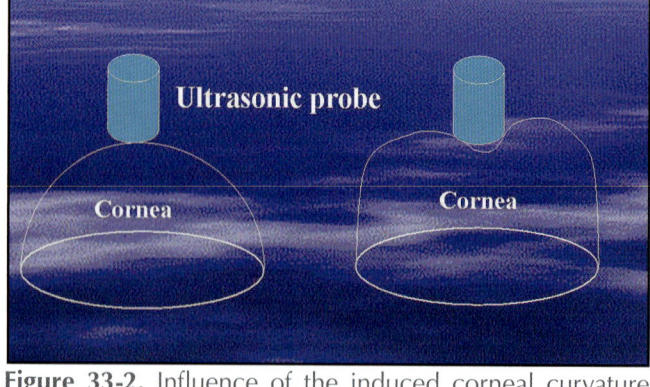

Figure 33-2. Influence of the induced corneal curvature change.

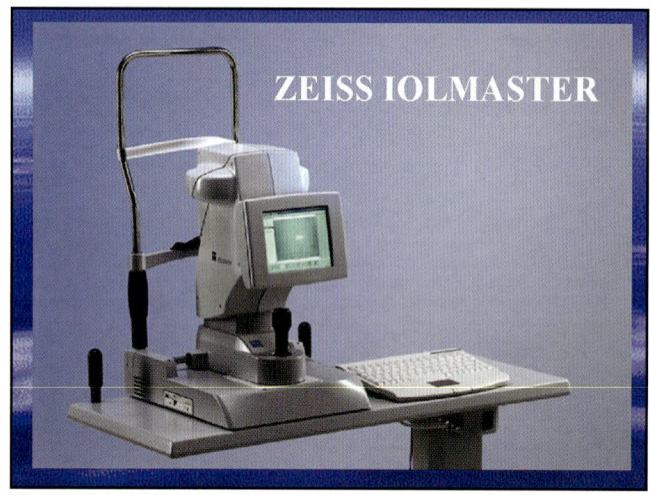

Figure 33-3. Zeiss IOLMaster.

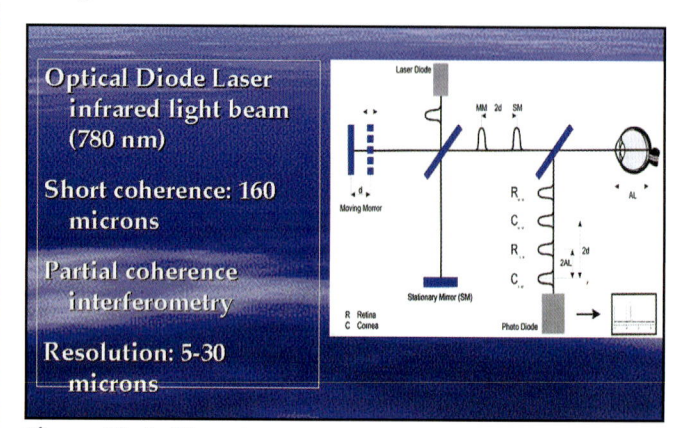

Figure 33-4. Biometry.

Table 33-1

ACOUSTIC BIOMETRY VS OPTICAL BIOMETRY

Acoustic Biometry	Optical Biometry
Contact	Noncontact
Infection transfer	No infection transfer
Topical anesthesia	No local anesthesia
Time consuming	Measurement in 0.4 seconds
Less user friendly	User friendly
Less patient friendly	Patient friendly
Segment measurements possible	No segment measurements possible
Adjustment is critical	Defocus uncritical
No patient cooperation is necessary	Minimum transparency and cooperation necessary

of surgical aggression and complications using the smallest possible amount of ultrasounds have accelerated the indication for this procedure. Therefore, the decreasing frequency of highly developed cataracts reduces the limits of optical biometry (ie, the conditions limiting patient fixation, such as total lens opacity [hypermature cataract]; nystagmus; severe maculopathy or vitreal hemorrhage; retinal detachment; or physical limitations such as tremor, respiratory problems, or patient immobility).[9,12,13]

The comparison between expected refraction and the refraction achieved after IOL implant, calculated by acoustic biometry on 2000 eyes, showed an average difference of +0.21 D with a range between -0.38 D and +0.6 D. The same comparison between values measured by optical biometry gave an average difference of +0.07 D.

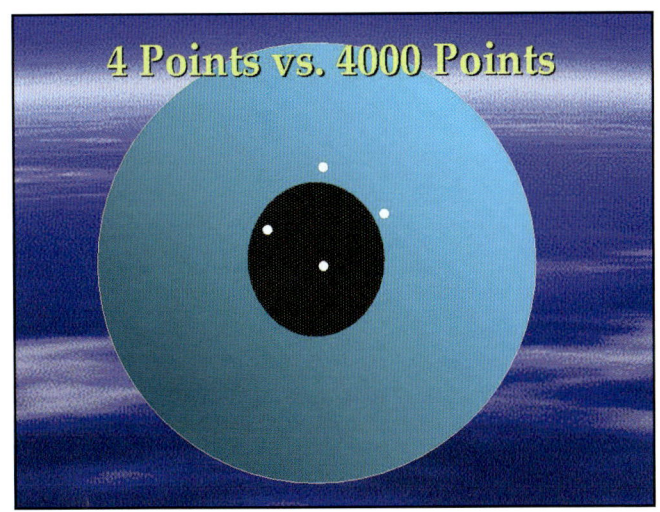

Figure 33-5. 4 points vs. 4000 points.

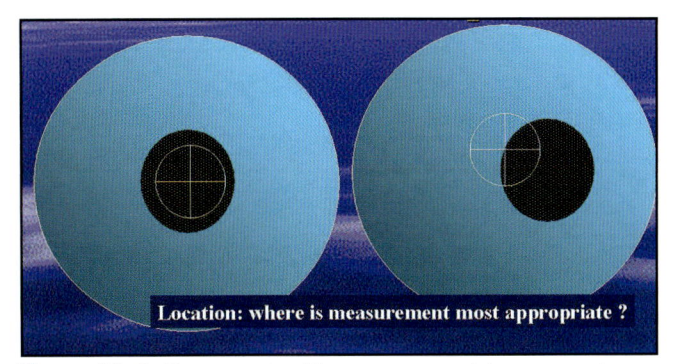

Figure 33-6. Keratometry (4 measurements) vs mean topographic pupil power (4000 real data points).

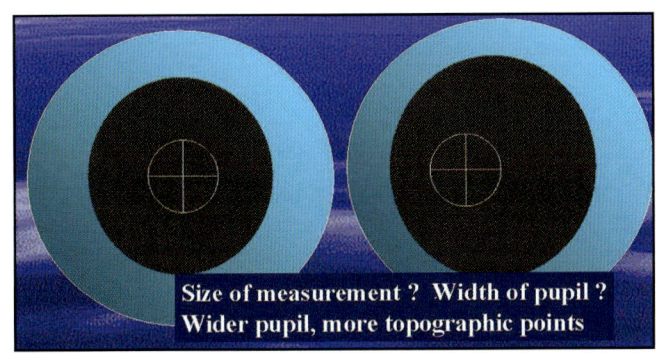

Figure 33-7. Keratometry (4 measurements) vs mean topographic pupil power (4000 real data points).

Measurement of the Anterior Chamber Depth

The average depth of the anterior chamber in the general population is 3.5 mm[14] and may range between 2 mm in hypothalamic patients (high hypermetropia, plateau iris) and 4.50 mm in patients with keratoconus. This variability plays an important role in impacting the reliability of the main calculation formulas, most of which do not take this factor into account. This is why it is recommended to use formulas requiring the preoperative measurement of anterior chamber depth[15] (eg, the Haigis formula). Optical biometry allows for this measurement; the eye is illuminated through a slit to produce an optical cross section; a charge-coupled device (CCD) camera records images of the anterior surface of the cornea and natural lens. The distance between optical cross sections is evaluated as the measurement of the anterior chamber depth. In a recent study, which compared different instruments for the measurement of this data, including AC-Master (Zeiss), Pentacam (Oculus, Lynnwood, Wash), and Jaeger slit-lamp pachymeter (Haag-Streit, Mason, Ohio), the results provided no evidence of significant differences.[16,17]

Measurement of the Corneal Curvature Power

The cornea's refractive power represents approximately 78% (about 45.0 D) of the eye's overall diopter power, with the natural lens accounting for the remaining 22% (approximately 13.0 D).[18] Clearly, an accurate evaluation of this information is key to obtaining the desired refraction when determining the IOL to be implanted. A 1.0 D error in assessing the average corneal power will lead to an IOL miscalculation of approximately 1.0 D; the extent of the evaluation error is significantly higher if the curvature of the corneal surface is markedly uneven. The number of points examined, the overall surface analyzed, and the relationship between the surface and the pupil area play a critical role.

Keratometry according to Javal is based on the measurement of the corneal curvature in four paracentral points, whose reference surface is very small, identified relative to the cornea's geometric center rather than to the point intersected by the visual axis (Figure 33-5). If there is a misalignment of the visual axis relative to the geometric center or the pupil center, the measurement's reliability is low (Figure 33-6).

In the case of large pupil diameters, the small size of the surface analyzed from the four points will only provide limited data assessment, unreliable if the pupil field curvature is uneven or decentered (Figure 33-7).

Often the presence of tear film supernatant, not detectable by the operator, reduces measurement reliability; also, because of the small number of points examined and the distance between them, an accurate measurement can only be obtained if the curvature is essentially even. Conversely, corneal topography on a patient with a 3.5-mm pupil involves the processing and analysis of some 4000 points, for the optical zone alone. In performing the topographic exam, the patient's fixation is obtained by identifying his or her visual axis; through this it is possible to evaluate the quality of the keratoscopic projection and verify the presence of any artifacts before processing the data, and it is possible to identify the visual axis centering on the pupil field. With corneal topography we can also measure the pupil diameter and assess its horizontal as well as vertical decentration.

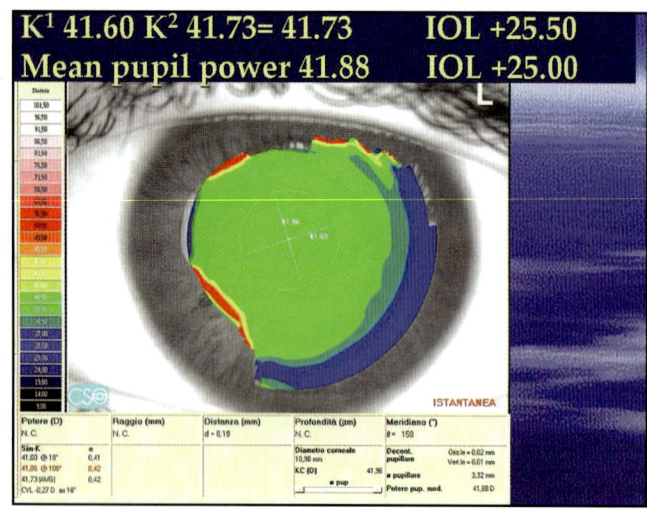

Figure 33-8. Emmetropia with IOL implant whose value was obtained using the average pupillary power. -0.5 D difference compared to the calculation made using keratometric values measured with Javal's keratometer.

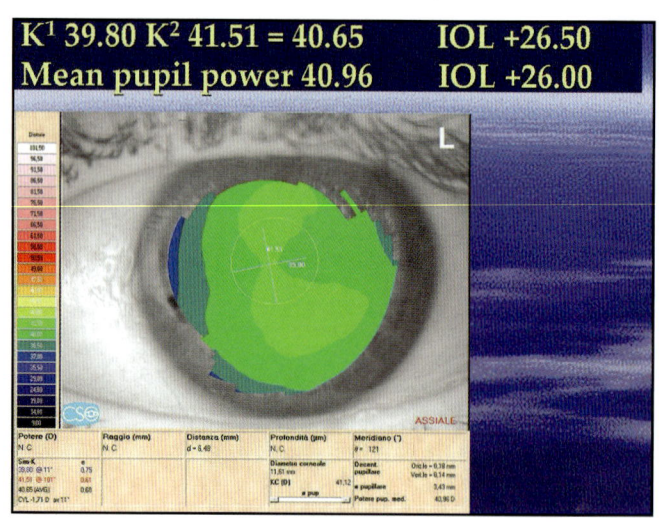

Figure 33-9. Emmetropia with IOL implant whose value was obtained using the average pupillary power. -0.5 D difference compared to the calculation made using keratometric values measured with Javal's keratometer (continued).

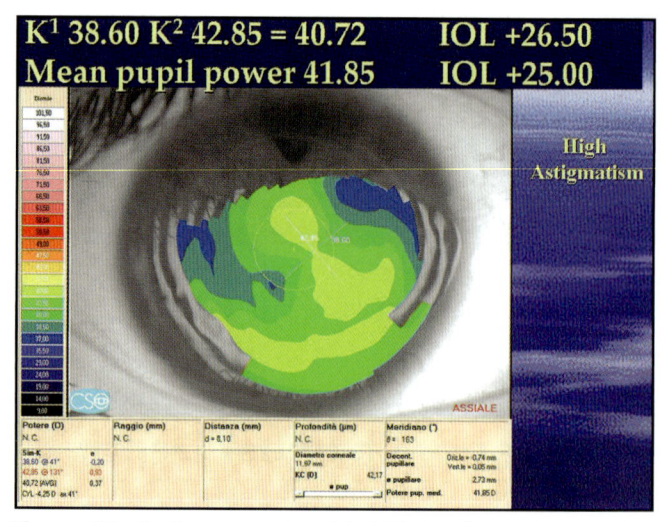

Additionally, the calculation is base on average pupillary power on the exact surface corresponding to the pupil. An increasing number of patients are treated with cataract surgery after refractive surgery. The cataract surgery performed in this case requires a special biometric evaluation.

Normal Condition

When the corneal curvature is essentially even, the difference between the IOL biometric calculation based on keratometry according to Javal and that obtained using the average pupillary power measured with corneal topography is fairly small (Figures 33-8 and 33-9).

It is important to note that in cataract surgery the desired refractive result can only be achieved through accurate selection of the IOL to be implanted and if the IOL positioning during the procedure is compliant with the biometric ratios of the natural lens. This principle is especially important in the case of eyes with short axial lengths: if the goal is postoperative emmetropia, a 1-mm IOL misplacement anteroposteriorly to the visual axis, in an eye with axial length of 20 mm, will cause a refractive error of 1.9 D.

Astigmatism

High astigmatism, high central corneal curvature, or irregular astigmatism results in a significant difference between the arithmetic average of the two keratometric values obtained using Javal's keratometer and the average corneal power derived from the topographic analysis of the corneal points corresponding to the pupil field. If the corneal curvature is high, with a markedly higher curvature peak at the apex, corresponding to the optical zone, the average pupillary power obtained using topography will be greater than the value measured with keratometry, and as a result the value of the IOL to be implanted will differ (Figures 33-10 through 33-12).

Figure 33-10. Emmetropia with IOL implant whose value was obtained using the average pupillary power. -1.5 D difference compared to the calculation made using keratometric values measured with Javal's keratometer.

Uneven Surface

Any surface unevenness due to scar revisions of the corneal stroma or pterygium cause this discrepancy in calculation to increase, to the detriment of accuracy. The greater number of points examined by the topograph better reflects the pupillary refractive power and the overall corneal morphology: consequently, the average pupillary power is more accurate even in the presence of marked surface unevenness (Figures 33-13 through 33-15).

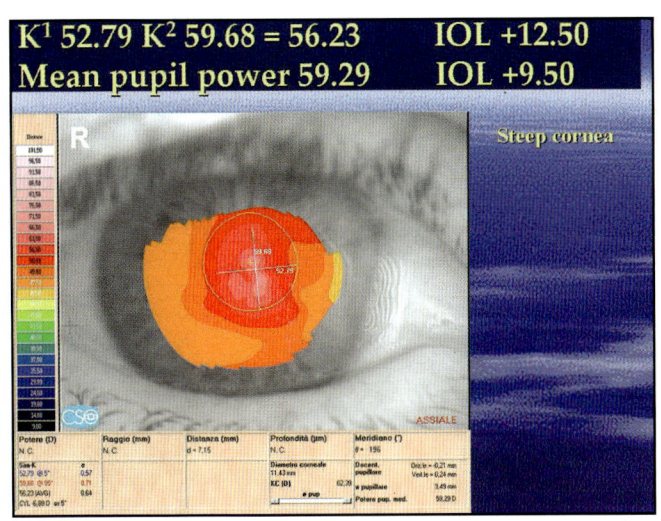

Figure 33-11. Emmetropia with IOL implant whose value was obtained using the average pupillary power. -3.0 D difference compared to the calculation made using keratometric values measured with Javal's keratometer.

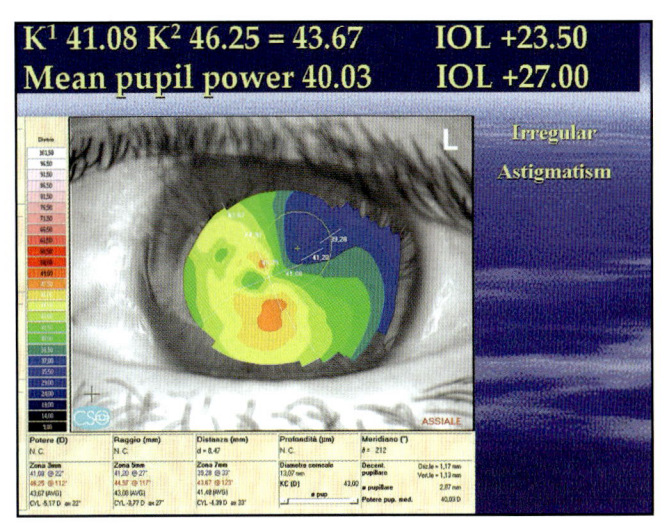

Figure 33-12. Emmetropia with IOL implant whose value was obtained using the average pupillary power. +3.5 D difference compared to the calculation made using keratometric values measured with Javal's keratometer.

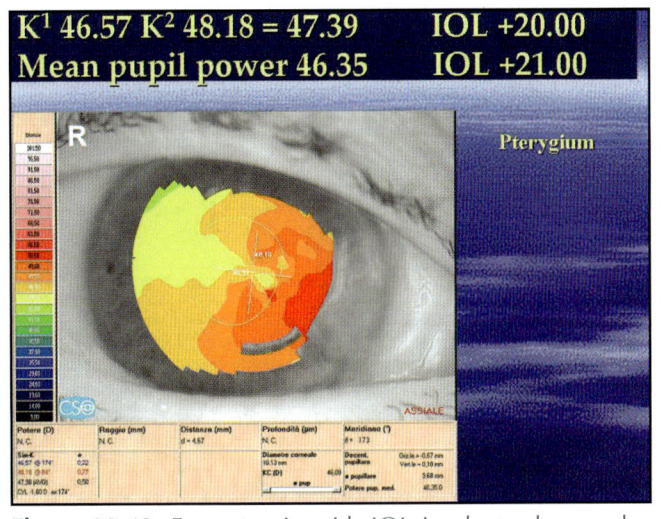

Figure 33-13. Emmetropia with IOL implant whose value was obtained using the average pupillary power. +1.0 D difference compared to the calculation made using keratometric values measured with Javal's keratometer.

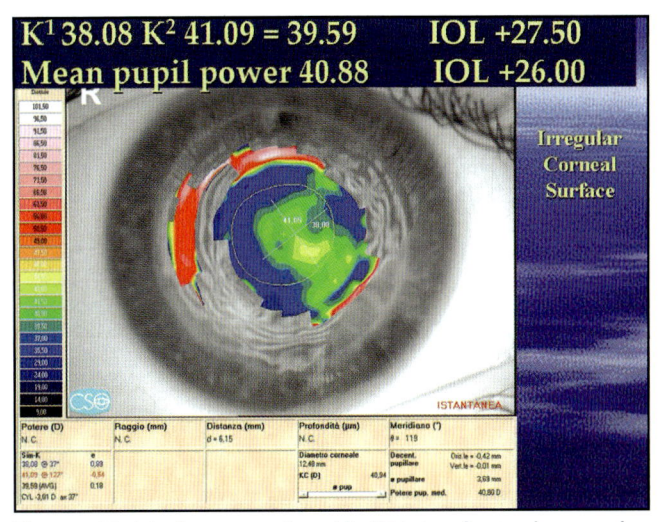

Figure 33-14. Emmetropia with IOL implant whose value was obtained using the average pupillary power. -1.5 D difference compared to the calculation made using keratometric values measured with Javal's keratometer.

IOL Implant in Patients With Ectatic Conditions Treated With Refractive Surgery

In the case of ectatic conditions, such as keratoconus or pellucid marginal degeneration (Figures 33-16 through 33-19), the geography of the hyperrefractive corneal surface, its diameter, and its ratio to the visual axis make it particularly difficult to measure the corneal curvature in order to determine the IOL to be implanted. In this case the average topographic pupillary power differs significantly, although it should be noted that, due to considerable surface unevenness and resulting optical aberrations, no guarantee can be offered as to refractive results. If the curvature at the apex corresponding to the optical zone is much higher than the rest of the corneal surface, keratometry may yield strongly diverging results (in this case, lower values) compared to the average pupillary value measured with the topograph.

A separate set of considerations should be made for corneal surfaces that were photoablated to treat a myopic defect. In this case the ablation profile characterized by central flattening and a transition area is an obstacle to the proper application of the ultrasound biometer probe, thus preventing the measurement to be performed at the central corneal portion, intersected by the optical axis, which has become thinner after the treatment (Figure 33-20). In addition to the biometric error (if ultrasound biometry is used), there will also be a significant difference between topographic average pupillary

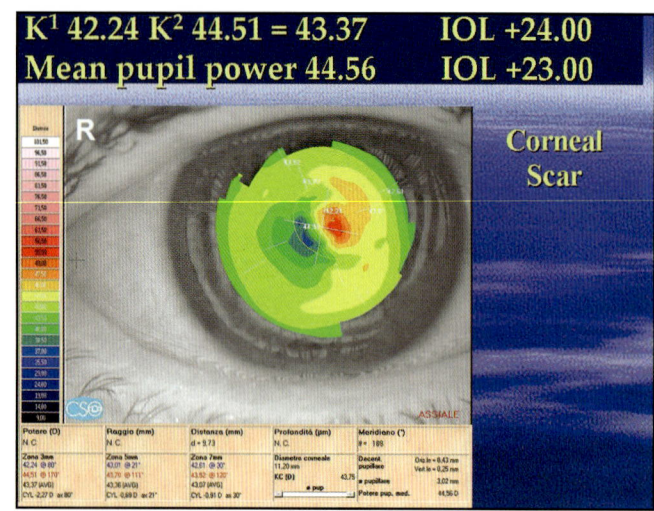

Figure 33-15. Emmetropia with IOL implant whose value was obtained using the average pupillary power. -1.0 D difference compared to the calculation made using keratometric values measured with Javal's keratometer.

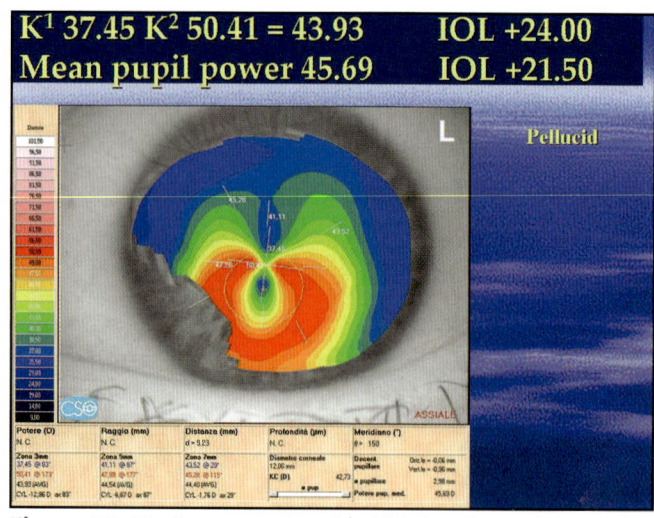

Figure 33-16. Emmetropia with IOL implant whose value was obtained using the average pupillary power. -2.5 D difference compared to the calculation made using keratometric values measured with Javal's keratometer.

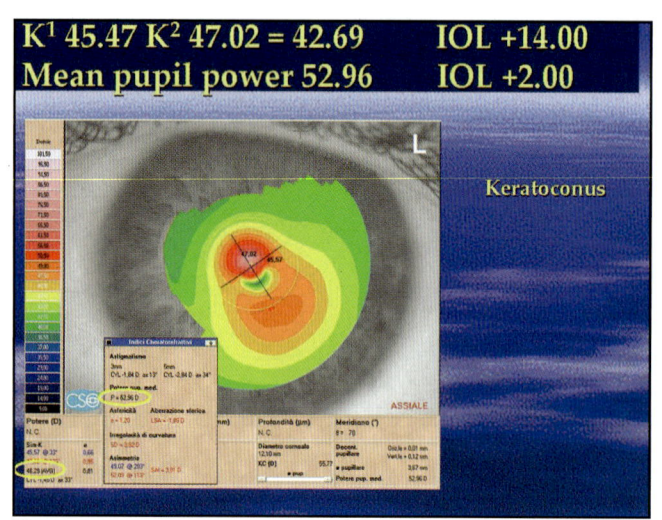

Figure 33-17. Emmetropia with IOL implant whose value was obtained using the average pupillary power. -12.0 D difference compared to the calculation made using keratometric values measured with Javal's keratometer.

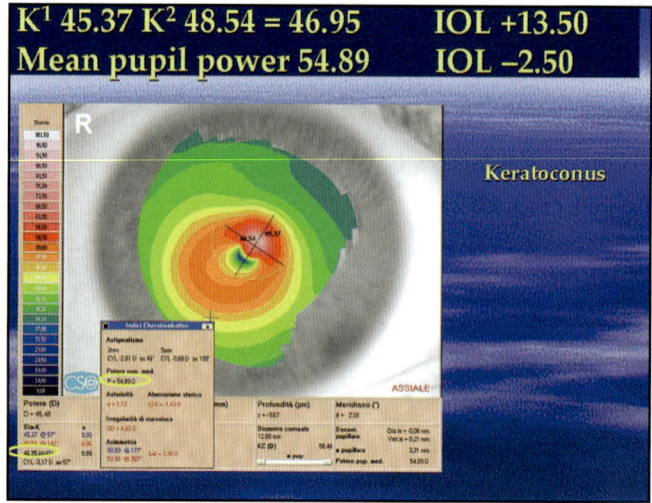

Figure 33-18. Emmetropia with IOL implant whose value was obtained using the average pupillary power. -16.0 D difference compared to the calculation made using keratometric values measured with Javal's keratometer.

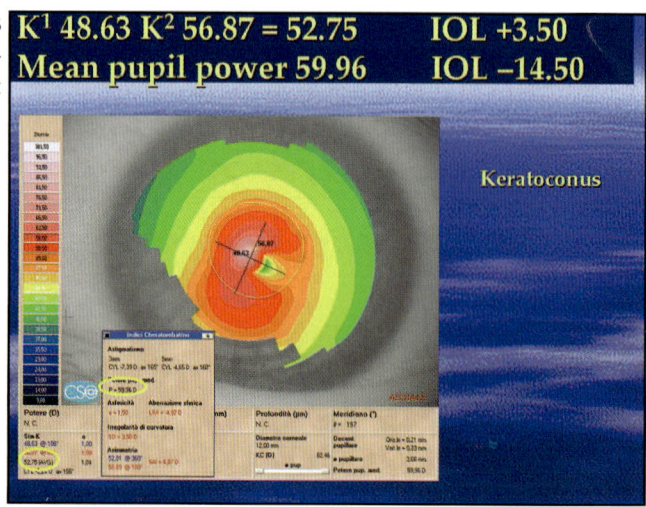

Figure 33-19. Emmetropia with IOL implant whose value was obtained using the average pupillary power. -18.0 D difference compared to the calculation made using keratometric values measured with Javal's keratometer.

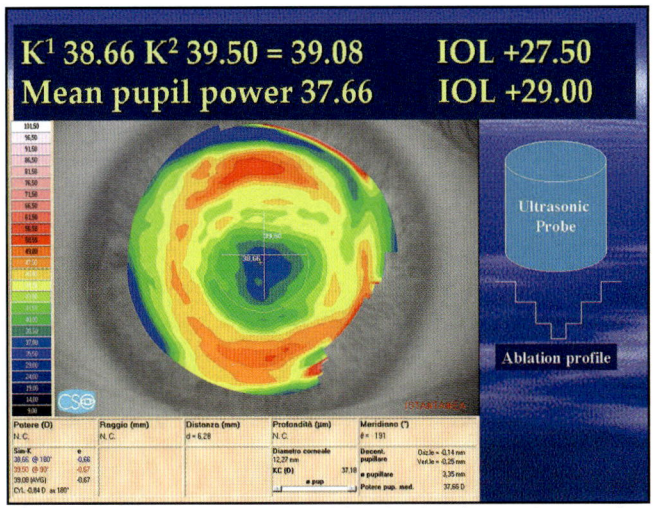

Figure 33-20. Emmetropia with IOL implant whose value was obtained using the average pupillary power. +1.5 D difference compared to the calculation made using keratometric values measured with Javal's keratometer.

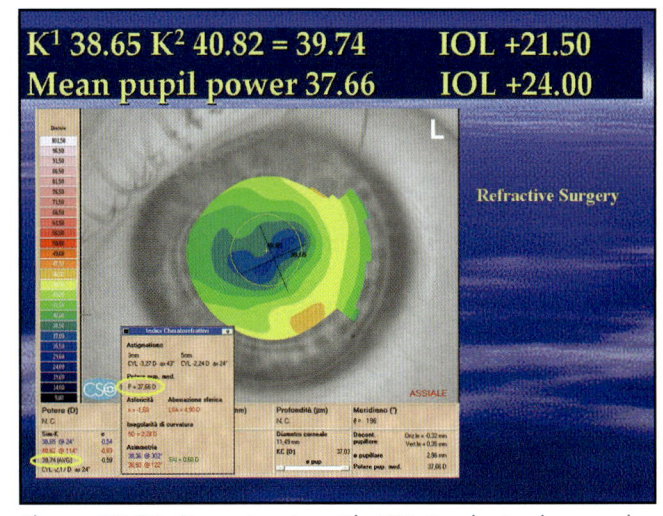

Figure 33-21. Emmetropia with IOL implant whose value was obtained using the average pupillary power. +2.5 D difference compared to the calculation made using keratometric values measured with Javal's keratometer.

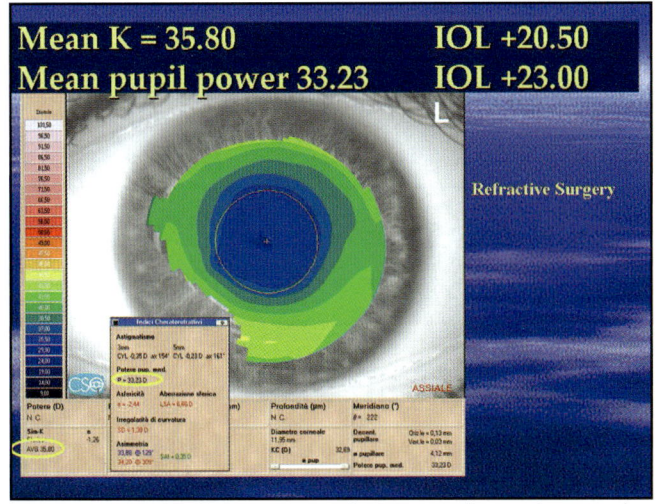

Figure 33-22. Emmetropia with IOL implant whose value was obtained using the average pupillary power. +2.5 D difference compared to the calculation made using keratometric values measured with Javal's keratometer.

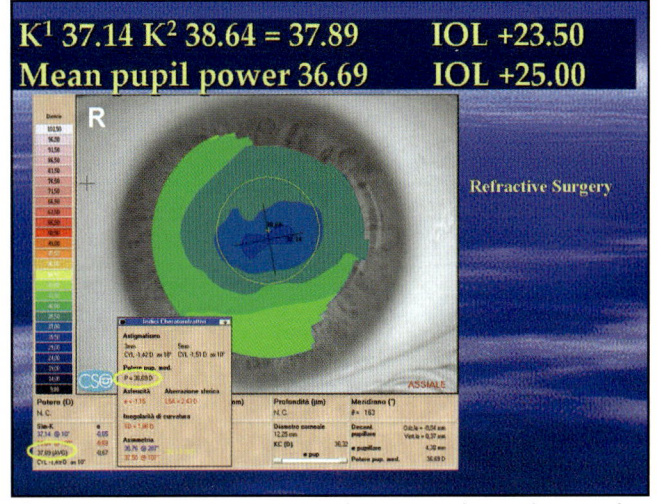

Figure 33-23. Emmetropia with IOL implant whose value was obtained using the average pupillary power. +1.5 D difference compared to the calculation made using keratometric values measured with Javal's keratometer.

power and keratometry, which is negatively impacted by the treatment diameter, centration, and refractive gradient at the transition area (Figures 33-21 through 33-25). For treatments with small-diameter optical zones, the average of the two keratometric values is higher than the average pupillary power determined with the topograph, due to the presence of a low-pupillary power optical zone. This also occurs in the case of substantially spherical corneas after refractive treatment or in treatments where the transition area is very wide, because the high number of points processed by the topograph ensures a more accurate evaluation of the total corneal curvature.

Currently, several solutions are suggested for biometric calculation, including the clinical history method; the contact lens method,[19] developed by Dr. Holladay; or the use of dedicated biometric formulas: Haigis-L, useful after a laser-assisted in situ keratomileusis (LASIK)/photorefractive keratectomy (PRK) procedure, does not require any knowledge of pre-LASIK refractive data or the Italian Camellin-Calossi formula (CSO),[20] which takes into account not only axial length and anterior chamber depth, but also type of keratorefractive surgery (incisional or lamellar), number of diopters treated, average postsurgery pupillary power, and thickness of the natural lens.[21-27]

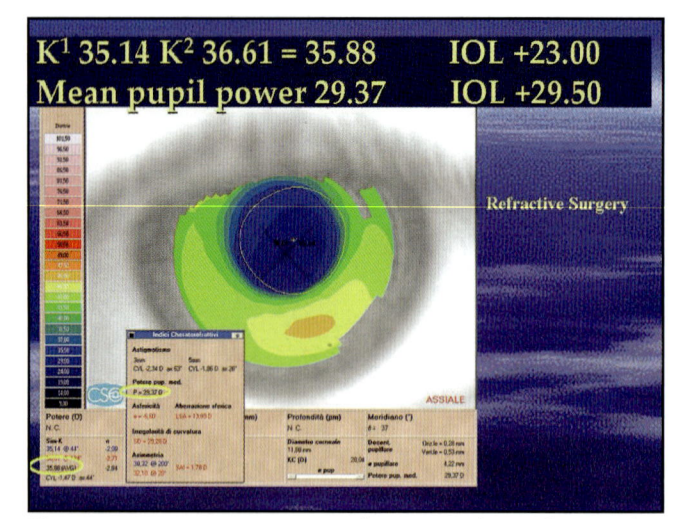

Figure 33-24. Emmetropia with IOL implant whose value was obtained using the average pupillary power. +6.5 D difference compared to the calculation made using keratometric values measured with Javal's keratometer.

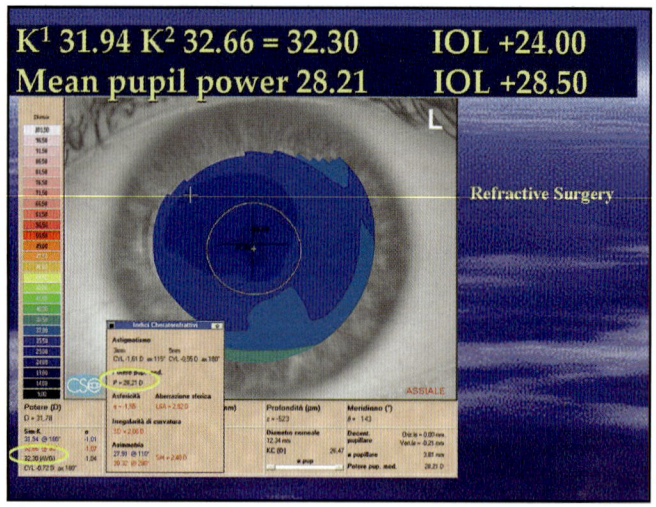

Figure 33-25. Emmetropia with IOL implant whose value was obtained using the average pupillary power. +4.5 D difference compared to the calculation made using keratometric values measured with Javal's keratometer.

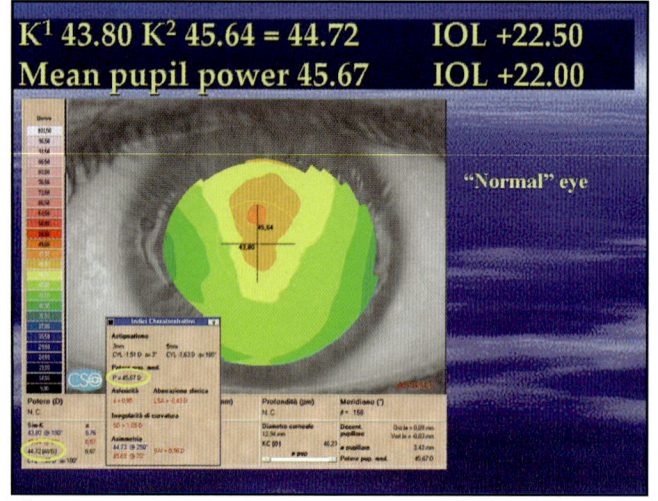

Figure 33-26. Emmetropia with IOL implant whose value was obtained using the average pupillary power. -0.5 D difference compared to the calculation made using keratometric values measured with Javal's keratometer.

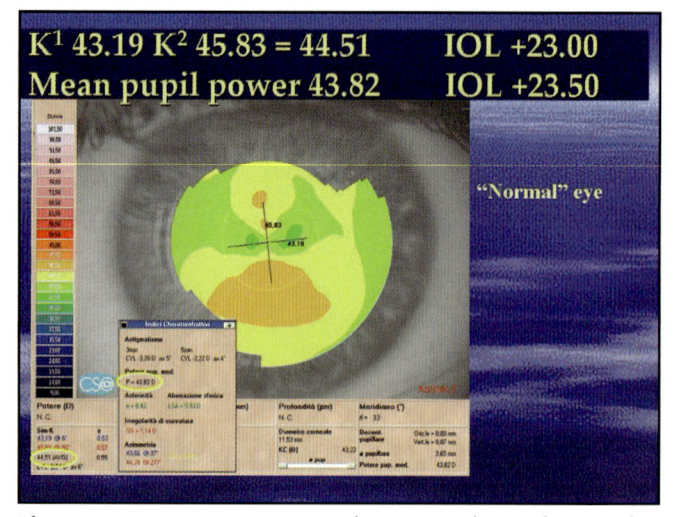

Figure 33-27. Emmetropia with IOL implant whose value was obtained using the average pupillary power. +0.5 D difference compared to the calculation made using keratometric values measured with Javal's keratometer.

Normal-Looking Eyes

There is also the possibility that normal-looking corneas, when examined with the slit-lamp equipment, exhibit a small amount of surface unevenness that causes measurement errors when assessed with Javal's keratometer, and therefore inaccuracies in IOL determination. Such unevenness, however, is detected by the topograph, providing a more accurate measurement of the average pupillary power and consequently a more accurate postoperative refractive result.

This is even more important when pseudoaccommodative IOLs are implanted: in this case, the accurate determination of the IOL to be implanted is crucial to ensure good natural visual acuity for close distances, and a small error in determining the IOL power may nullify the purpose for which these lenses were created (Figures 33-26 through 33-29).

In conclusion, an accurate determination of the IOL power in general, and particularly in the presence of abnormal corneal morphology, is a function of biometric accuracy, which must take into account the anterior chamber depth and must include the calculation of the corneal pupillary power, as obtained from a topographic analysis of the pupil area. The methods described in this chapter provide repeatable intra- and interoperator results; they are noninvasive, and, in cases of more severe unevenness of the corneal surface, they can be used to predict and limit any errors affecting the refractive result.

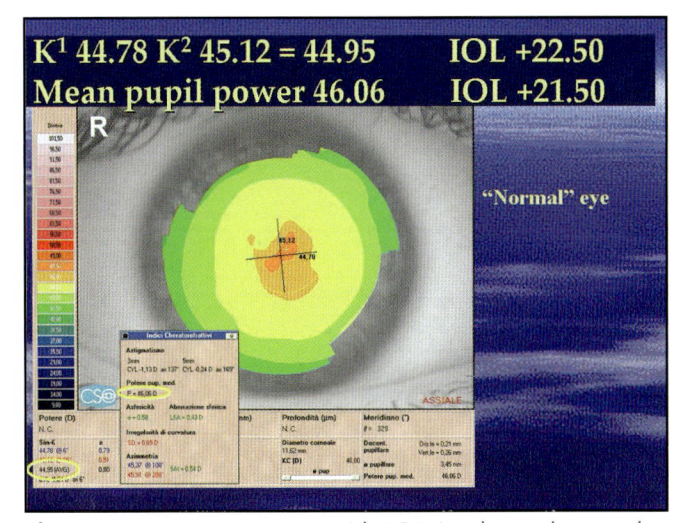

Figure 33-28. Emmetropia with IOL implant whose value was obtained using the average pupillary power. -1.0 D difference compared to the calculation made using keratometric values measured with Javal's keratometer.

Figure 33-29. Emmetropia with IOL implant whose value was obtained using the average pupillary power. -1.0 D difference compared to the calculation made using keratometric values measured with Javal's keratometer.

References

1. Olsen T. Sources of error in intraocular lens power calculation. *J Cataract Refract Surg*. 1992;18:125.
2. Mundt GH, Hughes WF. Ultrasonics in ocular diagnosis. *Am J Ophthalmol*. 1956;41:488.
3. Drexler W, Findl O, Menapace R, et al. Partial coherence interferometry: a novel approach to biometry in cataract surgery. *Am J Ophthalmol*. 1998;126:524.
4. Lackner B, Schmidinger G, Skorpik C. Validity and repeatability of anterior chamber depth measurements with pentacam and orbscan. *Optom Vis Sci*. 2005;82(9):858-861.
5. Goel S, Chua C, Butcher M, Jones CA, Bagga P, Kotta S. Laser vs ultrasound biometry—a study of intra- and interobserver variability. *Eye*. 2004;18(5):514-518.
6. Olsen T. Theoretical approach to intraocular lens calculation using Gaussian optics. *J Cataract Refract Surg*. 1987;13:141.
7. Haigis W, Lege B, Miller N, Schneider B. Optishe biometrie und IOL-Berechnung 97. *Tagung der Deutschen Ophthalmologischen Gesellschaft*. 1999.
8. Haigis W, Lege B. Optical and acoustical biometry. *ASCRS*. 1999.
9. Hitzenberger CK, Drexler W, Dolezal C, et al. Measurement of the axial length of cataract eyes by laser doppler interferometry. *Invest Ophthalmol Vis Sci*. 1993;6:1886.
10. Schmid GF, Papastergiou GI, Nickla DL, et al. Validation of laser Doppler interferopometry measurements in vivo of axial eye length and thickness of fundus layers in chicks. *Curr Eye Res*. 1996;15(6):691.
11. Haigis W, Lege B Ultraschallbiometrie und optische. *Biometrie: Erweiterung der Moglichkeiten Ophthalmologische Nachrichten*. 1999;S18.
12. Lege B, Haigis W. Optical biometry, first clinical experiences. *ASCRS*. 1999.
13. Hitzenberger CK. Optical measurement of the axial eye length by laser Doppler interferometry. *Invest Ophthalmol Vis Sci*. 1991;3:616.
14. Vogel A, Dick HB, Krummenauer F. Reproducibility of optical biometry using partial coherence interferometry: intraobserver and interobserver reliability. *J Cataract Refract Surg*. 2001;27(12):1961-1968.
15. Findl O, Drexler W, Menapace R, Hitzenberger CK, Fercher AF. High precision biometry of pseudophakic eyes using partial coherence interferometry. *J Cataract Refract Surg*. 1998;24:1087.
16. Meinhardt B, Stachs O, Stave J, Beck R, Guthoff R. Evaluation of biometric methods for measuring the anterior chamber depth in the non-contact mode. *Graefes Arch Clin Exp Ophthalmol*. 2005;15:1-6.
17. Lege BA, Haigis W. Laser interference biometry versus ultrasound biometry in certain clinical conditions. *Graefes Arch Clin Exp Ophthalmol*. 2004;242(1):8-12.
18. Saude T. The internal ocular media. In: *Ocular Anatomy and Physiology*. Oxford, UK: Blackwell Scientific. 1993;36-52.
19. Haigis W. Corneal power after refractive surgery for myopia: contact lens method. *J Cataract Refract Surg*. 2003;29(7):1397-1411.
20. Camellin M. Proposed formula for the dioptric power evaluation of the posterior corneal surface. *Refract Corneal Surg*. 1990;6(4):261-264.
21. Argento C, Cosentino MJ, Badoza D. Intraocular lens power calculation after refractive surgery. *J Cataract Refract Surg*. 2003;29(7):1346-1351.
22. Hoffer KJ. Intraocular lens power calculation for eyes after refractive keratotomy. *J Refract Surg*. 1995;11(6):490-493.
23. Kim JH, Lee DH, Joo CK. Measuring corneal power for intraocular lens power calculation after refractive surgery. Comparison of methods. *J Cataract Refract Surg*. 2002;28(11):1932-1938.
24. Randleman JB, Loupe DN, Song CD, Waring GO 3rd, Stulting RD. Intraocular lens power calculations after laser in situ keratomileusis. *Cornea*. 2002;21(8):751-755.
25. Seitz B, Langenbucher A. Intraocular lens calculations status after corneal refractive surgery. *Curr Opin Ophthalmol*. 2000;11(1):35-46. Review.
26. Latkany RA, Chokshi AR, Speaker MG, Abramson J, Soloway BD, Yu G. Intraocular lens calculations after refractive surgery. *J Cataract Refract Surg*. 2005;31(3):562-570.
27. Wang L, Booth MA, Koch DD. Comparison of intraocular lens power calculation methods in eyes that have undergone LASIK. *Ophthalmology*. 2004;111(10):1825-1831.

CHAPTER 34

Pharmacological Modulation of Corneal Wound Healing After Surface Ablation

Edoardo Midena, MD; Catia Gambato, MD; Alessandra Ghirlando, MD

Introduction

The physiologic process of wound healing has been described as a complex sequence of events that normally contributes to wound repair and to re-establish normal function. Biologic diversity in corneal wound healing response is a major factor in the outcome of all keratorefractive surgical procedures. It is an important determinant of overcorrection, undercorrection, regression, and other complications, such as haze and refractive instability, which occur with photorefractive keratectomy (PRK), laser-assisted subepithelial keratomileusis (LASEK), and laser-assisted in situ keratomileusis (LASIK) used in the treatment of myopia, hyperopia, or astigmatism.[1-4] In fact, these adverse events have partly been attributed to qualitative or quantitative variations in corneal keratocytes and their subsequent effects on corneal wound healing. Studies on corneal wound healing after PRK have shown epithelial hyperplasia and scarring by atypical glycosaminoglycans.[5-10] All these changes may influence refractive outcome and impair the transparency of the cornea. Variation in wound healing response of individual eyes cannot be entirely controlled, but it may be influenced by topical drugs.[11] Various drugs, such as corticosteroids, nonsteroidal anti-inflammatory agents (NSAIDs), interferon, plasmin and plasminogen activator inhibitors, collagenase inhibitors, vitamins, and antimetabolites, have been proposed for the modulation of the healing response after refractive surgery, frequently with poor or controversial results.[12-18] An objective evaluation of the changes of corneal epithelium and stroma may enhance our understanding of corneal wound healing process. Due to noninvasive optical sectioning ability, *in vivo* confocal microscopy is ideally suited for dynamic evaluation of corneal wound healing in three dimensions. Using this form of *in vivo* microscopy, high-resolution en face images can be obtained in real time from different layers within the intact living cornea without the need for staining or processing. Corneal confocal microscopy enables direct visualization of temporal changes in corneal wound healing in the same living eye at a high level of magnification (Figure 34-1). Cellular responses and structural changes can be correlated directly and sequentially over time to clinical observations.[19-32]

Corneal Wound Healing

The corneal wound healing response is a remarkably complex cascade mediated by cytokines, growth factors, and chemokines. Epithelial-stromal-neural-lacrimal gland-immune cellular interactions are interwoven in the corneal response to injury. The interactions between these cells orchestrate the corneal wound healing response and contribute to the maintenance and restoration of corneal anatomy and function.[1,3-6]

Like all squamous epithelium, the corneal epithelium is self-renewing, with epithelial cell turning over in approximately 5 to 7 days. Peripheral epithelium contains basal cells with *in vitro* higher proliferative capacity than central epithelium, which contributes to the gradual centripetal motion of epithelial cells during their maturation progress. Nevertheless, immediately after epithelial injury the wounded epithelium not only heals by migration, mitosis, and differentiation, but it contributes to healing process through the release of multiple cytokines and growth factors, such as interleukin (IL)-1, tumor necrosis factor (TNF) α, bone morphogenic proteins 2 and 4 (BMB), epidermal growth factor (EGF), and platelet-derived growth factor (PDGF). Release of collagenases, metalloproteinases, and other enzymes is also important. Impaired epithelial mechanical barrier function

Figure 34-1. Preoperative corneal confocal microscopy findings of the corneal layers (CS4 corneal confocal microscope, NIDEK Technologies, Italy).

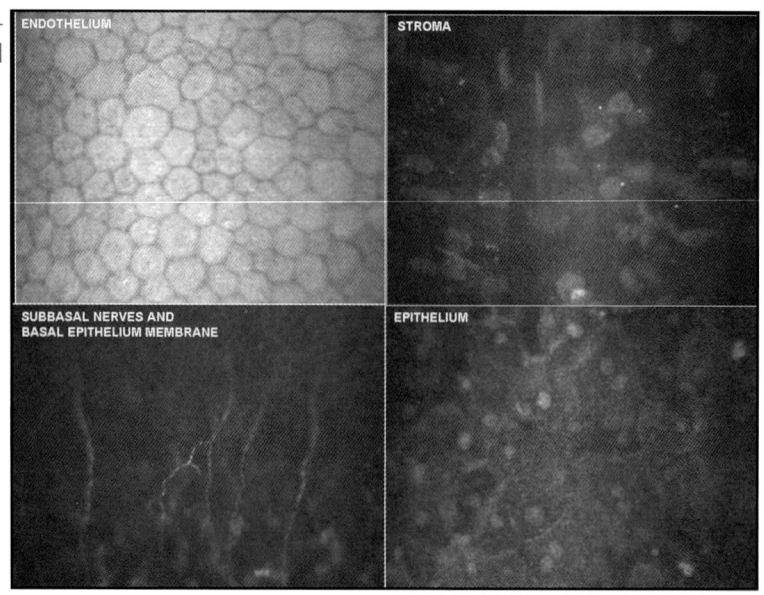

associated with the injury allows these mediators of cellular responses to reach the stroma and bind their respective receptors to the keratocyte cells, where they trigger a variety of biologic responses.

The cascade of responses to these cytokines leads to important changes in the stroma that contribute to wound healing, including keratocyte apoptosis and necrosis, keratocyte activation, keratocyte proliferation, and generation of myofibroblasts. These early changes contribute to other responses associated with stromal remodelling, epithelial healing, production of altered extracellular matrix, and wound contraction.[1,7,11]

Keratocyte apoptosis is a programmed form of cell death in response to an environmental stimulus that normally occurs without significant release of lysosomal enzymes or other intracellular components that could damage surrounding tissues or cells.

Multiple cytokines and intracellular pathways can induce apoptosis, but they ultimately merge in the activation of a family of proteases called caspases, which regulate the breakdown of DNA. The keratocyte apoptosis response peaks at approximately 4 hours after epithelial injury and may last 1 week or more after the initial insult. In addition to keratocytes, it is likely that other cells, such as inflammatory cells, also undergo apoptosis.

Proliferation (and migration) of residual activated keratocytes begin 12 to 24 hours after epithelial injury. The proliferating keratocytes are thought to give rise to activated keratocytes, fibroblasts, and myofibroblasts that repopulate the depleted stroma. The early phases of wound healing also involve the degradation and removal of damaged tissue orchestrated by the plasminogen-activator/plasmin system, collagenolytic metalloproteinases, and other enzymes. Moreover the cytokines released from the epithelial cells and keratocytes attract inflammatory cells (such as macrophages, monocytes, T-cells, and polymorphonuclear cells) into the stroma from the limbal vessel and tear film. Inflammatory cells may enter the wound, phagocytize residual cellular fragments, and secrete proteases that remove damaged extracellular matrix components.[1,33-36]

The myofibroblasts appear in the subepithelial stroma 1 to 2 weeks after surgery. They are probably derived from keratocytes under the influence of the TGFβ, and they may produce large amounts of growth factors, such as HGF and KGF, in addition to collagen, glycosaminoglycans, collagenases, gelatinases, and metalloproteinases, that are associated with remodelling of the extracellular matrix and stroma.[37,38]

Due to important differences in the cellular responses between different surgical procedures and between individuals, the complex cascading sequence of events constituting corneal wound healing can easily show changes leading to less organized corneal wound healing. This may induce loss of stromal transparency compromising refractive outcome and, sometimes, final visual function.[39]

Corneal Wound Healing After Surface Ablation

PRK, LASEK, and LASIK are the most common refractive surgery procedures performed for the correction of myopia, hyperopia, and astigmatism. Clinical outcome with these procedures is generally dependent on corneal wound healing response.[6,7]

In LASIK a lamellar flap is performed including epithelium, Bowman's layer, and approximately 100 μm of anterior stroma.

The stimulus for the cellular response to LASIK depends on many factors. These include the release of local cytokines, growth factors, and chemokines from injured epithelial cells and activated keratocytes. After a normal LASIK procedure, however, there is only minimal peripheral epithelial trauma corresponding to the edge of the flap. This minimizes the release of IL-1 and other mediators of the wound healing

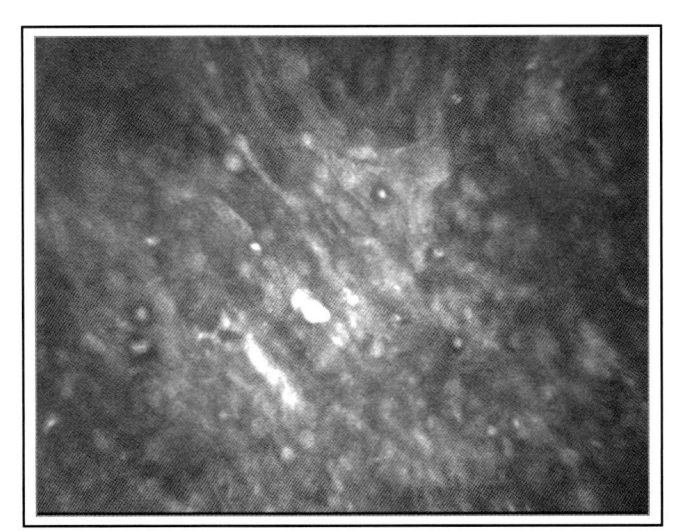

Figure 34-2. Epithelial flap 1 day after LASEK. Corneal confocal microscopy shows intact epithelial layer.

response. If there is significant epithelial trauma, however, such as with a large microkeratome-induced abrasion, the wound healing response is often markedly upregulated. However, even with normal LASIK procedure, there can be variability in epithelial thickness after surgery, and these changes may have significant effects on the long-term stability of the refractive correction. Furthermore, at the flap margins, there is direct contact between normal and activated keratocytes in the stromal tissue and epithelium at the incision site, and this can be associated with the higher healing response in the periphery of the cornea after LASIK. However, after LASIK procedure the basement membrane in the central cornea is intact and it is believed that this acts as a barrier to signaling molecules such as TGFβ from the epithelium or tear fluid.[2-4,40,41]

PRK technique involves the removal, chemical or mechanical, of the epithelium with exposure of the Bowman's membrane, which is ablated along with anterior stroma by the excimer laser beam. The recovery of the anterior corneal tissues is a very important phenomenon occurring after this kind of ablation, in which, moreover, the Bowman's layer is destroyed.

The removal of the epithelial basement membrane directly exposes anterior stromal keratocytes to the effect of cytokines and growth factors released by the injured epithelial cells and to factors present in the tear film. The corneal wound healing response that occurs after PRK is usually more intense than that after LASIK for the same level of correction. Probably the difference in response between anterior and posterior keratocytes is responsible of the more anterior stromal keratocyte apoptosis, keratocyte proliferation, and myofibroblast transformation. In fact, it is known that the distribution of keratocytes is heterogeneous, with a lower concentration at the posterior stroma, which could also contribute to the difference in wound healing between low and high PRK corrections.[2-4,39-41]

LASEK procedure is a modified PRK technique in which an epithelial flap is created and then repositioned after the ablation that occurs, as PRK, starting from the Bowman's layer and involving the most anterior stroma. The epithelial flap, especially with an intact Bowman's membrane, could serve as mechanical barrier that protects the stroma from direct exposure to growth factors in the tear film (Figure 34-2). The decrease in the release of cytokines and chemokines could result in a lower stimulus for myofibroblast differentiation. Some recent studies, however, questioned the theoretical advantages of LASEK.[42,43]

Pharmacologic Modulation of Corneal Wound Healing After Surface Ablation

Although in the past the studies on corneal wound healing have focused on controlling damage following trauma or infection, with the advent of refractive surgery the need to modulate corneal scarring and reduce complications such as regression, haze, visual glare, halos, and persistent epithelial defects has become extremely relevant. Significant progresses have been made in the technology used in refractive surgery, with great improvement in lasers and microkeratomes, but the final success of refractive surgery seems to be closely related to individual scarring response and modulation of corneal wound healing.[1,11,44]

Many studies have been performed to elucidate and control the wound healing cascade with the clinical purpose to improve this response, and many drugs or protective substances have been used to prevent altered corneal wound healing formation. Topical corticosteroids have been used to inhibit haze formation after PRK. The main mechanism through which corticosteroids may prevent haze is inhibition of collagen synthesis.[12,13] However, long-term corticosteroid treatment may cause relevant side effects: ocular hypertension, glaucoma, and cataract.[45,46] Moreover, controlled clinical trials have not demonstrated any significant role of topical corticosteroids in haze prevention.[12,13] Gartry and colleagues, and O'Brart and colleagues, after analyzing the effect of corticosteroids in prevention of corneal haze after PRK vs placebo, concluded that topical corticosteroids have no effects on corneal haze or visual performance after PRK. Otherwise, Chang et al reported the use on rabbit cornea of cyclosporin A (CSA) and inhibitors of metalloproteinase (SIMP). After 6 weeks of application (CSA 2% qid, SIMP every 2 hours), the authors demonstrated that SIMP can reduce significantly corneal haze, whereas CSA is not effective. Furthermore, using immunohistochemical methods they demonstrated that only SIMP can reduce type III collagen synthesis.[47] Several studies have evaluated the efficacy of vitamin C in haze prevention after PRK. It has been hypothesized that vitamin C may play a protective role in preventing UV damage produced by the excimer laser and in reducing keratocyte activation.[48] However, Corbett and colleagues found no evidence that ascorbate inhibits haze formation in rabbits.[49] Brancato and colleagues investigated, *in vivo*, whether ubiquinone Q10 associated with vitamin E protects rabbit corneas from keratocyte apoptosis after excimer laser irradiation. They demonstrated that the treatment of rabbit eyes before PRK with ubiquinone Q10 reduces the number of apoptotic events.[50] Vinciguerra et al documented improved reepithelialization when an increase of serum and tear film amino acids is obtained through oral administration.[51] Pakkar et al, considering that gamma interferon (IFN) is an immunoregulatory polypeptide modulating fibroblast function, investigated the *in vitro* effects of this substance on keratocyte proliferation and keratocyte-induced collagen gel contraction. They concluded that, *in vitro*, proliferation of keratocytes is not inhibited by gamma interferon and, at higher concentrations (≥10 U/ml), cellular proliferation has been stimulated by the drug.[52] Applying or suturing amniotic membrane onto injured corneas has been proposed as a therapeutic adjuvant for reconstructing corneal surface. Wang and colleagues showed that immediately covering the photoablated corneal surface with a preserved human amniotic membrane for 1 week may reduce corneal haze, epithelial hyperplasia, and stromal fibroblast cellularity in rabbits by 12 weeks postoperatively.[53] Tseng et al suggested that amniotic membrane has healing properties greater than that of a simple physical protective barrier, which may be due to suppression of TGFβ actions, thus decreasing the proliferation of fibroblasts and formation of corneal scar.[54] Recent investigations have been concentrated on inhibiting myofibroblast differentiation by targeting specific modulators such as TGFβ.[55,56] The TGFβ-system has become well established as playing a critical role in promoting scar formation in multiple tissue. The three TGFβ isoforms (TGFβ1, TGFβ2, and TGFβ3) produce similar actions on cultured fibroblasts, including stimulation of the synthesis of collagen, proteoglycans, elastin, and lysyl oxidase. In addition, TGFβ decreases the synthesis of metalloproteinase and increases the synthesis of tissue inhibitors of metalloproteinase by fibroblasts. TGFβ also appears to regulate key aspects of corneal wound healing. This protein was immunolocalized in corneal cells and lacrimal gland cells, and TGFβ levels in tears increased after PRK in patients. Levels of mRNA for all three isoforms of TGFβ, as well as its receptors, increased and remained elevated for 90 days in rat corneas following PRK ablation.[55,56] Unfortunately, previous studies aimed at modulate corneal wound healing through the use of exogenous factors, such as corticosteroids, CSA, IFN, vitamins, collagenase inhibitors, and amniotic membrane placement, were unsatisfactory because of long-term side effects, limited success, and additional adverse effects.[45,46,49,52] Among topical drugs evaluated to prevent or treat corneal haze, mitomycin C (MMC) has recently gained relevant interest.[8,9,14-18] MMC is an antibiotic antineoplastic agent that selectively inhibits the synthesis of DNA, RNA, and proteins. Although MMC was originally used as a systemic chemotherapeutic agent, it is now commonly used topically in ophthalmic surgery (mainly glaucoma surgery, pterygium excision) and in the treatment of conjunctival and corneal intraepithelial neoplasia and ocular cicatricial pemphigoid.[57,58] The rationale of using this cytostatic drug in refractive surgery is the long-term effect on prevention of hyperproliferation of keratocytes and on apposition of new, irregular generated material causing scars.[59,60] This use was originally proposed by Talamo et al in an experimental model.[61] Haze reduction following MMC administration was also documented by Xu et al in rabbit eyes.[62] Majmudar et al reported a successful series of 30 eyes treated using a 0.02% MMC solution to prevent recurrent haze after PRK and radial keratotomy.[14-16] Although this study was performed in a limited series, it assessed short-term safety of the use of 0.02% MMC. Recently, Carones et al reported the results of the prophylactic use of MMC to inhibit haze formation after PRK for medium and high myopia in eyes that were unsuitable to LASIK.[8] This study showed that the use of a single intraoperative application of MMC 0.02% after PRK leads to positive refractive and visual results over a 6-month period. The same authors also documented the absence of relevant corneal complications with this treatment modality.[8]

More recently, Gambato and colleagues performed a prospective study comparing long-term effects of topical intraoperative application of 0.02% MMC vs standard treatment in 36 patients. After 3 years follow-up, the authors documented that topical intraoperative application of 0.02% MMC can safely reduce haze formation in highly myopic eyes.[63] These results are encouraging, but, since MMC mimics radiation in long-term side effects, further investigations are mandatory to assess the safety and to elucidate the precise role of MMC in refractive surgery.[64-67]

Corneal Confocal Microscopy

Confocal microscopy is one of several emerging new imaging techniques and has provided an ever-increasing number of application both for studies of *in vivo* physiology, as well as clinical disease processes in the living eye. *In vivo* confocal microscopy provides the ability to section, optically, living tissues noninvasively over time at a magnification and a spatial resolution able to resolve cellular and subcellular structures in situ, in the living eye. Due to these characteristics, corneal confocal microscopy has shown to be the ideal technique to evaluate morphologically the corneal wound healing process after refractive surgery.[11,19,22,26,29-31] Erie and colleagues documented that the dense keratocyte population found in the preoperative anterior stroma is partially or completely removed during PRK, and this high keratocyte density is not reconstituted in the post-PRK anterior stroma.[32] Consequently, the distribution of keratocytes after PRK changes. After corneal photoablation, keratocytes are distributed uniformly, rather than nonuniformly, throughout the anterior-posterior stroma. Moreover, this research confirmed previous studies and documented a proliferation of keratocytes in the anterior stroma beginning at 1 month after PRK, peaking at 3 months, and returning to preoperative values by 6 months.[32] In a recent study, using a corneal confocal microscopy with a 40X surface-contact objective, a

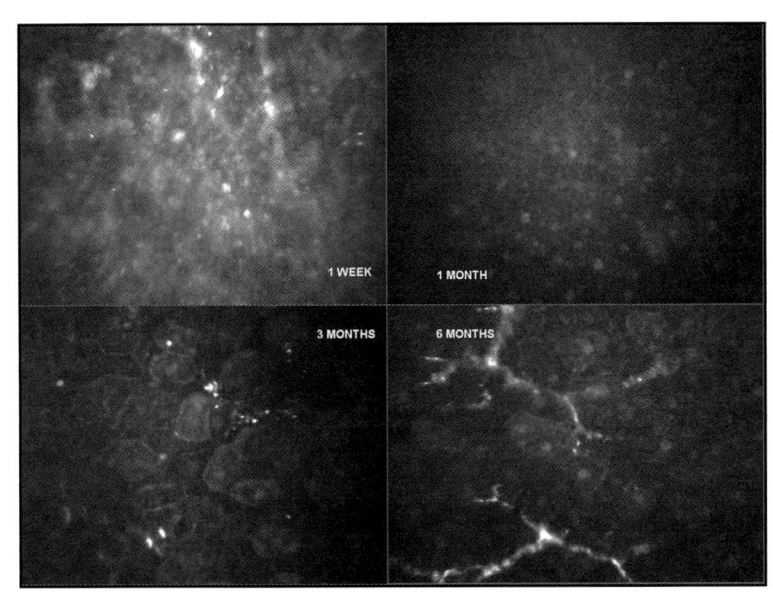

Figure 34-3. The progressive restoration of epithelium 1 week, 1 month, 3 months, and 6 months after LASEK. Note: higher central nuclei reflectivity during the earlier phases of follow-up.

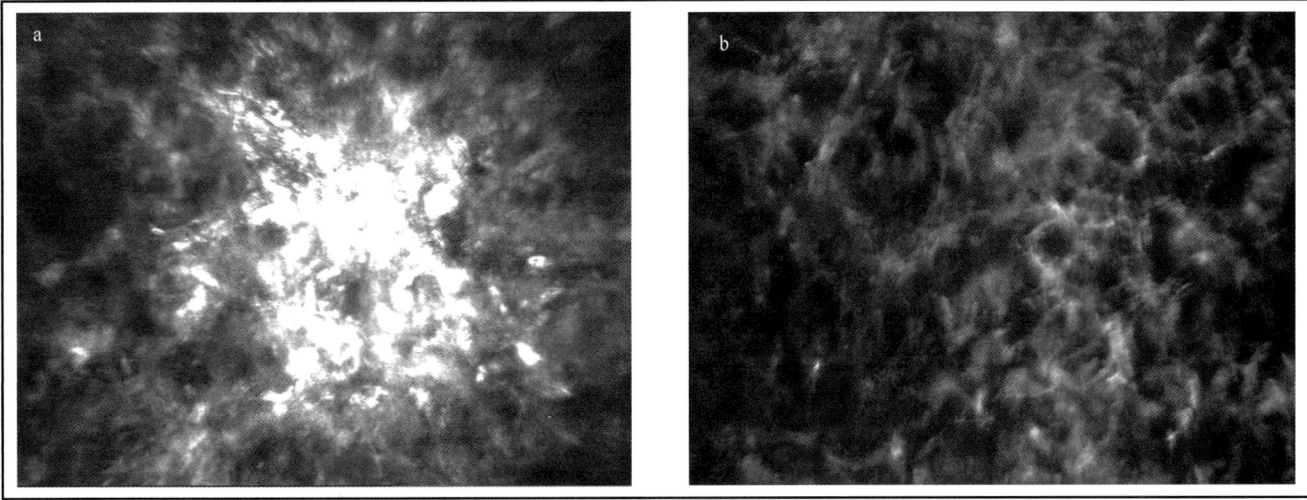

Figure 34-4. Modifications of corneal confocal reflectivity at 1 month (a) and 3 months (b) after PRK. In (a) increased anterior stromal reflectivity and increased cellular-based reflectivity of both nuclei and cell bodies of keratocytes is noted. At 3 months (b), progressive normalization of density and activity of keratocytes is observed.

field of view of approximately 340 x 255 µm and an optical slice thickness (z-axis resolution) of 10 µm, Ghirlando et al (unpublished data, 2006) compared LASEK and PRK for low to moderate myopia. Although these authors did not find any significant difference in visual acuity between the two treatment groups, they reported interesting findings using corneal confocal microscopy. Corneal epithelium fully restored to its preoperative thickness at 1 month after PRK or LASEK and remained in steady state throughout follow-up period, without any compensatory hyperplasia. At 1 month postsurgery, most of the patients regained normal epithelial morphology with individual superficial cells containing highly reflective central nuclei. No morphologic differences were visible between PRK- and LASEK-treated eyes. The evaluation of stromal wound healing showed preoperatively normal, quiescent keratocytes, with low-reflecting nuclei and invisible cell processes. In the very early phases of corneal wound healing, no morphologic differences were observed in LASEK- vs PRK-treated eyes. One month after treatment, in PRK-treated eyes anterior stromal keratocytes showed increased density and increased cellular-based reflectivity of both nuclei and cell bodies (Figure 34-3). More posteriorly located keratocytes remained quiescent. Anterior keratocytes reflectivity diminished by 3 months after PRK, because of normalization of density and activity of keratocytes located in this area (Figure 34-4). Therefore, at 1 and 3 months examination, LASEK eyes had less activated keratocytes and stromal extracellular matrix than PRK eyes, while no significant differences between the two treatment groups were found 6 and 12 months postoperatively (Figures 34-5 and 34-6).

Conversely, few days after LASIK, epithelial morphology already appears within normal limits, while the interface examination shows a hypocellular layer, with microfolds, hyperreflective particles, and increased background reflectivity without sign of keratocyte repopulation. At 1 month, a layer of repopulated stroma, in which keratocytes appear

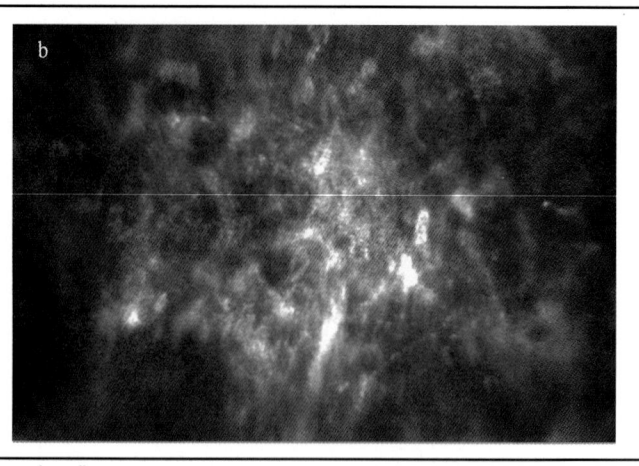

Figure 34-5. Corneal confocal microscopy shows higher stromal reflectivity in PRK (a) vs LASEK treated eyes (b).

as activated cells, is detectable under the interface. There is no evidence of subepithelial nerve fibers, but epithelium and posterior stroma appear unmodified. Six months postoperatively keratocytes show a decreased reflectivity because of diminished activity, while subepithelial nerve fibers, when detectable, present as thin nonbranched fibers with a lower density compared with preoperative nerve morphology. These findings confirm that the preservation of the integrity of the central corneal epithelium results in less epithelial-stromal interaction and subsequent lower rates of keratocyte apoptosis, proliferation, and myofibroblast differentiation.[28,68,69] Nevertheless the wound margin demonstrate excessive wound healing and distorted corneal tissue. Therefore, despite the preservation of the epithelial basement membrane and anterior stroma, wound healing and fibrosis still occur at the periphery, making regulation of wound healing important also in LASIK.

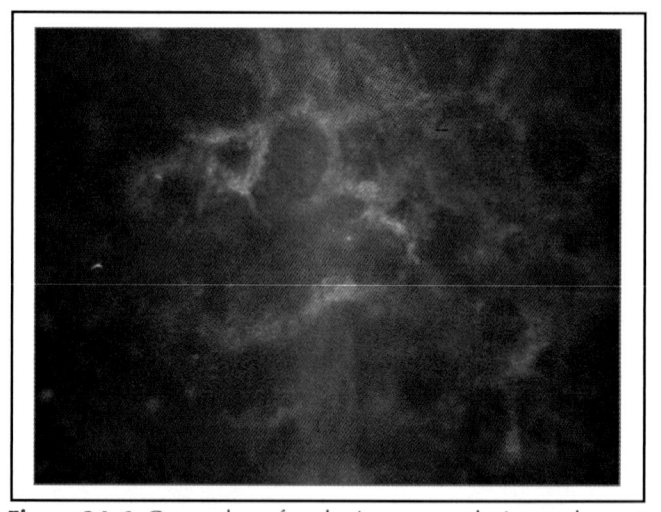

Figure 34-6. Corneal confocal microscopy during early postoperative examination after LASEK treatment: decreased keratocytes cellularity and enlarged spaces among nuclei in anterior stroma.

References

1. Netto MV, Mohan RR, Ambrosio R, et al. Wound healing in the cornea. *Cornea.* 2005;24:509-522.
2. Walker MB, Wilson SE. Incidence and prevention of epithelial growth within the interface after laser in situ keratomileusis. *Cornea.* 2000;19:173-3.
3. Amm M, Wertzel W, Winter M, et al. Histopathological comparison of photorefractive keratectomy and laser in situ keratomileusis in rabbits. *J Refract Surg.* 1996;12:758-766.
4. Wachtlin J, Laugenbeck K, Schrunder S. Immunohistology of corneal wound healing after photorefractive keratectomy and laser in situ keratomileusis. *J Refract Surg.* 1999;15:451-458.
5. Rawe IM, Zabel RW, Tuft SJ, et al. A morphological study of rabbit corneas after laser keratectomy. *Eye.* 1992;6:637-642.
6. Goodman GL, Trokel SL, Stark WJ, et al. Corneal healing following laser refractive keratectomy. *Arch Ophthalmol.* 1989;107:1799-1803.
7. Fantes FE, Hanna KD, Waring GO, et al. Wound healing after excimer laser keratomileusis (photorefractive keratectomy) in monkeys. *Arch Ophthalmol.* 1990;108:665-675.
8. Carones F, Vigo L, Scandola E, et al. Evaluation of the prophylactic use of mitomycin C to inhibit haze formation after photorefractive keratectomy. *J Cataract Refract Surg.* 2002;28:2088-2095.
9. Porges Y, Ben-Haim O, Hirsh A, et al. Phototherapeutic keratectomy with mitomycin C for corneal haze following photorefractive keratectomy for myopia. *J Cataract Refract Surg.* 2003;19:40-43.
10. Boote C, Dennis S, Newton RH, et al. Collagen fibrils appear more closely packed in the prepupillary cornea: optical and biomechanical implications. *Invest Ophthalmol Vis Sci.* 2003;44:2941-2948.
11. Tuli S, Goldstein M, Schultz GS. Modulation of corneal wound healing. In: Krachmer JH, Mannis MJ, Holland EJ, eds. *Cornea.* Elsevier Mosby Inc; 2005:133-150.
12. O'Brart DPS, Lohmann CP, Klonos G, et al. The effects of topical corticosteroids and plasmin inhibitors on refractive outcome, haze, and visual performance after photorefractive keratectomy. *Ophthalmol.* 1994;101:1565-1574.
13. Gartry DS, Kerr Muir MG, Lohmann CP, et al. The effect of topical corticosteroids on refractive outcome and corneal haze after photorefractive keratectomy. *Arch Ophthalmol.* 1992;110:944-952.
14. Majmudar PA, Forstot SL, Dennis RF, et al. Topical mitomycin C for subepithelial fibrosis after refractive corneal surgery. *Ophthalmol.* 2000;107:89-94.
15. Maldonado MJ. Intraoperative MMC after excimer laser surgery for myopia. *Ophthalmol.* 2002;109:826.
16. Raviv T, Majmudar PA, Dennis RF, et al. Mitomycin C for post-PRK corneal haze. *J Cataract Refract Surg.* 2000;26:1105-1106.
17. Azar DT, Jain S. Topical MMC for subepithelial fibrosis after refractive corneal surgery. *Ophthalmol.* 2001;108:239-240.

18. Vigo L, Scandola E, Carones F. Scraping and mitomycin C to treat haze and regression after photorefractive keratectomy for myopia. *J Refract Surg.* 2003;19:449-454.
19. Cavanagh HD, Petroll WM, Alizadeh H, et al. Clinical and diagnostic use of *in vivo* confocal microscopy in patients with corneal disease. *Ophthalmol.* 1993;100:1444-1454.
20. Petroll WM, Cavanagh HD, Jester JV. Three-dimensional imaging of corneal cells using *in vivo* confocal microscopy. *J Microsc.* 1993;170:213-219.
21. Petroll WM, Jester JV, Cavanagh HD. Quantitative three-dimensional confocal imaging of the cornea in situ and *in vivo*: system and design and calibration. *Scanning.* 1996;18:45-49.
22. Petroll WM, Jester JV, Cavanagh HD. *In vivo* confocal imaging: general principle and applications. *Scanning.* 1994;16:131-149.
23. Prydal JI, Dilly PN. Advances in confocal microscopy of the cornea. *Eye.* 1998;12:331-332.
24. Prydal JI, Kerr Muir MG, Dilly PN, et al. Confocal microscopy using oblique sections for measurement of cornea epithelial thickness in conscious humans. *Acta Ophthalmol Scan.* 1997;75:624-628.
25. Prydal JI, Franc F, Dilly PN, et al. Keratocyte density and size in conscious humans by digital image analysis of confocal images. *Eye.* 1998;12:337-342.
26. Moller-Pedersen T, Vogel M, Petroll WM, et al. Quantification of stromal thinning, epithelial thickness, and corneal haze after photorefractive keratectomy using *in vivo* confocal microscopy. *Ophthalmol.* 1997;104:360-368.
27. Li HF, Petroll WM, Moller-Pedersen T, et al. Epithelial and corneal thickness measurements by *in vivo* confocal microscopy through focusing (CMTF). *Curr Eye Res.* 1997;16:214-221.
28. Buhren J, Kohnen T. Stromal haze after laser in situ keratomileusis. Clinical and confocal microscopy findings. *J Cataract Refract Surg.* 2003;29:1719-1726.
29. Moller-Pedersen T. On the structural origin of refractive instability and corneal haze after excimer laser keratectomy for myopia. *Acta Ophthalmol Scand.* 2003;237:S6-S20.
30. Moller-Pedersen T. Keratocyte reflectivity and corneal haze. *Exp Eye Res.* 2004;78:553-560.
31. Moller-Pedersen T, Li HF, Petroll WM, et al. Confocal microscopy characterization of wound repair after photorefractive keratectomy. *Invest Ophthalmol Vis Sci.* 1998;39:487-501.
32. Erie JC, Patel SV, McLaren JW, et al. Keratocyte density in the human cornea after photorefractive keratectomy. *Arch Ophthalmol.* 2003;121:770-776.
33. Wilson SE, He YG, Weng J, et al. Epithelial injury induces keratocyte apoptosis: hypothesized role for the interleukin-1 system in the modulation of corneal tissue organization and wound healing. *Exp Eye Res.* 1996;62:325-327.
34. Wilson SE, Chen L, Mohan RR, et al. Expression of HGF, KGF, EGF and receptor messenger RNAs following corneal epithelial wounding. *Exp Eye Res.* 1999;68:377-397.
35. Helena MC, Baerveldt F, Kim WJ, et al. Keratocyte apoptosis after corneal surgery. *Invest Ophthalmol Vis Sci.* 1998;39:276-283.
36. Wilson SE. Role of apoptosis in wound healing in the cornea. *Cornea.* 2000;19:S7-S12.
37. Mohan RR, Hutcheon AE, Choi R, et al. Apoptosis, necrosis, proliferation, and myofibroblast generation in the stroma following LASIK and PRK. *Exp Eye Res.* 2003;76:71-87.
38. Baldwin HC, Marshall J. Growth factors in corneal wound healing following refractive surgery: a review. *Acta Ophthalmol Scand.* 2002;80:238-247.
39. Kang F, Tao J, Li Q, et al. Mechanism and treatments of regression and haze after photorefractive keratectomy. *Chung Hua Yen Ko Tsa Chih.* 2002;38:433-437.
40. Wang Z, Chen J, Yang B. Comparison of laser in situ keratomileusis and photorefractive keratectomy to correct myopia from −6.00 diopters. *J Refract Surg.* 1997;13:528-534.
41. Hersh PS, Brint SF, Maloney RK, et al. Photorefractive keratectomy versus laser in situ keratomileusis for moderate to high myopia: a randomized prospective study. *Ophthalmol.* 1998;105:1512-1522.
42. Litwak S, Zadok D, Garcia-de Quevedo V, et al. Laser-assisted subepithelial keratectomy versus photorefractive keratectomy for the correction of myopia. A prospective comparative study. *J Cataract Refract Surg.* 2002;28:1330-1333.
43. Lee JB, Seong GJ, Lee JH, et al. Comparison of laser epithelial keratomileusis and photorefractive keratectomy for low to moderate myopia. *J Cataract Refract Surg.* 2001;27:565-570.
44. Cennamo G, Rosa N, Breve MA, et al. Technical improvements in photorefractive keratectomy for correction of high myopia. *J Refract Surg.* 2003;19:438-442.
45. Becker B, Mills DW. Corticosteroids and intraocular pressure. *Arch Ophthalmol.* 1963;70:500-507.
46. Yablonski ME, Burde RM, Kolker AE, et al. Cataracts induced by topical dexamethasone in diabetics. *Arch Ophthalmol.* 1978;96:474-476.
47. Chang JH, Kook MC, Lee JH, et al. Effects of synthetic inhibitor of metalloproteinase and cyclosporine A on corneal haze after excimer laser photorefractive keratectomy in rabbits. *Exp Eye Res.* 1998;66:389-396.
48. Kasetsuwan N, Wu FM, Hsieh F, et al. Effect of topical ascorbic acid on free radical tissue damage and inflammatory cell influx in the cornea after excimer laser corneal surgery. *Arch Ophthalmol.* 1999;117:649-652.
49. Corbett MC, O'Brart DPS, Patmore AL, et al. Effect of collagenase inhibitors on corneal haze after PRK. *Exp Eye Res.* 2001;72:253-259.
50. Brancato R, Fiore T, Papucci L, et al. Concomitant effect of topical ubiquinone Q10 and vitamin E to prevent keratocyte apoptosis after excimer laser photoablation in rabbits. *J Refract Surg.* 2002;18:135-139.
51. Vinciguerra P, Camesasca FI, Ponzin D. Use of amino acids in refractive surgery. *J Refract Surg.* 2002;18(Suppl):374-377.
52. Pakkar A, Rofougaran R, Lu K, et al. Effects of gamma-interferon on keratocyte-induced collagen gel contraction and keratocyte proliferation. *J Refract Surg.* 1998;14:152-155.
53. Wang MX, Gray TB, Park WC, et al. Reduction in corneal haze and apoptosis by amniotic membrane matrix in excimer laser photoablation in rabbits. *J Cataract Refract Surg.* 2001;27:310-319.
54. Tseng SCG, Prabhasawat P, Barton K, et al. Amniotic membrane transplantation with or without limbal allografts for corneal surface reconstruction in patients with limbal stem cell deficiency. *Arch Ophthalmol.* 1998;116:431-441.
55. Jester JV, Barry-Lane PA, Petroll WM, et al. Inhibition of corneal fibrosis by topical application of blocking antibodies to TGF beta in the rabbit. *Cornea.* 1997;16:177-187.
56. Thom SB, Myers JS, Rapuano CJ, et al. Effect of topical antitransforming growth factor-beta on corneal stromal haze after photorefractive keratectomy in rabbits. *J Cataract Refract Surg.* 1997;23:1324-1330.
57. Beretta G, Cartei G, Giraldi T. *Mitomicina C. Farmacologia e Clinica.* Torino, Italy: Edizioni Minerva Medica; 1989.
58. Beretta G. *Mitomycin C. Current Clinical Status.* Torino, Italy: Edizioni Minerva Medica; 1998.
59. Sadeghi HM, Seitz B, Hayashi S, et al. *In vitro* effects of mitomycin C on human keratocytes. *J Refract Surg.* 1998;14:534-540.
60. Schipper I, Suppelt C, Gebbers JO. Mitomycin C reduces scar formation after excimer laser (193 nm) photorefractive keratectomy in rabbits. *Eye.* 1997;11:649-655.
61. Talamo JH, Gollamudi S, Green R, et al. Modulation of corneal wound healing after excimer laser keratomileusis using topical mitomycin C and steroids. *Arch Ophthalmol.* 1991;109:1141-1146.
62. Xu H, Liu S, Xia X, et al. Mitomycin C reduces haze formation in rabbits after excimer laser photorefractive keratectomy. *J Refract Surg.* 2001;17:342-349.
63. Gambato C, Ghirlando A, Moretto E, et al. Mitomycin C modulation of corneal wound healing after photorefractive keratectomy in highly myopic eyes. *Ophthalmology.* 2005;112:208-218.
64. Tae-im Kim, Hungwon Tchah, Seung-ah Lee, et al. Apoptosis in keratocytes caused by mitomycin C. *Invest Ophthalmol Vis Sci.* 2003;44:1912-1917.
65. Safianik B, Ben-Zion I, Garzozi HJ. Serious corneoscleral complication after pterygium excision with mitomycin C. *Br J Ophthalmol.* 2002;86:357-358.

66. Rubinfeld RS, Pfister RR, Stein RM, et al. Serious complications of topical mitomycin C after pterygium surgery. *Ophthalmol.* 1992;99:1647-1654.
67. Yi-Yu Tsai, Jane-Ming Lin, Jium-Dar Shy. Acute scleral thinning after pterygium excision with intraoperative mitomycin C. *Cornea.* 2002;21:227-229.
68. Mastropasqua L, Nubile M, Carpineto P, et al. *In vivo* investigation of corneal response after excimer laser surgery (PRK, LASEK, and LASIK): the role of confocal microscopy. In: Midena E, ed. *Myopia and Related Disease.* Ophthalmic Communications Society, Inc; 2005:432-442.
69. Linna TU, Perez-Santonja JJ, Tervo KM, et al. Recovery of corneal nerve morphology following laser in situ keratomileusis. *Exp Eye Res.* 1998; 66:755-763.

CHAPTER 35

CORNEAL SURFACE ANALYSIS AFTER PHOTOREFRACTIVE KERATECTOMY

Sebastiano Serrao, MD, PhD; Marco Lombardo, MD

Introduction

During the last decade, photorefractive surgery has undergone rapid technological development. Modern excimer laser systems permit a very accurate surgical correction of low-grade aberrations of the corneal surface. The individualized correction of the eye optical aberrations will be the next golden standard of refractive surgery allowing all the patients treated to achieve their optimal individual visual perception.[1-3] Indeed, although standard laser refractive surgery eliminates conventional refractive errors, high-order errors are typically induced.[4] The Rayleigh and Maréchal criterions suggested that if the ocular wavefront aberration exceeded a quarter-wavelength ($\lambda/4$: about 0.14 µm for green light), the image would be significantly degraded with respect to the diffraction-limited case.[5] Ocular and corneal wavefront sensors are capable of measuring with extreme precision sub-wavelength errors of the eye optics, and we are already aware that the ocular wavefront typically exceeds this quarter-wave limit.[6] Hence, it is reasonable to expect that the individualized correction of the wavefront aberration will almost definitely lead to significant improvements in optical image quality.

At present, the outcome of corneal refractive surgery largely depends on the biophysical response of the corneal tissue.[7-11] Hence, a better understanding of the biological response of the cornea to laser treatment may allow the prediction and modulation of the biophysical response for more precise correction: both the biomechanical changes of the cornea induced by the ablation as well as the epithelial and stromal remodeling.

It is well known that the final corneal profile (and thus the corneal optical quality) after surgical reshaping of the cornea is a function of the biomechanical response of the tissue to a change in its structure. Therefore, an accurate ablation algorithm has to take into account the expected corneal mechanical changes induced by the surgery in order to achieve the aim that this surgery has set: quite totally eliminate the optical aberrations of the eye. Predicting the biomechanical response is one of the major challenges of customized, aberration-reducing ablative procedures.[12]

Additionally, it is widely held that a smooth post-ablation surface is mandatory if refractive surgery is to be considered effective: an abnormal epithelial-stromal reaction of the ablated corneal surface is the consequence of an imperfectly polished ablated surface, which in itself has been proven to retard the healing process of the epithelium and stroma.[13] A better smoothened stromal surface is at the basis of an improved refractive result, and it is associated with an increased predictability and stability of the final outcome, as well as with an improved visual performance.[14] Several variables depending on the ablation parameters may vary the regularity of the corneal surface: the homogeneity of the laser beam,[15] the shape and dimensions of the laser spot and the overlapping of different impulses,[16] the ejected molecular ablated debris deposited back on the corneal surface,[17] the angle between corneal surface and the laser beam,[18] and the not negligible heating effect associated with photoablation.[19,20] The surgical technique itself[21,22] and ocular movements may additionally influence the corneal surface remodeling after ablation.

While great efforts have been made by laser constructors to improve the quality of the light emitted, ophthalmic surgeons are currently developing techniques to improve the results of current laser refractive surgery[13,23,24] in order to not induce new high-order aberrations of the eye.[25]

In this chapter we will present both the clinical and experimental results of a standardized surface ablation procedure using a flying-spot excimer laser (Technolas 217C excimer laser, Bausch & Lomb Chiron Technolas, Germany) in order to obtain a smoother and tapered ablated surface.

A power corneal topographic analysis tool has been developed to investigate the change of the first corneal surface induced by laser ablation.

Corneal Epithelial Renewal

The first corneal surface[26] is the interface between the ambient environment and the ocular tissues and it is the main refractive surface of the eye. It is in the interface between the corneal surface and air (ie, the tear film) that the main modification of the refractive index of the eye occurs, since the optical properties of the first corneal surface represent the primary element in the high-quality visual performance of the eye.

From experimental observations of corneal surface healing, we know that the epithelium migrates toward depressions on the corneal surface, thus compensating the irregularity of the underlying surface. By masking such irregularities, the epithelium confirms the capability of smoothing the optical quality of the eye.[27] In the past few years, reepithelialization kinetics have been investigated in detail. Light microscope evaluations and immunohistochemistry analysis studies have shown that a large number of molecules are involved in this process.[28] Every corneal abrasion, with no damage to the Bowman's layer or stroma, heals in a symmetric fashion, indicating that the rate of cellular migration is equivalent at all points along the wound border.[29,30] In the renewal process the epithelial cells are immediately able to establish appropriate connections with adjacent cells, maintaining the epithelial integrity and reducing the corneal surface impermeability to external agents.[33] Thereafter, corneal epithelial cells secrete anchoring structures and basal membrane constituents that will come to complete organization once the epithelium has recovered its normal pluristratified architecture.[31]

At present, for a model of corneal epithelial regeneration to be accurate, it must include[32]:

* The density of the proliferative cells (ie, those of the epithelial basal layer)[33]
* The density of the quiescent cells (ie, those of the epithelial upper layers)
* The concentration of every molecule that interferes with cell proliferation and migration
* The time elapsed since surgery
* The geometric characteristics of the wound
  1. In a normal cornea, the proliferative cells are equally distributed from the center to the limbus. In case of a large wound, 24 hours after the injury, we find a large number of proliferative cells both in the periphery as well as in the limbus.[34]
  2. The density of the quiescent cells is a function of the newly differentiated cells and of the entity of cell desquamation.[35]
  3. Many molecules are implicated in the promotion of epithelial migration, in particular growth factors and their receptors.[36]
  4. The speed is clearly a function of space and time.
  5. Again, the speed is clearly a function of space and time.

Thereafter, the epithelial renewal process after excimer laser refractive surgery involves four fundamental phases: cellular division, cellular migration, adhesion to the epithelial basal membrane, and epithelial-stromal interaction.[37,38] Clinical and experimental studies have previously demonstrated that a smooth and tapered anterior stromal ablated surface hastens epithelial adhesion and migration with a faster epithelial wound closure than a more irregular ablated stromal bed.[39] Furthermore, a rapid and noncomplicated epithelial healing has been correlated to the reduction in epithelial-stromal remodeling processes,[40] with less haze and refractive regression, allowing us to predict the refractive outcome and its stability more accurately.[41]

To clarify the relation between the epithelial migration velocity and the profile of the ablated cornea we took a series of digital photographs of fluorescein-stained corneas at 20 and 40 hours after photorefractive keratectomy (PRK) performed on three groups of patients subdivided depending on the preoperative spherical equivalent refraction (low-spherical ablation group, high-spherical ablation group, and cross-cylinder ablation group). We also took corneal topographies (Keratron Scout, Optikon 2000, Rome, Italy) before and 1 month after surgery to relate the epithelial renewal to the corneal curvature.

We created a color scale as a function of time and all the images of fluorescein-stained corneas were centered on the pupil and superimposed in such a way as to create an epithelial migration map. Edge detection of the fluorescein stain in each digital photograph revealed the contour of the wound (Figure 35-1).[13,42]

All the images were imported into custom-made software in order to place them in the same reference frame (the center of the reference frame was the center of the pupil) and to convert the contour of the wound into numerical data. These data permitted us to calculate the epithelial migration along the meridians centered on the pupil (Figure 35-2). The migration velocity was calculated as the ratio between the epithelial migration and the time interval between two sequential photographs

Between 20 and 40 hours after surgery an asymmetrical distribution of the radial epithelial progression was observed in all the eyes. Figure 35-3 shows, for all the cases in the study, the mean progression of migration for each of the following quadrants: 50 to 130 degrees, 140 to 220 degrees, 230 to 310 degrees, 320 to 40 degrees. One may readily note the differences between the quadrants. These differences are less consistent in the low-spherical ablation group.

According to our study results, the dynamics of the reepithelialization process are asymmetrical. In fact, we found: 1) a faster epithelial migration in the temporal quadrant and 2) a slower one in the superior quadrant.

The explanation for the first point could be the nasal decentralization of the pupillary axis with a wound shifted to the nasal quadrant and with more proliferative cells alive

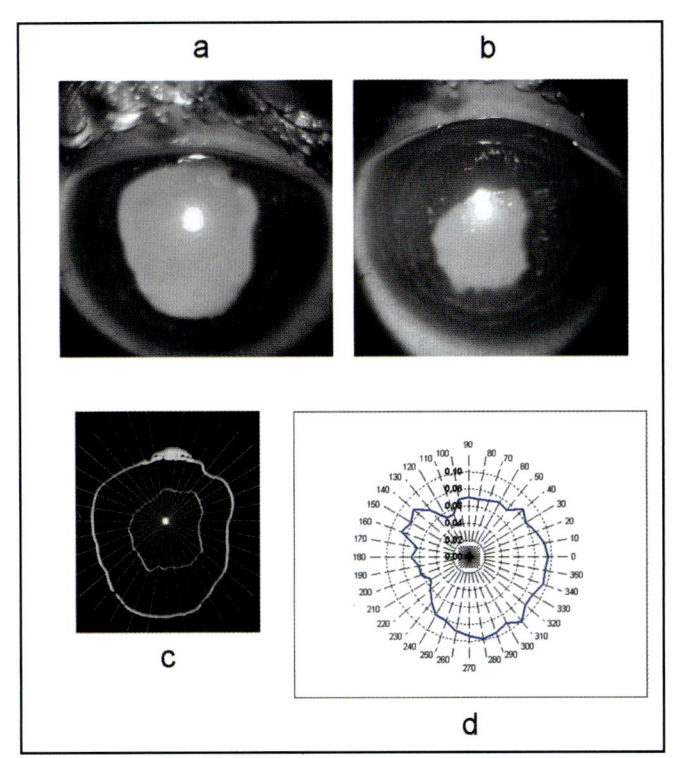

Figure 35-1. The figure shows one of the right eyes of the low-spherical ablation group. (a) The green channel of the RGB standardized photograph of the fluorescein-stained cornea shows 20 hours following surgery, the ablated stroma without the epithelial layer. (b) The same cornea 40 hours from surgery. (c) The epithelial leading edge after surgery respectively at the 40th hour (internal white line) and at the 20th hour (external with line) obtained by digital analysis processing of photographs a and b. (d) The graph shows the output of the model we customized in order to calculate the epithelial migration velocity distribution after surgery for 36 corneal meridians.

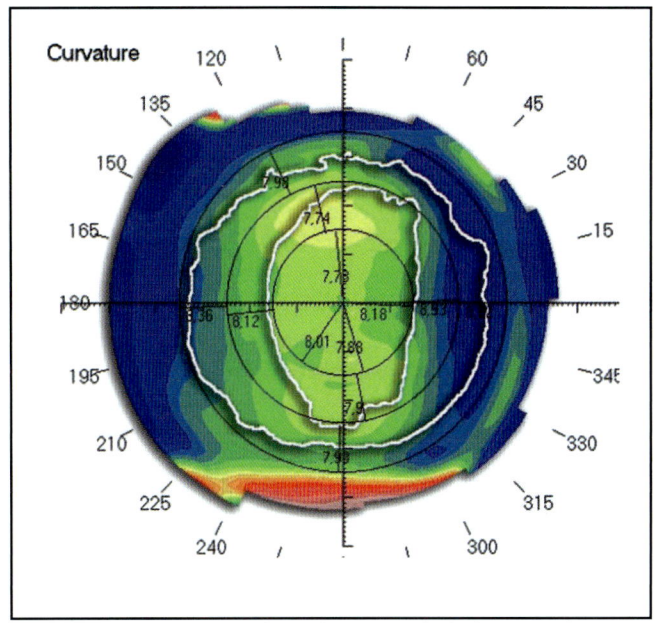

Figure 35-2. To correlate the reepithelialization kinetics to the regional variations in curvature, we imported in the same reference frame the first month postoperative topography and the epithelial leading edge, centered on the pupil center. The figure shows one of the right eyes of the cross-cylinder ablation group.

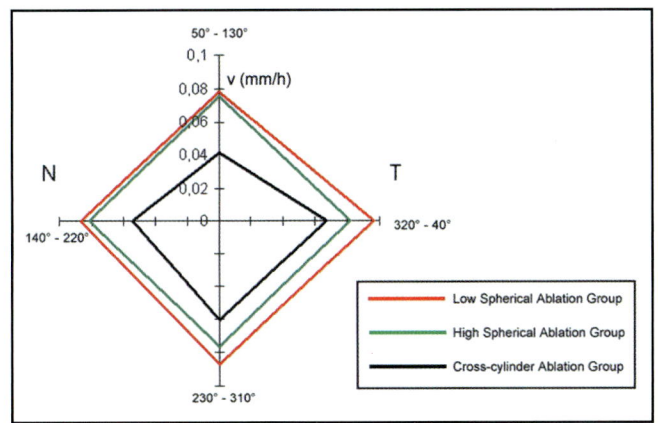

Figure 35-3. The graph shows the mean radial epithelial migration velocity in the three study groups. The 0 degree was sited on the temporal side for every eye. This, in order to compare the right to the left eye using the same criteria as those employed when evaluating the temporal/nasal asymmetry. The two spherical ablation groups show an homogeneous epithelial migration along all the corneal meridians, whereas the cross-cylinder group shows an inhomogeneous pattern.

in the temporal periphery of the cornea. As for the second point, the reason could lie in the mechanics of the superior lid closure on post-myopic PRK cornea.[43]

Thereafter, all the topographic tangential maps were considered as numerical output and imported into the same reference frame of the epithelial maps. They were evaluated using a new parameter: "the differential circular profile." The Keratron topographer offers the possibility of displaying a group of data referred to a circular zone with a variable diameter on a graph. This tool allows us to visualize two groups of data referred to two circles in the same graph. We chose two circles with a diameter of 6 and 3 mm and the pupil as center to understand the difference in curvature that the progressing epithelium encounters between 20 and 40 hours after PRK. We had previously observed that the epithelial edge migrates along this corneal region during this time and we simplified the migration dynamics by using a linear mathematical model.[13]

Different ablation corneal profiles proved to significantly modify the epithelial migration speed between groups (ANOVA, $p<0.001$). The mean speed of radial migration in the low-spherical ablation group was 0.087 ± 0.008 mm/h. This was significantly higher than that found in the high-spherical ablation group (0.078 ± 0.007 mm/h) and in the cross-cylinder ablation group (0.055 ± 0.014 mm/h).

The differences in curvature between 6 and 3 mm from the center of the pupil is higher in the high-spherical ablation group than in the low-spherical ablation group. This is not surprising given the deeper laser ablation. The cross-cylinder ablation group shows a negative difference in the corneal horizontal meridians (0 to 180 degrees) which corresponds to the hyperopic ablation pattern for the correction of the astigmatism with-the-rule. Thereafter, the variation in the curvature values between the corneal quadrants was smaller in the two spherical ablation groups than in the astigmatic group. In the cross-cylinder ablation group the distribution of the curvature along the meridians is not homogeneous; in particular, at 6 mm the correction of the astigmatism is less consistent than that of the 3-mm circle. Figure 35-4 shows the differential circular profiles between 6 and 3 mm for one eye of the cross-cylinder ablation group.

The results showed a significantly slower progression of the epithelium in the higher spherical and in cross-cylinder ablation groups than in the low-spherical ablation group, probably due to a more rapid and steeper change of the corneal profile in the ablation zone. However, the high-spherical ablation group showed a significantly faster epithelial migration than that observed in the cross-cylinder ablation group. The marked asymmetry of the stromal bed in the medium corneal periphery may explain the lesser migration of the epithelial edge in astigmatic ablation as compared with spherical ablation.

In conclusion, following excimer laser ablation the corneal epithelium does not heal in a symmetric manner, and the epithelial migration is strongly dependent on local variations in the curvature of the postoperative corneal surface. Hence, a postoperative more regular ablation profile is necessary to achieve an optimal surgical outcome after PRK

Refractive Results

In spite of the fact that the results following PRK performed using the Technolas 217C are satisfactory, all users have to include some hypercorrection in the planning treatment (about 5% to 10% of the spectacle correction) in order to avoid the hypocorrection consequent to the regression of the refractive outcome occurring in the months after surgery. We believe that this regression is due to the irregularity of the ablated corneal surface.[44]

In experimental settings, it has been found that a phototherapeutic keratectomy (PTK) type treatment at the end of PRK allows for a smoother ablation.[45,46] Smoothing of the corneal surface involves the use of a fluid that, when applied to the cornea, masks deeper tissues while at the same time leaves protruding irregularities exposed;[47] subsequent ablation of the irregular anterior stromal surface should therefore focally excise elevated corneal tissue, thereby reducing the surface irregularities. Which is the ideal fluid to be used in this technique has not yet been established.[48] The 0.25% sodium hyaluronate masking fluid is a moderately viscous solution with an ablation rate similar to that of corneal tissue. Thanks to these properties it can cover the irregular surface uniformly and not run off too quickly. The viscous masking solution formed a stable and uniform coating on the surface of the eye. In particular, it filled the depressed areas on the cornea and efficaciously masked the tissue to be protected against ablation by the laser pulses. Hence, only the stromal peaks are left exposed.

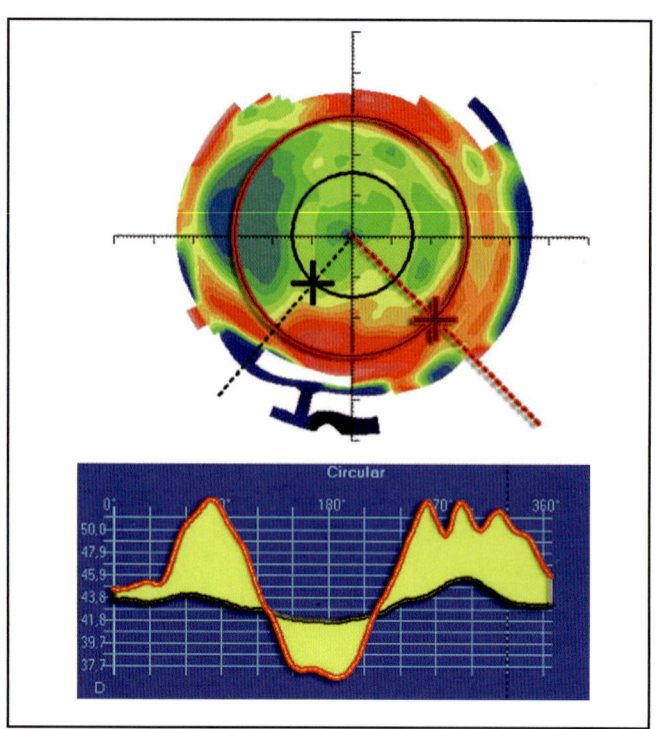

Figure 35-4. Between the 20th and 40th hours after PRK, the epithelium has reached an area between 3 mm (black circle) and 6 mm (red circle) in diameter from the center of the reference frame (pupil center). We created the circular differential profile (CDP) in order to analyze the profile of this region. The figure shows a CDP of a cross-cylinder case where the variation in curvature is high and inhomogeneous along the meridians.

Fifty-four patients aged between 22 and 50 years for a total of 100 eyes were included in a prospective study. We randomized the eyes into two groups: in one group PRK alone was performed whereas in the second group smoothing was performed immediately after PRK. The aim of the study was to relate the refractive and corneal topographic results to the laser technique.

The Technolas 217C is equipped with an active eyetracker device and utilizes a 2-mm laser beam (flying-spot). The fluency at the corneal plane was 120 mJ/cm^2, the ablation rate was 0.25 µm per pulse, and the repetition rate (frequency) was 50 Hz. The diameters of the ablation zone and of the transition zone were 6.0 mm and 9.0 mm respectively. The final smoothing was performed with the same laser in PTK mode. The maximum diameter of the ablation zone was 9.00 mm. We standardized the smoothing procedure using the Technolas 217 C laser: the ablation depth was set at 10 µm (divided into four intervals for a total of 428 spots) and a spatula was used to spread out the masking fluid on the corneal surface.

At 1 year of follow-up, the mean cycloplegic spherical equivalent refraction in the PRK group was -0.61 ± 0.50 D whereas that in the smoothing group was +0.02 ± 0.32 D. The safety index was 1.02 in the PRK group and 1.06 in the

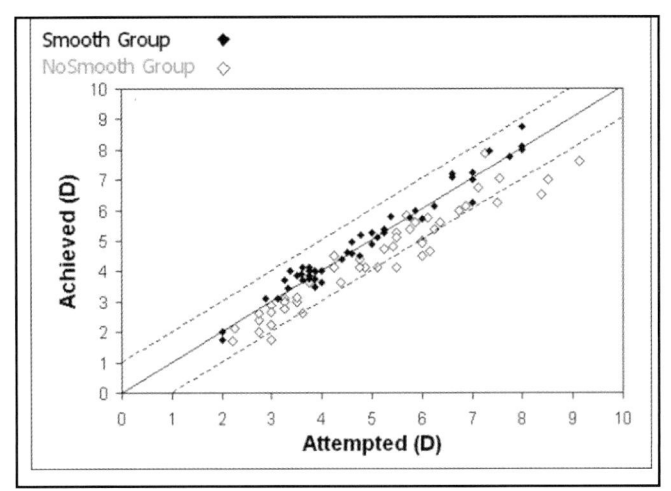

Figure 35-5. The 1-year postoperative scattergram shows the slight hypocorrection of the refractive target in the PRK alone group and the high predictability of the refractive result in the smoothing group. The *p* value was <0.05 (student's paired *t*-test).

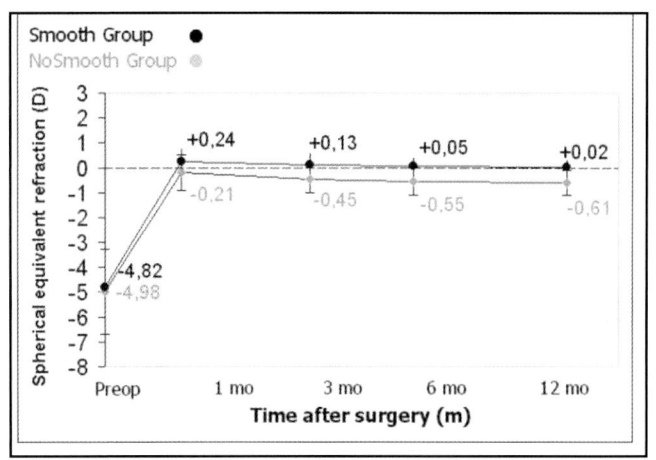

Figure 35-6. The graph shows the refractive changes of the cycloplegic refraction during the year of follow-up in the two study groups. There was a slight hyperopic shift in the smoothing group during the early postoperative period. A regression of the refractive data occurred in the PRK alone group between the first and third postoperative months. The *p* value was statistically significant (*p*<0.05) at each follow-up examination.

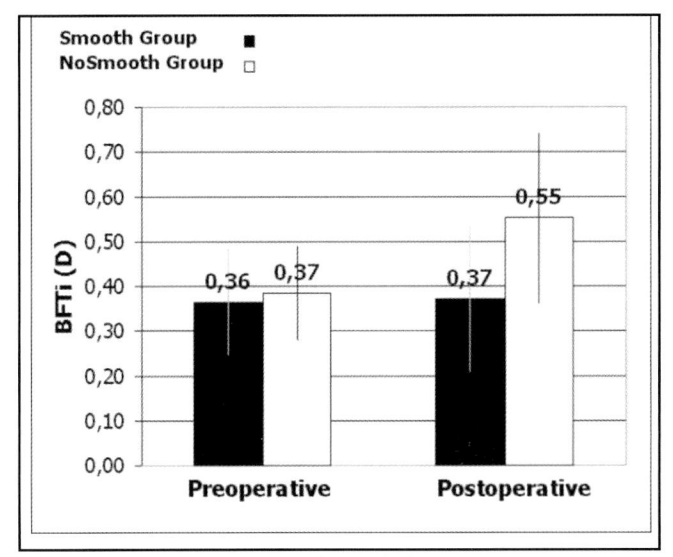

Figure 35-7. At the end of the follow-up an increase in the postoperative topographic irregularity index (BFTI) was observed in both study groups. The increase in the BFTI was much more marked in the PRK alone group. The regression observed in this group may be explained by the more marked irregularity of the ablated corneal surface. The *p* value was <0.05.

smoothing group. In the smoothing group 10 eyes (20%) gained one or more lines of Snellen visual acuity with an efficacy index of 1.03 vs 0.97 in the PRK where only two eyes (4%) gained one or more Snellen visual acuity.[49] In only two eyes (4%) of the smoothing group and in six eyes (12%) of the PRK group was the haze >1.[10]

The scattergram of the attempted vs the achieved correction of both groups is shown in Figure 35-5. Twenty-six eyes (52%) had a manifest spherical equivalent refraction within ±0.50 D of emmetropia in the PRK group whereas this result was achieved in 46 eyes (92%) included in the smoothing group; 41 eyes (81%) were within ±1.0 D in the PRK group and 50 eyes (100%) in the smoothing group. Figure 35-6 shows the mean spherical equivalent refraction during follow-up in the two study groups.

The regularity of the first corneal surface was determined using two topographic indexes: the Best Fit Topographic Irregularity (BFTI)[50] and the high-order root mean square (RMS) wavefront error. The BFTI is measured in diopters and is fitted to the central 4-mm-diameter circle at the center of the videokeratograph so as to approximate the size and location of the entrance of the pupil; it is defined as the RMS sum of the differences between the measured cornea and the best-fit spherocylinder that minimizes the distance between the two surfaces.

High-order RMS is measured in microns and represents the difference between the measured corneal wavefront and an aberration-free wavefront. We calculated the RMS over a 4-mm-diameter pupil and for third to sixth Zernike orders.

Figures 35-7 and 35-8 show the preoperative and 1-year postoperative values of the BFTI and RMS in the two study groups. The postoperative values were greater than the preoperative ones, showing that ablation causes an increase in irregularity; the increase was less consistent in the smoothing group and the difference was very significant. A postoperative reduction in the RMS was observed in nine eyes (18%) of the smoothing group but only in two (4%) of the no-smoothing group.

A correct and rapid reepithelialization is the principal process regulating epithelial and stromal remodeling after PRK. Postablation irregularities induce a more pronounced healing reaction when compared to a smooth ablation surface;[21] besides, it is well known that an altered wound healing is the first step toward the onset of haze and a worsened refractive outcome.[51,52]

The smoothing technique performed with a scanning-spot excimer laser showed to be safe and effective, the only complication was the induction of a slight hyperopic shift. Many published papers reported the induction of a hyperopic shift of the attempted correction as the major complication of PTK.[53] Various techniques have been proposed to minimize the refractive shift: the use of a masking agent to reduce the real depth of tissue ablation, the use of a large ablation zone with a transition zone and the setting of a low ablation depth.[54-57]

Topography analysis can identify whether or not the better result was due only to the hyperopic shift. The BFTI and the RMS over a pupil 4 mm in diameter and for third to sixth Zernike orders showed the difference between the two groups: the smoothing group had a result closer to emmetropia but it was also associated with better topographic indexes. The eyes in which smoothing was performed postoperatively were found to have a higher predictability of the refractive target and a more regular first corneal optical surface.

Microscopic Corneal Topographic Analysis

Since the publication of the first article on photorefractive surgery by Trokel et al[58] in 1983, numerous experimental studies documenting the efficacy of this procedure and the ultramicroscopic characteristics of the corneal surface on which excimer laser ablation had been performed have been published.[59,60]

To assess the regularity of the ablated corneal surface, we analyzed five fresh pig eyes on which laser ablation was performed using the Technolas Keracor 217C. The laser light output was the same we are used to set in clinical procedures. A laser technique was employed to excise the corneal epithelium. A -10.0 D ablation, with ablation zone and transition zone diameters of 6.0 mm and 9.0 mm respectively, was performed on all the eyes. The depth of ablation was chosen on the basis of data from previous literature that proved that the deepest stroma presents more marked irregularities and more accurately highlights the differences in the outcomes of the various types of surgery.[61]

The final standard smoothing was performed immediately after the photokeratectomy, masking half the cornea with a thin plate of aluminum on the five corneas using the same lasers. The maximum diameter of the ablation zone was 9.0 mm. A viscous solution of 0.25% sodium hyaluronate was used to mask the cornea.

To assess the smoothness of the corneal surface, the five corneas were immediately prepared in an identical fashion for scanning electron microscopy (SEM). Specimens were fixed in situ by topical application and anterior chamber injection of a 2.5% glutaraldehyde solution. Within 10 minutes, these corneas were excised near the limbus and placed in fixative for up to 12 hours. The samples for SEM were dehydrated in a graded alcohol series. Alcohol was exchanged for anhydrous carbon dioxide in a critical point drying apparatus. The mounted samples were then sputter-coated with gold and viewed using a Philips XL-30 unit (Philips Electronic Optics, Eindhoven, Holland).

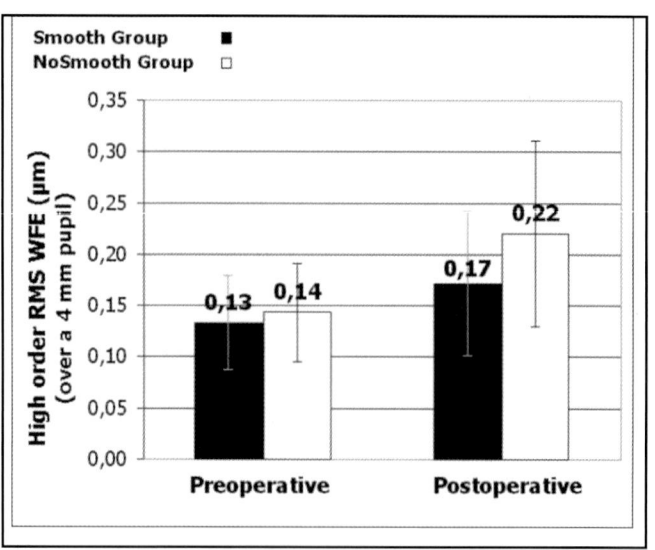

Figure 35-8. At 1-year of follow-up, the ablated first corneal surface showed an increase of the third to sixth high-order optical aberrations. The smoothing technique performed at the end of the PRK procedure reduced the postablation stromal irregularities allowing for a more even surface with respect to standard PRK alone. The induced high-order optical aberrations in the smoothing group were less marked. The p was <0.05.

Examination of the corneal surfaces revealed the presence of numerous artifacts in some specimens. As already described by other authors,[16,45] these artifacts are associated with water loss during the dehydration and critical point drying processes. Electron microscopy confirmed the increased smoothness of the corneal surfaces treated with the smoothing technique compared to that of the corneas in which PRK alone was performed (Figure 35-9).

However, preparation of the sample for SEM imaging may cause shrinkage of soft tissue specimens after fixation, dehydration, and critical point drying, and moreover, the surface roughness may be masked by the often required metal coating. For these reasons, in order to minimize the alterations of the corneal surface during the specimens preparation, we chose a noninvasive technique of imaging such as atomic force microscopy (AFM).[62,63] The most significant advantage of the AFM technique is that samples may be examined with little preparation and hence with a low risk of altering the surface features. AFM provides extraordinary topographic contrast, direct height measurements, clear views of the surface features (no coating is necessary) and the possibility of imaging in liquids. Further, an AFM allows a three-dimensional topographic reconstruction of the investigated sample on a nanometric scale.

In the AFM the sample is scanned by a tip, also called probe, which is mounted on a flexible cantilever. While scanning, the forces between the tip and the sample cause the bending of the cantilever. The deflection is monitored

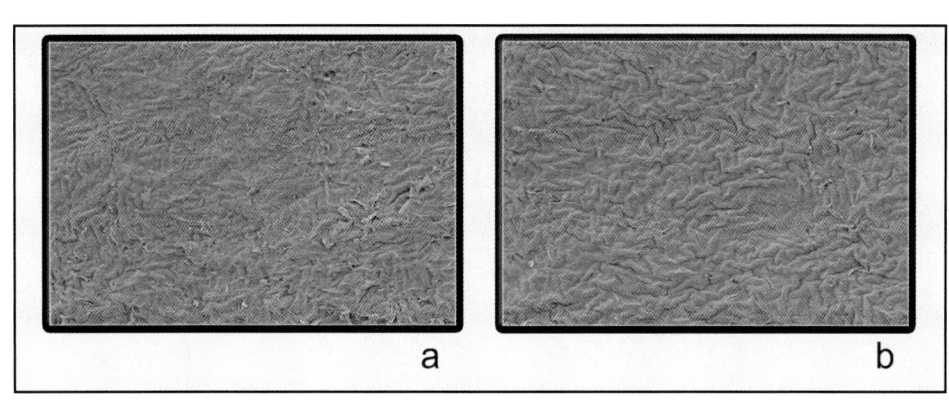

Figure 35-9. (a) High magnification (250x) of a porcine corneal surface ablated plus smoothing and (b) of the ablated surface without smoothing. SEM confirmed that a PTK-style treatment after initial ablation reduced the irregularity of the stromal surface.

through an optical system, composed by a laser diode and a position sensitive photodetector. The laser beam hits the reflective back of the cantilever and it is reflected in the two-segmented photodiode. The topography of the sample is obtained by plotting the deflections of the cantilever as a function of its position on the sample. Several forces typically contribute to the deflection of the cantilever. The force most commonly associated with AFM is an interatomic force called the van der Waals force, the magnitude of which is in the range of nN. There are also involved electrostatic forces and capillary forces between the tip and the sample. Capillary force arises from the condensation, between the tip and the sample, of water vapor present in air when working at room temperature, in particular capillary force could reach a magnitude of the order of μN and can be disruptive when analyzing soft biological samples. The capillary force can be significantly reduced if both the tip and the sample are completely immersed in liquid. Hence, the capillary force is extremely important when imaging biological structures in air. As we know, the adhesion properties of many substances are sensitive to the presence of water vapor in the atmosphere, and this is due to the water capillary condensation in the contact points between surfaces. The capillary forces strongly depend on the percentage of humidity in air and they may exceed 10^{-6} N. This is quite a huge value, and considering that the contact point between the tip and the sample is a very small one (of the order of tenths of Angstroms), such a force leads to a very high pressure exerted by the tip on the sample. For "hard" samples this is not a problem, but for "soft" samples, such as biological ones, this could cause an irreversible damage of the surface. To avoid disruption of the sample, it is possible to work with the tip and the sample completely immersed in a fluid medium; such a procedure largely neutralizes the capillary forces too. In case of biological structures the necessity of reducing the interaction forces between the tip and the surface goes hand in hand with that of creating the natural conditions of hydration of such structures.

The AFM can operate in several modes; in contact mode, the tip is held less than a few Angstroms from the sample surface.[64] When the microscope operates in contact mode the tip scans the sample in close contact (a few Angstroms) with the surface. The force on the tip is repulsive and has a magnitude of 10^{-7} to 10^{-6} N. In no-contact mode, the tip is held at about 100 Angstroms from the surfaces. Hence, the forces between the tip and the sample are weaker than the ones in contact mode and approximate 10^{-12} N. Therefore, this mode is particularly appropriate for the evaluation of mechanically delicate structures.

Ten enucleated porcine fresh globes were used for this study, six of which were ablated. A laser technique was employed to excise the corneal epithelium. A -8.0 D ablation with ablation zone diameter of 4.0 mm, which corresponds to a maximum ablation depth of 80 μm, was performed on all the eyes. The final standard smoothing was performed immediately after the photokeratectomy, with an ablation zone of 4.0 mm on three of the ablated eyes. A viscous solution of 0.25% sodium hyaluronate was used to mask the cornea.[65]

All the corneal specimens, both natural as well as ablated, were immediately fixed in situ by topical application and anterior chamber injection of a 2.5% glutaraldehyde solution. All the eyes were kept at a temperature of 4° C for 24 hours in the glutaraldehyde solution. Before AFM observations, the corneas were excised using a Hessburg-Barron trephine in order to obtain corneal specimens with a diameter of 8.0 mm. This procedure minimizes any possible alteration in the structure of the specimens themselves.[66] The specimens were carefully placed on the microscope sample holder with the endothelial side facing downward. Previous works[66,67] stated that the fixation procedure we used does not alter the surface of specimens compared to fresh unprepared ones and also facilitates the acquisition of high-resolution images.

The specimens were observed in balanced salt solution using the contact AFM imaging mode, as previously reported.[66,68,69] The images were obtained using a commercial AFM (Autoprobe CP, Veeco, Sunnyvale, Calif), and V-shaped silicon nitride gold coated cantilevers with a nominal spring constant of 0.01 N/m (Veeco). All images were acquired with a 256 x 256 point resolution with scan rates of 1 Hz per line. The vertical resolution of the instrument is of the order of 0.1 nm. A single area on the cornea was imaged repeatedly obtaining the same results, in order to ensure that the force exerted was not sufficient to damage the sample surface causing artifacts. We have investigated different areas near the center of the ablation zone of the single specimen in order to minimize the possibility that artifacts introduced by fixation would be misinterpreted as surface features. High-quality images were obtained within a wide range of image magnifi-

Figure 35-10. Contact mode AFM imaging of a fixed corneal epithelial surface. In (a) parts of six cells, covered by microprojections, are shown. (scale image: 30 x 30 μm; magnification 7500x). In (b) high-magnification of the previous image. The arrows show crater-like structures of the epithelial cells' surface. The significance of such features is unknown. (Scale image: 20 x 20 μm; magnification 10,000x.)

Figure 35-11. Section analysis of the surface of an ablated porcine cornea. In the color map, black corresponds to the lowest features and white to the highest ones (a). The AFM analysis module allows analysis along a line (b) or on a selected region (c and d) of the acquired images, providing a quantitative characterization of the surface roughness; graphs are used to display the measurement results.

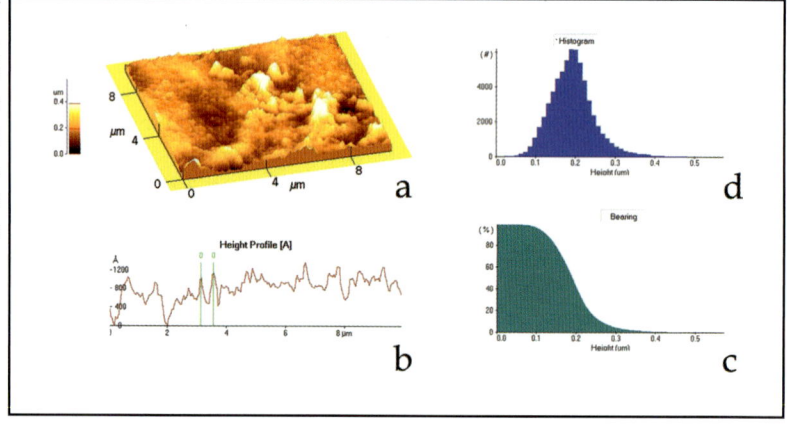

cation. The area scanned was limited to a maximum of 50 x 50 μm owing to the gross curvature of the corneal surfaces.

All images were processed and analyzed using the specific AFM software: we removed from all the pictures the background slope, due to the nonlinearities of the piezoelectric AFM scanner, and we performed surface analysis of the scanned images to measure the surface roughness. The surface morphology was evaluated to obtain information on the mean square root of the roughness within a given area (RMS rough), that is the standard deviation of the height data. AFM data are displayed using color mapping for height representation; dark areas represent depressions on the surface whereas brighter areas represent protrusions.

AFM evaluation of the nonablated corneas revealed the typical polygonal epithelial cells covered by numerous characteristic microprojections (Figure 35-10). The microprojections' density and length are the characteristic of the epithelium viewed at SEM.[70-72] One function of the microplicae may be to assist in stabilizing the tear film; another function may be to facilitate the transport of molecules such as oxygen by increasing the cell surface.[73] In our opinion, knowing that the reepithelialization edge cells have a smooth surface during wound healing and a rough surface after healing and stratification,[74] the difference is due to the variable degree of growth of the cells themselves. Doubtlessly, the microprojections are fundamental for the stability of the epithelial-lachrymal film interface which is in turn necessary for the homogeneity of the first corneal surface.[75]

Following ablation, the corneal surface was relatively rough showing undulations and microgranular structures (Figure 35-11). The changes occurring in the topography of the corneal plane after the ablation may be directly due to the effects of the impact of the laser beam on the surface: the pseudomembrane is considered to be a thin superficial zone of damage specific to 193-nm ArF laser irradiations that results in coagulation of the collagen fibrils.[76,77] Additionally, during ablation fragments of materials induced by boiling water solutions of the tissue are ejected from the ablated surface into the gaseous state meaning that a thermal loading is produced during the photorefractive procedure.[17]

The AFM observations showed differences in the roughness on the smoothed and nonsmoothed ablated surfaces. We performed several scans of the specimens at different magnifications, showing a different configuration of the surface architecture which varied according to the observation scale. In large scale images (from 35 x 35 μm up to 50 x 50 μm) surface granules were observed; we think they can be related to the pseudomembrane we had observed with the SEM. In the medium scale images (from 10 x 10 μm up to 30 x 30 μm) (Figure 35-12) we noticed pools of fibers oriented in the same direction; moreover, there were several microgranules on the surface.

The AFM images analysis has provided results similar to those obtained with SEM showing that the surface on which smoothing is performed is more regular than that on which PRK alone is performed.

Measurements confirm that AFM is an accurate tool for the analysis of biological structures; this explains why, in recent years, this instrument has been increasingly used in experimental research.[78] AFM allows the acquisition of

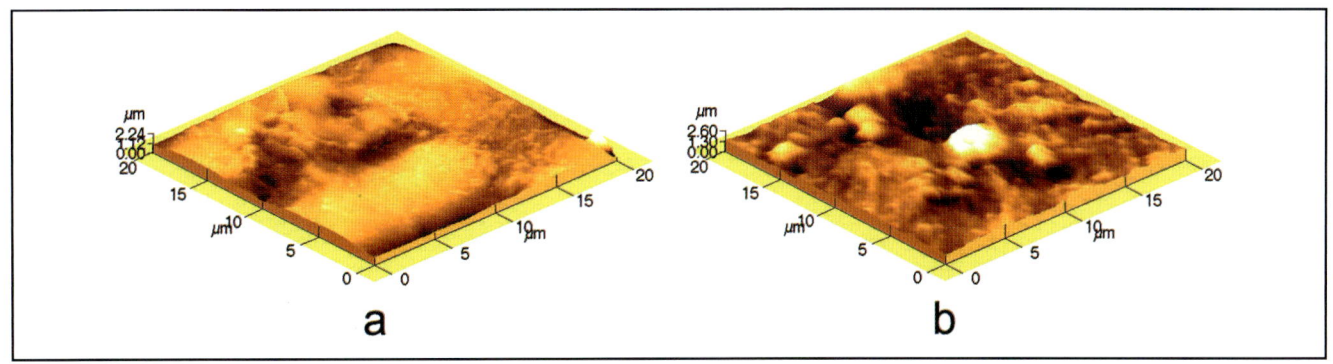

Figure 35-12. The AFM three-dimensional representation provides a topographical map of the anterior stromal features. (a) AFM image of the ablated corneal surface with smoothing (RMS rough: 0.112 μm). (b) AFM image of the ablated corneal surface without smoothing (RMS rough: 0.132 μm). Granules may be observed in both images. The standard ablated surface appeared less regular than the one on which smoothing was performed. (Image scale: 20 x 20 μm.)

three-dimensional images of the surface of biological samples with a resolution in the nanometer range and performance of a quantitative surface analysis. Possible artifacts caused by technical factors are still being investigated. Therefore, because of the ability in detecting differences in height of the order of Angstroms, AFM could be a useful instrument to test lasers as well as different techniques in applying an ablation beam.

Macroscopic Corneal Topographic Analysis

Since their introduction, radial keratotomy and refractive corneal laser surgery have been developed empirically without detailed knowledge of the intrinsic corneal behavior.[79] Refractive surgery, however, stimulated ophthalmologists and researchers in the understanding of the biomechanical properties of the human cornea. It is now held that there are only certain shapes that the cornea will accept and this can be achieved by respecting the normal cornea regional properties.[7]

The detailed knowledge of the corneal biomechanics will help us to understand how some of the biomechanical changes of the cornea can be determined and hence be more easily predictable allowing ophthalmic researchers and laser manufacturers to develop new ablation algorithms in order to predict and correct both unwanted biomechanical as well as optical changes.

Studies of the microstructure of the normal cornea demonstrated its highly heterogeneous nature[80] and that this tissue shows different regional properties. The collagen fibrils have a different orientation depending on the specific region and corneal layer being evaluated. At the limbus the fibrils have a circular arrangement, tangential to the limbus and give rise to a ring-shaped structure. In the stroma the collagen fibrils run preferentially in a vertical and horizontal direction, thus giving rise to a grid-like structure.[81] This arrangement is more regular in the posterior stroma than in the anterior one. Furthermore, the anterior stroma is less hydrated than the posterior stroma and appears to be stiffer than the latter with stronger junctions between collagen lamellae.[82] The various parts of the human cornea strained differently when exposed to the same IOP load. The differences in regional corneal strain may either be due to a real difference in corneal elasticity or to regional differences in the corneal stress level.[83] Interlamellar cross-links, which are preferentially distributed in the anterior one third and periphery of the stroma have been postulated to contribute to the regional differences in lamellar shearing strength and interlamellar cohesive strength in the human cornea.[84,85]

In addition to the regional biomechanical differences, there are also anatomic differences. The regional corneal thickness measurements and relationships between refractive and topographic parameters were previously reported[86,87]: the authors stated that the thinnest site on the cornea is most commonly located in the inferotemporal quadrant, followed by the superotemporal, inferonasal, and superonasal quadrants and that high levels of myopia correlate with steeper central corneal curvature.

To date, a single identical ablation pattern has been employed to treat both the right as well as the left eye. The assumption was to treat the cornea as a symmetric lens, subtracting tissue with the widest ablation zone possible.[88] However, the corneal topography of normal eyes shows a mirror symmetry[89,90] and while it is well known that the corneal plane is normally a prolate asphere,[91] nevertheless it is not borne in mind that the eccentricity values along the nasal and temporal meridians of the cornea are not identical.[92] The degree of flattening from the center to the periphery of the corneal surface (negative asphericity)[93] is greater along the nasal meridians than along the temporal ones.[94] Proceeding along the corneal nasal or temporal meridians, the eccentricity varies; the increase in flattening is more consistent along the nasal zones of the cornea. The laser ablation pattern does not take these nasal/temporal differences in the increase in flattening from the apex to the periphery into account, therefore, we have to consider that it could be necessary to maintain this natural binocular geometrical and optical structure of the cornea in the algorithm treatment plan. We specifically

Table 35-1. Numerical Results for Each Corneal Zone

Anterior tangential average regional differences, 1-year postoperative minus preoperative, both for the right and the left eye (D, Mean ± DS) for the four study groups at 1 year after surgery*

Eye—Corneal Zones**	Low-Myopia Group	Moderate-Myopia Group	High-Myopia Group	Astigmatism Group
Right—C-N	-1.03 ± 1.27	-2.81 ± 2.45	-3.29 ± 4.80	-3.34 ± 1.38
Right—C-T	-1.36 ± 1.05	-2.25 ± 2.48	-3.07 ± 3.35	-2.45 ± 1.32
Right—O-N	3.16 ± 3.14	5.44 ± 2.01	5.90 ± 6.90	5.38 ± 7.04
Right—O-T	1.99 ± 1.97	4.09 ± 1.10	5.10 ± 6.10	1.92 ± 3.77
Left—C-N	-1.25 ± 1.10	-2.81 ± 2.03	-3.09 ± 3.34	-3.43 ± 1.37
Left—C-T	-1.06 ± 0.87	-2.60 ± 1.74	-3.27 ± 4.61	-2.52 ± 1.19
Left—O-N	2.96 ± 2.29	4.22 ± 1.73	6.65 ± 5.50	2.36 ± 5.13
Left—O-T	2.06 ± 1.35	3.86 ± 1.67	5.90 ± 6.95	1.78 ± 3.53

*ANOVA $p < 0.05$
** N = nasal; T = temporal; C = inner region; O = outer region

---

noted that the corneal response in the nasal zones was different to that of the temporal zones, with a greater increase in curvature outside the area of ablation in the nasal peripheral regions as compared with the temporal ones.

A custom software (written in MATLAB, The Mathworks, Inc) was developed in order to characterize the corneal changes of a group of 70 eyes on which PRK has been performed.[95] Corneal topographies were subdivided in four groups: the low-myopia group (20 eyes), the moderate-myopia group (20 eyes), the high-myopia group (20 eyes), and the astigmatism group (10 eyes). The astigmatism group was treated with a cross-cylinder technique.[96]

The mathematical algorithm software computed the average tangential curvature map and the average elevation map for each study group both preoperatively as well as postoperatively, with respect to the reference axis. The average differences in the maps obtained at 1, 3, 6, and 12 months after the surgery as well as the preoperative state were also calculated.

The software permitted us to obtain, during follow-up, an average tangential curvature map for each group in the study both for the right and the left eyes as well as an average tangential curvature difference map (postoperatively at 1, 3, 6, and 12 months minus preoperative) and an average elevation difference map.

The central flattening and the peripheral steepening, as expected, well correlated with the degree to which the refractive error was corrected.[97] Table 35-1 summarizes the numerical results for each corneal zone both for the right and the left eyes in the four study groups. Figure 35-13 represents the average composite map of the right and the left eyes both before surgery as well as 1 year after for the moderate-myopia group.

At each follow-up evaluation, we observed a typical asymmetry between the nasal and temporal eccentricities. In case of cross-cylinder treatment, the hyperopic toric ablation cuts tissue in a more peripheral zone of the cornea and the differences in local curvature asymmetry between the nasal and temporal peripheral regions after the ablation prove to be more consistent than in spherical ablations. Further, at the end of follow-up, the astigmatism was quite fully corrected in the inner region of the cornea while a more marked asymmetry was created in the outer region. Figure 35-14 shows the average tangential composite maps and the average composite difference maps for the astigmatism group.

Figure 35-15 shows the color data analysis of the corneal regions performed by the software for the high-myopia group. The central region emphasizes the changes that were observed in the ablation zone, while the outer region emphasizes the changes outside the area of ablation. These changes were thus related to the biomechanical response of the cornea.

Nevertheless, in the ablated corneas the eccentricity values decreased to oblate values and the nasal zones changes were more pronounced than the temporal ones, the differences in regional peripheral curvature were quite similar to the preoperative values, with the nasal peripheral zones showing a lower radius of curvature than the temporal ones. Furthermore, the deeper and the more peripheral was the laser ablation, the greater was the increase in the curvature difference between the nasal and temporal peripheral zones.

In the low-myopia group the nasal-temporal difference changed softly after the laser ablation. A marked induced asymmetry was observed in the astigmatism group. We could consider that the greater induced asymmetry observed after the astigmatic ablation may be correlated to the more peripheral ablation pattern and to the different biomechanical properties of the periphery of the corneal plane. The more peripheral the ablation, as in hyperopic treatments, the more corneal surface asymmetry the laser will encounter and the greater the difference in the regional response of the cornea.

In conclusion, we consider that the local differences of the normal human cornea could influence our surgical technique as well as the calculation of the ablation algorithm; hence, they have to be included in the preoperative data. Furthermore, the

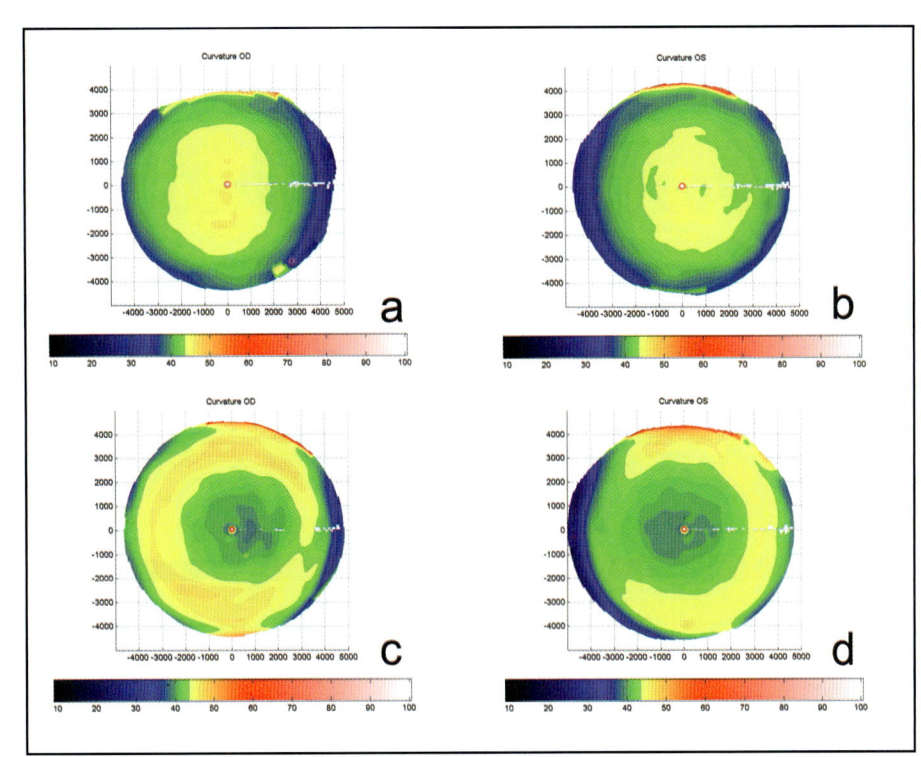

Figure 35-13. Tangential curvature maps of the moderate-myopia group. The preoperative average composite maps both for the right (a) as well as for the left eye (b) show the differences in corneal flattening from center to periphery between the nasal and the temporal meridians. The 1-year postoperative average composite maps (c and d) maintain the similar asymmetric surface pattern in compare with the preoperative state. (Color scale bar: diopters.)

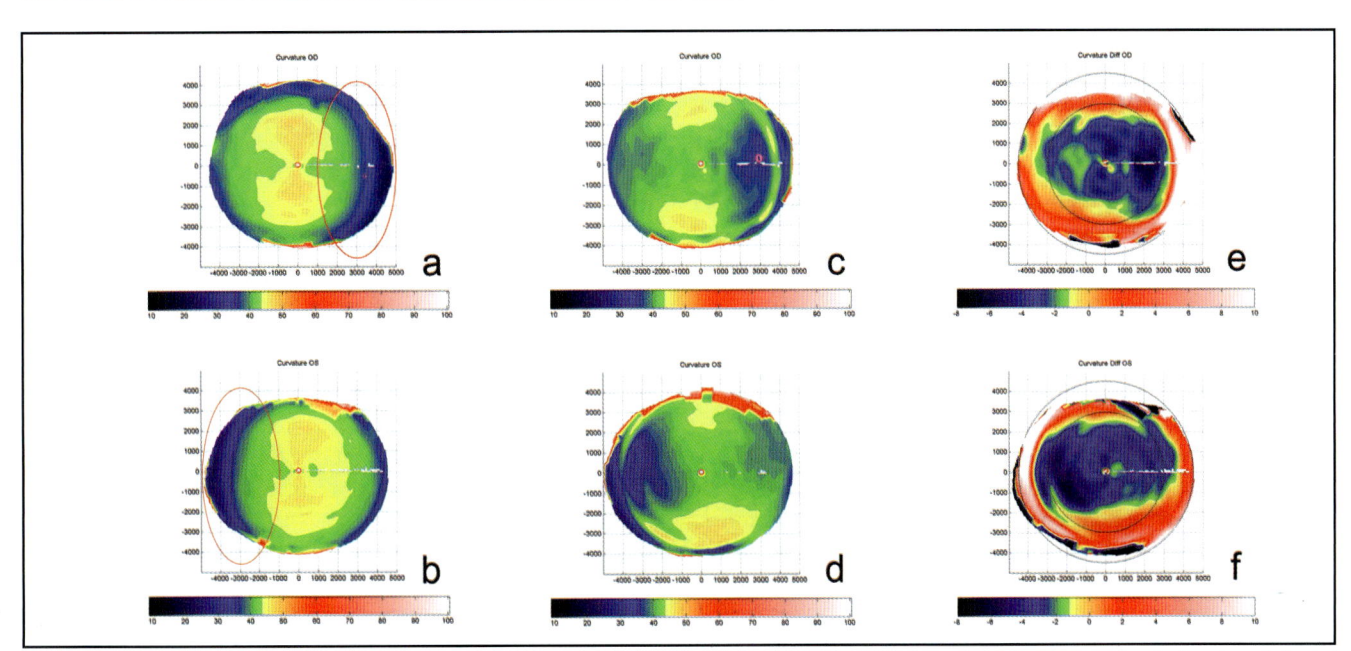

Figure 35-14. Average composite curvature maps of the astigmatism group. The preoperative maps both for the right (a) and the left eye (b) show a regular astigmatism with-the-rule pattern. Differences in corneal flattening from the apex to the periphery between the nasal and the temporal meridians are also observed (red circles). The 1-year postoperative average composite maps both for right (c) and left eyes (d) show the correction of the astigmatism in the inner region due to the cross-cylinder ablation and the increase in curvature differences between the nasal and the temporal peripheral zones in comparison with the preoperative state. In (e) and (f) the difference maps (1-year postoperative minus preoperative) for the right and the left eye respectively. Note the decreased curvature along the horizontal peripheral meridians due to the hyperopic toric ablation and how the nasal region is flatter than the temporal one. Note also the more marked increased curvature of the nasal region outside the ablation in compare with the temporal region. (Color scale bar: diopters.)

Figure 35-15. Average tangential curvature maps of the right and left eye of the high-myopia group. The software system permitted us to divide corneal topography into two concentric regions for analysis: the inner region has a radius of 3.0 mm from the corneal apex and the outer region has a radius of 4.5 mm from the apex. (Color scale bar: diopters.)

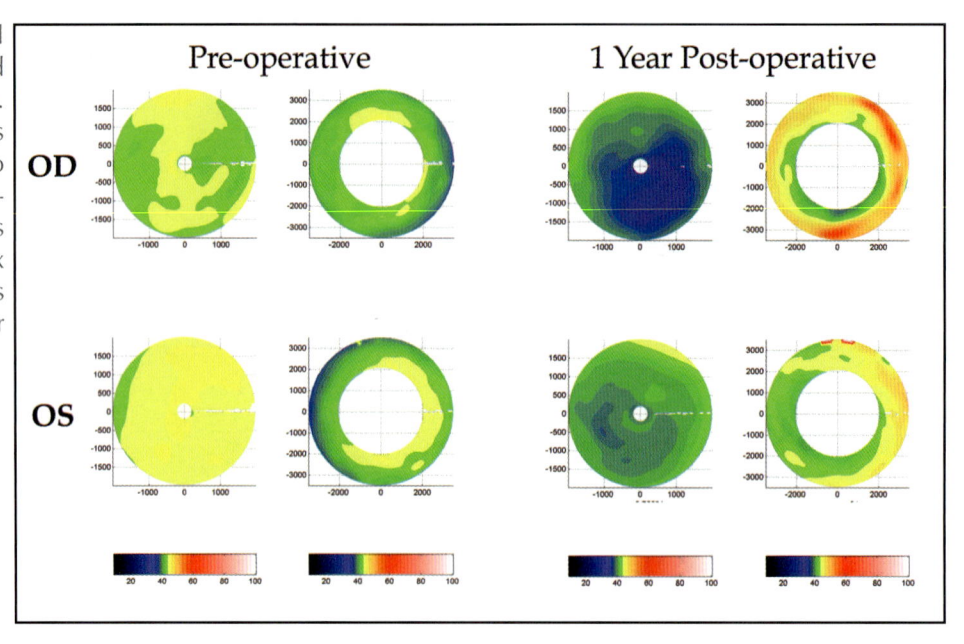

ablation algorithm has to consider the different degree of corneal flattening along the nasal meridians in comparison with the temporal ones and also the mirror symmetrical curvature of the right and left eye. Performing an axis-symmetric ablation on the normal cornea invariably leads to an asymmetry similar to or greater than that of the preoperative cornea. In addition, a difference in the nasal-temporal eccentricity between the right and left eyes resolves in a mirror symmetry of high-order aberrations. Not to consider this optical asymmetry between eyes in the treatment plan could mean to underestimate a variable of induction of high-order aberrations and of an unpredictable biomechanical response.

Conclusion

During the past few years we investigated the role of a smooth and tapered corneal profile in achieving a high-quality result after a standard surface laser refractive procedure. We observed that the outcome of refractive surgery is influenced primarily by the final optical qualities of the ablated corneal surface.

The corneal epithelial surface is continuously renewed[35] and the interaction between the epithelium and the stroma is driven by a complex number of variables. This renewal process is necessary for the maintenance of the smooth optical properties of the corneal epithelial surface. PRK gives rise to epithelial-stromal remodeling that may ultimately influence the surgical results. A smooth post-ablation surface is the principal issue to prevent an abnormal remodeling of the ablated surface.[38,98] A smoother anterior stromal ablated surface hastens epithelial adhesion and migration with a faster epithelial wound closure than a more irregular ablated stromal bed.[13,56]

In this chapter, we evaluated epithelial regeneration on the post-myopic PRK corneal surface. We focused our attention on the wound area, on the time necessary for healing, and on a new operative variable: the ablation pattern. We defined the circular differential profilometry as the variation in curvature along the topographic meridians: the greater this variation the slower the epithelial migration along the corneal surface. We reported a significant slower progression of the epithelium in higher spherical and in cross-cylinder ablations than in the low-spherical ablation group, probably due to a more rapid and steeper change of the corneal profile in the ablation zone.

Thereafter, a power computation of the corneal topographic maps, by means of custom software, was performed in order to characterize the changes of the corneal profile in response to the surface ablation. The corneal response to the laser ablation in the nasal zones was different to that of the temporal zones, with a greater increase in curvature outside the optical zone in the nasal peripheral regions as compared with the temporal ones. Hence, the asymmetric corneal response may increase the paracentral asymmetrical aberrations thus reducing the visual performance of the individual over a dilated pupil. In conclusion, a better understanding of the biological response of the cornea to laser treatment may allow the prediction and modulation of the biophysical response for more precise correction. The local differences of the normal human cornea have to be included in the preoperative data and could influence our surgical technique as well as the calculation of the ablation algorithm. Future nomograms cannot be based only on factors such as refractive error and age. To further refine the surgical procedure and to improve visual outcomes corneal topography is already recommended as an essential component of the treatment plan. The incorporation of the morphological changes induced in the cornea after ablation is the next step in the evolution of refractive surgery. In addition, future refinement of the ablation parameters may improve the surface regularity achieved after initial ablation.[4,99] This should enable us to obtain a clear surface following excimer laser ablation of the corneal stroma.

Disclosure: The authors have no financial interest in the materials described in this chapter.

Acknowledgments

The authors wish to express their gratitude to Fabio Mondini, Eng and Giuseppe Lombardo, Eng, PhD, for their collaboration with the analysis of data; Maria De Santo, PhD, and Mauro Barbieri, PhD, for their kind collaboration with the microscope studies.

References

1. Thibos LN. The prospects for perfect vision. *J Refract Surg*. 2000;16:S540-S546.
2. Applegate RA. Limits to vision: can we do better than nature? *J Refract Surg*. 2000;16:S547-S551.
3. Kanjani N, Jacob S, Agarwal A, et al. Wavefront-and topography-guided ablation in myopic eyes using Zyoptix. *J Cataract Refract Surg*. 2004;30:398-402.
4. Lipshitz I. Thirty-four challenges to meet before excimer laser technology can achieve super vision. *J Refract Surg*. 2002;18:740-743.
5. Charman WN, Chateau N. The prospects for super-acuity: limits to visual performance after correction of monochromatic ocular aberration. *Ophthal Physiol Opt*. 2003;23:479-493.
6. Porter J, Guirao A, Cox IG, Williams DA. The human eye's monochromatic aberrations in a large population. *J Optom Soc Am A*. 2001;18:1793-1803.
7. Roberts C. The cornea is not a piece of plastic. *J Refract Surg*. 2000;16:407-409.
8. Weiss RA, Liaw LHL, Berns M, Amoils SP. Scanning electron microscopy comparison of corneal epithelial removal techniques before photorefractive keratectomy. *J Cataract Refract Surg*. 1999;25:1093-1096.
9. Fiore T, Carones F, Brancato R. Broad beam vs. flying spot excimer laser: refractive and videokeratographic outcomes of two different ablation profiles after photorefractive keratectomy. *J Refract Surg*. 2001;17:534-541.
10. Fantes FE, Waring GO III. Effect of excimer laser radiant exposure on uniformity of ablated corneal surface. *Lasers Surg Med*. 1989;9:533-542.
11. Huang D, Arif M. Spot size and quality of scanning laser correction of higher-order wavefront aberrations. *J Cataract Refract Surg*. 2002;28:407-416.
12. Roberts C. Biomechanics of the cornea and wavefront-guided laser refractive surgery. *J Refract Surg*. 2002;18:S589-S592.
13. Serrao S, Lombardo M, Mondini F. Photorefractive keratectomy with and without smoothing: a bilateral study. *J Refract Surg*. 2003;19:58-64.
14. Serrao S, Lombardo M. One-year results of photorefractive keratectomy with and without surface smoothing using the Technolas 217C Laser. *J Refract Surg*. 2004;20:444-449.
15. Van Horn SD, Hovanesian JA, Maloney RK. Effect of volatile compounds on excimer laser power delivery. *J Refract Surg*. 2002;18:524-528.
16. Taylor ST, Fields CR, Barker FM, Sanzo J. Effect of depth upon the smoothness of excimer laser corneal ablation. *Opt Vis Sci*. 1994;71:104-108.
17. Hahn DW, Ediger MN, Pettit GH. Dynamics of ablation plume particles generated during excimer laser corneal ablation. *Lasers Surg Med*. 1995;16:384-389.
18. Ginis HS, Katsanevaki VJ, Pallikaris IG. Influence of ablation parameters on refractive changes after phototherapeutic keratectomy. *J Refract Surg*. 2003;19:443-447.
19. Maldonado-Codina C, Morgan PB, Efron N. Thermal consequences of photorefractive keratectomy. *Cornea*. 2001;20:509-515.
20. Ishihara M, Arai T, Sato S, Morimoto Y, Obara M, Kikuci M. Measurement of the surface temperature of the cornea during ArF excimer laser ablation by thermal radiometry with a 15-nanosecond time response. *Lasers Surg Med*. 2002;30:54-59.
21. Fasano AP, Moreira H, McDonnel PJ, Sinbawy A. Excimer laser smoothing of a reproducible model of anterior corneal surface irregularity. *Ophthalmology*. 1991;98:1782-1785.
22. Vinciguerra P, Azzolini M, Airaghi P, Radice P, De Molfetta V. Effect of decreasing surface and interface irregularities after photorefractive keratectomy and laser in situ keratomileusis on optical and functional outcomes. *J Refract Surg*. 1998;14:S199-S203.
23. Pallikaris IG, Naoumidi II, Kalyvianaki MI, Katsanevaki VJ. Epi-LASIK: comparative histological evaluation of mechanical and alcohol-assisted epithelial separation. *J Cataract Refract Surg*. 2003;29:1496-1501.
24. Camellin M. Laser epithelial keratomileusis for myopia. *J Refract Surg*. 2003;19:666-670.
25. Lombardo M, Serrao S. Smoothing of the ablated porcine corneas using the Technolas Keracor 217C and Nidek EC-5000 excimer lasers. *J Refract Surg*. 2004;20:450-453.
26. Applegate RA, Hilmantel G, Howland HC, Tu EY, Starck T, Zayac EJ. Corneal first surface optical aberrations and visual performance. *J Refract Surg*. 2000;16:507-514.
27. Lu L, Reinach PS, Kao WWY. Corneal epithelial wound healing. *Exp Biol Med*. 2001;226:653-664.
28. Zagon IS, Sassani JW, McLaughlin P. Reepithelialization of the human cornea is regulated by endogenous opioids. *Invest Ophthalmol Vis Sci*. 2000;41:73-81.
29. Crosson CE, Klyce SD, Beuerman RW. Epithelial wound closure in the rabbit cornea. A biphasic process. *Invest Ophthalmol Vis Sci*. 1986;27:464-473.
30. Estil S, Kravik K, Haaskjold E, Refsum SB, Bjerkness R, Wilson G. Pilot study on the time course of apoptosis in the regenerating corneal epithelium. *Acta Ophthalmol Scand*. 2002;80:517.
31. Gipson IK, Spurr-Michaud S, Tisdale A, Keough M. Reassembly of the anchoring structures of the corneal epithelium during wound repair in the rabbit. *Invest Ophthalmol Vis Sci*. 1989;30:425-434.
32. Gaffney EA, Maini PK, Sherratt JA, Tuft S. The mathematical modelling of cell kinetics in corneal epithelial wound healing. *J Theor Biol*. 1999;197:15-40.
33. Daniels JT, Dart JKG, Tuft SJ, Khaw PT. Corneal stem cells in review. *Wound Rep Reg*. 2001;9:483-494.
34. Sandvig KU, Nicolaissen Jr B, Haaskjold E. Morphology and proliferation of human corneal epithelium in organ culture. *Acta Ophthalmol*. 1991;69:234-240.
35. Ren H, Wilson G. The cell shedding rate of the corneal epithelium—a comparison of collection methods. *Curr Eye Res*. 1996;15:1054-1059.
36. Zieske JD, Hutcheon AEK, Guo X, Chung EH, Joyce NC. TGF-β receptor types I and II are differentially expressed during corneal epithelial wound repair. *Invest Ophthalmol Vis Sci*. 2001;42:1465-1471.
37. Wilson S, Mohan RR, Hong JW, Lee JS, Choi R, Mohan RR. The wound healing response after laser in situ keratomileusis and photorefractive keratectomy. *Arch Ophthalmol*. 2001;119:889-896.
38. Weber BA, Gan L, Fagerholm P. Wound healing response in the presence of stromal irregularities after excimer laser treatment. *Acta Ophthalmol Scand*. 2001;79:381-388.
39. Steele JG, Johnson G, McLean KM, Beumer GJ, Griesser HJ. Effect of porosity and surface hydrophilicity on migration of epithelial tissue over synthetic polymer. *J Biomed Mater Res*. 2000;50:475-482.
40. Moller-Pedersen T, Vogel M, Li HF, Petroll WM, Cavanagh HD, Jester JV. Quantification of stromal thinning, epithelial tickness, and corneal haze after photorefractive keratectomy using in vivo confocal microscopy. *Ophthalmology*. 1997;104:360-368.
41. Detorakis ET, Siganos DS, Kozobolis VP, Pallikaris IG. Corneal epithelial wound healing after excimer laser photorefractive and photoastigmatic keratectomy (PRK and PARK). *Cornea*. 1999;18:25-28.

42. Serrao S, Lombardo M. Corneal epithelial healing after photorefractive keratectomy: analytical study. *J Cataract Refract Surg.* 2005;31:930-937.
43. Lemp MA, Mathers WD. Corneal epithelial cell movement in humans. *Eye.* 1989;3:438-445.
44. Thomas JW, Mitra S, Chuang AZ, Yee RW. Electron microscopy of surface smoothness of porcine corneas and acrylic plates with four brands of excimer laser. *J Refract Surg.* 2003;19:623-628.
45. Fasano AP, Moreira H, McDonnel PJ, Sinbaway A. Excimer laser smoothing of a reproducible model of anterior corneal surface irregularity. *Ophthalmology.* 1991;98:1782-1785.
46. Horgan SE, McLaughlin-Borlace L, Stevens JD, Munro PMG. Phototherapeutic smoothing as an adjunct to photorefractive keratectomy in porcine cornea. *J Refract Surg.* 1999;15:331-333.
47. Kornmehl EW, Steinert RF, Puliafito CA. A comparative study of masking fluids for excimer laser phototherapeutic keratectomy. *Arch Ophthalmol.* 1991;109:860-863.
48. Tadmor R, Chen N, Israelachvili JN. Thin film rheology and lubricity of hyaluronic acid solutions at a normal physiological concentration. *J Biomed Mater Res.* 2002;61:514-523.
49. Koch DD, Kohnen T, Obstbaum SA, Rosen ES. Format for reporting refractive surgical data. *J Cataract Refract Surg.* 1998;24:285-287.
50. Maloney RK, Bogan SJ, Waring GO III. Determination of corneal image-forming properties from corneal topography. *Am J Ophthalmol.* 1993;115:31-41.
51. Wilson SE. Molecular cell biology for the refractive corneal surgeon: programmed cell death and wound healing. *J Refract Surg.* 1997;13:171-175.
52. Lee YC, Wang IJ, Hu FR, Kao WWY. Immunohistochemical study of subepithelial haze after phototherapeutic keratectomy. *J Refract Surg.* 2001;17:334-341.
53. Amano S, Oshika T, Tazawa Y, Tsuru T. Long-term follow-up of excimer laser phototherapeutic keratectomy. *Jpn J Ophthalmol.* 1999;43:513-516.
54. Dogru M, Katakami C, Yamanaka A. Refractive changes after excimer laser phototherapeutic keratectomy. *J Cataract Refract Surg.* 2001;27:686-692.
55. Liu C. Hyperopic shift and the use of masking agents in excimer laser superficial keratectomy. *Br J Ophthalmol.* 1992;76:62-63.
56. Fagerholm P. Phototherapeutic keratectomy: 12 years of experience. *Acta Ophthalmo Scand.* 2003;81:19-32.
57. Schipper I, Senn P, Lechner A. Tapered transition zone and surface smoothing ameliorate the results of excimer-laser photorefractive keratectomy for myopia. *Ger J Ophthalmol.* 1995;4:368-373.
58. Trokel SL, Srinivasan R, Braren B. Excimer laser surgery of the cornea. *Am J Ophthalmol.* 1983;96:710-715.
59. Lui MM, Silas MA, Fugishima H. Complications of photorefractive keratectomy and laser in situ keratomileusis. *J Refract Surg.* 2003;19(2 Suppl):S247-S249.
60. Kerr-Muir MG, Trokel SL, Marshall J, Rothery S. Ultrastructural comparison of conventional surgical and argon fluoride excimer laser keratectomy. *Am J Ophthalmol.* 1987;103:448-453.
61. Moller-Pedersen T, Cavanagh HD, Petroll WM, Jester JV. Corneal haze development after PRK is regulated by volume of stromal tissue removal. *Cornea.* 1998;17:627-639.
62. Fullwood NJ, Hammiche A, Pollock HM, Hourston DJ, Song M. Atomic force microscopy of the cornea and sclera. *Curr Eye Res.* 1995;14:529-535.
63. Meller D, Peters K, Meller K. Human cornea and sclera studied by atomic force microscopy. *Cell Tissue Res.* 1997;288:111-118.
64. Jaschke M, Butt HJ, Manne S, et al. The atomic force microscope as a tool to study and manipulate local surface properties. *Biosensors & Bioelectronics.* 1996;11:601-612.
65. Alio JL, Belda JI, Shalaby AM. Correction of irregular astigmatism with excimer laser assisted by sodium hyaluronate. *Ophthalmology.* 2001;108:1246-1260.
66. Tsilimbaris MK, Lesniewska E, Lydataki S, Le Grimellec C, Goudonnet JP, Pallikaris IG. The use of atomic force microscopy for the observation of corneal epithelium surface. *Invest Ophthalmol Vis Sci.* 2000;41:680-686.
67. Sinniah K, Paauw J, Ubels J. Investigating live and fixed epithelial and fibroblast cells by atomic force microscopy. *Curr Eye Res.* 2002;24:188-195.
68. Lydataki S, Lesniewska E, Tsilimbaris MK, Panagopoulou S, Le Grimellec G, Pallikaris IG. Excimer laser ablated cornea observed by atomic force microscopy. *Single Mol.* 2002;2-3:141-147.
69. Nogradi A, Hopp B, Revesz K, Szabo G, Bor Z, Kolozsvari L. Atomic force microscopic study of the human cornea following excimer laser keratectomy. *Exp Eye Res.* 2000;70:363-368.
70. Doughty MJ. Morphometric analysis of the surface cells of rabbit corneal epithelium by scanning electron microscopy. *Am J Anat.* 1990;189:316-328.
71. Renard G, Patey A, Savoldelli M, Montanez-Mendoza M, Pouliquen Y. Morphologic and quantimetric study of the surface of the corneal epithelium. *J Fr Ophthalmol.* 1983;6:777-783.
72. Amemiya T, Yoshida H, Yoshida M, Kawaji H. Ultrastructures of the normal surface of corneal epithelium of the heterozygous rhino mouse with special reference to so-called epithelial holes. *Albrecht Von Graefes Arch Klin Exp Ophthalmol.* 1980;213:101-107.
73. Ojeda JL, Ventosa JA, Piedra S. The three-dimensional microanatomy of the rabbit and human cornea. A chemical and mechanical microdissection-SEM approach. *J Anat.* 2001;199:567-576.
74. Brewitt H. Sliding of epithelium in experimental corneal wounds. A scanning electron microscopic study. *Acta Ophthalmol.* 1979;57:945-958.
75. Liotet S, Van Bijsterveld OP, Kogbe O, Laroche L. A new hypothesis on tear film stability. *Ophthalmologica.* 1987;195:119-124.
76. Betney S, Morgan PB, Doyle SJ, Efron N. Corneal temperature changes during photorefractive keratectomy. *Cornea.* 1997;16:158-161.
77. Puliafito CA, Steinert RF, Deutsch TF, Hillenkamp F, Dehm EJ, Adler CM. Excimer laser ablation of the cornea and lens. *Ophthalmology.* 1985;92:741-748.
78. Ushiki T. Atomic force microscopy and its related techniques in biomedicine. *Ital J Anat Embryol.* 2001;106(2 Suppl 1):3-8.
79. Buzard KA. Introduction to biomechanics of the cornea. *Refract Corneal Surg.* 1992;8:127-138.
80. Komai Y, Ushiki T. The three-dimensional organization of collagen fibrils in the human cornea and sclera. *Invest Ophthalmol Vis Sci.* 1991;32:2244-2258.
81. Meek KM, Blamires T, Elliot GF, Gyi TJ, Nave C. The organization of collagen fibrils in the human corneal stroma: a synchroton x-ray diffraction study. *Curr Eye Res.* 1987;6:841-846.
82. Muller LJ, Pels E, Vrensen GF. The specific architecture of the anterior stroma accounts for maintenance of corneal curvature. *Br J Ophthalmol.* 2001;85:437-443.
83. Hjortdal JØ. Regional elastic performance of the human cornea. *J Biomechanics.* 1996;29:931-942.
84. Smolek MK, McCarey BE. Interlamellar adhesive strength in human eyebank corneas. *Invest Ophthalmol Vis Sci.* 1990;31:1087-1095.
85. Smolek MK. Interlamellar cohesive strength in the vertical meridian of human eyebank corneas. *Invest Ophthalmol Vis Sci.* 1993;34:2962-2699.
86. Liu Z, Huang AJ, Pflugfelder SC. Evaluation of corneal thickness and topography in normal eyes using the Orbscan corneal topography system. *Br J Ophthalmol.* 1999;83:774-778.
87. Budak K, Khater TT, Friedman NJ, Holladay JT, Koch DD. Evaluation of relationships among refractive and topographic parameters. *J Cataract Refract Surg.* 1999;25:814-820.
88. Munnerlyn CR, Koons SJ, Marshall J. Photorefractive keratectomy: a technique for laser refractive surgery. *J Cataract Refract Surg.* 1988;14:46-52.
89. Wang L, Dai E, Koch DD, Nathoo A. Optical aberrations of the human anterior cornea. *J Cataract Refract Surg.* 2003;29:1514-1521.
90. McKendrick AM, Brennan NA. The axis of astigmatism in right and left eye pairs. *Optom Vis Sci.* 1997;74:668-675.
91. Bogan SJ, Waring GO 3rd, Ibrahim O, Drews C, Curtis L. Classification of normal corneal topography based on computer-assisted videokeratography. *Arch Ophthalmol.* 1990;108:945-949.

92. Preussner PR, Wahl J, Kramann C. Corneal model. *J Cataract Refract Surg.* 2003;29:471-477.
93. Eghbali F, Yeung KK, Maloney RK. Topographic determination of corneal asphericity and its lack of effect on the refractive outcome of radial keratotomy. *Am J Ophthalmol.* 1995;119:275-280.
94. Rowsey JJ, Balyeat HD, Monlux R, Holladay J, Waring GO 3rd, Lynn MJ. Prospective evaluation of radial keratotomy. Photokeratoscope corneal topography. *Ophthalmology.* 1988;95:322-334.
95. Mahmoud AM, Roberts C, Herderick EE. The Ohio State University corneal topography tool. *Invest Ophthalmol Vis Sci.* 2000;41(Suppl): S677.
96. Vinciguerra P, Sborgia M, Epstein D, Azzolini M, MacRae S. Photorefractive keratectomy to correct myopic or hyperopic astigmatism with a cross-cylinder ablation. *J Refract Surg.* 1999;15:S183-S185.
97. Dupps WJ, Roberts C. Effect of acute biomechanical changes on corneal curvature after photokeratomy. *J Refract Surg.* 2001;17:658-669.
98. Møller-Pedersen T, Cavanagh HD, Petroll WM, Jester JV. Stromal wound healing explains refractive instability and haze development after photorefractive keratectomy. *Ophthalmology.* 2000;107:1235-1245.
99. Manns F, Ho A, Parel JM, Culbertson W. Ablation profiles for wavefront-guided correction of myopia and primary spherical aberration. *J Cataract Refract Surg.* 2002;28:766-774.

CHAPTER 36

VERY HIGH FREQUENCY DIGITAL ULTRASOUND: ARTEMIS 2 SCANNING IN CORNEAL REFRACTIVE SURGERY

Dan Z. Reinstein, MD, MA(Cantab), FRCSC; Ronald H. Silverman, PhD; Timothy J. Archer, BA(Oxon)

Introduction

THE ARTEMIS VHF DIGITAL ULTRASOUND ARC B-SCANNER

Digital signal processing of ultrasound backscatter was pioneered by Coleman and coworkers at the Bio-Acoustic Research Facility in the Department of Ophthalmology of Cornell University in the 1980s. In the early 1990s, we began integration of very high-frequency (VHF) probes originally designed for quality control in the metallurgical industry into the Cornell University three-dimensional (3-D) ultrasound scanning prototype. Pavlin, Sherar, and Foster at the University of Toronto, also produced a VHF ultrasound scanner, but it was based only on conventional analog signal processing[1]; the Toronto prototype became a commercial unit called the Ultrasound Biomicroscope (UBM) manufactured by Humphrey Zeiss (Dublin, Calif). The Cornell prototype and patents were assigned to Ultralink LLC (St Petersburg, Fla). They have subsequently developed and commercialized the first VHF *digital* ultrasound arc B-scanner.

The Artemis (Figure 36-1) was created in conjunction with Cornell University researchers Reinstein, Silverman, Coleman, and colleagues and is based on their intellectual property and patents from the Bio-Acoustic Research Facility in the Department of Ophthalmology of the Weill Medical College of Cornell University, New York. Reinstein and Silverman focused on anterior segment refractive surgical applications, while Coleman, Silverman, and colleagues continued to apply the technology to the study of accommodation, ocular tumors and imaging, and analysis of the posterior pole.[2,3]

The Artemis was designed to help ophthalmologists in all disciplines, but particularly in refractive, cataract, and presbyopic surgery, to improve anatomical diagnosis for surgical planning and postoperative diagnostic monitoring. The Artemis' primary functions are to provide very high resolution ultrasound B-scan imaging of the anterior and posterior segment, high-precision 3-D mapping of individual corneal layers, and 3-D mapping of anterior segment dimensions and axial length by a combined additional immersion A-scan probe. The Artemis is designed to scan in an arc of adjustable radius, thus following the curved surfaces of either the cornea, the iris plane, or the globe, and enabling wide segments (up to 15 mm) to be imaged within one scan sweep.

The resolution of the Artemis, when set to scan cornea, is sufficient to distinguish individual corneal layers such as the epithelium, stromal component of the flap, residual stromal bed, and others, all in 3-D, thanks to multimeridional scanning. The Artemis VHF digital ultrasound technology is able to consistently detect internal corneal lamellar interfaces (such as the keratectomy track) because of the permanent "mechanical" interface present, even years after surgery, and despite total optical transparency. Analog UBM is not able to image the interface consistently because analog processing does not produce a high enough signal-to-noise ratio between interface echo complex and the surrounding tissue. Optical coherence tomography (OCT) has been shown to be capable of detecting the interface in laser-assisted in situ keratomileusis (LASIK) in the early postoperative period, but this ability diminishes with time as edema subsides in the cornea and the optical properties of the corneal lamellar interface homogenize. We have scanned former nonfreeze keratomileusis patients more than 10 years after surgery and have been able to clearly delineate, end-to-end, the lamellar interface.

The development of digital VHF ultrasound corneal scanning technology was first reported in 1991, where digital signal processing was used to identify and analyze the epithelium and scar layers formed in an experimental rabbit model.[1,2] In

Figure 36-1. Artemis 2: VHF digital ultrasound 50 MHz 3-D arc B-scan (Ultralink, LLC).

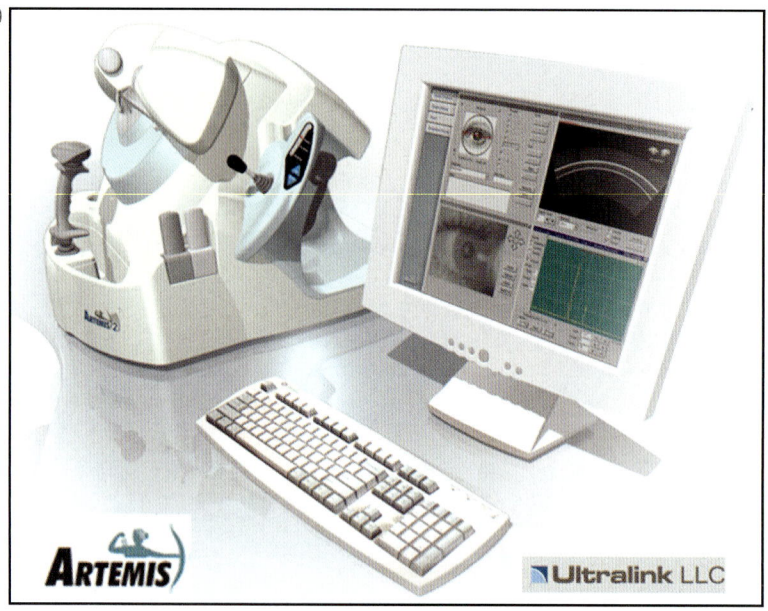

1993, we reported the first confirmed measurement of the epithelium of the cornea *in vivo*, using VHF ultrasound, demonstrating that acoustic interfaces that were being detected were indeed located spatially at the epithelial surface and at the interface between epithelial cells and the surface of Bowman's layer.[4] We also reported the first high-precision 3-D thickness mapping of the corneal epithelium and flap.[5] This system, acquiring a series of parallel, rectilinear B-scans, was capable of mapping the epithelial layer thickness within the central 3- to 4-mm area. By using digital signal processing techniques (the I-scan), a 2.0 µm reproducibility for epithelial thickness measurements was obtained.[6] The I-scan is an A-scan-like trace produced by digital processing of the stored radiofrequency ultrasonic data. The trace represents the instantaneous energy intensity with time as opposed to the average amplitude as is represented by the conventionally employed A-scan. Previous studies demonstrated that the I-scan more than doubles the measurement precision afforded by the analog A-scan process.[6] We further improved epithelial thickness measurement precision to 1.3 µm by increasing the fidelity of the digitized signal.[7] Measurement precision within the cornea in LASIK has been formally tested and published. The axial measurement precision within 9-mm-wide corneal scans is of approximately 1 µm.[8] When scans are expanded to include the entire anterior segment (15-mm width), the axial precision remains similar, while the lateral precision for measuring angle-to-angle is 0.15 mm and from sulcus-to-sulcus is 0.20 mm.[9] (Note: Axial measurement precision will be higher than lateral measurement precision because axial measurements are made from analysis of data within scan lines [pulse-echo axis] while lateral measurements are made from analysis of data between adjacent scan lines.)

This VHF digital ultrasound system has been used to characterize central epithelial lenticular anatomy and to demonstrate that the power of the epithelium is not constant from eye to eye.[10] We have also examined the shape of Bowman's layer,[11] the measurement of anterior corneal scars for planning therapeutic keratectomy,[12-14] the quantitative analysis of corneal scarring (haze) after photorefractive keratectomy (PRK),[15] and the measurement of the depth of radial keratotomy incisions.[16] In 1999, we were the first to publish on the analysis of epithelial and stromal changes after lamellar corneal surgery, demonstrating significant epithelial changes after uncomplicated LASIK and the masking of stromal surface irregularities that were producing optical complications.[7] This chapter will be focused on this application.

Artemis Technology

Details of the scanning and signal processing technology have been described comprehensively elsewhere.[4,8,12,17] Briefly a broadband 50 MHz VHF ultrasound transducer (bandwidth approximately 10 to 60 MHz) is swept by a reverse arc high-precision mechanism to acquire B-scans as arcs that follow the surface contour of anterior or posterior segment structures of interest. The Artemis possesses a unique scan-arc adjustment mechanism to enable maximum perpendicularity (and signal-to-noise ratio) to be obtained for scanning any of the different curvatures within the globe (cornea, iris plane, retina). Ultrasound data are first digitized and stored. The digitized ultrasound data are then transformed, using Cornell digital signal processing technology. Digital signal processing significantly reduces noise and enhances signal-to-noise ratio. We have demonstrated that using digital signal processing on 50 MHz ultrasound data doubles resolution and increases measurement precision by a factor of three when compared to conventional analog processing of the same very high-frequency data.[6] Scanners produced by Paradigm (UBM), OTI (35 MHz), and others employ only analog ultrasound processing. As a result of a unique, coaxial, simultaneous video image capture at each scan position (Figure 36-2), a correlation of measurements

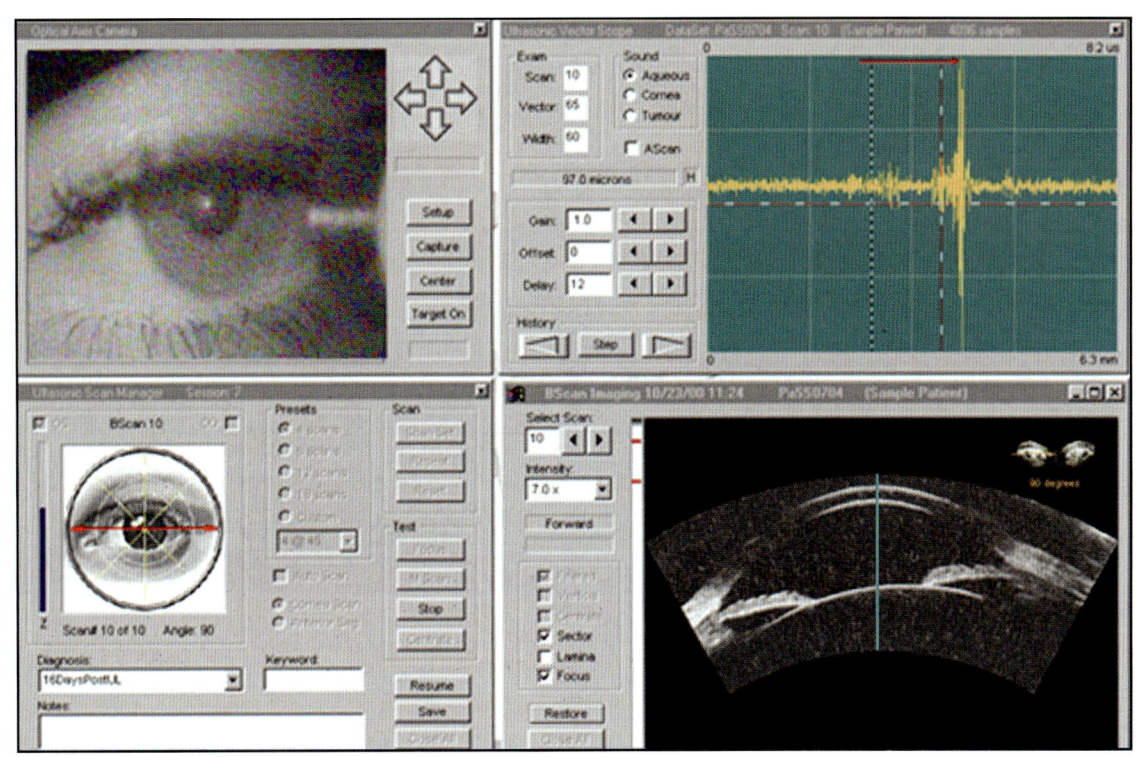

Figure 36-2. Artemis advanced control display panel. The upper left quadrant shows an infrared real time video image of the eye being scanned in which eye position can be verified and monitored during scanning. The lower left panel is used for scan motion control, while the upper right panel displays the raw ultrasound echo data. In this screen-shot, the lower right anterior segment scan was known to have been taken in the horizontal plane when the eye was fixating on a light source coaxial with an alignment beam that is centered on the corneal vertex (corneal reflex visible). The patient's angle kappa produces a geometrical tilt of the anterior segment compared to the visual axis (green line). The corneal reflex is an excellent landmark for correlating scans taken before and after anatomy by subtraction imaging.

made from the ultrasound scans can be formed into visible ocular landmarks (such as the corneal reflex) and enables accurate 3-D reconstructions made from multiple meridional scans and the production of corneal mapping. Simultaneous optical and ultrasound imaging also enables the anterior segment sulcus-to-sulcus distance to be determined in a verified plane, such as the visual axis for surgical planning in phakic intraocular lens (IOL) surgery. For the first time, it also enables localization of the optimum implantation site for devices, such as scleral expansion bands, which need to be positioned based on internal (invisible) landmarks. The Artemis possesses a software application that will give the surgeon external landmarks, identifiable under the operating microscope, that identify the location of lens equator based on a caliper measurement from the corneal reflex (Figure 36-3).

While Artemis scanning is a noncontact test, it does require an ultrasonic standoff medium, and thus provides the advantages of immersion scanning. The Artemis 2 was designed specifically to enable quick setup of this immersion scanning by a novel (patented) reverse-immersion technique. The patient sits and positions his or her chin on a three-point forehead and chin rest, while placing the eye into a soft-rimmed eye-cup akin to a swimming goggle (Figure 36-4).

The sterile coupling fluid fills the compartment in front of the eye and the scanning is performed via an ultrasonically transparent (sterile) membrane, without the need for a speculum. Thus, there is no contact by the scanner probe with the eye. Performing a 3-D scan set with the Artemis requires 2 to 3 minutes for each eye.

Clinical Utility

Two-Dimensional B-Scan Imaging

Figure 36-5 demonstrates an arc B-scan taken along the horizontal plane of the cornea of a patient 4 months after LASIK. The interfaces of saline-epithelium (E), epithelium-Bowman's (B), the keratectomy interface (K), and the posterior surface (endothelial-aqueous) (P) are clearly visualized along the 9-mm chord-length of the B-scan preoperatively. The keratectomy interface can be seen with an entrance track nasally (S), coursing temporally to a stop at the hinge (H). Magnification of the keratome entrance position shows that the flap was not fully distended and Bowman's was not fully apposed, potentially inducing astigmatism and/or increasing the risk of epithelial ingrowth. The interface track has a

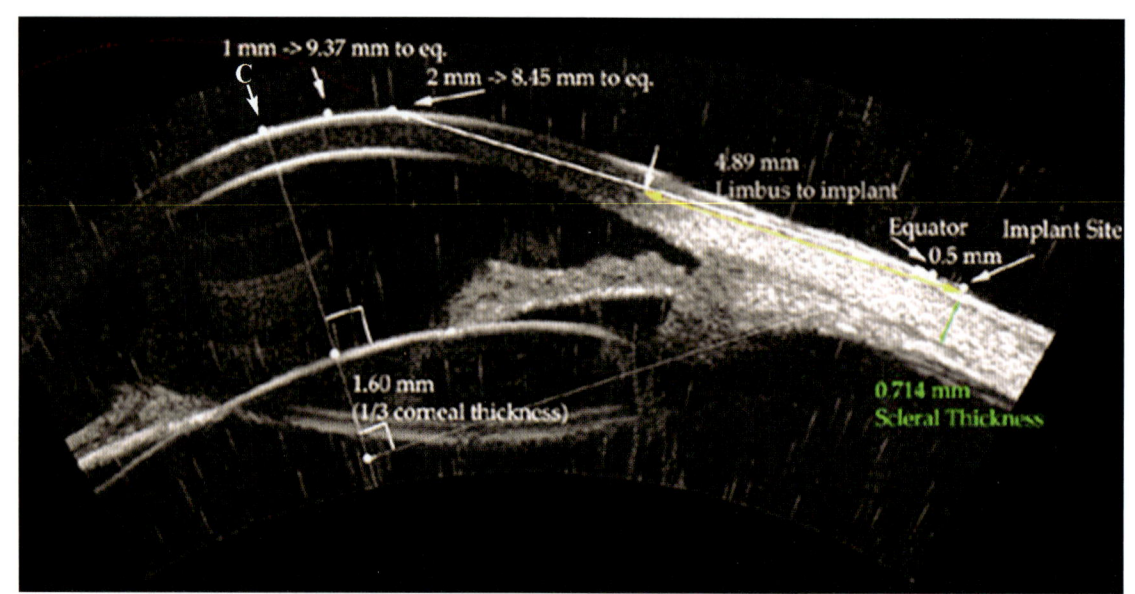

Figure 36-3. Annotated arc B-scan ultrasound image showing all measurements required for the accurate implantation of a scleral expansion band. The intersection of the cornea with the line-of-sight is indicated by arrow and "C." The lens equator plane is localized based on the ultrasound image, and the eternal intersection of this plane at the scleral surface is localized. The distance from C to the equatorial plane is identified for exact localization of the scleral implant to achieve maximum effect. The thickness of the sclera is provided in order to maximize depth without intraoperative exposure of the choroid.

small irregularity (I) (magnified insert), perhaps caused by a patient squeeze during passage of the keratome. The flap can be seen to be thicker temporally and thinner (T) nasally.

THREE-DIMENSIONAL REINSTEIN C12 DIAGNOSTIC DISPLAY

This display configuration and format forms the mainstay, and state-of-the-art, in anatomical diagnosis after LASIK. Figure 36-6 shows such a display created from scans of the right cornea of a patient scanned before and 6 months after LASIK for myopia of -4.75 -0.25 x 55. Uncorrected visual acuity (UCVA) was 20/16 with a residual subjective manifest refraction of plano. Videokeratographic examination showed the customary central flattening with a small surface with-the-rule astigmatism. The lamellar interface was only faintly detectable in places by slit-lamp examination.

This display of 12 pachymetric maps was designed as a standardized layered pachymetric summary of corneal anatomical changes following LASIK. We have chosen to name this presentation a Reinstein "C12" diagnostic display, for it consists of 12 corneal pachymetric topographical maps of the same cornea before and after LASIK. Each map depicts the local thickness of a given corneal layer represented on a color scale in microns (µm). The Reinstein C12 display was designed as a layout of map groupings by time, anatomic depth, and calculation. Columns 1 and 2 depict maps pre- and postoperatively respectively. Within these two columns, the rows represent depth within the cornea. Thus the first column depicts the thickness profiles of the preoperative

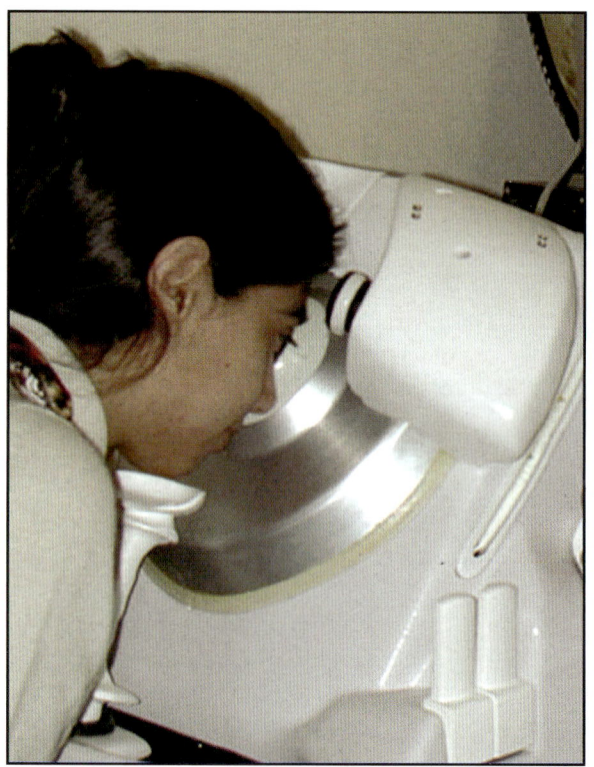

Figure 36-4. Patient demonstrating the simple set up of the reverse immersion scanning system. Head stabilization is achieved by the patient resting against a tripod of support points: an adjustable chin rest and two adjustable forehead rests. The eye rests comfortably in a sterile cushioned eye-seal that produces a separate sterile compartment for the eye, from the fluid-filled scanner mechanism compartment.

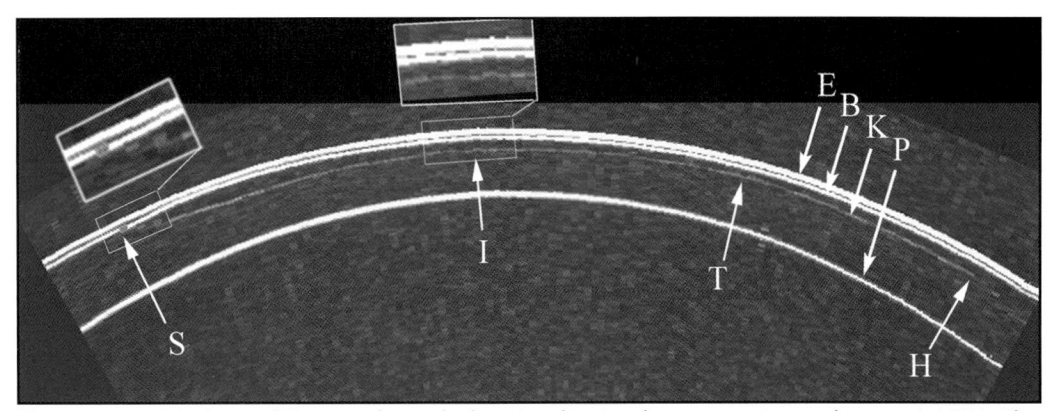

Figure 36-5. Horizontal B-scan through the visual axis of a cornea 4 months post-LASIK. The interface is clearly visualized throughout the length of the keratectomy. See text for annotations.

corneal epithelium (Figure 36-6: map 1), full stroma (Figure 36-6: map 2), and full cornea (Figure 36-6: map 3) respectively. The second column demonstrates the postoperative thickness profiles of the corneal epithelium (Figure 36-6: map 4), stroma (Figure 36-6: map 5), and full cornea (Figure 36-6: map 6). Epithelium, full stroma, and full cornea color scales are identical for pre- and postoperative stages to allow direct color (thickness) comparison. The third column consists of calculated maps representing topographical epithelial change (Figure 36-6: map 7) (derived by subtraction of the preoperative from postoperative epithelial map), the stromal change (Figure 36-6: map 8) (derived by subtraction of the postoperative from preoperative stromal map), and the (calculated) original flap produced at the time of surgery a Reinstein Flap Profile[18] (Figure 36-6: map 9). The Reinstein Flap Profile is calculated by adding the stromal component of the flap (Figure 36-6: map 12) to the preoperative epithelial thickness. The fourth column represents postoperative corneal layers: the thickness profile of the flap at 6 months (including epithelial changes) (Figure 36-6: map 10), the 3-D thickness profile of the residual stromal layer (stroma excluding the flap), and the postoperative stromal component of the flap (Figure 36-6: map 12).

The profile map of the preoperative epithelium OS was approximately 9.25 mm in diameter (Figure 36-6: map 1). The epithelial change map (Figure 36-6: map 7) shows the pattern of epithelial thickening and thinning. The epithelium thickened between 15 and 20 µm centrally, with a concentric decrease in thickening progressing toward the 7.5-mm diameter zone. It is interesting to note that within a 1-mm annulus at the 8-mm diameter zone there was circumferential epithelial thinning after LASIK. We also note in this case that the pattern of epithelial change increased anterior corneal power (greater tissue addition centrally), but the patient had a plano refraction postoperatively. This indicates that the optical power shift produced by the epithelium in this case was exactly as expected by the nomogram setting used.

The stromal change map (see Figure 36-6) shows a well-centered difference about the center (0,0 coordinate) of the cornea. The difference in stromal thickness after surgery is 70 µm centrally, decreasing to zero at the 7.5-mm diameter zone. Thus, the zone depicted on the color scale from green to red represents the effective volume of tissue change in the cornea (the predicted central ablation depth by the Nidek EC5000 readout was 73 µm for a 6.5-mm optical zone, transition to 7.5 mm). Within the peripheral 8- to 9-mm zone there is annular stromal *thickening* of between 10 and 20 µm. We were the first to publish this finding,[8] and Roberts has proposed a mechanism to account for it.[19] It is also interesting to note that this annulus of stromal thickening coincides with the annulus of epithelial thinning described above, consistent with the Reinstein's law of epithelial compensation (see below).

Examination of the anatomy of the calculated original flap (Figure 36-6: map 9) by the Moria LSK-One microkeratome (predicted mean 160 µm) reveals a central thickness of 158 µm. Within the 4-mm diameter zone, the flap thickness was generally homogeneous between 160 and 165 µm although irregularity is evident. Note that direct measurement of the flap thickness at 6 months (Figure 36-6: map 10) would not provide an accurate description of the flap anatomy at the time of creation due to the epithelial thickness changes present after LASIK. The stromal component of the flap (Figure 36-6: map 12) can be seen to possess a thickness profile of approximately 110 to 120 µm within the central 6-mm diameter zone, except for the quadrant superotemporally within the 4-mm diameter zone, where this is decreased to approximately 95 µm. This area may have been thinner due to the presence of thicker epithelium preoperatively in the corresponding quadrant and the passage of the microkeratome parallel to the surface of the cornea during applanation by the microkeratome head.

The 3-D thickness profile of the residual stromal layer (Figure 36-6: map 11) shows a thinnest point of 280 µm approximately 1 mm inferior to the center of the cornea. This is an example of why intraoperative handheld ultrasound residual stromal pachymetry can be misleading; Lateral position variations of only a few hundred microns could completely alter the course of an ablation by providing a residual stromal thickness that is not the minimum.

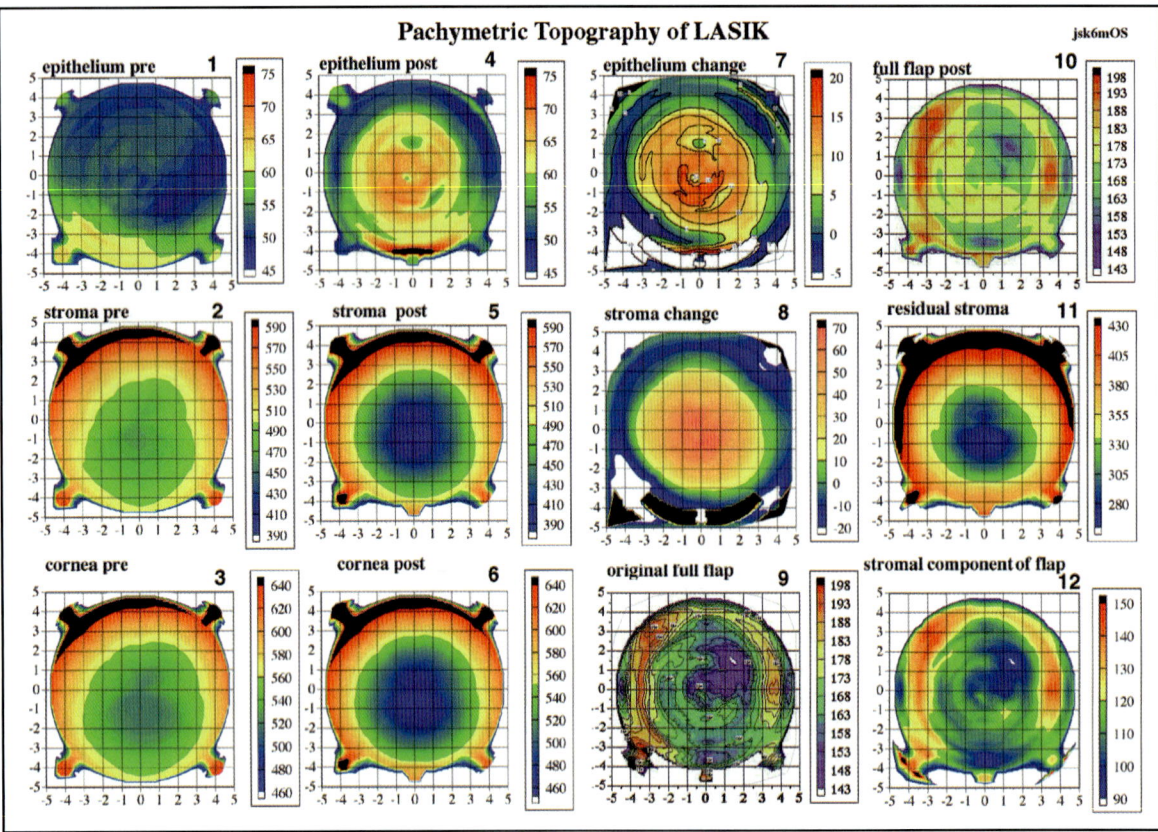

Figure 36-6. Reinstein "C12" display of the cornea of a patient pre- and 6 months post-LASIK OS. All 12 maps are pachymetric representations of particular corneal layers depicted on a color scale in microns. The preoperative epithelial (1), stromal (2), and full corneal (3) thickness maps appear in the first column. To the right of each of these maps (column two) are the post-LASIK pachymetric maps of epithelium (4), stroma (5), and full cornea (6) on identical color scales for direct comparison to preop. The third column depicts calculated maps only. The calculated epithelial change map (7, third column, first row) is derived through point-by-point subtraction of the preoperative from the postoperative epithelial pachymetric map. Thus the epithelial change map shows the number of microns increase due to surgery on a color scale. Note that the pattern of epithelial thickness change is such that it is greatest centrally, with a decrease in a symmetrical centrifugal fashion thus producing an increase in outer curvature of the postoperative cornea. Note that the area of epithelial thickening is confined to the ablation zone or the zone of surgical corneal flattening. The calculated stromal change map (8, third column, second row) is derived in point-by-point subtraction of the postoperative from the preoperative stromal pachymetric map. Thus the stromal change map shows on a color scale the number of stromal microns decrease due to surgery in a topographic fashion and hence represents the ablation volume of tissue. The calculated map of the "original flap" (9, third column, third row) is derived by addition of the preoperative epithelial thickness profile (1) to the postoperative "stromal component of the flap" (12, third column, third row). It is necessary to perform a temporally displaced addition of epithelial and stromal components of the flap separately because of the epithelial changes present post-LASIK, leading to a flap anatomy post-LASIK (10, third column, first row) that is different from that at the time of creation by the keratome. Finally, the pachymetric topography of the "residual stromal layer" comprising all stroma beneath and around the flap is shown in map 11 (third column, second row). This map can be critically important in the determination of adequacy of the stromal bed for further LASIK enhancement surgery under the flap in that the thinnest point is not always located centrally and may be missed by any form of intraoperative single-point measurement of the bed. Thus the "C12" display is set out to be read by temporal grouping (columns) or anatomical grouping (rows). See text for further descriptive analysis.

Preoperative Assessment: Corneal Thickness Profile, Minimum Thickness, and Screening for Keratoconus

The importance of accurate preoperative corneal thickness profile determination is now generally accepted as an aid in the determination of candidacy for safe LASIK with avoidance of ectasia.[20] Concentricity of the thickness profile about the corneal center is also a contributor in screening for keratoconus. Because of the significant, added expense to the patient for Artemis scanning, at present we offer to, but do not routinely use this preoperatively in every patient. Current indications for Artemis scanning in our practice include a greater than 15 μm discrepancy between Orbscan and handheld ultrasound pachymetry and a predicted residual stromal thickness of less than 300 μm based on whichever is the thinnest of Orbscan or handheld ultrasound pachymetry.

The *accuracy* of measurement is defined as the concordance between the measured and the true value. A theoretical error analysis to estimate the accuracy of Artemis pachymetry has been published.[8] The accuracy of Artemis thickness measurements within the cornea was found to be at worst ± 1.8%. This means that the 95% confidence interval for concordance between the measured and the true value is expected to be within ±5 μm for corneal thickness measurements (mean thickness 515 μm by VHF digital ultrasound[6]).

Optical methodology for the determination of corneal back surface shape and hence 3-D corneal thickness mapping, although possessing the convenience of in-air data acquisition, suffers from variable accuracy[21-23] almost certainly due to the variable optical properties of the cornea before and after corneal refractive surgery.[24] But variations in refractive index of the cornea probably also exist between normal, unoperated individuals. To test the difference in accuracy between Orbscan and 3-D VHF digital ultrasound scanning, we determined the thinnest point of the cornea in 52 eyes using the two devices. The variance of pachymetry measurements was 25 μm greater for Orbscan measurements than for VHF digital ultrasound measurements (95% confidence interval ±35 μm). This implies that VHF digital ultrasound measurements are 7% more accurate.

Postoperative Assessment with Artemis Technology: True Diagnosis After LASIK and Optimal Treatment Planning

While LASIK and PRK are already relatively safe procedures today, we are constantly striving to make them even safer. We need to prevent complications, and when these do occur we need methods for correcting them and restoring visual function. In keeping with basic principles of surgery, accurate imaging and biometry will be the cornerstone of these goals, since accurate diagnosis enables optimal treatment planning.

Surface topography has been the mainstay of diagnostic testing in complicated LASIK. Recently, the introduction of aberrometry has greatly enhanced our diagnostic capabilities in being able to understand in a quantitative way how irregular astigmatism and other shape irregularities produce visual complaints. However, neither the understanding of the optical defect or the surface shape of the cornea will necessarily provide a *diagnosis* for the cause of the problem.[7] The anatomical cause of a surface abnormality may only be understood at an internal corneal level (eg, irregularities in the flap vs the stromal bed). With burgeoning surgical rates of PRK and LASIK worldwide, it is becoming increasingly evident that there is a distinct need for a method of determining the layered anatomy of the changes induced. Without an accurate anatomical diagnosis, topography or wavefront-guided treatments may lead to a suboptimal treatment plan.

In clinical application, analysis of epithelial and stromal changes after lamellar corneal surgery using digital VHF ultrasound scanning has demonstrated significant epithelial changes after uncomplicated LASIK and the masking of stromal surface irregularities that were producing optical complications.[7] The importance of epithelial changes in corneal refractive surgery has probably been underestimated. Significant changes in epithelial thickness profiles in both PRK[25,26] and LASIK[27-29] have been demonstrated and implicated in regression as well as the inaccuracy of topographically guided excimer laser ablation.[7] The curvature of Bowman's layer in the center of the normal cornea is on average greater than that of the epithelial surface.[11] As the refractive index of epithelium and stroma are sufficiently different (1.401 vs 1.377),[30] the epithelial-stromal interface constitutes an important refractive interface within the cornea, with a mean power contribution estimated at approximately -3.60 D.[11] Thus, unpredicted changes in the epithelial lenticule after surgery will result in unplanned refractive shifts. This is one of the reasons why current ablation depths and profiles ("nomograms") differ from theoretical ablation profiles—they incorporate the average change of epithelial power for a given level of stromal surface flattening (level of myopia treated). Thus the understanding of epithelial dynamics and their patterns begin to unfold,[28,29] and these factors may potentially be used to improve the accuracy of corneal refractive outcomes.

Artemis scanning will significantly contribute to LASIK accuracy and safety. Accuracy in LASIK translates to the chances of an eye achieving target refraction. Safety relates to achieving this target without loss of best spectacle corrected visual acuity (BSCVA) or other visual disturbance.

Ectasia is one of the most devastating potential consequences of LASIK and it behooves us to prevent it from happening in every possible way. The thickness of the flap determines at what level stromal tissue removal commences, and hence is directly related to the amount of stromal tissue remaining in the posterior cornea under the flap after

Figure 36-7. Horizontal VHF digital ultrasound corneal B-scan through the visual axis of the left cornea of a patient in whom a slightly short flap was created, and the ablation was carried out. The surface of epithelium (E), Bowman's (B), the keratectomy interface (I), and the endothelium (P) are labeled. The abrupt termination of the keratectomy producing a short hinge is shown (SH). Lack of ablation nasal to this has produced a large step in the cornea. The stromal surface step is partially compensated for by epithelial remodeling: the epithelium characteristically thins over the "bump" while thickening in the crevice produced. This cross-section clearly demonstrates why topography-guided ablations (or even wavefront-guided ablations, which are 70% biased to the front surface) will not be fully successful in correcting the stromal irregularity.

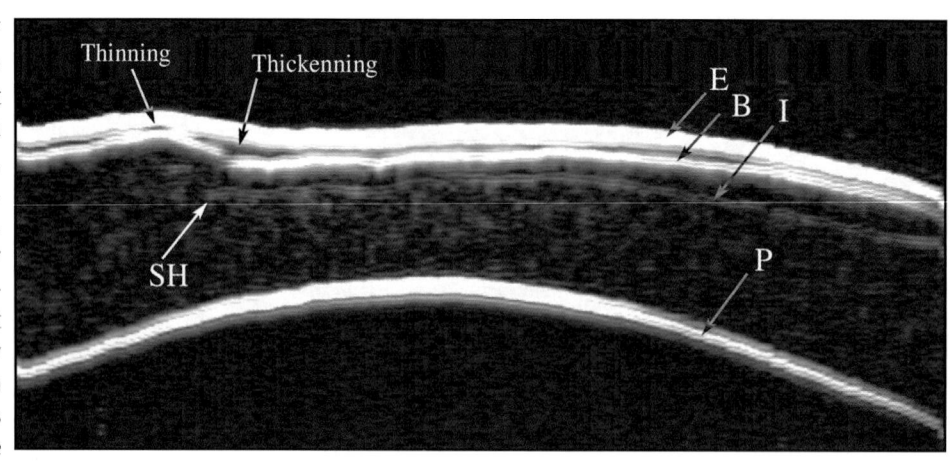

surgery. The thinner the flap the more difficult it is to handle surgically, however the thicker the flap, the less tissue remains for the correction of ametropia by LASIK. Below are some clinical examples demonstrating the importance of distinguishing biomechanical from epithelial components of ametropia after an initial treatment.

Despite all the advances in corneal topography and ocular wavefront measurement, it is not always possible to diagnose the cause of subjective visual complaints by these means alone.[7] This is due to the fact that internal corneal refractive interfaces (such as the epithelial-stromal interface) are not being measured independently. In fact, topography is often not, strictly speaking, a *diagnostic* test, but rather a descriptive one. For the diagnosis and correction of complications, identifying the anatomical cause of a corneal surface abnormality—front or back—may only be possible by understanding the layered internal corneal anatomy. For example, the distinction between irregularities in the flap profile (microkeratome), flap positioning (surgeon) vs the stromal bed (laser) will aid in planning further surgical correction. In addition, further surgery on the cornea should always be based on a full knowledge of the remaining tissue available.

Below are several examples of cases referred to our practice for Artemis anatomical evaluation after complicated LASIK in which Artemis provided essential information for further treatment planning.

In 1994, we coined *Reinstein's Law of Epithelial Compensation* for irregular astigmatism[31]: "Irregular astigmatism results in irregular epithelium." The epithelium often compensates fully for stromal surface irregularities, keratoconus being an excellent example of this. Everyone knows that as cone formation in keratoconus progresses, the epithelium overlying the cone becomes progressively thinner. This is because the epithelium becomes invaginated by the underlying bulging stromal surface while its outer surface is kept as regular as possible by the action of 10,000 blinking events a day. In fact, this is why keratoconus can be detected earlier by looking at the back surface topography of the cornea rather than the front surface. We

are investigating whether examination of epithelial thickness profiles may provide an even earlier and therefore more sensitive screening tool for keratoconus. According to *Reinstein's Law of Epithelial Compensation*, if a patient presents with stable irregular astigmatism, by definition the epithelium has reached its maximum compensatory function.

In the following example, a 23-year-old patient underwent LASIK in 1998, in the left eye, using the Moria LSK One microkeratome in which a short, nasal hinged flap was obtained and the laser ablation was performed. VHF digital ultrasound scanning is shown in Figure 36-7. A large amount of epithelial compensation takes place in cases like this, in which there are large steps in the shape of the stromal surface. This is why neither topography-guided nor wavefront-guided ablations will be sufficient to correct such complications. In this case, the stromal surface is asymmetric. The epithelium has compensated as much as it can, but is still leaving asymmetry and the patient presents with topographic asymmetric astigmatism. If one were to base the corrective ablation profile on the topography or ocular wavefront now (70% epithelial surface shape dependent), there would clearly be ineffective correction of the stromal surface shape. Following such a case, the epithelium may or may not compensate fully for the remaining stromal surface asymmetry. If it does, the topography would become regular but the patient may still have symptoms, due to the significant refractive index difference between epithelium and stroma.[11]

The Topographic Diagnosis of Decentration: Is It Really a Laser Decentration?

Decentration is a diagnosis made postoperatively by inspection of topography. Decentration denotes off-center ablation. We have found that what appears to be decentration by topography is not always due to off-center ablation.

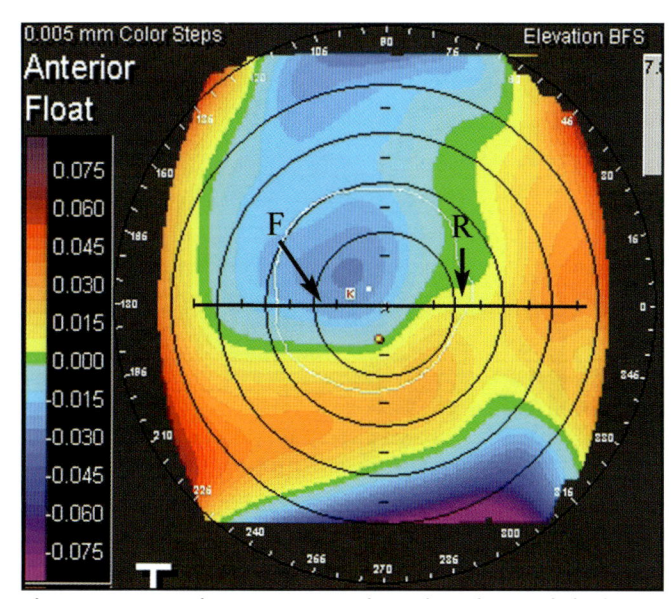

Figure 36-8. Orbscan anterior best fit sphere (default 10-mm zone fit) plot of the cornea in a patient presenting with monocular diplopia and a topographic diagnosis of "decentered ablation," proved incorrect by B-scan imaging in the plane represented by the horizontal black line. Flatter (F) and raised (R) areas are correlated to the ultrasound B-scan in Figure 36-13.

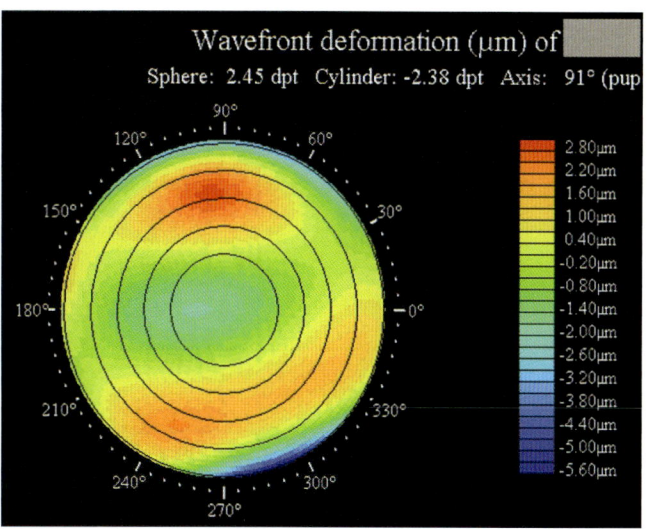

Figure 36-9. Zywave aberrometry displaying the higher-order wavefront plot of the eye represented in Figure 36-11 of a patient presenting with monocular diplopia and a topographic diagnosis of "decentered ablation." There is marked coma. Conventional wisdom would dictate ablation that would involve relatively more removal of tissue in the yellow-to-red zones. B-scan imaging (Figure 36-13) proves this to be inappropriate for this case.

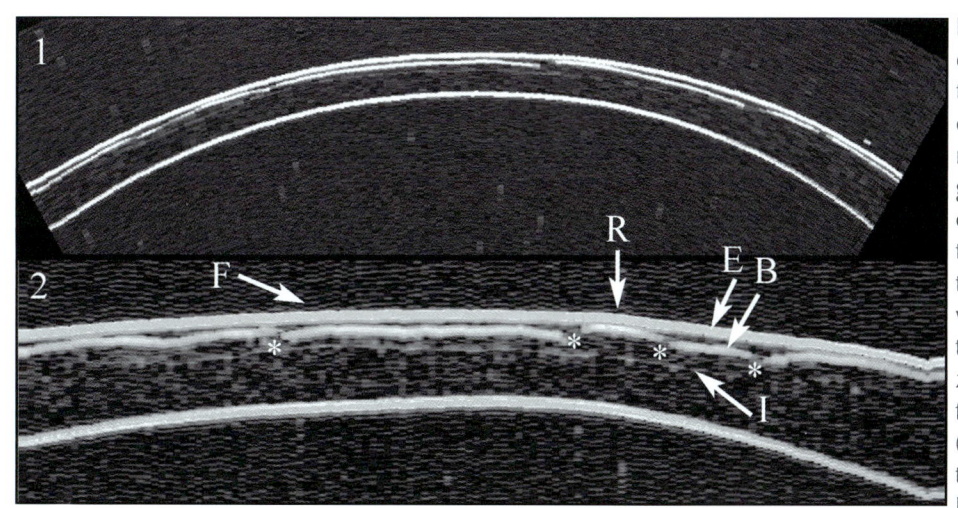

Figure 36-10. Horizontal VHF digital ultrasound corneal B-scan through the visual axis of the right cornea of a patient presenting with monocular diplopia and a topographic and wavefront diagnosis consistent with "decentered ablation." The upper image (1) shows the geometrically corrected image, while the lower image (2) shows the raw ultrasound data with axial zoom to better appreciate the interfaces. The surface of epithelium (E), Bowman's (B), and the keratectomy interface (I) are labeled. It is clearly noted that Bowman's surface is highly irregular, with numerous true microfolds (*) which were only very faintly visible on slit-lamp examination, due to the impressive epithelial compensation producing excellent smoothing of the corneal surface. The diagnosis of "decentered ablation" is clearly less likely than that of an inadequately distended flap, producing surface asymmetry. Appropriate management would most likely involve flap distension and repositioning, not further laser ablation.

In the following example, a patient presented to us complaining of monocular double vision after LASIK. The initial refraction was -6.5 D. Treatment was carried out with the Moria LSK-One microkeratome and the NIDEK EC-5000. Preoperative corneal thickness by Orbscan was measured as 516 µm. With an ablation depth of 90 µm, the predicted postoperative residual stromal thickness was 266 µm. On examination, his UCVA was 20/70. Manifest refraction was +3.00 -3.75 x 96 yielding a BSCVA of 20/40 +2. Slit-lamp examination showed a clear cornea, with an unremarkable flap possessing a few very faint, faded shallow-appearing vertical microfolds. Orbscan anterior best fit sphere mapping is shown in Figure 36-8, providing a differential diagnosis of decentration of the ablation zone, or ectasia. Figure 36-9 shows Zywave (Bausch & Lomb, Rochester, NY) aberrometry of the same eye, demonstrating coma like higher-order aberrations.

Horizontal 3-D VHF digital ultrasound B-scan cross-section of the cornea revealed anatomical features that provided further diagnostic information. Figure 36-10 shows the B-

Figure 36-11. Reinstein "C6" corneal pachymetric map display of the thickness in microns (color scale) of the epithelium, stroma, full cornea, stromal component of the flap, and residual stromal bed in the case of monocular diplopia with a topographic diagnosis of "decentered ablation." The residual stromal thickness minimum is 223 µm (third row, second column). Inspection of the epithelial thickness profile (first row, first column) demonstrates the error introduced by epithelial compensation if one were to attempt topography-guided or wavefront-guided ablation to correct the optical defect. B-scan imaging (see Figure 36-13) confirms that laser ablation would be a less optimal management strategy in this case, in which there is extreme flap bunching due to inadequate distension.

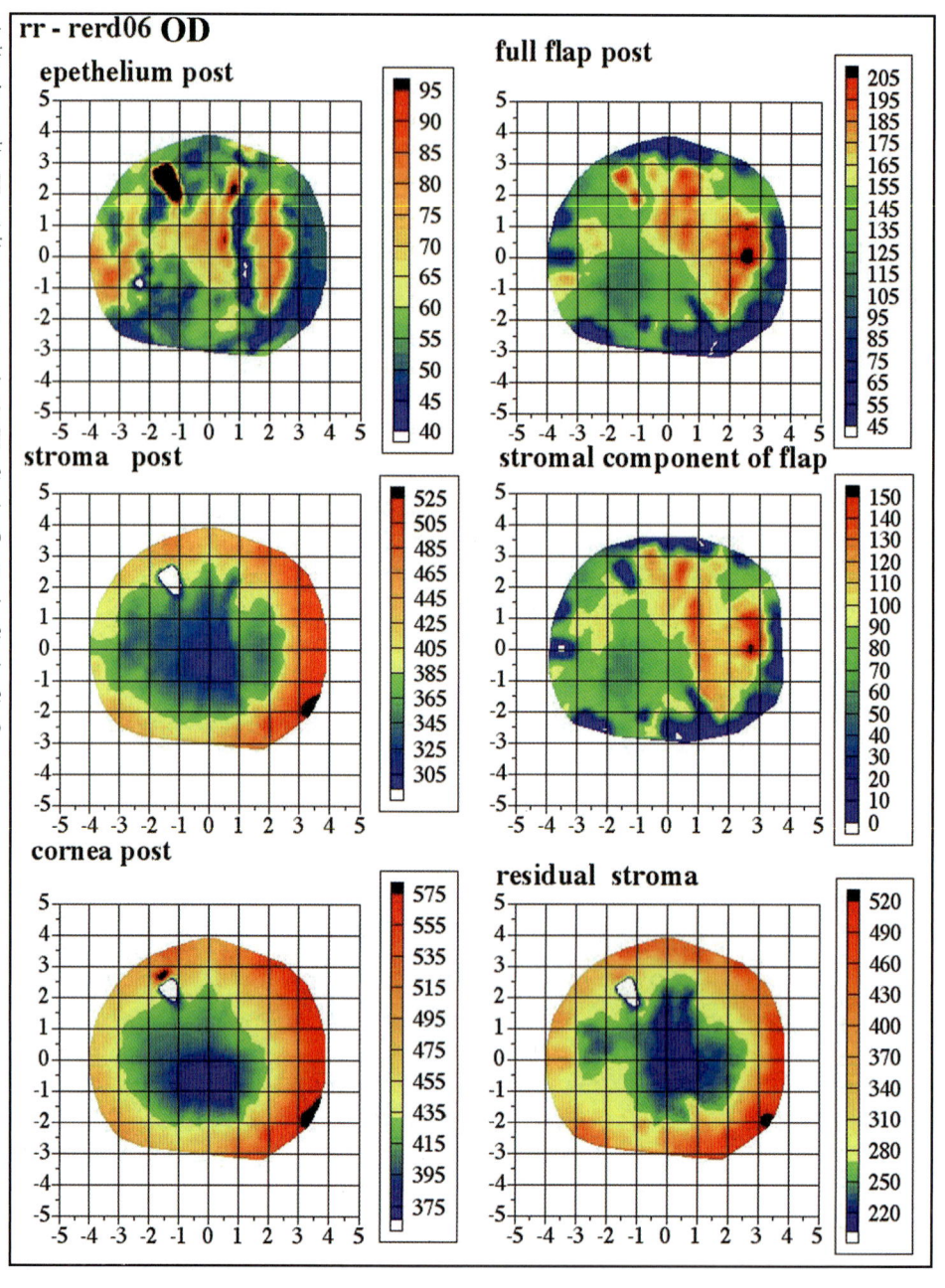

scan demonstrating a flatter (F) nasal side of the cornea, with a raised (R) surface temporally as found also on the Orbscan best fit sphere surface shape map. Beneath the raised (R) area the epithelial thickness is seen to be reduced, due to invagination by the underlying Bowman's layer (B). Bowman's (B) is highly irregular, showing three major ultrasonic discontinuities (*) representing either cracks or microfolds in the flap surface. 3-D pachymetric topography of this cornea is shown in Figure 36-11. The epithelial thickness profile is seen to vary continuously, filling in and smoothing out the surface of Bowman's layer. The thinnest point within the residual stromal bed, as determined by 3-D thickness mapping in a Reinstein C6 (post-LASIK with no preoperative data for subtraction maps) display (see Figure 36-11), is 223 µm. The residual stromal layer thickness profile appears slightly asymmetric or decentered in the nasal direction. Inspection of the stromal component of the flap map (see Figure 36-11, second column, second row) shows the reason for this—the stromal component of the flap was thicker temporally than nasally. The central stromal component of the flap was 80 µm, thus implying that the central flap thickness was originally approximately 130 µm (80+50). The original surgeon had calculated that the patient would still have 266 µm under the flap after treatment. Given that this is 43 µm less than observed, and that the flap was 30 µm thinner than intended, it is probable that his preoperative pachymetry (by Orbscan) was underestimated by approximately 43 µm, and the original corneal thickness must have been closer to 473 µm.

A diagnosis was made of flap malposition and possible asymmetric biomechanical shift. In addition, the residual stromal thickness was noted to be too thin for further under-the-flap ablation, despite the fact that the preopera-

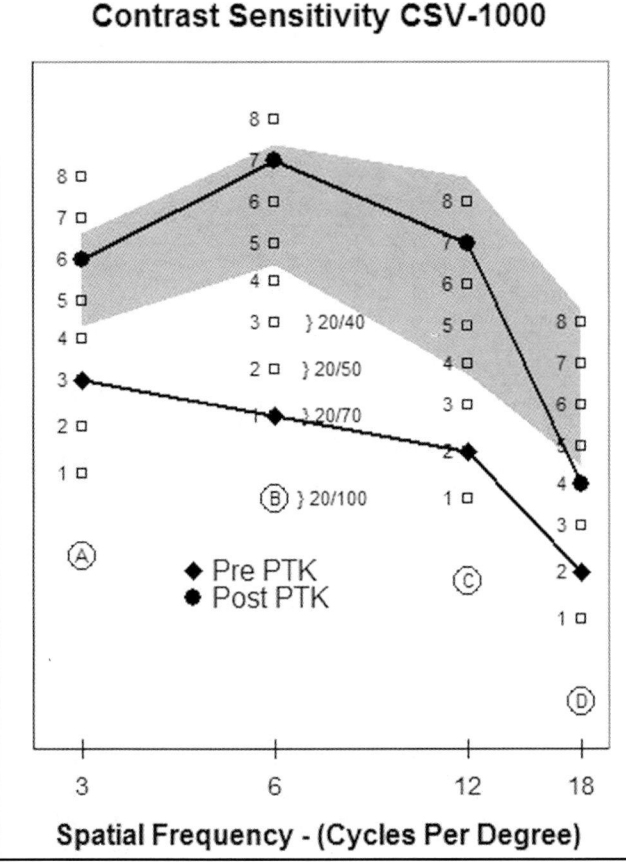

Figure 36-12. Contrast sensitivity chart (CSV-1000, VectorVision, Greenville, Ohio) showing the contrast sensitivity across four frequency levels before and after a Artemis-guided transepithelial PTK treatment for a patient suffering severe visual difficulties due to an irregular stromal surface.

tive parameters would have implied that there was room for further treatment.

This case clearly illustrates the importance of anatomical diagnosis as in contrast to a topographical description, in planning the management of the complications of LASIK. By topography alone, this case may well have been diagnosed as a decentration. The eye may well have then undergone a topographically guided treatment under the flap. Given the low residual stromal thickness, it is conceivable that further tissue removal would have led to further mechanical shifts, and an unpredictable result, with a high possibility of inducing progressive ectasia.[32]

Ultrasound-Guided Phototherapeutic Keratectomy

Many have advocated PTK as a means of smoothing an irregular cornea. Transepithelial ablation and/or masking agents have been advocated for this purpose. Controversy exists as to the effectiveness of transepithelial techniques.

We believe that this is because knowledge of the epithelial thickness profile is necessary in order to appropriately plan trans-epithelial ablation. Without this prior knowledge, break-through of the epithelial layer in certain parts of the cornea while not others can lead to a new irregularity being induced on the surface. The following case demonstrates how an accurate preoperative epithelial map can aid in the smoothing of even highly complex surfaces.

In May 2005, a 60-year-old male NASA Space Shuttle Program employee was referred to our clinic with severe visual difficulties in his dominant left eye. The patient complained that the vision in the left eye was not compatible with that of the right eye. The vision was described as if "everything is coming in from the side." The patient also complained of reduced contrast sensitivity (Figure 36-12). These symptoms meant that the patient preferred to keep his left eye closed, sometimes resorting to wearing an eye patch.

In his refractive surgical history, his original manifest refraction (MR) in his left eye was 6.25/-0.50 x 180. In 1994, he underwent automated lamellar keratoplasty (ALK), which resulted in a residual astigmatism of -1.5 D. Later in 1994 and again in 1995, the left eye was treated by arcuate keratotomy (AK) procedures. In May 2000, he underwent LASIK with a newly created flap to treat residual compound hyperopic astigmatism of +2.50/-1.75 x 95. In September 2000, he underwent a second LASIK procedure with a further flap cut to treat 1.00/-0.75 x 75. Finally, in June 2001, he underwent a LASIK enhancement by relifting of a flap to treat a refraction of +1.00/-1.00 x 65.

On presentation to the London Vision Clinic in May 2005, his UCVA in the left eye was 20/32, improving to 20/25 with -0.50/-0.50 x 80. His UCVA in the right eye was 20/32, improving to 20/20 with plano/-0.50 x 70.

Further testing included Orbscan II (Bausch & Lomb, Rochester, NY) and Tomey (Tomey Corp, Nagoya, Japan) topography, wavefront using the WASCA aberrometer (Carl Zeiss Meditec, Jena, Germany) both undilated and after cycloplegia using Tropicamide 1% (Alcon UK, Hemel, Hempstead), pupillometry (Procyon Instruments, London, UK), ultrasonic pachymetry (Corneo-Gauge Plus, Sonogage, Cleveland, Ohio) and tonometry. His left eye was his dominant eye. Vertical sinusoidal grid contrast sensitivity testing was obtained at 3, 6, 12, and 18 cpd using the CSV-1000 (VectorVision, Greenville, Ohio). Artemis VHF digital ultrasound arc-scanning technology (Ultralink LLC, St Petersburg, Fla) was used to determine the thickness profile for each corneal layer.

The contrast sensitivity was found to be well below the normal range with the patient not able to see more than two patches for 6, 12, and 18 cycles per degree (cpd) (see Figure 36-12). The placido topography exam showed an irregularly irregular surface (Figure 36-13). There was a central flattened optical treatment zone of approximately 4 mm in diameter. There was slight inferior displacement of the optical zone. Within this central zone, there was an outer ring of extreme flattening to a power of about 37.5 D surrounding

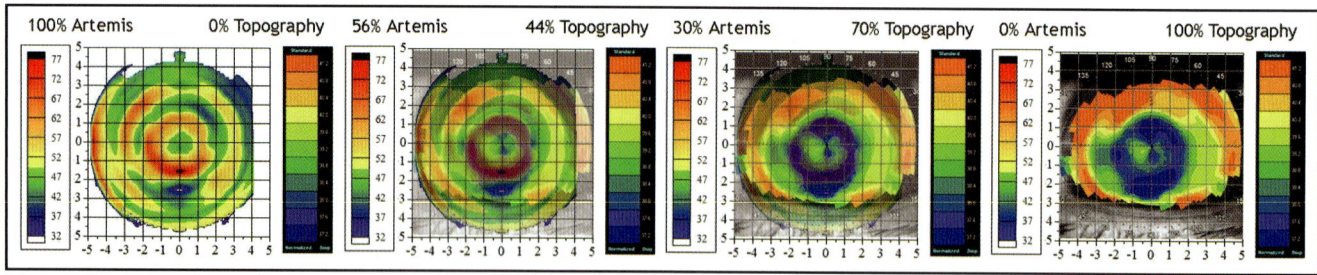

Figure 36-13. 3-D pachymetric map of the epithelium (top left map) digitally superimposed onto Tomey front surface topography (bottom right map). The topography map is shown at different levels of transparency to demonstrate the coincidence of the irregular topography with the epithelial irregularities.

Figure 36-14. Horizontal B-scans through the visual axis of a cornea before and 3 months after VHF digital ultrasound assisted transepithelial PTK. The concentric rings of epithelial thinning (a) and epithelial thickening (b) are marked on the pre-PTK B-scan. The epithelium has become significantly more regular as a consequence of the VHF digital ultrasound assisted PTK smoothing of the stromal surface irregularities.

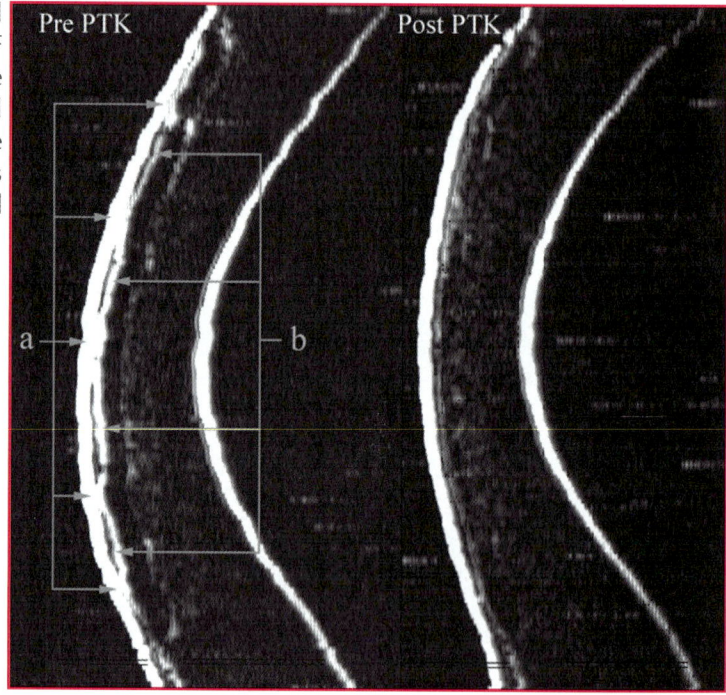

a central area with a power of about 39.0 D at a diameter of approximately 1.5 mm. The WASCA exam showed that the eye had significantly raised higher order aberrations (HOA) with Z (4,0) of 0.615 μm, Z (3,1) of 0.302 μm, Z (3,-1) of 0.483 μm (OSA notation) and higher order RMS of 0.96 μm.

The Artemis epithelial profile (see Figure 36-13) revealed a central area of thin epithelium (44 μm) covering a diameter of approximately 1 mm surrounded by concentric rings of thick (up to 75 μm) and thin (down to 32 μm) epithelium; a difference of 43 μm. The horizontal cross-sectional B-Scan (Figure 36-14) shows the undulations of the surface of Bowman's layer accompanied by (partial) epithelial compensation within the troughs. The epithelial thickness profile was digitally superimposed over the TMS-3 topography in Adobe Photoshop (Adobe Systems Incorporated, San Jose, Calif) and multiple snapshots were taken while adjusting the transparency of the superimposed epithelial thickness profile. It was found that each ring of thickened epithelium coincided with the rings of flattening on topography (see Figure 36-13). This is another example of the epithelium remodeling itself to try to regularize the front surface of the cornea;[25-29] it has become thicker to fill in troughs in the stromal surface and thinner over peaks in the stromal surface. However, the irregular topography shows that the epithelium had not been able to completely compensate for the stromal irregularities.

The epithelium profile matched to the topography provided a confident diagnosis of an irregular stromal surface introducing micro-optical scattering within the cornea combined with significant higher order aberrations as the cause of the visual symptoms. Current wavefront sensors are not sensitive enough to pick up such microirregularities, so the microoptical scattering effect would not be addressed by wavefront-guided treatment. Thus, the treatment plan was split into to two parts: 1) perform a transepithelial photo-therapeutic keratectomy (PTK) using the epithelium as a mask to focus the laser ablation on the areas of raised stroma in order to regularize the stromal surface, 2) remove any remaining epithelium and perform a wavefront guided ablation to attempt to correct the higher order aberrations also present. Following this treatment, if the stromal surface has been successfully regularized then the epithelium should remodel itself in a more regular pattern.

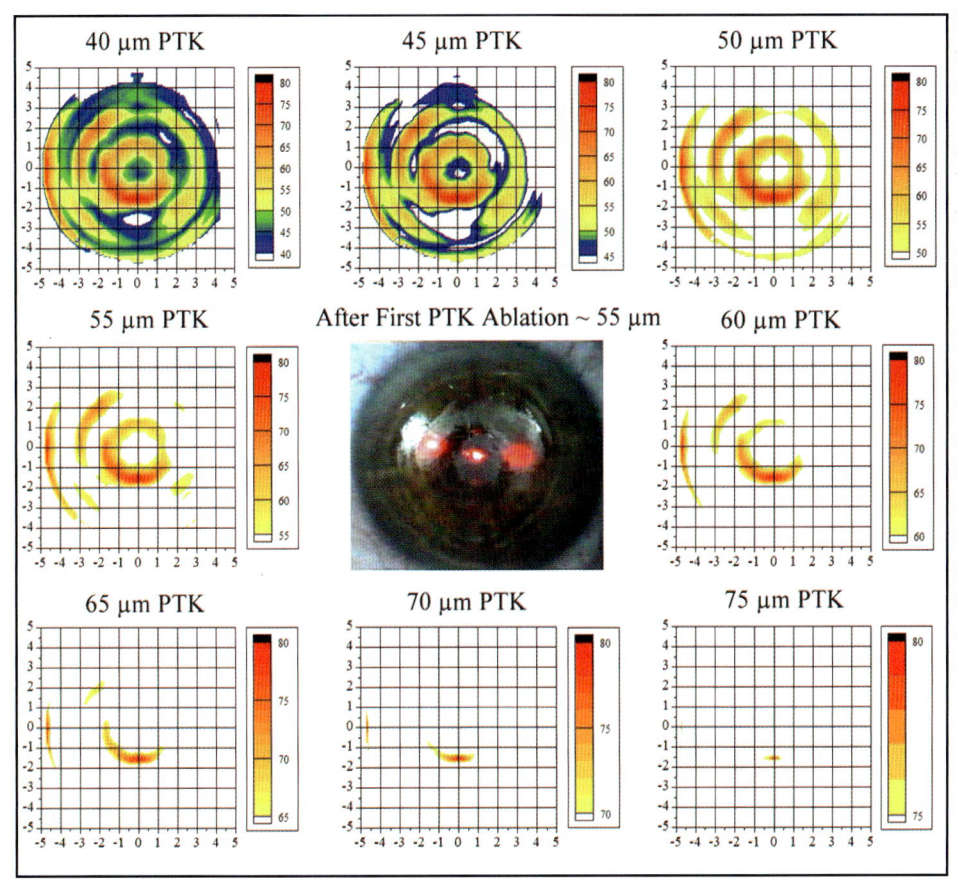

Figure 36-15. Artemis digital subtraction pachymetry simulation of the pattern of remaining epithelium after increasing amounts of epithelial tissue removal by PTK. The white areas indicate where the stromal surface is exposed and hence the areas where it is being ablated. The stromal surface is first exposed in these areas because the epithelium was thinner in order to compensate for the peaks on the irregular stromal surface. The central image shows the epithelial pattern after the first PTK ablation as seen under the microscope. On inspection, the pattern of remaining epithelium closely resembles the Artemis predicted pattern after an ablation of 55 μm.

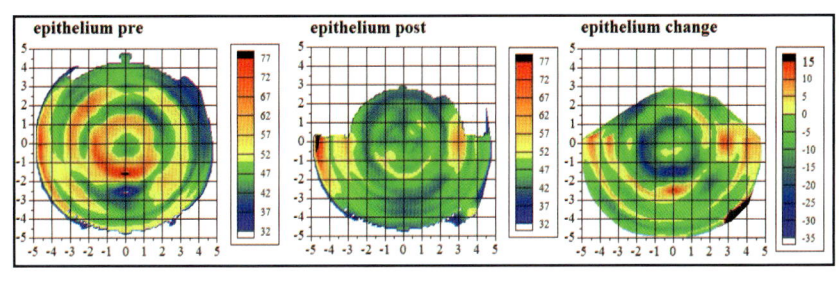

Figure 36-16. 3-D pachymetric map of the epithelium before and after Artemis-guided transepithelial PTK both plotted on the same scale to facilitate comparison. The concentric rings of thin and thick epithelium have been significantly regularized. The map on the right shows the change in the epithelium following the treatment.

The laser ablation was performed using the MEL80 and the wavefront treatment was prepared with the CRS-Master using the dilated WASCA exam analyzed at 7 mm. The PTK ablation was performed in a 7-mm zone. The Artemis epithelial profile was mapped to display the pattern of remaining epithelium after regular intervals of ablation (Figure 36-15). The PTK was performed in stages with the amount of ablation determined after comparing the remaining epithelium with the epithelial pattern predicted by the Artemis. In this way, the ablation depth could be revised to remove exactly the desired amount of ablation. The PTK was continued until the pattern of remaining epithelium matched the Artemis predicted pattern after 75 μm. The remaining epithelium was then removed using a spatula and the wavefront-guided ablation was performed.

On day 1, the patient's vision was subjectively significantly improved and he felt able to keep the left eye open all the time. The UCVA was 20/100 and the manifest spherical equivalent was +1.00 D. After 1 week, the UCVA had improved to 20/32 and the manifest refraction was -1.50/-0.75 x 55 (20/25). The WASCA exam at 1 week showed significant reduction in higher order aberrations; coma was reduced by 31% to 3.35 μm, spherical aberration was reduced by 78% to -1.83 μm and the higher order RMS was reduced by 35% to 0.62 μm.

The patient returned at 3 months and the UCVA had improved further to 20/25 and the manifest refraction was +0.50/-1.25 x 81 (20/20). The WASCA exam at 3 months showed significant reduction in higher order aberrations; Z (4,0) was reduced by 53% to 0.287 μm, Z (3,1) was reduced by 79% to 0.063 μm, Z (3,1) was reduced by 94% to 0.031 μm and the higher order RMS was reduced by 57% to 0.41 μm. The contrast sensitivity was vastly improved to the top end of the normal range (see Figure 36-12).

An Artemis VHF digital ultrasound exam was also taken at 3 months. The epithelial thickness profile was significantly more regular with the difference in thickness of the thick (up to 52 μm) and thin (down to 42 μm) concentric rings

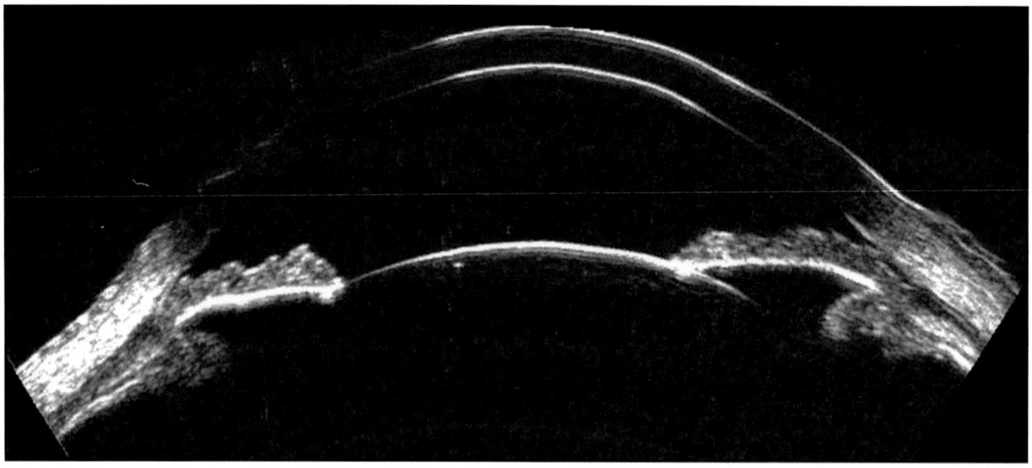

Figure 36-17. Full anterior segment horizontal VHF digital ultrasound B-scan encompassing a 15-mm wide sector. The anterior retina can be seen within this scan plane also. The angle-to-angle and sulcus-to-sulcus diameters are easily measured directly. Anterior chamber and posterior chamber volume and dimensions can be studied before insertion of phakic IOLs to predict the separation of such implants from the endothelium of the cornea or the crystalline lens. Predictive effects on the angle due to posterior chamber phakic IOLs could also be made prospectively to improve patient safety.

now only 10 µm compared to 43 µm before treatment The vertical cross-sectional B-Scans (see Figure 36-14) before and after the PTK treatment show the reduced undulations of the epithelial thickness profile due to the smoothing of the stromal surface. The epithelial profile at 3 months and the difference profile are shown in Figure 36-16.

This case demonstrated a method of diagnosing visual symptoms caused by irregular stromal surface masked by remodeling of epithelium using Artemis VHF digital ultrasound scanning. Using the Artemis we were able to produce 3-D thickness profiles of the irregularities in the epithelium and stroma. The irregularities in the epithelium were matched to those apparent on the topography. We also demonstrate a method of treating such irregularities of higher order than wavefront aberrations (up to the fourth order) using transepithelial PTK as well as correcting higher order aberrations by wavefront guided ablation.

Such anatomical analysis of corneal layers and diagnosis of complex refractive surgery complications is not possible with corneal topography alone. Topography does not provide information on the thickness profile of the epithelium and stroma, which proved essential to accurately diagnose the cause of the visual symptoms in this case. This case demonstrates how layered 3-D anatomical imaging and biometry can be a unique resource in the management of refractive surgery complications.

A Note on Phakic IOL Surgery

There are currently no phakic IOLs approved by the US FDA, and this is almost certainly contingent (for angle-supported and posterior chamber lenses) on the lack of adequate preoperative internal ocular biometry in surgical planning. Maximizing the safety of phakic IOLs is the honorous responsibility of surgeons who expect these devices to remain in normal eyes for several decades without causing serious side effects.

One of the most unique contributions to ophthalmology by the Artemis 2 will be in the sizing of IOLs, particularly phakic IOLs. Incorrect lens sizing or positioning can lead to long-term complications. One of the main safety hurdles encountered in anterior chamber, angle-supported phakic IOLs implantation has been defining the correct amount of haptic force in the angle. If the lens is too large, this can lead to ischemia of the iris, causing iris stromal scarring and pupil ovalization. If too small, the lens may become displaced in the anterior chamber, risking endothelial damage or decreased ability to correct astigmatism with toric lenses. Issues relating to the sizing of posterior chamber lenses exist as well. If the vault of such a lens in the posterior chamber is too large, it can lead to narrowing of the anterior chamber angle. It can also increase the chances of pigment dispersion from the pigment epithelium of the iris with subsequent glaucomatous consequences. If the posterior chamber phakic IOL is too small, excessive contact between it and the crystalline lens may decrease aqueous flow and lens nutrition, as well as directly traumatize the lens surface, leading to cataract.

By providing accurate sulcus-to-sulcus and angle-to-angle measurements, the Artemis 2 has the potential to increase the safety of both anterior and posterior chamber phakic IOLs by improving the accuracy of lens sizing—a crucial issue for long-term safety of these devices (Figure 36-17). Until recently, surgeons have been using the external white-to-white measurement to estimate the internal or sulcus-to-sulcus or angle-to-angle diameters.[39,40] A recent study revealed either none or insufficient statistical correlation between the external ocular measurements (including white-to-white) and the

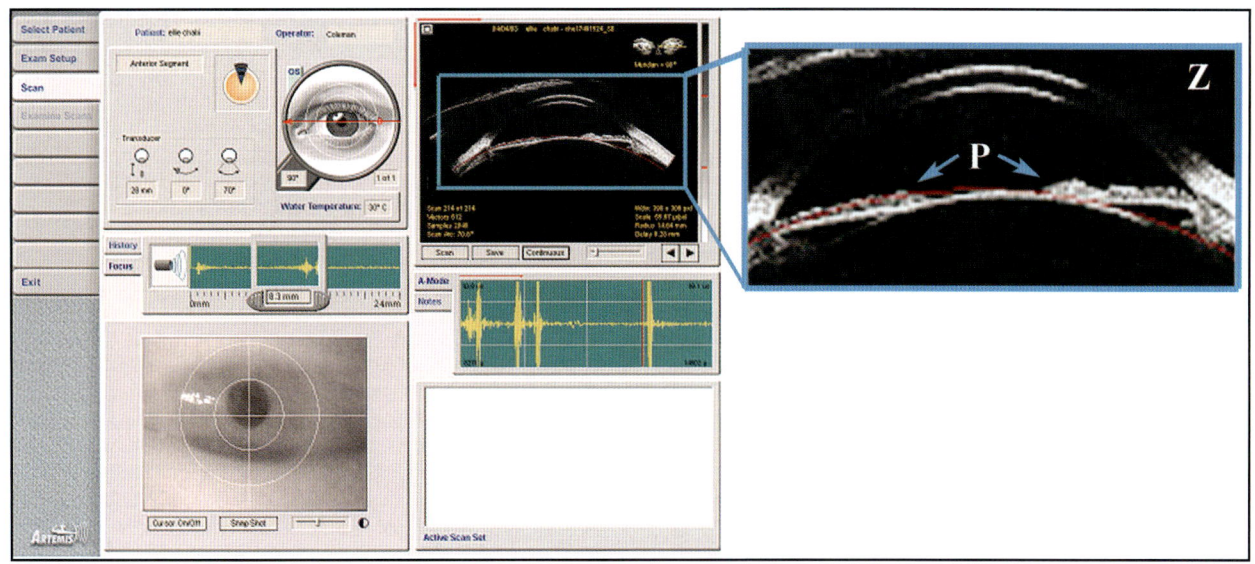

Figure 36-18. Screen capture from the Artemis during an anterior segment patient exam for direct measurement of the sulcus-to-sulcus. Real-time horizontal B-scans are displayed on the upper right quadrant of the screen. The infrared simultaneous video image shows that the position of the horizontal scanning plane is not central or axial. The zoom window (Z) of the B-scan shows a cross-sectional anterior segment representation containing pupil borders (P) that, in the absence of positional information, could have been interpreted as an axial scan, producing a false-low sulcus-to-sulcus diameter. Similarly the angle-to-angle would have been underestimated falsely. Simultaneous video control is paramount for maximizing the safety of phakic IOL sizing, as improper localization will lead to erroneous biometry and the potential for over-sizing of phakic IOLs.

Table 36-1

REINSTEIN CLASSIFICATION OF FLAP MICROFOLDS IN LASIK

Type	Anatomic Location	Loss of BSCVA	Fluorescein Pooling	Clinical Findings	Anatomical Basis	Management
Corrugation	Stroma	✔	✔	Gross folds, differential pooling of gutters, mixed-cylinder	Flap slip	Flap repositioning
True Microfolds	Bowman's	✔	✔	Grooves in Bowman's	Grooves in Bowman's	Flap repositioning and microfold distension
Bowman's Cracks	Bowman's	✔	Ø	Gray lines, no groove	Fractures in Bowman's	Observe only

These anatomical disturbances often change astigmatism and produce loss of BSCVA. Anatomical localization within the flap is important in designating the optimal management plan.

internal angle-to-angle or sulcus-to-sulcus measurements of the eye, even if other conventional measurements (such as sphere, axial length, anterior chamber depth) were included.[9] This means that the only alternative for ensuring the greatest sizing safety in phakic IOL surgery will be to determine angle-to-angle and sulcus-to-sulcus dimensions by direct measurement. To date, the Artemis 2 is the only technology available that can provide both these measurements directly, in 3-D, and under direct visualization for positional confirmation of the location of where measurements are taken. Without this feature, it would be relatively easy to measure internal ocular dimensions in the wrong plane (Figure 36-18).

Improving the safety of phakic IOLs by accurate anatomical surgical planning, and postoperative monitoring, could position phakic IOLs as a real alternative treatment for correcting lower refractive errors where, currently, extraocular corneal refractive surgery is the first-line approach.

Conclusion

Orthopedic surgery was practiced without pre- and postoperative anatomical imaging until the discovery of X-ray imaging in 1895, by Wilhelm Konrad Roentgen. Perhaps layer-by-layer anatomical imaging and biometry of the cornea and anterior segment will have a similar impact on refractive surgery.

References

1. Pavlin CJ, Sherar MD, Foster FS. Subsurface ultrasound microscopic imaging of the intact eye. *Ophthalmology.* 1990;97(2):244-250.
2. Cusumano A, Reinstein DZ, Silverman RH, Belmont S, Coleman DJ. Very high-frequency ultrasound analysis of lamellar corneal refractive procedures. *Invest Ophthalmol Vis Sci.* 1997;34(4):S698.
3. Coleman DJ, Woods S, Rondeau MJ, Silverman RH. Ophthalmic ultrasonography. *Radiol Clin North Am.* 1992;30(5):1105-1114.
4. Reinstein DZ, Silverman RH, Coleman DJ. High-frequency ultrasound measurement of the thickness of the corneal epithelium. *Refract Corneal Surg.* 1993;9(5):385-387.
5. Reinstein DZ, Silverman RH, Trokel SL, Coleman DJ. Corneal pachymetric topography. *Ophthalmology.* 1994;101(3):432-438.
6. Reinstein DZ, Silverman RH, Rondeau MJ, Coleman DJ. Epithelial and corneal thickness measurements by high-frequency ultrasound digital signal processing. *Ophthalmology.* 1994;101(1):140-146.
7. Reinstein DZ, Silverman RH, Sutton HF, Coleman DJ. Very high-frequency ultrasound corneal analysis identifies anatomic correlates of optical complications of lamellar refractive surgery: anatomic diagnosis in lamellar surgery. *Ophthalmology.* 1999;106(3):474-482.
8. Reinstein DZ, Silverman RH, Raevsky T, et al. A new arc-scanning very high-frequency ultrasound system for 3-D pachymetric mapping of corneal epithelium, lamellar flap and residual stromal layer in laser in situ keratomileusis. *J Refract Surg.* 2000;16:414-430.
9. Reinstein DZ, Silverman RH, Lloyd OH. Estimation of angle-to-angle or sulcus-to-sulcus from white-to-white and conventional ocular measurements: are there adequate correlations for safe phakic-IOL surgery? In: European Society of Cataract and Refractive Surgery Annual Meeting; 2002 September 7-11, Nice, France, 2002.
10. Reinstein DZ, Aslanides IM, Patel S, et al. Epithelial lenticular types of human cornea: classification and analysis of influence on PRK. *Ophthalmology.* 1995;102(Suppl):156.
11. Patel S, Reinstein DZ, Silverman RH, Coleman DJ. The shape of Bowman's layer in the human cornea. *J Refract Surg.* 1998;14(6):636-640.
12. Reinstein DZ, Polack PJ, McCormick S, Rondeau MJ, Coleman DJ. High frequency ultrasound scanning of corneal scar formation in vivo. *Invest Ophthalmol Vis Sci.* 1992;33(4):1233.
13. Reinstein DZ, Silverman RH, Trokel SL, Allemann N, Coleman DJ. High-frequency ultrasound digital signal processing for biometry of the cornea in planning phototherapeutic keratectomy. *Arch Ophthalmol.* 1993;111(4):430-431.
14. Aslanides IM, Reinstein DZ, Silverman RH, et al. High-frequency ultrasound spectral parameter imaging of anterior corneal scars. *Clao J.* 1995;21(4):268-272.
15. Allemann N, Chamon W, Silverman RH, et al. High-frequency ultrasound quantitative analyses of corneal scarring following excimer laser keratectomy. *Arch Ophthalmol.* 1993;111(7):968-973.
16. Lazzaro DR, Aslanides IM, Belmont SC, et al. High frequency ultrasound evaluation of radial keratotomy incisions. *J Cataract Refract Surg.* 1995;21(4):398-401.
17. Silverman RH, Reinstein DZ, Raevsky T, Coleman DJ. Improved system for sonographic imaging and biometry of the cornea. *J Ultrasound Med.* 1997;16(2):117-124.
18. Reinstein DZ, Sutton HFS, Srivannaboon S, Silverman RH, Coleman DJ. Microkeratome efficacy: 3-D thickness assessment of corneal lamellar flap accuracy and reproducibility by arc-scanning very high-frequency digital ultrasound. *J Refract Surg.* In press.
19. Roberts C. The cornea is not a piece of plastic. *J Refract Surg.* 2000;16(4):407-413.
20. Holland SP, Srivannaboon S, Reinstein DZ. Avoiding serious corneal complications of laser assisted in situ keratomileusis and photorefractive keratectomy. *Ophthalmology.* 2000;107(4):640-652.
21. Boscia F, La Tegola MG, Alessio G, Sborgia C. Accuracy of Orbscan optical pachymetry in corneas with haze. *J Cataract Refract Surg.* 2002;28(2):253-258.
22. Prisant O, Calderon N, Chastang P, Gatinel D, Hoang-Xuan T. Reliability of pachymetric measurements using orbscan after excimer refractive surgery. *Ophthalmology.* 2003;110(3):511-515.
23. Iskander NG, Anderson Penno E, Peters NT, Gimbel HV, Ferensowicz M. Accuracy of Orbscan pachymetry measurements and DHG ultrasound pachymetry in primary laser in situ keratomileusis and LASIK enhancement procedures. *J Cataract Refract Surg.* 2001;27(5):681-685.
24. Patel S, Alio JL, Perez-Santonja JJ. A model to explain the difference between changes in refraction and central ocular surface power after laser in situ keratomileusis. *J Refract Surg.* 2000;16(3):330-335.
25. Gauthier CA, Holden BA, Epstein D, Tengroth B, Fagerholm P, Hamberg-Nystrom H. Factors affecting epithelial hyperplasia after photorefractive keratectomy. *J Cataract Refract Surg.* 1997;23(7):1042-1050.
26. Lohmann CP, Reischl U, Marshall J. Regression and epithelial hyperplasia after myopic photorefractive keratectomy in a human cornea. *J Cataract Refract Surg.* 1999;25(5):712-715.
27. Srivannaboon S, Reinstein DZ, Sutton HFS, Silverman RH, Coleman DJ. Effect of epithelial changes on refractive outcome in LASIK. *Invest Ophthalmol Vis Sci.* 1999;40:S896.
28. Reinstein DZ, Srivannaboon S, Silverman RH, Coleman DJ. Limits of wavefront customized ablation: biomechanical and epithelial factors. *Invest Ophthalmol Vis Sci.* 2002;43:E-Abstract:3942.
29. Reinstein DZ, Srivannaboon S, Silverman RH, Coleman DJ. The accuracy of routine LASIK; isolation of biomechanical and epithelial factors. *Invest Ophthalmol Vis Sci.* 2000;S318.
30. Patel S, Marshall J, Fitzke FW. Refractive index of the human corneal epithelium and stroma. *J Refract Surg.* 1995;11(2):100-105.
31. Reinstein DZ, Aslanides IM, Silverman RH, et al. Epithelial and corneal 3-D ultrasound pachymetric topography post excimer laser surgery. *Invest Ophthalmol Vis Sci.* 1994;35(4):1739.
32. Reinstein DZ, Srivannaboon S, Sutton HFS, Silverman RH, Shaikh A, Coleman DJ. Risk of Ectasia in LASIK: revised safety criteria. *Invest Ophthalmol Vis Sci.* 1999;40(Suppl):S403.
33. Barraquer JI. *Queratomileusis y queratofakia.* Bogota: Instituto Barraquer de America; 1980.
34. Srivannaboon S, Reinstein DZ, Sutton HFS, Shaikh A, Silverman RH, Coleman DJ. Hansatome flap consistency analysis by 3-D VHF ultrasound pachymetric topography. *Invest Ophthalmol Vis Sci.* 1999;40(4).
35. Seitz B, Torres F, Langenbucher A, Behrens A, Suarez E. Posterior corneal curvature changes after myopic laser in situ keratomileusis. *Ophthalmology.* 2001;108(4):666-672, discussion 73.
36. Pallikaris IG, Kymionis GD, Astyrakakis NI. Corneal ectasia induced by laser in situ keratomileusis. *J Cataract Refract Surg.* 2001;27(11):1796-1802.
37. Seiler T, Koufala K, Richter G. Iatrogenic keratectasia after laser in situ keratomileusis. *J Refract Surg.* 1998;14(3):312-317.
38. Reinstein DZ, Cremonesi E. Ectasia in routine LASIK: occurrence rate is reduced by one third when consistently using a thinner flap. *Invest Ophthalmol Vis Sci.* 2001;42(4):S725.
39. Zaldivar R, Oscherow S, Ricur G. The STAAR posterior chamber phakic intraocular lens. *Int Ophthalmol Clin.* 2000;40(3):237-244.
40. Baikoff G. Intraocular phakic implants in the anterior chamber. *Int Ophthalmol Clin.* 2000;40(3):223-235.

CHAPTER 37

THE FRACTAL GEOMETRY OF HUMAN CORNEAL STROMA

Fabio Grizzi, PhD; Carlo Russo, PhD; Maria Ingrid Torres Munoz, MD; Francesco Saverio Dioguardi, MD; Nicola Dioguardi, MD

Introduction

Despite the fact that all anatomical forms are characterized by nonpolyhedral volumes, rough surfaces, and irregular outlines, a number of sophisticated computer-aided image analysis systems based on the Euclidean principles of regularity, smoothness, and linearity have been developed and applied in human quantitative anatomy. However, the more recently introduced fractal geometry has been demonstrated to be a powerful means of quantifying the spatial complexity of real irregularly shaped objects.

Here we introduce the human corneal stroma as a complex system made up of different but interrelated anatomical parts and describe its whole spatial structure as a natural fractal object. The application of this geometry has led us to first define a quantitative measure of the spatial complexity of the corneal stroma architecture by calculating the surface fractal dimension. Its behavior has been show during computer-simulated changes in keratocyte density and distribution and in the heterogeneous composition of the surrounding extracellular matrix (ECM).

Basic Principles of Fractal Geometry

The fundamental property of all the anatomical systems, macroscopic as well as microscopic level of observation, is their complexity in shape and behavior. This term, which was originally introduced in order to describe natural systems as consisting of parts differently interrelated each other, has become very important in theoretical biology.

The morphometry, based on the Euclidean concepts of perimeter, area, and volume, although largely used in the quantitative analysis of the anatomical entities, defines, in an extremely approximate way, the object in measurement. Such approximation derives from the rigidity of the reported linear measures of the natural objects for which, instead, the irregularity of their shape is the major qualitative feature.

We are used to thinking that natural objects have a certain form and that this form is determined by a characteristic scale. If we magnify the object beyond this scale, no new features are revealed. To correctly measure the properties of the object, such as length, area, or volume, we measure it at a resolution finer than the characteristic scale of the object. This simple idea is the basis of calculus, Euclidean geometry, and the theory of measurement.

However, the mathematician Benoit Mandelbrot (1924-) brought to the world's attention the fact that natural objects simply do not have this preconceived form.[1,2] Living things have structures in space that cannot be characterized by only one spatial scale.

A number of authors have applied fractal geometry for quantifying the irregularity of several biological systems, including human natural and pathological structures.[3-6]

The concepts of fractal geometry were introduced by Mandelbrot building on the works of Jules Henri Poincaré (1854-1912), George F. Cantor (1845-1918), and others and were expressed first in his book entitled *Les Objets Fractals, Form, Hasard et Dimension*, published in 1975, and subsequently in his book *The Fractal Geometry of Nature*, published in 1982.[1,2] He described a new universal code able to interpret the heterogeneous world of the natural forms. Unlike the most ancient and well-known Euclidean geometry, so rigid in the representation of the visible objects and so distant from the power to represent the natural forms, fractal geometry is able to represent the profiles of a mountain or a coast, the clouds and the crystalline or molecular structures. Fractal objects are characterized, mainly, by four "properties":

Figure 37-1. Examples of mathematical fractals showing geometrical self-similarity. The "curve" (A) and the "snowflake" (B), from Niels Fabian Helge von Koch, and the "Sierpinski's triangle" (C), described for the first time in 1915 by the mathematician Waclaw Sierpinski.

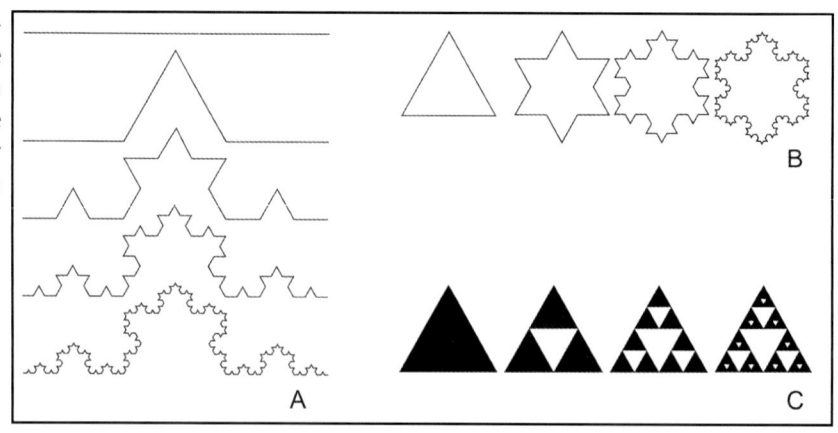

* Irregularity of their shape
* Self-similarity of their structures
* Their non-integer or fractional dimension
* Scaling, which means that measured properties depend on the scale at which they are measured

The most important property of fractal objects is that the schemes that characterize them are found again continually in orders of greatness decreasing, so that their component parts, in all the dimensions, have a form similar to the whole. This property was coined by Mandelbrot with the term "self-similarity."

The self-similarity can be geometrical or statistical. An object can be defined as geometrically self-similar, when every smaller piece of the object is an exact duplicate of the whole object. The classical examples of geometrically self-similar objects are the "curve" and the "snowflake," from Niels Fabian Helge von Koch (1870-1924), a Swedish mathematician who in 1904, for the first time, described these peculiar geometrical forms (Figure 37-1). Another important fractal form named "Sierpinski's triangle" was described for the first time in 1915 by the mathematician Waclaw Sierpinski (1882-1969) (see Figure 37-1).

The statistical self-similarity, also indicated with the term "self-affinity," concerns natural objects, including all the anatomical structures. This term means "to look alike," in other words "to remain statistically invariant by dilation or reduction." In fact, small pieces that constitute the natural objects are rarely identical copies of the whole object; usually alone like they are the object of affiliation. For example, if we consider a portion of a tree, it is not equal to the whole tree but it is representational to the same similarity and structural complexity (Figure 37-2).

Examples of statistically self-affine anatomical structures are the general circulatory system, the bronchial tree, the biliary tree of the liver, the dendritic structure of the neuronal cells, the ductal system of a gland, the cell membrane, the fibrous fragments deposited during the course of chronic liver disease, and the airways in the lung.[3-14]

A fundamental concept for the evaluation of the geometric spaces is that of dimension. Two definitions of dimension have been expressed. The first, named "topological dimension," was introduced by the Austrian mathematician Karl Menger

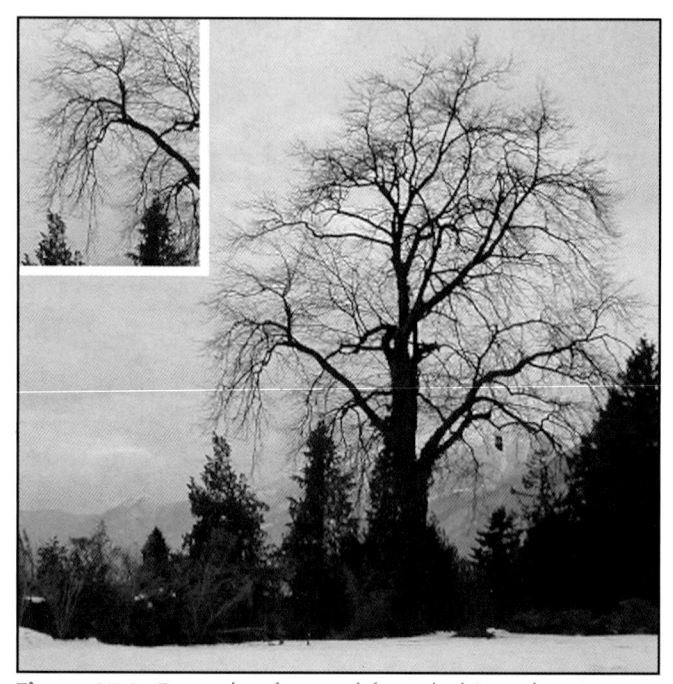

Figure 37-2. Example of natural fractal object showing statistical self-similarity. A portion of a tree is not equal to the whole tree but it is representational to the same similarity and structural complexity.

(1902-1985).[15] The topological dimension assigns an integer number to every point in the Euclidean space, indicated with the symbol E3, and attributes dimension 0 to the point (a point is defined by what has no part), dimension 1 to the straight line (a line is defined by a length without thickness), dimension 2 to the plain surface (a surface is defined by length and thickness), and dimension 3 to the three-dimensional (3-D) figures (a volume is defined by length, thickness, and depth).

The second definition is from mathematicians Felix Hausdorff (1869-1942) and Abram S. Besicovitch (1891-1970).[16] They attribute a real number to every natural object in E3, lying between topological dimension and 3.

Mandelbrot indicates the dimension of Menger with the symbol Dγ and that of Hausdorff-Besicovitch with the symbol D. For all the Euclidean figures, Dγ and D are coincident (Dγ=D). However, this equality is not valid for all the fractal natural objects since the inequality D>Dγ is verified. In

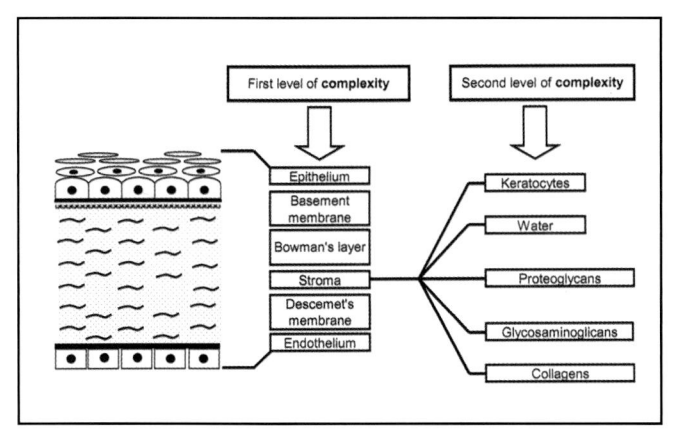

Figure 37-3. Schema showing the hierarchical complexity of the human cornea. The cornea is a complex system made up of different parts that are morphologically and functionally interconnected; the stroma subsystem can be divided into the subcomponents that determine its overall complexity. For example, the number of keratocytes, the composition of the ECM, and their intricate relations determine the degree of anatomical complexity of the corneal stroma, which may be geometrical when it regards the architecture of the whole structure or behavioral when it concerns the relationships among its components.

fact, none of the biological objects corresponds to a regular Euclidean figure (a tree resembles a cylinder, the sun is similar to a sphere, a mountain can be interpreted as a cone, but in the reality these shapes are not Euclidean figures).

As suggested by Mandelbrot in his famous contribution entitled "How Long Is the Coast of Britain—Statistical Self-Similarity and Fractional Dimension," and published in *Science* in 1967, it is possible to determine the Hausdorff-Besicovitch or fractal dimension of irregularly shaped objects through the covering procedure of the topological space of the object in measurement.[17] A number of different algorithms have been described for the estimation of the fractal dimension. The more widely used in the biological sciences is called "box-counting method."[18,19]

The box-counting method applies the following general formula:

$$D_B = \lim_{\varepsilon \to 0} \frac{Log N(\varepsilon)}{Log(1/\varepsilon)}$$

where, D_B is the box counting fractal dimension of the object, ε is the side length of the box, and $N(\varepsilon)$ is the smallest number of boxes of side ε required to cover the outline of the object completely. Since the zero limit cannot be applied to natural objects, the dimension was estimated by the formula:

$$D = d$$

where d is the slope of the graph of log $\{N(\varepsilon)\}$ against log $(1/\varepsilon)$. The linear segments of these graphs were identified using the least-squares method of regression and the gradients of these segments are calculated using an iterative resistant line method.[18,19]

In the past 20 years, fractal geometry has had a vast expansion as a quantitative method able to model a great number of natural phenomenon in a simple and efficient manner.[3-6] Fractal dimension has been applied in fields of investigation other than the biological sciences, including normal and pathological anatomy, radiological sciences, histology, botany, molecular biology, and zoology.

The Fractal Corneal Stroma

Like other biological entities, the human cornea is a complex anatomical system consisting of various interconnected parts. It has five histological layers:

1. The epithelium, consisting of basal cells, wing cells, and squames
2. Bowman's layer, an acellular zone of the anterior stroma located just beneath the basement elastic membrane
3. The stroma, which constitutes about 90% of the depth of the cornea and consists of keratocytes and a heterogeneous ECM
4. Descemet's membrane, which forms the basement membrane of the endothelium
5. The endothelium, which pumps excess water out of the stroma, thus preventing corneal edema and maintaining stroma transparency[20-24]

These anatomical subsystems are morphologically and functionally interrelated to each other (Figure 37-3) and form a whole anatomical system that has a inhomogeneous structure[25] and complex behavior. It is well known that the cells in the cornea define an intricate framework that is critical during development, homeostasis, and wound healing; it has also been established that disordered cell communications contribute to various corneal diseases.[26]

The mathematical definition of the measure of complexity as "the number of species or connections in the interaction environment" designates the cornea as the first level of anatomical complexity (see Figure 37-3) and the stroma as the second level.[27,28]

The complexity of any anatomical system can be geometrical when it regards the architecture of the system or behavioral when it concerns the intricate relationships of the system's components.

Complexity can reside in the structure of a system (eg, the existence of many different component parts with varying interactions or an intricate architecture) or its nonlinear functions (ie, physiological rhythms are rarely strictly periodic but fluctuate irregularly over time).[27-29]

The cornea that provides our window on the world is a complex anatomical system made up of different anatomical entities that are morphologically and functionally continuous. The stroma consists of intercalated layers of collagens and other ECM components and cells, called keratocytes, that are known to maintain the stroma by aiding its repair and probably in other critical roles.[30,31] Emerging evidence

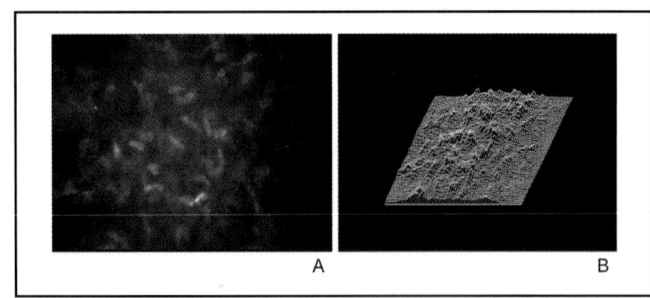

Figure 37-4. Computer-aided procedures used to quantify the surface fractal dimension of a 2-D image of the corneal stroma. (A) Prototypical digitized confocal microscopy image of the corneal stroma. (B) The generation of an (x, y) matrix with z values derived from the grey-intensity values of the filtered image. The matrix is used to create a 3-D surface representing the spatial complexity of the stroma at a particular depth level.[38]

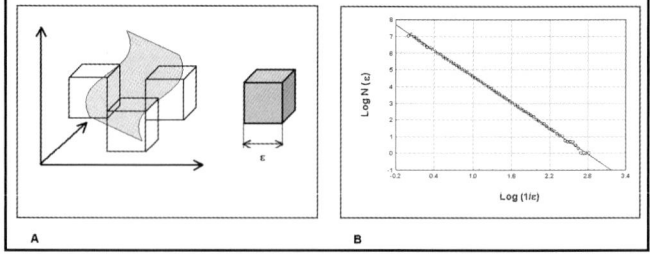

Figure 37-5. Mathematical estimate of the surface fractal dimension. (A) Covering an irregular surface requires triplets of intersections of contiguous and nonoverlapping 3-D box, of side length ε. That is, we count N(ε), the number of boxes that contain at least one point of the object for different box sizes ε and then determine the fractal dimension D_B from Equation 1. (B) A typical N(ε) vs ε plot (log-log scale) and determined by the box-counting method. The slope of the straight line which could be plotted within the scale window (ε_{MIN}-ε_{MAX}) is used to calculate the surface fractal dimension (D_B).[38]

suggests that keratocytes may interact directly by means of intercellular communication channels and act cohesively throughout the cornea, or at least within variable 3-D functional groups.[20,30,32-34] Such an integrated cell system provides an anatomical network for the coordinated maintenance of the corneal stroma, cohesive reactions to injury or disease, and programmed cell death (apoptosis) and replacement.

Despite confocal microscopy techniques that have been developed as a means of investigating the microanatomy of the corneal stroma,[35] no computer-aided quantitative approaches for measuring its geometrical complexity have yet been investigated.

The need to reduce complications and suboptimal refractive outcomes has led to the early detection and beneficial management of potentially aberrant reactions to photorefractive keratectomy (PRK) and laser-assisted in situ keratomileusis (LASIK) by modifying those that are unsatisfactory.[35] However, in order to achieve this, we need to improve our knowledge of the microanatomy and function of human keratocytes under normal and pathological conditions.[21,36,37] Moreover, the introduction of quantitative methods suitable for measuring the geometrical structure of the corneal stroma requires the replacement of subjective qualitative and semiquantitative evaluations that are insufficient for statistical purposes with quantitative methods that are statistically effective and appropriate for comparing different microarchitectures under physiological and diseased conditions. It is also necessary to emphasise that quantitative methods that do not rely on human skills are diagnostically advantageous.

Recently, we introduced a computer-aided method that uses the surface fractal dimension (D_B) as a quantitative estimator of the spatial complexity of the corneal stroma (Figures 37-4 and 37-5).[38] Comparative analyses of the data obtained from eight patients has revealed an intersubject variability, thus indicating that D_B makes it possible to measure smaller differences in the geometrical complexity of the corneal stroma.

The theoretical concepts underlying D_B were abstracted from the theory of the fractal geometry, which has recently been applied to quantitative ophthalmology.[38-40]

The most noticeable properties of any anatomical form are the irregularity of their shapes or the distribution patterns of a set of forms (ie, the arrangement of unconnected cells in the surrounding ECM) and their dissimilarity to smooth Euclidean figures. As the space filled by a set of objects is geometrically irregular, its dimension cannot be expressed by integers of zero, 1, 2, and 3 (the Euclidean or topological dimensions), but the space-filling property of a set of irregularly shaped objects can be measured using nonintegers (the fractal dimension) falling between two Euclidean dimensions. In our case, D_B falls between 2 (corresponding to the Euclidean dimension of a plane) and 3 (the dimension of a 3-D Euclidean object). The more D_B tends to 3, the more the analyzed configuration (spatial conformation) tends to fill a 3-D space and the greater its geometrical complexity.

The concept of spatial conformation has assumed a fundamental role in the study of biological macromolecules in biochemistry since the early 1950s. However, in the science of morphology, it has only been introduced in theoretical morphology, which studies extant organismal forms (complex structures of interdependent and subordinate elements whose relationships and properties are largely determined by their function in the whole) as a subset of the range of theoretically possible morphologies.[38,41]

As the corneal stroma consists of different but interconnected anatomical parts (keratocytes and the different components of the ECM) whose relationship and properties are largely determined by their function in the whole, its geometrical complexity can be defined on the basis of its whole spatial architecture. The significance of D_B also comes from the fact that, like any other complex system, the microanatomy of the corneal stroma cannot be correctly quantified by measuring its individual components (ie, cell density).[38]

D_B is a parameter that depends on the spatial relationships between the cellular component itself and the surrounding heterogeneous ECM. In other words, its estimate is "ecologically" important because it provides a quantitative index of the "habitat structure."

It is interesting to underline that analysis of the images of corneal stroma sections taken by means of in vivo confocal microscopy has revealed differences in D_B that can be ascribed not only to cell density, but also to the spatial distribution of the cellular component.[38]

As computer-aided models are crucial for scientific procedures[42] and the modeling process itself represents the hypothetic-deductive approach in science,[42] we have recently developed a computer-aided model capable of generating an unlimited number of two-dimensional (2-D) images of corneal stroma sections.[38]

The model was simplified by using a minimum amount of mathematical complexity and only three parameters:

1. The number of cells
2. The concentrations of the four components of the ECM
3. The distribution of the cells and components

It is necessary to emphasize that although the corneal stroma is a complex system any mathematical model is aimed to simplify this complexity in order to better understand the general behavior of the system. A large number of corneal stroma images showing a variable number of unconnected keratocytes randomly distributed on a planar surface and separated from each other by a heterogeneous ECM were automatically generated and, interestingly, the model shows that D_B increases in accordance with the number (ie, density) of keratocytes making up the system. Furthermore, its value changed when an equal number of cells were distributed differently in the surrounding ECM. These results confirm that a primary role in the quantitative analysis of the microanatomy of the corneal stroma is played by its whole architecture. In other words, it is plausible that an equal number of cells have different space-filling properties depending on their distribution pattern. This may have important implications for the measure of all of the biological processes that involve keratocytes, their interrelationships, and their relationships with the surrounding ECM.

Conclusion

The investigation of the human corneal stroma as fractal natural object has led us to develop a new quantitative index for quantifying its complex architecture. The application of this parameter has shown that:

* It quantifies the geometric complexity arising from the intricate relationships of the components of the corneal stroma.
* It not only depends on the number of keratocytes and their different degrees of contiguity and continuity (the two characteristics determining the connectivity of the cellular component, ie, from isolated cells to the continuous cell network), but also on differences in the composition of the ECM.
* It might help to quantify morphologic attributes over the entire anterior-posterior stromal thickness, as has previously been shown in the porcine cornea.[30,34] The differences in spatial complexity at different depths of the corneal stroma may not only be related to dissimilarities in cell density, but also to dissimilarities in the cell distribution pattern and type of ECM environment. It is important to point out that these differences can be recognized by D_B estimates and that they may be related to a specific pathological state. Two further findings are that D_B is suitable for recognizing variations in spatial structure in both the normal and diseased corneal stroma and assessing drug-related changes in keratocyte density,[43] and that it can be usefully evaluated by means of computer-aided simulations in which the parameter values of a geometrical model of form are systematically varied.

Although the present knowledge is limited to give the first steps in developing a useful method that enable specific morphological analyses of the human corneal stroma, the broad applicability of this quantitative index makes it possible to explore the possible range of morphological variability that can be produced in nature, thus increasing its diagnostic importance in ophthalmology.

References

1. Mandelbrot BB. *Les Objets Fractals: Forme, Hasard et Dimension*. Paris, France: Flammarion; 1975.
2. Mandelbrot BB. *The Fractal Geometry of Nature*. San Francisco, Calif: Freeman; 1982.
3. Nonnemacher TF, Losa GA, Weibel ER. *Fractals in Biology and Medicine*. Vol 1. Basel, Germany: Birkhauser-Verlag; 1994.
4. Losa GA, Merlini D, Nonnemacher TF, Weibel ER. *Fractals in Biology and Medicine*. Vol 2. Basel, Germany: Birkhauser-Verlag; 1998.
5. Losa GA, Merlini D, Nonnemacher TF, Weibel ER. *Fractals in Biology and Medicine*. Vol 3. Basel, Germany: Birkhauser-Verlag; 2002.
6. Losa GA, Merlini D, Nonnemacher TF, Weibel ER. *Fractals in Biology and Medicine*. Vol 4. Basel, Germany: Birkhauser-Verlag; 2005.
7. Losa GA. Fractals in pathology: are they really useful? *Pathologica*. 1995;87:310-317.
8. Cross SS. Fractals in pathology. *J Pathol*. 1997;182:1-8.
9. Muzzio PC, Grizzi F. Fractal geometry: its possible applications to radiologic imaging. *Radiol Med*. 1999;98:331-336.
10. Grizzi F, Ceva-Grimaldi G, Dioguardi N. Fractal geometry: a useful tool for quantifying irregular lesions in human liver biopsy specimens. *Ital J Anat Embryol*. 2001;106:337-346.
11. Losa GA. Fractal morphometry of cell complexity. *Riv Biol*. 2002;95:239-258.
12. Dioguardi N, Grizzi F. Fractal dimension exponent for quantitative evaluation of liver collagen in bioptic specimens. In: Losa GA, Merlini D, Nonnemacher TF, Weibel ER, eds. *Fractals in Biology and Medicine*. Vol 3. Basel, Germany; Birkhauser-Verlag; 2002.
13. Dioguardi N, Franceschini B, Aletti G, Russo C, Grizzi F. Fractal dimension rectified meter for quantification of liver fibrosis and other irregular microscopic objects. *Anal Quant Cytol Histol*. 2003;25:312-320.

14. Dioguardi N, Grizzi F, Franceschini B, Bossi P, Russo C. Liver fibrosis sand tissue architectural changes measurement using fractal-rectified metrics and Hurst's exponent. *World J Gastroenterol*. In press.
15. Menger K. What is dimension? *Am Math Monthly*. 1943;50:2-7.
16. Hausdorff GS. Dimension und äueres. *Maas Math Ann*. 1919;79:157-179.
17. Mandelbrot BB. How long is the coast of Britain—statistical self-similarity and fractional dimension. *Science*. 1967;155:636-638.
18. Bassingthwaighte JB, Liebovitch LS, West BJ. *Fractal Physiology*. New York, NY: Oxford University Press; 1994.
19. Hastings HM, Sugihara G. *Fractals: A User's Guide for the Natural Sciences*. New York, NY: Oxford University Press; 1998.
20. Hogan MJ, Alvarado JA, Weddel JE. *Histology of the Human Eye*. London, England: WB Saunders; 1971.
21. Bron AJ. The architecture of the corneal stroma. *Br J Ophthalmol*. 2001;85:379-381.
22. Hodson S, Miller F. The bicarbonate ion pump in the endothelium which regulates the hydration of rabbit cornea. *J Physiol*. 1976;263:563-577.
23. Daniels JT, Dart JK, Tuft SJ, Khaw PT. Corneal stem cells in review. *Wound Repair Regen*. 2001;9:483-494.
24. Meek KM, Fullwood NJ. Corneal and scleral collagens—a microscopist's perspective. *Micron*. 2001;32:261-272.
25. Langefeld S, Reim M, Redbrake C, Schrage NF. The corneal stroma: an inhomogeneous structure. *Graefes Arch Clin Exp Ophthalmol*. 1997;235:480-485.
26. Green CR. Keratocytes: more than a framework for the window. *Clin Exper Ophthalmol*. 2003;31:91-92.
27. Lumsden CY, Brandts WA, Trainor LEH. *1997. Physical Theory in Biology. Foundations and Explorations*. London, England: World Scientific; 1997.
28. Grizzi F, Franceschini B, Chiriva-Internati M, et al. The complexity and the microscopy in the anatomical sciences. In: A. Méndez-Vilas, ed. *Science, Technology and Education of Microscopy: An Overview*. Badajoz, Spain: Formatex; 2003.
29. Waddington CH. *Tools for Thought*. Frogmore, St Albans: Paladin; 1977.
30. Poole CA, Brookes NH, Clover GM. Confocal imaging of the human keratocyte network using the vital dye 5-chloromethylfluorescein diacetate. *Clin Exper Ophthalmol*. 2003;31:147-154.
31. Muller LJ, Pels L, Vrensen GF. Novel aspects of the ultrastructural organization of human corneal keratocytes. *Invest Ophthalmol Vis Sci*. 1995;36:2557-2567.
32. Watsky MA. Keratocyte gap junctional communication in normal and wounded rabbit corneas and human corneas. *Invest Ophthalmol Vis Sci*. 1995;36:2568-2576.
33. Hahnel C, Somodi S, Weiss DG, Guthoff RF. The keratocyte network of human cornea: a three-dimensional study using confocal laser scanning fluorescence microscopy. *Cornea*. 2000;19:185-193.
34. Poole CA, Brookes NH, Clover GM. Keratocyte networks visualised in the living cornea using vital dyes. *J Cell Sci*. 1993;106:685-691.
35. Vinciguerra P, Torres-Munoz I, Camesasca FI. Applications of confocal microscopy in refractive surgery. *J Refract Surg*. 2002;18:S378-S381.
36. Ojeda JL, Ventosa JA, Piedra S. The three-dimensional microanatomy of the rabbit and human cornea. A chemical and mechanical microdissection-SEM approach. *J Anat*. 2001;199:567-576.
37. Moller-Pedersen T. A comparative study of human corneal keratocyte and endothelial cell density during aging. *Cornea*. 1997;16:333-338.
38. Grizzi F, Russo C, Torres-Munoz I, et al. Computer-aided estimate and modelling of the geometrical complexity of the corneal stroma. In: Losa GA, Merlini D, Nonnemacher TF, Weibel ER, eds. *Fractals in Biology and Medicine*. Vol 4. Basel, Germany: Birkhauser-Verlag; 2005.
39. Misson GP, Landini G, Murray PI. Fractals and ophthalmology. *Lancet*. 1992;339:872.
40. Misson GP, Landini G, Murray PI. Size dependent variation in the fractal dimensions of herpes simplex epithelial keratitis. *Curr Eye Res*. 1993;12:957-961.
41. McGhee GR. *Theoretical Morphology: The Concept and Its Applications*. New York, NY: Columbia University Press; 1998.
42. Massoud TF, Hademenos GJ, Young WL, Gao E, Pile-Spellman J, Vinuela F. Principles and philosophy of modeling in biomedical research. *FASEB J*. 1998;12:275-285.
43. Torres-Munoz I, Grizzi F, Russo C, Camesasca FI, Dioguardi N, Vinciguerra P. The role of amino acids in corneal stromal healing: a method for evaluating cellular density and extracellular matrix distribution. *J Refract Surg*. 2003;19:S227-S230.

APPENDIX A

Pre- and Intraoperative Instrumental Diagnostics

Paolo Vinciguerra, MD; Fabrizio I. Camesasca, MD

This appendix illustrates how to perform an intraoperative control of the corneal surface and thickness. Since they are mainly used during PTK, this technique will be mostly addressed in the text, even if the same principles are valid for smoothing.

1. **Keratoscopy**. This exam uses the projection of light rings on the cornea and the study of their morphology to allow a precise evaluation of the shape and regularity of the corneal surface. It is the mainstay of PTK strategy and pre-, intra-, and postoperative evaluation. Together with pachymetry, it provides information on the progress of PTK surgery and aids surgeons in defining when the planned surgical goal has been achieved. Since it is a dynamic examination, it is mandatory to perform it preoperatively in the presence of a regular tear film. Therefore, the surgeon must ask the patient to blink several times and acquire the image without tear pools, surface irregularities or irregular tear distribution. Intraoperatively, when the flap is lifted, the surgeon must lightly wet and evenly distribute the fluid on the stromal bed.

    Several features of the keratoscopic rings must be considered. For the sake of completeness, description of these features will refer to keratoscopy performed on the corneal surface before flap lifting.

    a. Shape regularity. Keratoscopic rings regular in shape indicate a corneal surface with good optical features and regular lamination of tear fluid. The rings are well delineated with no deformations, interruptions, or irregularities. A good contrast between light and dark rings is present.

    b. Continuity. Regularly continuous rings are typical of regular corneal surface and tear film distribution. Interruptions indicate irregular corneal areas with poor optical quality (ie, leukomas) as well as the presence of secretion or breaks in tear film. Blinking permits differentiation between surfactant that may be removed and corneal irregularities that will persist.

    c. Circularity. Regularly, circular and concentric rings are present when the surface is spherical. In the case of astigmatism, the rings will appear oval-shaped along the axis of greatest curvature. Elliptical or pear-shaped rings are present in the case of regular or irregular astigmatism, asymmetric astigmatism, and with small or large bow ties.

    d. Symmetry. Symmetry is typical of a homogeneous distribution of dioptrical power in the different sectors. Asymmetry indicates an important difference in dioptrical power in the different sectors (ie, in irregular astigmatism).

    e. Deformations. These may be observed in the presence of irregular astigmatism, which cannot be corrected with a lens and often induces marked reduction in visual acuity.

    f. Edges. These are interruptions in the regularly circular shape of the keratoscopic ring and can be observed in the case of a full-thickness corneal structure interruption (ie, perforating wounds or radial keratotomy).

    g. Inter-ring distance. Smaller or greater distance between rings indicates, respectively, greater or smaller curvature. Flat areas display spaced-out rings, and curve areas display close rings. When the distance is homogeneous, the dioptrical power is evenly distributed. On the contrary, relevant variations in distance among rings indicate irregular surface dioptrical power.

h. Width. Highlights the focal dioptrical power. A thinner ring indicates a steeper area; a wider ring indicates a flatter area.
i. Absence. Rings are absent in cases of marked surface anatomical changes, large epithelial defects, or relevant changes in the tear film.
j. Focus. When nearby areas are on planes markedly distant one from another, focusing of rings is not homogeneous. It indicates a marked surface anomaly. It is normal in transplants because graft and recipient areas lie on different planes.
k. Centering. If the rings appear off-center, it is probable that the patient was not staring directly at the target light.

When keratoscopic rings appear irregular, off center, or jagged, PTK may eliminate the irregularities, thus improving visual acuity. Conversely, when keratoscopy shows well-centered, round, and regular rings, there is no indication for PTK. When keratoscopy is regular, other causes for vision reduction must be carefully investigated. A 20/30-vision patient with irregular, jagged, and asymmetrical rings will probably see more and with better quality vision after PTK.

2. **Topography.** Derived from processing keratoscopy, topography aids the surgeon in the preoperative evaluation of the PTK patient. Topography offers great accuracy in the determination of axis and power of astigmatism, thus permitting precise determination of visual acuity and a more exact prognosis. The commonly used algorithms are axial, tangential, altitudinal, pachymetric, and wavefront with the Zernicke polynomials analysis. The latter two provide different information and are both necessary and important for preoperative evaluation.

a. Axial. This scale closely represents the refractive situation on the corneal surface. The dioptrical value of each point is calculated according an algorithm that accounts for the distance of the point from an axis positioned on the center of the cornea. With this scale, corneal topography is built from the center (visual axis) to the periphery and represents the visual situation of the patient. It must be remembered, however, that the dioptrical power of astigmatism is underestimated in this scale.
b. Tangential. According to the algorithm of this scale, each point of the corneal surface is calculated by creating a circle tangential to that point. The reference axis connects the point with the center of the circle, and is, therefore, different for each considered point. A morphological representation of the cornea is thus generated.

Neither of these two scales shows the real morphology of the cornea, even if both provide a reliable interpretation. For this reason, several other algorithms and scales have been developed.

c. Altimetric. The altimetric map is defined by subtracting the values of the cornea that is being examined from a ideal reference sphere. In this way, differences are defined in altimetric position, above (steeper) or below (flatter) the surface of the ideal sphere.
d. Gaussian. This algorithm considers several different parameters, thus providing an evaluation that can be considered intermediate between the tangential and altimetric algorithms, thus closer to the real corneal shape.
e. Pachymetric. This map can be obtained with the Orbscan topographer (Bausch and Lomb, Rochester, NY). This instrument, using light scanning of the anterior and posterior corneal surfaces, provides topographic examination with axial or tangential algorithms. It also provides a pachymetric map with details of the stromal thickness in each analyzed point. These three different maps are shown simultaneously, permitting an estimate of possible coincidence between topographical and pachymetric irregularities.
f. Aberrometry. The aberrometric evaluations of the anterior corneal surface simultaneously shows the position and extent of the different sources of aberration. With the Seidel calculation, areas where the wavefront is altered are highlighted, providing an indication of the corneal areas that require regularization with PTK.

Sometimes, altered keratoscopic rings induce an omission in topographical analysis of the area involved, causing incomplete or erroneous topographical calculation with false flat or steep corneal areas. Topographers such as the CSO (Florence, Italy) and the Keratron Scout (Optikon 2000, Rome, Italy) permit manual identification and correction of each ring course, providing complete and detailed topography. These two topographers can be portable or applied to a movable arm and therefore can be used intraoperatively.

3. **Pachymetry.** Based on ultrasound, pachymetry permits determination of corneal thickness. It is recommended that this should be considered in relation to the irregularity requiring treatment. When stromal irregularities are limited, it is possible to smooth even very thin corneas. When defects are very severe (eg, inducing 20.0 D of astigmatism), treatment is not possible even with almost normal corneal thickness.

APPENDIX B

LASEK Information for Patients

Thomas V. Claringbold II, DO; Lee Shahinian Jr, MD

Sample LASEK Consent Form

1. This consent form is provided as a sample only, on the assumption that each surgeon will develop a personal written consent.
2. This written consent does not replace the physician's responsibility surrounding the informed consent process, which includes discussions with the patient.
3. In both discussion and written consent, the surgeon may need to address patient-specific risks and benefits not covered in this sample consent.
4. There may be specific state requirements for informed consent that are not covered in this sample consent.
5. The surgeon's professional liability insurance carrier should be consulted for further input regarding what to include in the written consent form.

INFORMED CONSENT FOR LASER-ASSISTED SUB-EPITHELIAL KERATECTOMY

Introduction

Laser-assisted sub-epithelial keratectomy (LASEK) is a relatively new laser procedure to correct myopia, hyperopia, and astigmatism. The excimer laser has not been approved by the Food and Drug Administration (FDA) for use in LASEK. The FDA considers LASEK an "off-label" use of the excimer laser, an approved medical device. The FDA clearly states that it will not regulate the practice of medicine or the performance of the procedure by a physician. "Off-label" usage of FDA-approved devices and drugs is commonly practiced by physicians without interference from the FDA and allows physicians to practice medicine in a manner they feel is most beneficial to their patients.

This consent form describes the diagnosis, procedure, alternative treatments, fees, possible risks, and benefits of LASEK. Because LASEK is a relatively new surgery, there may be long-term effects not yet known or anticipated at this time. The material provided will help you make an informed decision on whether to choose LASEK. This information accompanies but does not replace our discussions before and after LASEK. You are encouraged to ask questions about the diagnosis, procedure, alternative treatments, fees, risks, benefits, descriptions, medical terms, and language in this consent form.

The Normal Eye, Myopia, Hyperopia, and Astigmatism

The cornea is the clear, dome-shaped window that forms the front wall of the eye. It acts as a lens to focus incoming light rays onto the retina, the light-sensitive tissue in the back of the eye.

In the normal eye, light rays are brought to a single sharp focus directly on the retina, resulting in clear vision without glasses or contact lenses. Any deviation from this normal focusing is called a "refractive error." Myopia, hyperopia, and astigmatism are different types of refractive errors.

In myopia, or nearsightedness, the eye is longer than normal. The light rays come together at a point in front of the retina and, thus, are out of focus on the retina. Distant objects appear blurry, whereas near objects may be seen clearly. Myopia affects approximately one-fourth of adults in the United States.

In hyperopia, or farsightedness, the eye is shorter than normal. The light rays come together at a point behind the retina and, thus, are out of focus on the retina. Both distant and near objects appear blurry.

In astigmatism, the curvature of the cornea (and, therefore, its focusing power) is not the same in the horizontal and vertical directions. Therefore, light rays entering the eye do not focus at a single point, causing distorted vision. Many people with myopia or hyperopia also have some degree of astigmatism.

Correction of Refractive Errors— Alternative Treatments

Eyeglasses remain the most common method of correcting vision. In myopia, a concave or "minus" lens causes the incoming light rays to diverge before they reach the cornea. The cornea, in turn, focuses these divergent light rays directly onto the retina, and vision becomes clear once again. In hyperopia, a convex or "plus" lens causes the incoming light rays to converge, bringing their focus onto the retina. Glasses are safe, relatively inexpensive, and usually well tolerated. To correct large refractive errors, glasses must be thick and may reduce or increase the size of the visual image by up to 25%.

Contact lenses correct myopia and hyperopia much like glasses. If fitted and used properly, they are effective and relatively safe for correcting myopia, hyperopia, and astigmatism. However, complications such as allergic reactions, infections, and mechanical injury to the cornea can sometimes occur with the use of hard or soft contact lenses.

Radial keratotomy (RK) is an incisional procedure to correct myopia and astigmatism. Deep (90% of corneal thickness) radial cuts, like the spokes of a wheel, are made in the cornea with a hand-held surgical knife. These incisions cause the peripheral cornea to bulge and the central cornea to flatten, thus correcting up to 6 D of myopia. Unstable results and other problems have caused this procedure to be largely abandoned.

Photorefractive keratectomy (PRK) uses an excimer ("x'-i-mur") laser to reshape the front surface of the cornea. This argon fluoride laser was developed by IBM in the early 1980s to etch silicon chips. It was subsequently discovered that the laser can be used to cleanly and precisely reshape the cornea. The laser's ultraviolet-light pulses evaporate tissue without burning or cutting. The distribution of laser energy on the cornea is computer-controlled. With multiple laser pulses, the cornea is reshaped, making it optically correct for the eye. For every diopter of correction, approximately 10 μm of corneal tissue are removed. For example, correcting 5 D of myopia requires the removal of roughly 50 μm of tissue, about 10% of the corneal thickness (less than the thickness of a human hair!).

Laser-assisted in situ keratomileusis (LASIK) is a modification of excimer laser PRK that is particularly effective for correcting moderate to high myopia, astigmatism, and hyperopia. In this procedure, a miniature precision-cutting device called a microkeratome is used much like a carpenter's plane to create a hinged flap on the front surface of the cornea. This flap is folded back, and the underlying corneal tissue is reshaped with the same excimer laser used for PRK. The corneal flap is then replaced in its original position.

The main difference between LASIK and PRK is that the former does not disrupt the front surface of the cornea. LASIK may have several advantages. First, haze and regression (loss of effect) appear to be less of a problem with LASIK than with PRK in patients with high myopia and hyperopia. Second, steroid drops are only needed for 1 week instead of 4 months or longer after surgery. Third, vision recovers more quickly after LASIK than after PRK, and patients usually have less pain after LASIK. However, the use of a microkeratome in LASIK carries risks that do not occur with PRK. Complications with the creation and healing of the corneal flap can affect visual outcome.

LASEK—A Hybrid Procedure

In LASEK, the excimer laser treatment is applied to the cornea under a flap of the superficial epithelium, or surface cells, of the cornea. The epithelial flap can be lifted without using a microkeratome. Thus, unlike LASIK, no deep cut is made in the cornea. LASEK is a hybrid procedure which creates less haze and regression than PRK and avoids the deep corneal flap complications of LASIK.

Epi-LASIK is the newest addition to the family of refractive procedures. This procedure is identical to LASEK, except that the epithelial flap is created with a special microkeratome, making the application of a dilute alcohol solution (see "The Procedure" on the next page) unnecessary.

Preoperative Consultation and Patient Selection

The preoperative consultation with Dr. _____ and his staff provides an explanation of LASEK, its benefits, risks, and alternatives. Specialized testing determines your suitability for treatment. To allow accurate measurements, soft contact lenses must not be worn for at least 1 week prior to this appointment (3 weeks for toric soft contact lenses and gas permeable lenses).

LASEK is appropriate for individuals with myopia, hyperopia, and astigmatism who wish to be less dependent on glasses or contact lenses and are willing to assume the risks associated with the procedure. Minimum age is 21 years. There should be no significant change in glasses or contact lens prescription for the previous 12 months.

Contraindications

The treatment should not be performed on persons:
* With herpes eye infection
* With severely dry eyes
* With excessive corneal scarring, keloid formation
* With keratoconus
* With autoimmune disease, rheumatoid arthritis, systemic lupus erythematosis
* With uncontrolled diabetes
* Taking Accutane or amiodarone (Cordarone)
* Who are pregnant or are nursing, or who expect to become pregnant within 6 months following the LASEK procedure
* Who are not available for postoperative care
* Who have unrealistic expectations or a poor understanding of the procedure and its risks

Fees

The fee for LASEK is per eye. This fee includes preoperative assessment, the LASEK procedure, laser center charges, a royalty payment to the laser company, initial postoperative medications, and 1 year of postoperative care. Additional eye medications and postoperative glasses or contact lenses are not included and are the patient's responsibility. Patients should be prepared to pay for LASEK, as it is not usually covered by health insurance or Medicare.

If a retreatment is performed by Dr. _____ within 18 months of the original surgery, the fee is ____ (depending on the laser used), payable to the laser center.

Preparation for Treatment

If you qualify and opt for LASEK, we will schedule the procedure. We recommend that patients take a few days off from work or school. We also recommend that you do not drive for a few days after the procedure. **Three days prior to surgery**, contact lenses must be removed and makeup and perfume discontinued.

The Procedure

LASEK is an outpatient procedure. Eye drops given a few minutes before treatment provide suitable anesthesia. No injections are necessary.

The patient is positioned under the operating microscope. The eyelids are held gently open with a speculum. The patient is asked to look at a fixation light in the microscope. The eye not being treated is covered during the procedure.

With the eye well anesthetized by drops, a trephine (circular marker) outlines the area of epithelium to be lifted. A dilute alcohol solution is then applied to the marked area for about 30 seconds. This allows the epithelium, or superficial cells of the cornea, to be lifted. The epithelial flap is then folded to one side, and laser energy is delivered through the microscope to reshape the front surface of the remaining cornea. The patient may hear a ticking sound as each laser pulse removes a small amount of tissue. A computer controls the distribution and number of laser pulses, based on the amount of myopia (or hyperopia) and astigmatism to be corrected. The actual laser treatment lasts about 30 to 90 seconds, during which time the patient must look at the fixation light. At the end of the laser treatment, the epithelial flap is returned to its original position. A thin soft contact lens is placed on the eye.

After the Procedure

There is usually mild to moderate irritation or foreign body sensation for 1 to 2 days after surgery. Serious pain is less likely after LASEK than after PRK. Pain medicine is provided as needed. Steroid and antibiotic drops are used for the first week, and steroid drops are used for several months in some cases. **To avoid dislodging the epithelial flap, it is extremely important not to poke or rub your eye in the first week after LASEK.** Cosmetics and strenuous exercise, gardening, and dusty environments should be avoided for 1 week after the procedure, swimming for 2 weeks.

The eye is examined the first day after LASEK, and on the fourth day, the contact lens is usually removed. The eye is then checked typically at 1 month, 3 months, 6 months, and 1 year. Additional visits may be necessary. Vision is initially blurry after surgery but typically shows marked improvement in the first week. Stable vision is usually achieved within 1 to 3 months.

Possible Benefits

The purpose of LASEK is to reduce your level of nearsightedness, farsightedness, and/or astigmatism in order to provide better vision than you now have without eyeglasses or contact lenses. Often, the procedure allows people to function most or all of the time without eyeglasses or contact lenses. However, excellent uncorrected vision cannot be guaranteed, especially when high degrees of myopia, hyperopia, or astigmatism are being treated, and some correction with glasses may still be necessary. The visual improvement may also have psychological benefits if you feel that you look better, or can function better, without glasses or with thinner glasses.

Potential Risks and Other Considerations

No surgical procedure is completely free of risk. It is not possible to list every complication that can occur, and there may be adverse reactions that are unknown at this time. Since glasses or contact lenses in general safely correct myopia, hyperopia, and/or astigmatism, you need to consider thoroughly if the risks of having the LASEK procedure outweigh the possible benefits.

1. **Undercorrection or Overcorrection**. It is not possible to completely predict how your eye will respond to this procedure. As a result, you may not achieve acceptable vision without glasses. In some cases, contact lenses may not be tolerated. In many cases, but not all, a second procedure can be done. It is also possible that your myopia may be overcorrected, resulting in farsightedness. If you are farsighted after LASEK, you may need eyeglasses for close as well as far viewing.

2. **Presbyopia and Reading Glasses.** Even if LASEK is successful in correcting your vision, you may require reading glasses sooner than you would otherwise. As a person grows older, the lens of the eye is less able to focus, and near vision becomes more difficult. This normal aging process is called presbyopia, a condition that can be alleviated with reading glasses or bifocal lenses. An advantage of being myopic, or nearsighted, is that it generally takes longer to be affected by presbyopia. The myopic person can usually remove his distance glasses to read. Therefore, if you do not have LASEK and remain myopic, you may not need additional reading glasses or bifocals until age 50 or older. If you have LASEK, you may need reading glasses in your early 40s, as do most individuals who are not myopic. For farsighted patients, even if the laser corrects your distance vision, you will still need reading glasses typically in your early 40s, as do most people with good distance vision.

3. **Decrease of Best Corrected Vision.** After LASEK, some patients find that their vision with the best eyeglass or contact lens correction is not as good as it was before the procedure with eye glasses or contact lenses.

4. **Regression.** In some patients, the effect of LASEK treatment is partially lost over a few weeks to several months. In some, but not all cases, significant regression can be retreated.

5. **Excessive Corneal Haze.** Mild corneal haze occurs as part of the normal healing process after LASEK. In most cases, it has little or no effect on the final vision and can only be seen by the ophthalmologist with a microscope. Rarely, excessive haze could permanently decrease your vision. In some cases, a retreatment may be successful in removing the corneal haze.

6. **Halo/Glare/Sensitivity to Light.** Halo is an optical effect that is noticed primarily in dim light. As the pupil enlarges, a second faded image is produced by the untreated peripheral cornea. Some patients who have undergone LASEK notice this effect especially while driving at night, and this can interfere with night driving. Some patients notice glare and increased or decreased sensitivity to light, usually improving with time. These symptoms may not completely go away.

7. **Decentration.** Significant decentration of the zone of treatment (the laser beam not centered on the pupil) can occur when the patient does not fixate correctly during surgery. Halo and blurry vision can result.

8. **Irregular Laser Ablation.** The excimer laser may not create a smooth tissue removal, leaving the vision distorted. In some cases, the distortion clears with time, and in others, retreatment may be possible.

9. **Flap Damage or Loss.** During the creation of the hinged flap of epithelium on the central cornea, the entire flap could come off. If this occurs, the flap can usually be repositioned at the end of the procedure. However, there might be more postoperative haze, similar to PRK.

10. **Dry Eye.** Dry eye is common following laser vision correction. It may be necessary to use artificial tears or to have punctal plugs inserted, a simple 5-minute office procedure.

11. **Inconvenience Between Procedures.** In the time between LASEK on the first and second eye, the two eyes may not work well together because of their temporary difference in refraction (glasses strength). If a contact lens is not tolerated on the unoperated eye, work and driving may be awkward or impossible until the second eye has had LASEK.

12. **Steroid Side Effects.** Steroid eye drops are often needed for a few weeks to several months after LASEK to reduce corneal haze and prevent regression. Potential side effects of these steroid eye drops include clouding of the lens inside the eye (cataract), drooping of the eyelid (ptosis), and increased eye pressure, resulting in optic nerve damage (glaucoma) in rare cases. The occasional pressure rise can usually be treated with additional eye drops. The pressure returns to normal when the steroid eye drops are discontinued. Cataract is extremely rare with this steroid dosage. Ptosis has occasionally persisted for several months after steroid treatment.

13. **Rare Complications and Unknown Risks.** Other reported complications include endothelial cell loss (loss of cell density in the inner layer of the cornea), possibly leading to corneal swelling and poor vision; ptosis (droopy eyelid); contact lens intolerance; unstable corneal shape; fluctuating vision; and allergic reaction to drops or oral medications. If the cornea is severely damaged, a corneal transplant using a donor cornea might be necessary. As with any eye procedure, there is a remote possibility of severe infection, drug reaction, or other rare complication, which could cause chronic pain, an unsightly eye, or partial or complete loss of vision. Because LASEK is a relatively new procedure, there may be other risks to vision and health that are still unknown and unanticipated.

Summary

I have read this Informed Consent for LASEK and I fully understand it, including the possible risks, complications, and benefits that can result from the treatment.

Specifically, I understand the following (a summary of this Informed Consent):

1. That laser-assisted sub-epithelial keratectomy (LASEK) is an "off-label" surgical procedure that reshapes the cornea with an excimer laser under an epithelial flap to reduce or eliminate myopia, hyperopia, and astigmatism.

2. That the results of the procedure cannot always be predicted, nor the safety guaranteed. I may still need corrective eyeglasses or contact lenses to achieve satisfactory vision after LASEK. Contact lens fit may not be possible in some cases.

3. That alternative treatments such as PRK and LASIK have been explained to me.

4. That complications from the procedure, such as under- or overcorrection, decrease of best-corrected vision, dry eye, corneal haze or swelling, regression, haloes, glare, change in sensitivity to light, fluctuating vision, and ptosis (droopy eyelid) can occur. Retreatment may be possible to attempt to achieve satisfactory uncorrected vision. As with any eye procedure, there are remote risks such as severe infection and partial or complete loss of vision. Because LASEK is a relatively new procedure, there may be other unknown and unanticipated risks.

5. That if LASEK is reducing my myopia, I may need reading glasses sooner than I would if I were to remain nearsighted. If LASEK corrects my hyperopia for distance vision, I will still need reading glasses, usually by my early 40s.

6. That LASEK is an elective procedure. I do not have to have this operation.

7. That it is important to protect the operated eye from rubbing and poking.

8. That I am expected to return for scheduled follow-up visits 1 day, 4 days, 1 month, 3 months, 6 months, and 12 months after the procedure. Additional visits may be necessary. Beyond this 1-year follow-up, routine eye check-ups are important to help assure good vision.

9. That if there is a time interval between LASEK on my first and second eye, inconvenience and visual discomfort may result from having a temporary difference in refraction in my two eyes as a result of having had LASEK on one eye.

10. That I will be charged a fee for LASEK, which includes postoperative care for 1 year. There will be additional charges for medications, contact lenses, and glasses after the procedure and for postoperative visits after 1 year. Health insurance and Medicare do not usually cover LASEK.

The procedure of LASEK, along with the alternative treatments, advantages and disadvantages, risks, and possible complications of this procedure have been explained to me by the doctor. Although it is impossible for the doctor to inform me of every possible complication that may occur, the doctor has answered all my questions to my satisfaction.

I understand that information gathered about my procedure and postoperative course may be used to further study the safety and efficacy of the procedure. I give permission for my case to be presented at scientific meetings or published in scientific journals, as long as I am not identified by name.

I give permission to be photographed by a still camera, movie camera, or videotape and for these photographs to be shown at scientific meetings or published in scientific journals, as long as I am not identified by name.

I wish to have laser-assisted sub-epithelial keratectomy (LASEK) performed on my _____ eye (s).

Patient's Signature: _____

Patient's Name (printed): _____

Date, Time, Place: _____

Witness's Signature, Date: _____

Witness's Name (printed): _____

LASEK Instruments

E. Janach SRL

Address: via Borgovico 35, Como 22100, Italia. Tel: 011-39-031-574-088, Fax: 011-39-031-572-055, Web site: www.janach.it, Email: international@janach.it

We also highly recommend their CD-ROM by Dr. Camellin, an excellent introduction to LASEK.

Instruments can be ordered directly from Janach or from: MAXWELL MEDICAL exclusive US reseller: Mr. Mack Maxwell, 316 Daylily Drive, Lexington SC 29072, Tel: 803-356-3188, Fax: 803-356-0400, Email: mmax@usit.net.

Janach LASEK Instruments (Selected)

* Camellin Epithelial Trephine 8 mm (J2900) and 9 mm (J2901)
* Shahinian Alcohol Well 9 mm (J2907) and 10 mm (J2908)
* Camellin Epithelial Microhoe J2915A
* Camellin Epithelial Detaching Spatula J2910A
* Camellin Bow Dissector J2930A
* Camellin Flap Replacement Spatula J2920A
* LASEK Sterilization Tray J4715

Katena Products, Inc

Address: 4 Stewart Court, Denville, NJ 07834, Tel: 800-225-1195, Fax: 973-989-8175, Web site: www.katena.com.

Katena LASEK Instruments (Selected)

* K2-7810 LASEK Epithelial Trephine, 8 mm
* K2-7812 LASEK Epithelial Trephine, 9 mm
* K3-1830 Shahinian LASEK Alcohol Well, 9 mm
* K3-1832 Shahinian LASEK Alcohol Well, 10 mm
* K3-1840 Sloane LASEK Micro Hoe
* K3-1845 Sloane LASEK Epi Peeler
* K3-1855 Sloane LASEK Flap Repositor
* K7-3805 LASEK Alcohol Cannula, Olive Tip
* K9-2026 Sterilizing Case for LASEK Instrument Set
* Shahinian LASEK Alcohol Well. Features dual fixation rings for a tight seal and is cone-shaped to provide maximum visibility for the surgeon while centering the instrument over the precut flap. The handle is mounted at a 55-degree angle for applying direct pressure on the ring to ensure a secure seal.

Preparation of 20% Autologous Serum Eye Drops

1. Draw 10 cc of patient's blood using plastic BD Vacutainer tube with clot activator. (The clot activator consists of silica beads sprayed over the inside of the tube. The interior of the tube is sterile.)
2. Gently invert the tube 5 times to expose the blood to the clot activator. Do not shake anything (eg, like a cocktail) to avoid hemolyzing the red cells.
3. Allow Vacutainer tube to sit upright for 30 to 60 minutes, until clot forms. As clot retracts, it pulls the silica into the clot. Serum is free of silica.
4. Spin the red top tube down to obtain the serum.
5. Using sterile technique, pop the nipple off a new 15-cc bottle of BSS (Alcon), and draw off 3 cc of solution.
6. Remove the stopper from the red top tube and draw off 3 cc of serum.
7. Inject this serum into the BSS bottle. Reinsert the nipple of the BSS bottle.
8. This procedure creates a 20% solution of autologous serum in BSS, which can be used as an eye drop.

Index

aberrometry. *See* corneal aberrometry
ablation zone, 122
absolute scale, 14, 52
accommodation
    Schachar theory, 129
    wavefront error and, 21–22
acoustic biometry, 282
adjustable scale, 14, 52
AFM (atomic force microscopy), 63–64, 66, 304–307
aging. See elderly population
AIDS (acquired immunodeficiency syndrome), 43
alcohol, toxic effect on cells, 184
aliasing, 24–25
allergies, 44
amino acids, effects on corneal healing, 143–147
ANSI (American National Standard Institute)
    ANSI Z80.28 standard, 20–21
    keratometric diopter measurement, 9
anterior chamber depth, 283
apoptosis, 220
Artemis VHF digital ultrasound arc B-scanner, 315–320
asphericity, 15, 53–54
astigmatism
    astigmatic bow-tie, 13
    cataracts and, 284
    characteristics, 107–111
    congenital, 6
    effect on surface ablation, 15
    hyperopic astigmatism, 126–127
    irregular, 27
    keratorefractive indices, 53
    treatment
        corneal eccentricity (Q value), 111
        cross-cylinder ablation technique, 111
        custom ablation, 113–114
        cyclotorsion, 116–117
        locating the true cylinder axis, 114–116
        smoothing, 117–118
        "splitting" technique, 111–113
        surface ablation, 107–111
    types of, 118–119
autologous serum eye drops, 344
autorefractometry, 48–49
average pupillary power, 15, 53
axial length measurement, 281–283
axial mapping, 10, 28, 37
axis variation, 127
AZ (ablation zone), 76

B-complex vitamins, role in epithelial turnover, 41–42
band keratopathy, 269
basal epithelial cell hypertrophic modifications, 67
BCVA (best corrected visual acuity), 243
BFS (best fit sphere), 13, 55
BFTI (Best Fit Topographic Irregularity), 303
biomechanical customization, 62–63
biometric exam, 281–282
blanket effect, 78
blur, 33
Bowman's layer, 67, 183
BSCVA (best spectacle corrected visual acuity), 170–171, 195, 247
butterfly LASEK, 159–161, 222

cataracts
    caused by steroids, 43
    extraction with IOL implants
        anterior chamber depth, 283
        astigmatism, 284
        axial length measurement, 281–283
        corneal curvature power, 283–284

ectatic conditions, 285–288
normal condition, 284
normal-looking corneas, 288–289
uneven surface, 284–285
CATZ ablation, 79, 166
CCA (cone for controlled atmosphere), 133
cell death, 292
cell-matrix and cell-cell interactions, 66–67
central corneal curvature, 130–131
central topical irregularity, 103
chromatic aberrations, 33
colimetric scale types, 14
collagen disorders, 43
colorimetric corneal map, 7
colorimetric scale types, 52
compound hyperopic astigmatism, 119
confocal microscopy, 294–296
congenital astigmatism, 6
contrast, 3
contrast visual acuity, 173–174, 325–328
cornea, objective examination, 46–47
corneal aberrometry
   consequences of higher-order aberrations, 24–25
   diffraction, 18–19
   high-order wavefront error, 21–22
   instrumental examinations, 54
   measuring principle, 28
   modulation transfer function, 22–23
   neural limits, 23–24
   optical quality of the retinal image, 17–18
   in refractive surgery, 169
   topography and, 49–50
   treatments, 257–258
   visual acuity, 17
   wavefront corrections, 25
   wavefront error, 19–20
   whole eye vs corneal wavefront error, 22
corneal curvature, 65, 283–284
corneal eccentricity (Q value), 122–123
corneal ectasy, 54–55
corneal elasticity, 61–62
corneal epithelium stratification, 258
corneal flattening, 5, 307–310
corneal haze. See haze formation
corneal healing, effects of amino acids, 143–147
corneal hypercurvature, 7
Corneal Hysteresis, 62
corneal morphology, 15
corneal onlays, 67
corneal opacities, 257, 262
corneal stroma, effects of amino acids, 145
corneal stroma, fractal geometry, 331–335
corneal surface irregularities, 63–65, 84–85
corneal thickness, 55, 321
corneal topography
   algorithms, 9
   instrumental examinations, 52–53

interpretation, 37–38
keratoscopy, 338
measuring principle, 28–29
corneal transparency, 66
corneal wound healing
   after LASEK, 220–221
   after refractive surgery, 219–220
   Epi-LASIK as an alternative to LASEK, 223
   lamellar procedures and, 220–221
   pharmacological modulation after surface ablation
      clinical results, 291, 293–294
      considerations, 292–293
      corneal confocal microscopy, 294–296
CPK (custom phototherapeutic keratectomy)
   clinical results, 259–262
   demographical data, 257
   indications for, 256
   pre- and postoperative refraction, 258
   selection criteria, 256
   surgical techniques, 255–257
   topography-based, 257
   treatment of ultrathin corneas after surface retreatment
      efficacy and stability parameters, 266–267
cross-cylinder technique, 111, 127
crystalline lens optics, 22–23
curvature
   induced, 77
   mapping, 55
   parameters, 10
custom ablation. *See also* LASEK
   efficacy and safety, 169–171
   wavefront error, 171
CVP (variation of corneal power), 14, 53
cylinder power and axis, 114
cytokines, 67, 292
cytokines, produced by keratocytes, 219–220
cytoskeletal dynamics, 66

D index, 147
data acquisition, 3
decentration, 124–125, 127, 243–246, 322–325
dermatological disorders, 44
diabetic patients, 42
differential topographical maps, 104
diffraction effects, 24
diffraction-limited pupil, 22
diffraction phenomena, 33
digitized retroillumination, with Scheimpflug camera, 84–85
diopter scale for wavefront display, 37
diplopia, monocular, 323
distance between rings, 3
DLK (diffuse lamellar keratitis), 211, 211–212
dry eye, 44
dynamic skiascopy, 27

ECM (extracellular matrix), 220
ectasia, 6, 62, 237–240, 244, 268, 321–322

EDTA (ethylenediaminetetraacetic acid), 262
EGF (epidermal growth factor), 219, 232
elderly population
    high-order wavefront error, 21–22
    lenticular defects, 33
    loss of low contrast mesopic acuity, 17
emmetropia, 110
employment history, 45–46
EMR (electronic medical record), 277
endocrine system disorders, 42–43
endothelial microscopy, 56
Epi-LASIK. See also LASEK
    alcohol-assisted epithelial removal, 183
    clinical results, 177–178
    complications, 185–186
    effect of alcohol on epithelial cell survival in vitro, 184
    electron microscopy, 184
    histological findings of mechanically separated epithelial sheets, 175–176
    indications and contraindications, 181
    in vivo confocal microscopy, 211–216
    postoperative management, 182–183
    surgical technique, 176–177
    surgical techniques, 181–182
epithelial cell survival *in vitro*
    effect of alcohol on, 184
epithelial flap-based surface ablation techniques, 215
epithelial healing, 300–302
epithelial hyperplasia, 67, 78, 109–110
epithelial thickening, 319
epithelial variability, in LASEK, 222–223
ethanol, 222–223
Ex vivo confocal microscopy, 67
excimer laser
    historical perspectives, 76–81
    refractive surgery, 205, 207–208
eye adnexa, 46
eye bank cornea study, 143–144
eye motility, 46
eye pressure
    objective examination, 47
eye prosthesis, 44

foveolar cones
    diameter, 23
fractal geometry, 331–335
fractal surface dimension, 147

G-CSF (granulocyte colony stimulating factor), 220
Gaussian profile, 200
ghosting, 33
glandular disorders, 42–43
glaucoma
    caused by steroids, 43
    objective examination, 47
Goldmann tonometry, 61–62
grating acuity, measuring, 17

growth factors, 67
GTP-binding proteins, 66

habitat structure, 335
haze formation
    characteristics, 247
    following PRK, 44, 134, 234–235
    following PRK and LASIK, 65–68
    in late re-epithelialized eyes, 231
    mitomycin C treatment, 247–251
    postoperational, 118
    undercorrection and overcorrection, 104
height
    mapping, 10–15
    parameters, 10
height mapping, 52
height tomography, 54–55
Helmholtz theory, 129
hemisphere test, 91–93
herpes infection, 43
herpetic leukomas, 43
HGF (hepatocyte growth factor), 219–220
high compound myopic astigmatism, 118
high contrast mesopic acuity, 17
high contrast photopic letter acuity, 17
high contrast photopic visual acuity, 17
high contrast scotopic acuity, 17
high-order wavefront error, 21–22
higher order aberrations, 54
histopathology, 67
HIV virus, 43
HO (higher order) aberrations, 33–34, 38, 59
hyperopia
    hyperopic astigmatism, 126–127
    treatment
        analyzing, 122–124
        complications, 124–127
        considerations, 121–122
        cross-cylinder technique, 127
        retreatment, 126
hyperopic shift, 60–61
hyperopic white scar, 125–126
hyperplasia, 63
hypolacrimia, 42
hysteresis, 62

iatrogenic ectasia. *See* ectasia
IL-1 (interleukin-1), 219
immunofluorescence, 222
immunohistochemistry, 221
immunological disorders, 43
in vivo confocal microscopy, 205–207
in vivo studies, 144–145
infectious diseases, 43
infective keratitis, 233–234
inflammation, 220, 229–231
informed consent, 56

instrumental diagnostics, 337–338, 343
instrumental examinations, 50–56
interstitial keratitis, 43
intraoperative topography, 256–257
IOLs (intraocular lenses)
    in patients with ectatic conditions, 285–288
        phakic surgery, 329–329
        surgical planning, 317
IOP (intraocular pressure)
    after PRK, 234–235
    after refractive surgery, 61–62
irregular astigmatism, 322
irregularity of curvature, 15, 54

Janach LASEK instruments, 343

Katena LASEK instruments, 343
keloid formation, 43
keratectasia, 268. *See also* ectasia; CPK; PTK
keratoconus
    changes in curvature, 4
    corneal hypercurvature, 7
    LASIK and, 238
    peripheral, 8
    screening for, 321
    spatial relationships, 15
    warpage, 9
keratocyte activation, 67, 220
keratocyte apoptosis, 222, 292
keratocyte cell function, 63
keratocyte proliferation, 67
keratomalacia, 41–42
keratometry, 48
keratorefractive indices, 53–54
keratoscopy
    advantages, 7
    instrumental diagnostics, 337–338
    instrumental examinations, 50–51
    morphological information, 3
    topography, 3–7
KGF (keratinocyte growth factor), 219–220

lachrymal film
    colorimetric corneal map, 7
    instrumental examinations, 51
    lamination of, 3–4
    objective examination, 46
lagophthalmos, 42–43
lamellar procedures, 220–221
LASEK (laser-assisted sub-epithelial keratectomy). *See also* corneal wound healing; Epi-LASIK
    alcohol-assisted epithelial removal, 183
    butterfly LASEK, 159–161
    clinical outcomes, 184–185
    clinical results, 156
    complications, 185–186, 291
    corneal wound healing
        component processes, 219–220
    correction of hyperopia, 124
    effect of alcohol on epithelial cell survival *in vitro*, 184
    electron microscopy, 184
    epithelial variability, 222–223
    final corneal curvature gradient, 79
    historical perspectives, 151
    indications and contraindications, 181
    in vivo confocal microscopy, 211–216
    keratocyte apoptosis, 222
    no alcohol LASEK vs PRK, 199–204
    pain management, 155–156
    patient information
        alternative treatments for correcting refractive errors, 223, 340
        autologous serum eye drops, 344
        sample consent form, 339–343
    postoperative management, 154, 182–183, 341
    preoperative evaluation and preparation, 152, 341
    rationale for, 151–152
    smoothing techniques, 88–89
    surgical technique, 153–154, 163–165
    surgical techniques, 181–182
laser decentration, 322–325. *See also* decentration
laser modality, 65
laser photoablation, 171–173
laser sculpting, 37–38
LASIK (laser in situ keratomileusis). *See also* Epi-LASIK
    biomechanics of the flap, 60–61
    complications, 177–178, 291, 321–322
    confocal microscopy and, 208–209
    correction of hyperopia, 124
    Reinstein classification of flap microfolds, 329
    risk for post-LASIK ectasia
        clinical examples, 239–240
        clinical findings, 237–238
        learning from keratoconus, 238
        pachymetry maps, 238–239
    smoothing techniques, 89
lens, objective examination, 47
lenticular defects, 33
leukoma, formation, 3
light scatter, 33
low compound myopic astigmatism, 118
low contrast mesopic acuity, in the elderly, 17
low contrast photopic acuity, 17
lupus erythematosus, 43

macromechanics, 59–63
macrophages, 220
Maréchal criterion, 299
Marfan's syndrome, 44
masking fluid, 65, 88
MCAF (monocyte chemotactic activating factor), 220
MDNCF (monocyte-derived neutrophil chemotactic factor), 220
mediators, produced by stromal cells, 219–220
metabolic disorders, 42
micron scale for wavefront display, 36–37
midriasis, 44

minimal thickness, 321
mixed astigmatism, 118–119
MMC (mitomycin C), for treatment of haze, 247–251
monochromatic light, 33–34
monocytes, 220
MTF (modulation transfer function), 22–23, 29–30
Munnerlyn approach, 59, 172
musculoskeletal apparatus, 44
myopia, treatment. *See also* Epi-LASIK
    ablation profile in, 98–100
        follow up and complications, 103–104
        selection criteria and planning, 97–98

nanoscale topography, 66–67
NAVEX (Node Advanced Vision Excimer Laser Platform), 27
necrosis, 220
neural limits, 23–24
neurological disorders, 43
neutrophil activating peptide, 220
nomograms for surface laser correction
    advances, 273
    considerations, 271–272
    development and refractive results, 273–277
    improving accuracy of laser refractive surgery, 272–273
normalized scale, 14, 52
NSAIDs (nonsteroidal anti-inflammatory drugs), 230
Nyquist sampling theorem, 23

OCT (optical coherence tomography), 315
Ocular Response Analyzer, 62
off-center ablation. *See* decentration
OPD-HO (OPD higher-order maps), 29
OPD (optical path difference) scanning, 27–31
optical aberrations, 54
optical biometry, 282
Optical Society of America, 19–21, 35–36
Orbscan keratoconus maps, 238, 240
OZ (optical zone), 76, 100, 102, 110, 122, 123–124, 243

pachymetry maps, 338
pain management, 155–156, 229–231
patient interview, 56
PCI (partial coherence light), 281
PDGF (platelet-derived growth factor), 134, 219
pentacam evaluation, 9–13
peripheral keratoconus, 8
phacoemulsification, 281–282
pharmacological history, 44–45
phlyctenules, 43
photoablation, 169, 205
photopic conditions, 55
phototherapeutic keratectomy, 136–137
PKPs (penetrating keratoplasties), 237–240
PMD (pellucid marginal degeneration), 30
PMMA (polymethyl methacrylate), 64, 91–93
polymorphonuclear cells, 220
presbyopia, 129–132

prism aberrations, 54
PRK (photorefractive keratectomy), 79–81. *See also* corneal wound healing; CPK; LASEK
    alcohol-assisted epithelial removal, 183
    clinical outcomes, 184–185
    complications, 291
        delay in re-epithelialization, 231–233, 303
        infective keratitis, 233–234
        postoperative pain and control of inflammation, 229–231
        of the stromal healing phase, 234–235
        subepithelial fibrosis, 247
        ultrathin corneas, 265
    confocal microscopy and, 208–209
    corneal surface analysis
        considerations, 299–300
        epithelial renewal, 300–302
        macroscopic topographic analysis, 307–310
        microscopic topographic analysis, 304–307
        refractive results, 302–304
    correction of hyperopia, 124
    decentration and, 243–246
    following LASIK complication, 137–141
    IVCM after, 210
    topographically guided transepithelial PRK
        equipment and software, 133–135
        phototherapeutic keratectomy, 136–137
        surgical techniques, 135–136
        TOSCA characteristics, 135
    vs no alcohol LASEK, 199–204
PSF (point spread function, 18–19, 33–34, 38
pterygium, 6
PTK (phototherapeutic keratectomy). *See also* CPK; LASIK
    after PRK, 302
    alcohol-assisted epithelial removal, 183
    central flattening in, 59
    complications, 262
    corneal opacities and, 257
    excimer laser trials, 63–64
    on herpetic leukomas, 43
    MMC (mitomycin C) treatment, 247
    retreatments, 270
    study on eyes with ultrathin corneas, 267–270
    surface ablation for, 55
    surgical technique, 135–137
    treatment of ultrathin corneas after surface retreatment, 265–266
    ultrasound-guided, 325–328
pupil, evaluation, 15
pupil size, high-order wavefront error, 21–22
pupillary foramen, 6
pupillometry, 55
Purkinje images, 30

Q value (corneal eccentricity), 122–123

Rayleigh criterion, 299
re-epithelialization, 42, 44–45, 231–233, 303

red ring, 76–77, 79–80, 110
reflection topography, 54–55
refractive surgery, 173–174
refractometry, 34
Reinstein classification of flap microfolds, 329
residual keratocytes, 220
retina, objective examination, 47–48
retinal image, optical quality, 17–18
retinoscopy, 27
Rho protein, 66
RMS (root mean square), 171, 303
RMS wavefront error, 22
RSVP (Refractive Status and Vision Profile, 170–171

SAI (surface asymmetry index), 14, 15, 53, 54
Schachar theory of accommodation, 129
Scheimpflug camera, 84–85
scotopic conditions, 55
SDP (standard deviation of corneal power), 14, 53
Seidel series, wavefront data analysis, 35–36
SEM (scanning electron microscopy)
    drawbacks, 63–65
    surface irregularities and, 66
Shack-Hartmann approach, wavefront sensors, 34
Sim-K (simulated keratometry), 15, 53
Sjögren's syndrome, 42–43
skiascopy, 49
skin disorders, 44
slope, parameters, 10
smoothing. *See also* LASEK
    after ablation, 164
    after CPK, 256
    after PRK, 232
    clinical study, 86–88
    complications, 117
    in excimer refractive surgery, 83–87
    with masking fluid, 260
    questions about, 89–90
    surgical technique, 88–89, 117–118
spatial dynamic skiascopy, 27
spatial information, 22
spherical aberration, 15, 54, 123, 129–130
staphyloma, 28
Stickler's syndrome, 44
stroma structure, measuring, 145–147
stromal cell apoptosis, 220
stromal keratocyte differentiation, 63
stromal remodeling, 220
subepithelial fibrosis, 247
submicron-scale irregularities, 63–65
surface ablation. *See also* astigmatism; hyperopia; myopia; presbyopia; smoothing
    astigmatism, 107–111
    biomechanics and LASIK
        macromechanics, 59–63
        micromechanics, 63–68
    corneal curvature gradient, 76–81

historical perspectives, 75–76
mitomycin C for treatment of haze, 247–251
patient selection
    examining patients for refractive surgery, 41–46
    instrumental examinations, 50–56
    objective examination, 46–50
topography
    corneal, 7–15
    keratorefractive indices, 15
    keratoscopy, 3–7
surface irregularities
    haze and, 67–68
    laser ablation and, 65–65
symmetry of rings, 5
systemic collagenopathy, 42–43

T cells, 220
tangential mapping, 10–15, 52
Taylor Series, wavefront data analysis, 35–36
TdT {terminal deoxyribonucleotidyl transferase), 220
TE (transepithelially) technique, 134
TEM (transmission electron microscopy), 64, 66, 220
TGFß (transforming growth factor-ß), 220, 234–235
thyroid disorders, 42–43
TNF (tumor necrosis factor), 219
topical steroids, 43
topography. *See* corneal topography
TOSCA (Topography Supported Customized Ablation), 133, 135
Tracey ray tracing system, 34
TSA (Tissue Save Ablation) software, 133–134
TUNEL assay, 220
TZ (transition zone), 97, 101, 111, 121, 125, 163, 243

UCVA (uncorrected visual acuity), 170–171, 195, 200, 243, 318
ulcerative keratitis, 43
ultrastructure response, 63–65

very high frequency digital ultrasound
    Artemis VHF digital ultrasound arc B-scanner, 315–320
    phakic IOL surgery, 328–329
    postoperative assessment, 321–322
    preoperative assessment, 321
    ultrasound-guided PTK, 325–328
videokeratographic outcomes, 65
visual acuity
    in eyes with ultrathin corneas, 266
    high contrast photopic visual acuity, 17
    high-order wavefront error, 21–22
    refraction and, 48
VISX laser, 62, 64, 153
Vitamin A, role in epithelial metabolism, 41–42
vitrectomy, re-epithelialization following, 42
vitreous body, objective examination, 47–48
VSIA (Vision Science and Its Applications), 35

warpage, 8–9
wavefront corrections, 25

wavefront customized PRK, 190–196
wavefront data analysis, 35–38
wavefront error
    after customized treatment, 171
    characteristics, 19–21
    clinical implications, 22
    corneal, 22
wavefront sensors, 33–34
WF (wavefront analyzer), 29
whole eye wavefront error, 22

xerophthalmia, 41–42

Zernike decomposition, 37
Zernike expansion, 20–21
Zernike method, wavefront data analysis, 35–36
Zernike polynomial approximation, 37–38
Zernike tree affect, 22
Zyoptix
    data acquisition and ablation files, 190–191
    historical perspectives, 190
    indications and limitations, 194–196
    wavefront-guided treatments, 191–194
Zywave aberrometry, 323

WAIT ...*There's More!*

SLACK Incorporated's Health Care Books and Journals offers a wide selection of products in the field of Ophthalmology. We are dedicated to providing important works that educate, inform and improve the knowledge of our customers. Don't miss out on our other informative titles that will enhance your collection.

Corneal Topography in the Wavefront Era: A Guide for Clinical Application
Ming Wang, MD, PhD
336 pp., Hard Cover, Pub. Date: 2006, ISBN 10: 1-55642-718-2, ISBN 13: 978-1-55642-718-3, Order# 67182, **$174.95**

Corneal Topography in the Wavefront Era: A Guide for Clinical Application delivers the information needed to develop an understanding of the state-of-the-art corneal topographic technology and its relationship to keratorefractive surgery. Dr. Ming Wang has organized a team of over 30 of the field's leading professionals to produce this informative, comprehensive, and clinically oriented text.

Refractive Surface Ablation: PRK, LASEK, Epi-LASIK, Custom, PTK and Retreatment
Paolo Vinciguerra, MD
376 pp., Hard Cover, Pub. Date: 2006, ISBN 10: 1-55642-713-1, ISBN 13: 978-1-55642-713-8, Order# 67131, **$124.95**

Wavefront Customized Visual Correction: The Quest for Super Vision II
Ronald Krueger, MD; Raymond Applegate, OD, PhD; Scott MacRae, MD
416 pp., Hard Cover, Pub. Date: 2004, ISBN 10: 1-55642-625-9, ISBN 13: 978-1-55642-625-4, Order# 66259, **$196.95**

Handbook of Ophthalmology
Amar Agarwal, MS, FRCS, FRCOphth
752 pp., Soft Cover, Pub. Date: 2006, ISBN 10: 1-55642-685-2, ISBN 13: 978-1-55642-685-8, Order# 66852, **$64.95**

LASIK: Advances, Controversies, and Custom
Louis E. Probst, MD
528 pp., Hard Cover, Pub. Date: 2004, ISBN 10: 1-55642-654-2, ISBN 13: 978-1-55642-654-4, Order# 66542, **$195.95**

Refractive Surgery Nightmares: Conquering Refractive Surgery Catastrophes
Amar Agarwal, MS, FRCS, FRCOphth
250 pp., Hard Cover, Pub. Date: 4/07, ISBN 10: 1-55642-788-3, ISBN 13: 978-1-55642-788-6, Order# 67883, **$169.95**

Dr. Amar Agarwal explains all there is to know about refractive surgery techniques in *Refractive Surgery Nightmares* to help you stay in control when facing unique surgical challenges. More than 300 illustrations and clinical photographs supplement the important information presented, providing visual as well as textual references. An accompanying video CD-ROM with 60 minutes of live video techniques supplements the text.

The Little Eye Book: A Pupil's Guide to Understanding Ophthalmology
Janice K. Ledford, COMT; Roberto Pineda II, MD
160 pp., Soft Cover, Pub. Date: 2002, ISBN 10: 1-55642-560-0, ISBN 13: 978-1-55642-560-8, Order# 65600, **$19.95**

Quick Reference Dictionary of Eyecare Terminology, Fourth Edition
Janice K. Ledford, COMT; Joseph Hoffman
424 pp., Soft Cover, Pub. Date: 2004, ISBN 10: 1-55642-711-5, ISBN 13: 978-1-55642-711-4, Order# 67115, **$28.95**

Intraocular Lens Power Calculations
H. John Shammas, MD
240 pp., Hard Cover, Pub. Date: 2004, ISBN 10: 1-55642-652-6, ISBN 13: 978-1-55642-652-0, Order# 66526, **$74.95**

Please visit

www.slackbooks.com

to order any of these titles!
24 Hours a Day...7 Days a Week!

Attention Industry Partners!
Whether you are interested in buying multiple copies of a book, chapter reprints, or looking for something new and different — we are able to accommodate your needs.

Multiple Copies
At attractive discounts starting for purchases as low as 25 copies for a single title, SLACK Incorporated will be able to meet all your of your needs.

Chapter Reprints
SLACK Incorporated is able to offer the chapters you want in a format that will lead to success. Bound with an attractive cover, use the chapters that are a fit specifically for your company. Available for quantities of 100 or more.

Customize
SLACK Incorporated is able to create a specialized custom version of any of our products specifically for your company.

Please contact the Marketing Manager of Health Care Books and Journals for further details on multiple copy purchases, chapter reprints or custom printing at 1-800-257-8290 or 1-856-848-1000.

*Please note all conditions are subject to change.

CODE: 328

SLACK
INCORPORATED

SLACK Incorporated • Health Care Books and Journals
6900 Grove Road • Thorofare, NJ 08086

1-800-257-8290 or 1-856-848-1000

Fax: 1-856-853-5991 • E-mail: orders@slackinc.com • Visit www.slackbooks.com